Bladder Cancer: Diagnosis and Clinical Management

Bladder Cancer: Diagnosis and Clinical Management

Editor: Trinity Schell

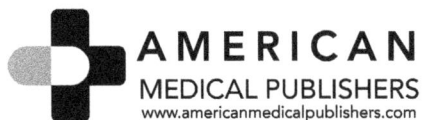

AMERICAN
MEDICAL PUBLISHERS
www.americanmedicalpublishers.com

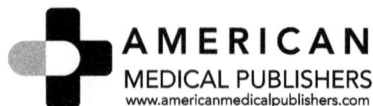

AMERICAN
MEDICAL PUBLISHERS
www.americanmedicalpublishers.com

Cataloging-in-Publication Data

Bladder cancer : diagnosis and clinical management / edited by Trinity Schell.
    p. cm.
Includes bibliographical references and index.
ISBN 978-1-63927-604-2
1. Bladder--Cancer. 2. Bladder--Cancer--Diagnosis. 3. Bladder--Cancer--Treatment.
4. Bladder--Diseases. I. Schell, Trinity.
RC280.B5 B53 2023
616.994 62--dc23

© American Medical Publishers, 2023

American Medical Publishers,
41 Flatbush Avenue,
1st Floor, New York,
NY 11217, USA

ISBN 978-1-63927-604-2 (Hardback)

Contents

Preface

Bladder cancer is referred to as a form of cancer which develops in the bladder cells. The bladder is a hollow muscular organ in the human body that retains urine in the lower belly. Bladder cancer typically starts in the urothelial cells that line the inner part of the bladder. There are various signs and symptoms of bladder cancer such as painful urination, blood in urine, back pain and frequent urination. Chronic bladder inflammation, smoking, family or personal history of cancer and increasing age are risk factors for bladder cancer. The most common method of diagnosis is cystoscopy with tissue biopsies. Treatment for bladder cancer includes intravesical therapy, surgery, radiation therapy and chemotherapy. It can be prevented by quitting smoking and taking a diet which is rich in vegetables and proteins. This book elucidates the innovative models around prospective developments with respect to the study of bladder cancer. Such selected concepts that redefine the diagnosis and clinical management of bladder cancer have been presented herein. Those with an interest in this disease would find this book helpful.

The information contained in this book is the result of intensive hard work done by researchers in this field. All due efforts have been made to make this book serve as a complete guiding source for students and researchers. The topics in this book have been comprehensively explained to help readers understand the growing trends in the field.

I would like to thank the entire group of writers who made sincere efforts in this book and my family who supported me in my efforts of working on this book. I take this opportunity to thank all those who have been a guiding force throughout my life.

Editor

Present Status, Limitations and Future Directions of Treatment Strategies using Fucoidan-based Therapies in Bladder Cancer

Yasuyoshi Miyata *[iD], **Tomohiro Matsuo** [iD], **Kojiro Ohba** [iD], **Kensuke Mitsunari** [iD], **Yuta Mukae,**
Asato Otsubo, Junki Harada, Tsuyoshi Matsuda, Tsubasa Kondo and **Hideki Sakai**

Department of Urology, Graduate School of Biomedical Sciences, Nagasaki University, Nagasaki 852-8501, Japan;
tomozo1228@hotmail.com (T.M.); ohba-k@nagasaki-u.ac.jp (K.O.); ken.mitsunari@gmail.com (K.M.);
ytmk_n2@yahoo.co.jp (Y.M.); a.06131dpsc@gmail.com (A.O.); harada-junki@nagasaki-u.ac.jp (J.H.);
matsudatsuyoshi9251@gmail.com (T.M.); t-udonko@nagasaki-u.ac.jp (T.K.); hsakai@nagasaki-u.ac.jp (H.S.)
* Correspondence: yasu-myt@nagasaki-u.ac.jp

Simple Summary: Prognosis of bladder cancer patients is often poor despite various intensive treatments are performed. Therefore, many investigators pay attention to the efficacy of natural product-based treatments to avoid additional adverse events in these patients. Here, we review the anti-cancer effects of fucoidan-based treatments and the protective effects against cancer-related disorders and cisplatin-induced toxicities.

Abstract: Bladder cancer (BC) is a common urological cancer, with poor prognosis for advanced/metastatic stages. Various intensive treatments, including radical cystectomy, chemotherapy, immune therapy, and radiotherapy are commonly used for these patients. However, these treatments often cause complications and adverse events. Therefore, researchers are exploring the efficacy of natural product-based treatment strategies in BC patients. Fucoidan, derived from marine brown algae, is recognized as a multi-functional and safe substrate, and has been reported to have anti-cancer effects in various types of malignancies. Additionally, in vivo and in vitro studies have reported the protective effects of fucoidan against cancer-related cachexia and chemotherapeutic agent-induced adverse events. In this review, we have introduced the anti-cancer effects of fucoidan extracts in BC and highlighted its molecular mechanisms. We have also shown the anti-cancer effects of fucoidan therapy with conventional chemotherapeutic agents and new treatment strategies using fucoidan-based nanoparticles in various malignancies. Moreover, apart from the improvement of anti-cancer effects by fucoidan, its protective effects against cancer-related disorders and cisplatin-induced toxicities have been introduced. However, the available information is insufficient to conclude the clinical usefulness of fucoidan-based treatments in BC patients. Therefore, we have indicated the aspects that need to be considered regarding fucoidan-based treatments and future directions for the treatment of BC.

Keywords: fucoidan; molecular mechanisms; combination therapy; nanoparticles; bladder cancer

1. Introduction

Bladder cancer (BC) is a common malignancy of the urinary system. Generally, the prognosis of BC is relatively good if cancer cells do not invade the muscle layer and disseminate to lymph nodes or distant organs. On the other hand, outcomes for patients with advanced forms of this disease, including muscle invasion and/or metastasis, is poor despite various treatments such as radical cystectomy, chemotherapy, immune therapy, and radiotherapy. Moreover, most therapies for such advanced BC lead to a decrease in the quality of life (QoL) owing to complications and adverse events. Therefore, information on additional therapeutic strategies that use safe and low-cost agents is important for maintaining the QoL and improving prognosis in patients with advanced BC. Consequently, many investigators have paid special attention to the preventive effects against adverse events and anti-cancer properties of natural products in the treatment of BC [1–4].

Fucoidan is a marine sulfated carbohydrate derived from marine brown algae. It is a heparin-like molecule with an α-1,3-linked fucose and an α-1,4-linked fucose with branches attached at the C2 position [5]. It is known to have various biological activities, including antibacterial, anti-inflammatory, antioxidant, and immunomodulatory effects [6–8]. Additionally, fucoidan has been favored owing to its low toxicity in vivo, including in humans [9,10]. Furthermore, there is a general agreement that fucoidan exerts anti-cancer effects by regulating tumor growth, cancer cell apoptosis, invasion, metastasis, cell cycle, tumor angiogenesis, and immune reactivities in various types of malignancies [5,11–15]. Numerous factors and molecules have been reported in in vivo and in vitro studies as part of the molecular mechanisms underlying the anti-cancer properties of fucoidan. These include the phosphatidylinositol-3-kinase (PI3K)/AKT signaling pathway in hepatocellular carcinoma and colon cancer [16,17], Bcl-2 family in lung cancer [18], caspases in breast cancer [19], cyclins in cervical cancer [20], and cytochrome c in osteosarcoma [21]. Excellent reviews are available on the structure, biological activity, and interactions of fucoidan under various physiological and pathological conditions [6,8,10,14]. On the other hand, there are only a few systematic reviews depicting the pathological significance of fucoidan and the molecular mechanisms of its anticancer effects in BC, although some previous studies have shown and discussed these factors in original articles.

Various pathological steps are necessary for tumor growth, invasion, and metastasis in solid tumors. Furthermore, many factors are associated with these processes, such as cancer cell proliferation, apoptosis, cell cycle, cell migration, invasion, and angiogenesis. In addition, at the molecular level, numerous cancer-related molecules modulate these pathological processes as stimulators or suppressors. Importantly, several natural foods and their extracts can alter such malignant processes at the molecular level in BC, as observed in in vivo and in vitro studies [22–25]. Thus, understanding the influence of fucoidan on malignant behavior and its regulatory mechanisms at the molecular level is essential to formulate treatment strategies in patients with BC. Various treatment strategies using nanoparticles with fucoidan have been reported in various types of malignancies. In this review, we highlight and discuss the following aspects: (1) pathological roles of fucoidan in malignancies, (2) effects of combination therapies of fucoidan and conventional anti-cancer agents, (3) trials of nanoparticles including fucoidan, (4) differences in biological and pharmacological activities of fucoidans according to species and molecular weight, and (5) protective effects of fucoidan in cancer-related disorders. Lastly, we discuss the future directions and limitations of fucoidan-based therapies in malignancies, including BC.

2. Biological Effects of Fucoidans in Bladder Cancer Cells

2.1. Effect on Cell Proliferation and Tumor Growth

One of the most important determinants of tumor growth and development is the regulation of cell survival, which comprises cell proliferation and cell death. In fact, several studies have focused on the relationship between fucoidan and tumor growth, cancer cell proliferation, and/or apoptosis in BC [26–30]. To the best of our knowledge, the anti-tumor effects of fucoidan in BC, including suppression of cancer cell proliferation and induction of apoptosis, were first reported in two papers published in 2014 [26,27]. In both the studies, the fucoidan used was obtained from the same company (Sigma-Aldrich Chemical Co., St. Louis, MO, USA) and the studies were performed by the same research group in Korea. However, in one of the studies, the researchers used 5637 cells (originating from grade 2 carcinoma) and T24 cells (undifferentiated grade 3 carcinoma), whereas in the other, they used T24 cells [26,27]. Cho et al. [26] reported that 5637 cell viability was inhibited in a concentration-dependent manner when cultured in a standard medium containing various concentrations (0–400 µg/mL) of fucoidan for 24 h. Similarly, the other report showed that fucoidan inhibited T24 cell viability in a concentration- and time-dependent manner [27]. However, it should be noted that the anti-proliferative effects of fucoidan, when examined in detail, were different between them, despite the fact that the source of fucoidan was the same and cell viability was measured using the same method (3-(4,5-dimethyl-2-thiazolyl)-2,5-diphenyl-2H tetrazolium; MTT assay). Briefly, although 5637 cell viability was inhibited by ≥50 µg/mL of fucoidan for 24 h, T24 cell viability was inhibited by ≥100 µg/mL of fucoidan for 48 h, but not by 50 µg/mL [26,27]. Furthermore, in 2017, the same study group showed that treatment of 5637 cells with 25 µg/mL of fucoidan for 24 h (purified from *Fucusvesiculosus* (purchased from Sigma-Aldrich Chemical Co., St. Louis, MO, USA) significantly inhibited cell viability (measured via MMT assay) [30]. Thus, the anti-proliferative effect depended on the type of cancer cells, and it was speculated that high-grade BC was able to tolerate fucoidan. Subsequently, such fucoidan-induced anti-proliferative effects in 5637 and T24 cells have been reported in other studies [28,30]. Additionally, a dose-dependent anti-proliferative effect (50–150 µg/mL) of fucoidan was observed in other human bladder cancer cells (EJ cells) [29].

On the other hand, there are no in vivo studies regarding the anti-proliferative effects of fucoidan on BC. However, Chen et al. [28] reported that low-molecular-weight fucoidan (LMWF) inhibited tumor growth in vivo. Briefly, when 80, 160, and 300 mg/kg/day LMWF (molecular weight was mainly 760 Da) was orally administered for 30 days to BALB/c nude mice that were injected with T24 cells, the tumor size and weight decreased significantly in mice treated with 160 and 300 mg/kg/day LMWF but not in those administered a fucoidan dose of 80 mg/kg/day [28].

2.2. Effect on Apoptosis

Like the anti-proliferative effects, the pro-apoptotic effects of fucoidan were first reported in an in vitro study in 2014 [27]. In this study, the authors evaluated apoptosis in T24 cells using three methods, namely, nuclear morphological change, DNA fragmentation, and annexin V staining. Increase in nuclear chromatin condensation, DNA fragmentation, and annexin V-stained cells was observed in a dose-dependent manner after treatment with various concentrations of fucoidan (50, 100, and 150 µg/mL) for 48 h [27]. The number of apoptotic cells measured by the percentage of annexin V-positive/propidium iodide-negative cells in cells treated with 100 and 150 µg/mL fucoidan (approximately 20 and 26%, respectively) were remarkably higher than that in control cells (0 µg/mL, approximately 2%) [27]. Additionally, dose-dependent pro-apoptotic activity was observed using similar methods in other types of EJ cells [29]. On similar lines, another study in 2017 investigated the relationship between fucoidan and apoptosis in in vitro studies using 4,6-diamidino-2-phenylindole (DAPI) staining and flow cytometry in 5637 cells [30]. In this study, BC cells were treated with 0, 10, 25, or 100 µg/mL of fucoidan for 24 h; nuclear fragmentation and chromatin condensation were found to increase in a concentration-dependent manner. Furthermore, flow cytometry results showed that the percentage of cells with sub-G1 DNA content, which is a parameter of apoptosis, was also increased in a concentration-dependent manner (0 µg/mL = 2.97%, 10 µg/mL = 3.17%, 25 µg/mL = 6.47%, 50 µg/mL = 19.87%, and 100 µg/mL = 40.12%) [30]. Thus, the pro-apoptotic effect of fucoidan was confirmed in BC cells using various methods. However, in vivo studies regarding these effects of fucoidan, including LMWF, have not been performed yet. Moreover, there are no data on the relationship between fucoidan and non-apoptotic cell death, such as necrosis and ferroptosis in BC, despite their correlation being studied in other malignancies [21].

2.3. Effect on Cell Migration and Invasion

To our knowledge, only one study has investigated the relationship between fucoidan and BC cell migration/invasion [26]. This study used scratch assay and cell invasion assay to show that fucoidan inhibited the migration and invasion of two different BC cell lines (5637 and T24 cells) [26]. Interestingly, the healing area (% of control) in 5637 cells treated with 100 µg/mL of fucoidan after 24 h was 45 ± 5.05%, similar to that in T24 cells treated under similar conditions (46 ± 5.26%) [26].

Additionally, the cell invasion assay showed that the proportion of invasive cells (% of control) in 5637 cells was similar to that in T24 cells (15 ± 7.53 and 17 ± 6.12%, respectively) under similar culture conditions (100 µg/mL fucoidan after 24 h) [26]. This study demonstrated that the inhibitory effects of fucoidan on cell migration and invasion might be dependent on the malignant potential of BC cells [26]. In addition, there was a report that LMWF inhibited cell migration and invasion of T24 cells in a dose-dependent manner [28]. However, it should be noted that these analyses were performed under hypoxic conditions of 1% O_2.

2.4. Effects on Angiogenesis

Metastasis is the most important predictor of survival, and angiogenesis is recognized as an important step in disseminating cancer cells from the primary tumor mass. Therefore, many investigators have reported the relationship between tumor angiogenesis and crude fucoidan or fucoidan extracts in various types of cancers [13,31,32]. For example, abalone glycosidase-digested fucoidan extracts derived from the seaweed, Mozuku (Cladosiphon novae-caledoniae Kylin), inhibited vascular tube formation, including the number, total length, and total area of tubes in human cervical cancer cells (HeLa cells) in an in vitro study [31].

Unfortunately, the relationship between fucoidan and angiogenesis in BC is not fully understood. One study investigated the anti-angiogenic activities of LMWF using in vivo and in vitro studies [28], wherein LMWF suppressed capillary tube-formation in human umbilical vein endothelial cells (HUVECs) under hypoxic conditions. Notably, such anti-angiogenic activity was not observed under normoxic conditions, implying that LMWF may suppress only hypoxia-induced angiogenesis. Generally, hypoxia in the tumor microenvironment is one of the most representative characteristics of solid tumors and plays crucial roles in malignant potential, tumor development, and outcomes in various types of malignancies [33–35]. Consequently, it is possible that the specific anti-angiogenic activity of LMWF under hypoxic conditions is advantageous for increasing anti-cancer effects and decreasing adverse events in cancer patients because it leads to stronger biological effects of fucoidan in cancer tissues compared to that in normal tissues. On the other hand, more detailed information, especially the correlation of LMWF with cell proliferation and migration of endothelial cells, is essential to discuss its anti-cancer effects via regulation of angiogenesis in malignant tumors. Chen et al. [28] also analyzed the microvessel density after staining using the anti-CD31 antibody in matrigel plug and injecting T24 cells in nude mice (BALB/c). Results showed that the amount of CD31 in matrigel and tumor tissues under stimulation by vascular endothelial growth factor (VEGF) was suppressed in a dose-dependent manner by the administration of LMWF (matrigel plug: 0, 25, 50, and 75 µg, T24 tumors: 0, 80, 160, and 300 µg/kg/day). Specifically, CD31-positive vessel density under VEGF stimulation in matrigel plugs with 50 and 75 µg of fucoidan was significantly lower than that in the control group plugs (0 µg). On the other hand, CD31-stained capillaries were remarkably decreased in tumor tissues in mice treated with 160 and 300 µg/kg/day of fucoidan.

Thus, the cell lines used and the species, types, and doses of fucoidans are closely associated with the biological effects of fucoidans in BC. A summary of the pathological roles of fucoidans in BC cells according to these parameters is given in Table 1.

Table 1. Anticancer effects of fucoidans in bladder cancer cells.

Pathological Feature	Cell Line	Design	Species	Type	Dose	Year/References
Tumor growth	5637	In vitro	Not tested	Crude	50–400 *	2014/[26]
	T24	In vitro	Not tested	Crude	100–150 *	2014/[27]
	T24	In vivo	Sargassum hemiphyllum	LMWF	160–300 **	2015/[28]
	EJ	In vitro	Fucusvesiculosus	Crude	50–150 *	2015/[29]
	5637	In vitro	Fucusvesiculosus	Crude	25–100 *	2017/[30]
Apoptosis	T24	In vitro	Not tested	Crude	50–150 *	2014/[27]
	EJ	In vitro	Fucusvesiculosus	Crude	50–150 *	2015/[29]
	5637	In vitro	Fucusvesiculosus	Crude	50–100 *	2017/[30]

Table 1. *Cont.*

Pathological Feature	Cell Line	Design	Species	Type	Dose	Year/References
Migration/invasion	5637	In vitro	Not tested	Crude	100 *	2014/[26]
	T24	In vitro	Not tested	Crude	100 *	2014/[26]
	T24	In vitro	*Sargassum hemiphyllum*	LMWF	25–100 *	2015/[28]
Angiogenesis	T24	In vitro	*Sargassum hemiphyllum*	LMWF	25–100 *	2015/[28]

LMWF: low molecular weight fucoidan (760 Da), Doses: * μg/mL, ** mg/kg/day.

3. Molecular Mechanisms of Fucoidans Underlying Their Anti-Cancer Effects in Malignancies

3.1. Anti-Cancer Cell Growth and Survival

Cho et al. [26] reported that fucoidan inhibited the proliferation of 5637 cells (Cho 2014). They speculated that PI3K/AKT signaling played a crucial role in this fucoidan-induced anti-proliferative effect because fucoidan-induced activation of AKT was inhibited by a PI3K-specific inhibitor, and subsequent blockage of AKT signaling led to the inhibition of fucoidan-induced inhibitory effect [26].

A previous study reported fucoidan-induced apoptosis of T24 cells in a concentration-dependent manner [27]. In this study, the detailed molecular mechanisms of fucoidan-induced apoptosis in BC cells were investigated. The authors discovered that: (1) the initiator of the extrinsic apoptotic pathway (caspase-8) and the intrinsic apoptotic pathway (caspase-9) were associated with fucoidan-induced apoptosis; (2) the Fas/Fas ligand (FasL) system, which belongs to the extrinsic apoptotic pathway, is a key signaling transduction pathway in this system; (3) activation of caspase-3 and cleavage of the pro-form poly(ADP-ribose) polymerase (PARP) protein to its inactive form led to its pro-apoptotic activity; (4) fucoidan-induced apoptosis was positively associated with increase in Bax and decrease in Bcl-2 (increase in the Bax/Bcl-2 ratio, characterizing the intrinsic apoptotic pathway); (5) fucoidan treatment resulted in downregulation of inhibitors of apoptosis (IAP) family numbers, such as XIAP, cIAP-1, and cIAP-2, and full-length Bid (a BH3-only protein from the Bcl-2 family); and (6) fucoidan-induced apoptosis via regulation of mitochondrial function, such as, a significant decrease in cytochrome c in the mitochondria and loss of the mitochondrial membrane potential [27]. Thus, treatment with fucoidan induced apoptosis via complex mechanisms in T24 cells. A summary of fucoidan-induced changes of tumor growth- and/or apoptosis-related molecules was showed in Table 2.

Table 2. Fucoidan-induced changes of cell survival-related molecules.

Molecules	Change	Cell Line	Species	Year/Reference
Akt/PI3K	↓	5637	Not tested	2014/[26]
	↓	5637	*Fucusvesiculosus*	2017/[30]
Bax	↑	T24	Not tested	2014/[27]
	↑	5637	*Fucusvesiculosus*	2017/[30]
Bcl-2	↓	T24		2014/[27]
	↓	5637	*Fucusvesiculosus*	2017/[30]
Bid	↓	T24	Not tested	2014/[27]
truncated Bid	↑	T24	Not tested	2014/[27]
Caspase-3	↑	T24	Not tested	2014/[27]
Caspase-8	↑	T24	Not tested	2014/[27]
Caspase-9	↑	T24	Not tested	2014/[27]
cIAP-1	↓	T24	Not tested	2014/[27]
cIAP-2	↓	T24	Not tested	2014/[27]
DR4	NC	T24	Not tested	2014/[27]
DR5	↑	T24	Not tested	2014/[27]
Fas	↑	T24	Not tested	2014/[27]
XIAP	↓	T24	Not tested	2014/[26]

PI3K: phosphoinositide 3-kinase, Bax: Bcl-2 associated protein, Bcl-2: B-cell lymphoma 2, Bid: BH3 interacting domain death agonist, cIAP: cellular inhibitor of apoptosis, DR: death receptor, XIAP: X-chromosome-linked inhibitor of apoptosis.

Several investigators have shown that control of the cell cycle by fucoidan also plays an important role. Briefly, fucoidan induced G1 phase cell cycle arrest in 5637 cells via the upregulation of p21Waf1 expression and suppression of cyclins and CDK expression [26]. Additionally, these phenomena were negated when AKT signaling was blocked [26]. Therefore, the authors concluded that fucoidan had a significant inhibitory effect on tumor growth, followed by G1-phase-associated upregulation of p21Waf1 expression and suppression of cyclins and CDK expression in BC [26]. Similarly another study showed that the proportion of cells in the G1 phase in T24 cells treated with control medium (0 μg/mL of fucoidan) was 34.2%, and those in cells treated with 50, 100, and 150 μg/mL of fucoidan were 52.1%, 61.7%, and 67.8%, respectively [27]. Thus, the author corroborated the notion that fucoidan modulated the cell cycle in BC cells. Furthermore, the molecular mechanisms of fucoidan-induced cell cycle arrest in the G1 phase and decreased expression of cyclin D1, cyclin E, and CDK were reported in this study [27]. These results were supported by the findings of the above-mentioned report [26]. Additionally, Park et al. [27] demonstrated that the expression of CDK inhibitor p21 was increased at the transcriptional and translational levels in T24 cells treated with fucoidan.

Furthermore, Park et al. [27]. investigated the relationship between the phosphorylation of retinoblastoma (Rb) and the transcription factors E2Fs in T24 cells because Rb is an important checkpoint in the G1 phase [36]. They found that pRb expression was decreased after fucoidan treatment in a time-dependent manner, and a strong increase in the association of pRB and E2F-1 as well as E2F-4 post fucoidan treatment in T24 cells was observed [27]. The authors concluded that fucoidan inhibits the release of E2Fs proteins from pRb in T24 cells. Likewise, the same study group performed similar research in another kind of human bladder cancer (RJ) cells, and reported that fucoidan induced G1 arrest through downregulation of pRb via increased binding of pRb to E2Fs (1 and 4) [27].

Summary of fucoidan-induced changes of cell-cycle-related molecules was showed in Table 3.

Table 3. Fucoidan-induced changed of cell-cycle-related molecules.

Molecules	Change	Cell Line	Year/Reference
Cdk2	↓	5637	2014/[26]
	↓	T24	2014/[27]
	↓	RJ	2015/[29]
Cdk4	↓	5637	2014/[26]
	↓	T24	2014/[27]
	↓	RJ	2015/[29]
Cdk6	↓	T24	2014/[27]
	↓	RJ	2015/[29]
cyclin D1	↓	56372	2014/[26]
	↓	T24	2014/[27]
	↓	RJ	2015/[29]
cyclin E	↓	5637	2014/[26]
	↓	T24	2014/[27]
	↓	RJ	2015/[29]
E2F-1	No change	T24	2014/[27]
	No change	RJ	2015/[29]
E2F-4	No change	T24	2014/[27]
	No change	RJ	2015/[29]
p21	↑	T24	2014/[28]
	No change	RJ	2015/[29]
p21WAF1	↑	5637	2014/[26]
p27	No change	T24	2014/[27]
	No change	RJ	2015/[29]
pRb	↓	T24	2014/[27]
	↓	RJ	2015/[29]

Cdk; cyclin-dependent kinase, Rb, retinoblastoma.

3.2. Anti-Invasive and Migration Effects

Cancer cell migration and invasion are important steps in cancer cell dissemination into surrounding tissues, lymph nodes, and distant organs. In fact, muscle invasion is closely associated with dismal prognosis in patients with BC [37,38]. Although the invasive step of BC is regulated by many molecules, matrix metalloproteinases (MMPs) are considered to be one of the most important stimulators in BC tissues [39–41]. Among MMP members, the pathological significance and prognostic roles of MMP-2 and -9 have been investigated most widely in many types of cancers [42–44]. In 2005, Ye et al. [31]. reported that enzyme-digested fucoidan extracts inhibit cell invasion via the downregulation of MMP-2 and -9 in human fibrosarcoma (HT1080) cells. Subsequently, other investigators reported that a mixture of fucoidan and vitamin C suppressed HT1080 cell invasion via suppression of MMP-2 and -9 activities [45]. Furthermore, other investigators showed that the sulfated fucoidan (98% purity) obtained from *Sargassum fusiforme* suppressed cell migration and invasion of hepatocellular cancer cells (HCC SMMC-7721, Huh7, and HCCLM3 cells), and the decreased expression of MMP-2 was speculated to be associated with this outcome [11]. Similar anti-cancer effects of fucoidan via the regulation of MMP-2 have also been reported in lung cancer cells (Lee 2012) [46]. Thus, fucoidan is speculated to play crucial roles in cell migration and invasion via regulation of MMP-2 and -9 in several malignancies. Similar findings were reported in BC cells (5637 cells) [26]. This study also showed that fucoidan-related MMP-9 expression was mediated by activator protein (AP)-1 and NF-κB binding activity, and that treatment with wortmannin, a PI3K-specific inhibitor, abolished tumor suppressive effects by regulating MMP-9, NF-κB, and AP-1 in fucoidan-treated cells [26]. Lastly, the authors concluded that activation of AKT was closely associated with BC cell migration and invasion via inhibition of MMP-9 expression through reduction of AP-1 and NF-κB activities [26]. However, to our knowledge, there is no other report on the molecular regulatory mechanisms of fucoidan on MMP-2 and -9 expression in BC. Correspondingly, fucoidan suppressed cancer cell migration and invasion in human lung cancer cells (A549 cells) via inhibition of MMP-2, wherein blocking of the ERK1/2 and PI3K-AKT-mTOR pathways was associated with the MMP-2-related anti-cancer effects of fucoidan [46].

Thus, several reports have described the regulatory mechanism of fucoidan on MMP-2 and -9 at the molecular level in malignant cells. However, these results are not adequate to discuss fucoidan-based therapeutic strategies in patients with cancer. Fucoidan-induced changes in the expression levels and activities of other MMP members in malignant cells are not fully understood, even though MMPs other than MMP-2 and -9 also play important roles in malignant aggressiveness and prognosis in various types of cancers, including BC [47–51].

3.3. Role of Oxidative Stress

Oxidative stress plays an important role in the regulation of various biological activities, including cell survival and metabolism under physiological and pathological conditions [52,53]. Oxidative stress induces excessive production of reactive oxygen species (ROS), and increased intracellular ROS damages cell components such as proteins, lipids, and DNA [54]. Additionally, elevated ROS production is closely associated with malignant aggressiveness via regulation of various cancer-related molecules in many types of cancers, including BC [55–57]. However, fucoidan was reported to induce apoptosis via upregulation of intracellular ROS production in BC cells (5637 cells) [30]. This study also showed that the PI3K/AKT pathway and telomerase activity were associated with such fucoidan-induced apoptotic function.

4. Combination of Fucoidan and Conventional Chemotherapeutic Agents

Treatments with cisplatin (CDDP) and gemcitabine (GEM) are recognized as standard chemotherapeutic regimens in patients with advanced/metastatic BC [58]. Additionally, taxanes, including paclitaxel (PTX) and docetaxel (DTX), are often used as second- or third-line of therapy for platinum-resistant BC [59,60]. Some investigators have paid special attention to combination therapies of fucoidan and conventional anti-cancer agents, including CDDP, GEM, and taxanes. However, unfortunately, there is no report on anti-cancer effects of such a combination therapy on BC yet. Therefore, we have described the anti-cancer effects of combination therapy of fucoidan and these chemotherapeutic agents in other types of malignancies.

4.1. Cisplatin

Several investigators have shown that crude fucoidan enhances the cytotoxic effects of CDDP in several cancer cell types. For example, in head and neck squamous cell carcinoma cells, a combination of crude fucoidan (derived from *Fucusvesiculosus*) and CDDP showed synergistic anti-proliferative effects in all tested cancer cell lines (H103, FaDu, and KB cells) and synergistic pro-apoptotic effects in H103 and KB cells [61]. Interestingly, although regulation of ROS production and cell cycle were associated with a part of these fucoidan-induced anti-cancer effects, the influence of these cancer-related mechanisms was different among the three cancer cell lines. Briefly, ROS production was increased in H103 cells, was not significantly changed in FaDu cells, and was decreased in KB cells [61]. The cell cycle was arrested in the S/G2 phase in H103 and FaDu cells and in the G1 phase in KB cells. Finally, the authors speculated that KB cells showed the most sensitivity to the combination of fucoidan and CDDP treatment [61]. Similarly, the combination of fucoidan with CDDP, doxorubicin, and PTX displayed enhanced cytotoxic effects in breast cancer cells (MCF-7 cells) via regulation of apoptosis and cell cycle [62]. This study also showed that fucoidan did not have harmful effects, including apoptosis in normal cells (MCF-12 cells) [62]. Based on these findings, the authors of these two studies concluded that fucoidan was a promising candidate for combination therapy with conventional therapeutic agents in patients with breast cancer [61,62]. Moreover, in lung cancer cells (LLC1 cells), sequential treatment with CDDP and fucoidan was reported to have stronger anti-cell-growth effect than that with CDDP alone, through upregulated caspase-3 and PARP activities [63]. In addition to the above-mentioned in vitro studies, this study showed that fucoidan increased CDDP-induced cytotoxicity in an in vivo lung cancer model using LLC1-bearing C57BL/6 mice [63]. Briefly, the tumor volume in C57BL/6 mice subcutaneously injected with LLC1 cells, after the sequential treatment with CDDP (intraperitoneal injection of 1.0 mg/kg at day 1) followed by fucoidan (oral intake of 15 mg/kg/day for the duration of the treatment period), was significantly lower than that in mice treated with CDDP alone [63]. Thus, crude fucoidan has additional and synergistic anti-cancer effects with CDDP in various types of cancers.

Similarly, there was a report that extract from the seaweed *Cladosiphon novae-caledoniae* consisting of a digested small molecular weight fraction (72%; <500 Da) and a non-digested fraction (less than 28%; peak = 800 kDa) enhanced the anti-cancer effects of CDDP via inhibitory effects on cell growth (using 200 and 400 µg/mL fucoidan extract for 48 h) and the pro-apoptotic activity (using 200 µg/mL fucoidan extract for 24 and 48 h) in breast cancer cells (MDA-MB-231 and MCF-7 cells) [64]. Furthermore, in recent years, oligo-fucoidan (molecular weight: 92.1%; 500–800 Da) has been reported to promote the cytotoxic activity of CDDP in colon cancer cells [12]. Briefly, in primary C6P2-L1 cell lines derived from colorectal cancer patients, the number of apoptotic cells in the group treated with a combination of CDDP and oligo-fucoidan was significantly higher than those in groups treated with CDDP alone or oligo-fucoidan alone, and upregulation of PARP cleavage and caspase-3 activation were associated with these results [12]. This study also showed that oligo-fucoidan enhanced the anti-tumor effects of CDDP in colorectal cancer cells in vivo. Briefly, in a xenograft model with subcutaneous injection of HCT 116 cells, tumor volume in the group with a combination treatment of CDDP and oligo-fucoidan was significantly lower than that in the group with CDDP treatment alone [12]. Notably, such additional anti-tumor growth effects of fucoidan with CDDP were detected in p53$^{+/+}$ tumors only and not in p53$^{-/-}$ tumors [12].

4.2. Gemcitabine

To our knowledge, there are very few studies on the cooperative effects of fucoidan and GEM in cancer cells. In one such study, the anti-growth effects of a combination of GEM and fucoidan extracts derived from *Undaria pinnatifida* and *Fucusvesiculosus* were analyzed in various types of malignant cell lines [65]. Antagonistic interactive effects of GEM were observed with fucoidan derived from *Undaria pinnatifida* in breast cancer cells (HCC-38 cells) and tongue squamous cell carcinoma cells (CAL-27 cells), and with that from Fucusvesiculosus in HCC-38 cells, CAL-27 cells, ovarian cancer cells (SKOV-3), and melanoma cells (HS294T cells) [65]. Thus, several fucoidans may affect the biological and pharmacological activities of GEM in some malignant cells; however, their efficacy is not clear because there has been no in vivo study.

On similar lines, there was a report that combination therapy with fucoidan and GEM had additive and synergistic anti-tumor effects in uterine sarcomas and carcinosarcoma cells [61]. In this study, fucoidan from *Undaria pinnatifida* had an additive anti-tumor effect in combined treatment with GEM and fucoidan in ESS-1 cells (endometrial stromal sarcoma cells) and SK-UT-1 cells (carcinosarcoma cells), and the synergistic effect was detected in SK-UT-1B cells (carcinosarcoma cells) [61]. Additionally, this study showed that the combination of GEM and fucoidan displayed significant additional pro-apoptotic effects in ESS-1 cells; however, such a significant additive effect was not observed in carcinosarcoma cells (SK-UT-1 and SK-UT-1B cells) [61]. Contrastingly, there was hardly any merit of this combination therapy in uterine leiomyosarcoma cell line (MES-SA cells) [63]. Such information is important in understanding the specificity of combination therapy of GEM and fucoidan according to types of malignant cells and their limitations on anti-tumor effects.

4.3. Taxanes

Mathew et al. [65]. reported the anti-proliferative effects of a combination of crude fucoidans and various conventional chemotherapeutic agents, including PTX. In this study, two different fucoidan extracts derived from *Undaria pinnatifida* and *Fucusvesiculosus*, were investigated, and PTX demonstrated synergistic growth-inhibitory effects in combination with both the fucoidans in many types of cancer cell lines (cervical cancer: HeLa and SiHa, ovarian cancer: TOV-112D and SKOV-3, endometrial carcinoma: HEC-1A and Ishikawa, melanoma: HS294T, tongue squamous cell carcinoma: CAL-27, and prostate cancer: PC-3) [61]. Furthermore, the same study group confirmed the anti-tumor effects of these combined treatments in in vivo studies using human cancer orthotopic mouse models [66]. In contrast to the results of in vitro studies, combination of PTX and fucoidan extract derived from *Undaria pinnatifida* or *Fucusvesiculosus* showed no significant effects on tumor growth in human ovarian cancer orthotopic models with SKOV-3 as well as TOV-112D cell lines [66]. However, surprisingly, these combinations of fucoidans and PTX significantly enhanced tumor growth in mouse models of breast cancer, using MCF-7 and ZR-75 cells [66]. Although there is no similar study in BC, such information is extremely important to plan further studies on the anti-cancer effects of a combination treatment of fucoidans and PTX in BC. On the other hand, fucoidan extracts composed of LMWF (<50 Da) and HWMF (800 kDa) enhanced the anti-proliferative and pro-apoptotic effects of PTX in two breast cancer cell lines (MCF-7 and MDA-MB-231 cells) [67]. This study also reported that increase in oxidative stress was a crucial process in the anti-cancer effects of fucoidan extract and chemotherapeutic agents, including PTX, because enhanced intracellular ROS production and reduced antioxidant levels were detected in this process [67]. These findings support the hypothesis that regulation of oxidative stress may modulate the anti-cancer effects of fucoidan-based chemotherapy in cancer patients. In Table 4, we showed the summary of increased anti-cancer effects of fucoidan combined with CDDP, GEM, or PTX.

Table 4. Increased anti-cancer effects of fucoidan combined with chemotherapeutic agents.

Agents	Type of Malignancy	*Species*	Design	Reference
CDDP	Breast cancer	*Cladosiphonnavae-caledoniae*	In vitro	[64]
	Breast cancer	*Fucusvesicluosus*	In vitro	[62]
	Head and neck cancer	*Fucusvesicluosus*	In vitro	[61]
	Lung cancer	*Fucusvesiculosus*	Both	[63]
	Colorectal cancer	*Sargassum hemiphyllum* *	Both	[12]
GEM	Breast cancer	*Fucusvesiculosus*	In vitro	[65]
	Tongue	*Fucusvesiculosus*	In vitro	[65]
	Melanoma	*Fucusvesiculosus*	In vitro	[65]
	Ovarian cancer	*Fucusvesiculosus*	In vitro	[65]
	Breast cancer	*Undaria pinnatifida*	In vitro	[65]
	Tongue	*Undaria pinnatifida*	In vitro	[65]
	Uterine sarcoma	*Undaria pinnatifida*	In vitro	[61]
	Uterine carcinosarcoma	*Undaria pinnatifida*	In vitro	[61]
PTX	Breast cancer	*Cladosiphonnavae-caledoniae*	In vitro	[64]
	Cervical cancer	*Undaria pinnatifida/Fucusvesiculosus*	In vitro	[65]
	Endometrial cancer	*Undaria pinnatifida/Fucusvesiculosus*	In vitro	[65]
	Melanoma	*Undaria pinnatifida/Fucusvesiculosus*	In vitro	[65]
	Ovarian cancer	*Undaria pinnatifida/Fucusvesiculosus*	In vitro	[65]
	Prostate cancer	*Undaria pinnatifida/Fucusvesiculosus*	In vitro	[65]
	Tongue cancer	*Undaria pinnatifida/Fucusvesiculosus*	In vitro	[65]

CDDP: cisplatin, GEM: gemcitabine, PTX: paclitaxel.

5. Nanoparticles with Fucoidans

There is a general agreement that anti-cancer therapy employing a drug delivery system using nanoscale drug carriers is a useful and promising method in various types of cancers [68]. Accordingly, many investigators have focused on treatment strategies using fucoidan-based nanoparticles in various malignancies [69–71]. However, information on the anti-cancer effects of fucoidan-based nanoparticles in BC cells has not been reported yet. On the other hand, anti-cancer effects of fucoidan-based nanoparticles with CDDP, GEM, and taxans, which have been recognized as standard anti-cancer agents for BC, have been reported in various types of malignant cells. Therefore, in this section, we present this information to discuss the possibility of a promising treatment strategy for BC.

Hwang et al. [68] reported that CDDP–fucoidan (derived from *Fucusvesiculosus*) nanoparticles had stronger anti-cancer effects than CDDP alone, wherein the nanoparticles increased the anti-cancer immunity and cytotoxic effects in human ileocecal adenocarcinoma cells (HCT-8 cells). Interestingly, although various CDDP–fucoidan nanoparticles were prepared using different concentrations of CDDP (0.5, 1.5, 2.0, and 4.0 mg/mL) and fucoidan (2.5, 5.0, 7.5, and 10.0 mg/mL), nanoparticles made using 2 mg CDDP and 10 mg fucoidan exhibited the strongest anti-cancer effects [68].

Likewise, the cytotoxic effects of GEM drug delivery using nanoparticles made from fucoidan and chitosan have been reported [72]. Briefly, cytotoxic effects on breast cancer increased by 25% upon using GEM-loaded nanoparticles (around 115–140 nm in size) based on fucoidan- and chitosan-origin polymers [72].

The cytotoxic effects of DTX-encapsulated fucoidan-polymeric micelles poly(lactic-co-glycolic acid) nanocarriers against triple-negative breast cancer cells were reported earlier in 2020 [73]. In that study, fucoidan was derived from *Fucusvesicululos*, and MDA-MB-231 cells were used. The authors concluded that the nanoparticles effectively exerted better anti-cancer effects and were recognized as a competent drug delivery system [73]. Moreover, other investigators showed the synergistic effects of DTX and fucoidan in multifunctional nanoparticles encapsulated in green tea polyphenol and low-dose DTX within fucoidan-based nanoparticles against prostate cancer [74]. We concur with the concept of their treatment regimen using low-dose cytotoxic agents because we also reported the safety of chemotherapeutic regimens using low-dose PTX in patients with BC [75,76]. Correspondingly, a study group focused on new cancer treatment strategies using fucoidan nanoparticles loaded with PTX [77,78].

Briefly, the authors analyzed the loading efficiency and release patterns of fucoidan nanoparticles with curcumin and PTX to investigate their potential as promising anti-cancer agents [77,78]. We have a keen interest regarding the anti-cancer effects and safety of patients with BC because, in addition to fucoidan, these studies used natural products, including green tea polyphenol and curcumin, which have been widely reported to suppress tumor growth, progression, and treatment resistance in BC [1,79–81].

6. Protection against Cancer-Related Disorders and Adverse Events

In the earlier section, we focused on the biological and pharmacological roles of fucoidan and its anti-cancer effects in BC. However, in the care and treatment of patients with BC, especially in advanced/metastatic disease, management of tumor-related cachexia and/or treatment-induced decline in physical strength is also necessary to improve the prognosis and maintain the QoL of patients. In fact, in cases of unresectable advanced or recurrent colorectal cancer, patients treated with 4.05 g fucoidan for six months from the initial day of chemotherapy (FOLFOX or FOLFIRI) reported significantly reduced frequency of fatigue compared to those treated with chemotherapy alone [82]. In this section, we present the protective effects of fucoidan against cancer-related disorders and adverse events, especially with respect to skeletal muscle loss and CDDP-induced adverse events.

Skeletal muscle atrophy is one of the most representative features of cancer cachexia, and is often observed in cancer patients undergoing chemotherapy [83,84]. Skeletal muscle atrophy leads to a decrease in QoL owing to a reduction in social activity and exercise, along with clinical problems including poor tolerance to cancer therapy [85]. Therefore, many investigators have focused on the prevention of chemotherapy-induced anorexia, including skeletal muscle atrophy, via various nutritional supplements or medications [86–88]. In the case of BC, several investigators have opined that sarcopenia, which is defined as the degenerative and systemic loss of skeletal muscle mass, plays an important role in the prognosis and survival of patients treated with radical cystectomy, systematic chemotherapy, and radiotherapy [89–91]. Consequently, several chemical agents and natural products have been investigated to assess whether they suppress the chemotherapy-induced skeletal muscle atrophy in BC-bearing mice, including, anamorelin, a ghrelin receptor agonist, and magnolol, isolated from the Chinese herb, *Magnolia officinalis* [92,93]. Similarly, fucoidan was reported to inhibit tumor- and chemotherapy-induced skeletal muscle atrophy in BC-bearing mice [86]. Briefly, muscle atrophy in orthotopic mice transplanted with T24 cells and treated with a combination regimen of CDDP and GEM was remarkably suppressed by LMWF (mainly molecular weight was 760 Da) derived from *Sargassum hemiphyllum* [86]. The authors also showed that favorable control of inflammation, muscle proteolysis, and protein synthesis by myostatin/activin A/FoxO3/MAFbx/MuRF-1 cascade, NF-κB, and IGF-1 played crucial roles in the mitigation of chemotherapy-induced toxicity [86]. Additionally, this study demonstrated that fucoidan suppressed intestinal damage and function in a similar animal model [86]. Lastly, they speculated that LMWF is a promising and useful nutritional supplement and chemotherapeutic adjuvant for minimizing chemotherapy-induced toxicities in patients with BC, and we agree with their opinion.

As mentioned above, CDDP is a key drug in the treatment of BC. However, CDDP causes relatively severe adverse events in the gastrointestinal tract and kidneys. LMWF extracted from *Undaria pinnatifida* inhibits the chromic CDDP-induced weight loss and delayed gastrointestinal motility in a rat model [94]. Furthermore, in an in vitro study using proximal tubule epithelial (TH-1) cells, fucoidan suppressed CDDP-induced apoptosis and cell-cycle arrest via its anti-oxidative effects, including decreased ROS accumulation and excessive ER stress [95]. Accordingly, the authors suggested that fucoidan may be useful in protecting renal function in patients with cancer, who were treated with CDDP [95].

7. Issues Worth Considering and Future Direction of Fucoidan-Based Therapies

7.1. Points to Be Aware of Regarding Discussion of Fucoidan-Based Treatments

While discussing the anti-cancer effects and clinical usefulness of fucoidan in cancer therapy, special attention must be paid to its species, extraction methods, administration methods, and harvesting seasons. Briefly, bioactivities, including the anti-cancer effects of fucoidan, depend on these internal and external factors [10,15,63,96–98].

For example, although 50% cell proliferation of lung cancer cells (A549 cells) was inhibited by treatment for 48 h with 700 μg/mL fucoidan extracted from *Undaria pinnatifida* [97], a similar anti-cancer effect in A549 cells was shown by treatment for 48 h using only 100 μg/mL fucoidan extracted from *Fucusvesiculosus* [63]. Additionally, there is a report suggesting that fucoidans from *Macrocystis pyrifera* and *Undaria pinnatifida* at concentrations of 5–100 μg/mL display inhibitory effects on neutrophil apoptosis; however, this effect, in fucoidans obtained from *Ascophyllum nodosum* and *Fucusvesiculosus*, is observed at concentrations of 50–100 μg/mL [99]. Thus, the effective concentration of fucoidan extracts varies by the species of fucoidans.

The molecular weight of fucoidan has been suggested as another important determinant of its anti-cancer effects in various types of malignancies [8,10,21]. However, there is no general agreement on the relationship between the potency of anti-cancer effects and the molecular weight fractions of fucoidan. It was believed that the pro-apoptotic activity of high molecular weight fucoidan (HMWF) was significantly higher than that of LMWF and middle molecular weight fucoidan (MMWF) [10,21,100]. However, other investigators suggest the opposite and state that LMWF has greater anti-angiogenic and anti-metastatic effects [101]. In fact, LMWF treatment suppressed tumor growth in a dose-dependent manner in xenograft mice implanted with human BC cells (T24 cells) [28]. Furthermore, it is important to note that the molecular weight of fucoidan in the serum remains unchanged; however, molecular weight of fucoidan isolated from the urine is significantly lower than that of the ingested form [102]. This information is important to discuss the difference in anti-cancer effects of fucoidan in BC. Moreover, although detailed information on absorption, distribution, metabolism, and extraction of fucoidan in human subjects is not fully understood, several reports have shown that fucoidan is detected in the serum/plasma of healthy human volunteers after oral administration of this compound [102,103]. Thus, oral intake of crude fucoidan is recognized as a useful mode of administration in human subjects. However, it is generally agreed upon that the absorption rate of orally administered fucoidan is dependent on its molecular weight. Correspondingly, LMWF shows a better absorption rate than MMWF or HMWF in an in vivo study [10,104].

On the other hand, we should note an important fact that the criteria of molecular weights are not uniform across studies. For example, although several investigators have defined <10 kDa as LMWF, 10–10,000 kDa as MMWF, and >10,000 kDa as HMWF [10,100], another study classifies 10–50 kDa as LMWF, 50–100 kDa as MMWF, and >100 kDa as HMWF [21].

7.2. Future Directions

As mentioned above, various new treatment strategies, such as fucoidan-based combination therapies and nanoparticles have been suggested and developed using in vivo and in vitro studies. In recent years, immune therapies have been used as standard treatment methods in various types of malignancies, including BC, and many investigators have paid special attention to the development and modification of this therapy [105–107]. Fucoidans play significant roles in mutation of dendritic cells, activity of T and B lymphocytes, macrophages, and natural killer cells, and differentiation of macrophages in different experimental models, including cancer xenograft models [12,99,108–110]. Importantly, such an immune system is closely associated with malignant potential and outcome of BC cells [111–114]. Additionally, immune therapy is currently recognized as a major treatment in patients with BC [115,116]. Based on these facts, fucoidan may enhance the anti-cancer effects of immune therapy as an immunomodulator in BC. However, no in vivo studies have clarified this hypothesis yet.

On the other hand, while discussing the immunomodulatory effects of fucoidan, it is noteworthy to remember that its effects are dependent on the species from which it is extracted [99]. For example, the effect of activating the function of NK cells, T lymphocytes, and dendritic cells by fucoidan from *Macrocystis pyrifera* is stronger than those from others, such as *Ascophyllum nodosum, Undaria pinnatifida*, and *Fucus vesiculosus* [99]. Therefore, we emphasize that well-designed clinical studies are necessary to ascertain the anti-cancer effects of fucoidan as an immunomodulator in BC patients.

Currently, photodynamic therapy and thermal therapy are emerging as new treatment tools for patients with malignancies [117,118]. Furthermore, photodynamic and photothermal therapy based on nanoparticles have been suggested as novel anti-cancer treatments [119,120]. Moreover, the anti-cancer effects and molecular mechanisms of photothermal therapy using photosensitive polypyrrole nanoparticles and fucoidan have been reported in 2020 [121]. Thus, the development of new treatment strategies using fucoidan-based anti-cancer agents is expected in the near future. On the other hand, regulation of ROS and VEGF are associated with the pharmacological activity of photothermal therapy using photosensitive polypyrrole nanoparticles and fucoidan [121]. It is well known that both ROS and VEGF play crucial roles in tumor growth, progression, and survival in cancer patients [52,122–124]. Therefore, we agree with the opinion that this regimen may become a potential and promising treatment for many types of malignancies, including BC.

Currently, in most of the clinical trials on fucoidan, fucoidan is administered orally [125,126]. In contrast, a phase I clinical trial on imaging examination following intravenous injection of 99mTc-fucoidan has been reported [127]. Interestingly, this study showed that 99mTc-fucoidan did not have any drug-related adverse events [127]. Unfortunately, there is no clinical trial on the anti-cancer effects and safety of intravenously injected fucoidan in cancer patients. Conversely, although an effective fucoidan dose is dependent on the type of cancer, the effective dose for BC seems to be lower than that for other cancers [15,128]. For example, the effective dose of fucoidan derived from *Fucus vesiculosus* in hepatocellular carcinoma cell line and that of fucoidan supplied by Sigma-Aldrich Chemical Co. in prostate cancer cell line was reported to be 1,000 µg/mL. Thus, anti-cancer effects of fucoidan may be stronger in BC compared to those in the other types of cancers. In addition, there is the possibility that intravesical administration of fucoidan can suppress the recurrence of non-muscle invasive BC. We think a treatment strategy based on non-oral administration of fucoidan may have stronger biological effects in patients with malignancies including BC.

8. Conclusions

We reviewed the anti-cancer effects of fucoidan and fucoidan-based treatment strategies and their detailed molecular mechanisms. Accordingly, fucoidan is speculated to have clinical application and is a potential therapeutic for patients with malignancies, including BC. On the other hand, we should note that its biological and pharmacological activities are dependent on many internal and external factors, such as the species it is extracted from and its molecular weight. Unfortunately, there are very few clinical trials, including comparative and randomized studies in patients with BC. However, it is difficult to plan clinical trials with large populations in BC patients because basic information regarding the pharmacological characteristics of fucoidan, such as absorption, distribution, metabolism, and pharmacokinetics based on the molecular weight, is still unavailable. Nevertheless, we emphasize that fucoidan is a much sought-after compound, owing to its low in vivo toxicity, including that in humans. Lastly, we suggest that well-designed preclinical and clinical trials are needed to investigate the anti-cancer effects and safety of fucoidan-based therapies in patients with BC.

Author Contributions: Conceptualization: Y.M. (Yasuyoshi Miyata); Supervision: H.S.; Writing—original draft Preparation: Y.M. (Yasuyoshi Miyata), T.M. (Tomohiro Matsuo), K.M., K.O., Y.M. (Yuta Mukae), A.O., J.H., T.M. (Tsuyoshi Matsuda), T.K. All authors have read and agreed to the published version of the manuscript.

References

1. Yasuda, T.; Miyata, Y.; Nakamura, Y.; Sagara, Y.; Matsuo, T.; Ohba, K.; Sakai, H. High Consumption of Green Tea Suppresses Urinary Tract Recurrence of Urothelial Cancervia Down-regulation of Human Antigen-R Expression in Never Smokers. *In Vivo* **2018**, *32*, 721–729. [CrossRef] [PubMed]

2. Matsuo, T.; Miyata, Y.; Yuno, T.; Mukae, Y.; Otsubo, A.; Mitsunari, K.; Ohba, K.; Sakai, H. Molecular Mechanisms of the Anti-Cancer Effects of Isothiocyanates from Cruciferous Vegetables in Bladder Cancer. *Molecules* **2020**, *25*, 575. [CrossRef]

3. Rutz, J.; Janicova, A.; Woidacki, K.; Chun, F.K.-H.; Blaheta, R.A.; Relja, B. Curcumin—A Viable Agent for Better Bladder Cancer Treatment. *Int. J. Mol. Sci.* **2020**, *21*, 3761. [CrossRef] [PubMed]

4. Sherif, I. Uroprotective mechanisms of natural products against cyclophosphamide-induced urinary bladder toxicity: A comprehensive review. *Acta Sci. Pol. Technol. Aliment.* **2020**, *19*, 333–346. [CrossRef] [PubMed]

5. Hsu, H.-Y.; Hwang, P. Clinical applications of fucoidan in translational medicine for adjuvant cancer therapy. *Clin. Transl. Med.* **2019**, *8*, 15. [CrossRef]

6. Kusaykin, M.; Bakunina, I.; Sova, V.; Ermakova, S.; Kuznetsova, T.; Besednova, N.; Zaporozhets, T.; Zvyagintseva, T. Structure, biological activity, and enzymatic transformation of fucoidans from the brown seaweeds. *Biotechnol. J.* **2008**, *3*, 904–915. [CrossRef]

7. Ye, J.; Chen, D.; Ye, Z.; Huang, Y.; Zhang, N.; Lui, E.M.K.; Xue, C.; Xiao, M. Fucoidan Isolated from Saccharina japonica Inhibits LPS-Induced Inflammation in Macrophages via Blocking NF-κB, MAPK and JAK-STAT Pathways. *Mar. Drugs* **2020**, *18*, 328. [CrossRef]

8. Zhang, R.; Zhang, X.; Tang, Y.; Mao, J. Composition, isolation, purification and biological activities of Sargassum fusiforme polysaccharides: A review. *Carbohydr. Polym.* **2020**, *228*, 115381. [CrossRef]

9. Kim, K.-J.; Lee, O.-H.; Lee, H.-H.; Lee, B.-Y. A 4-week repeated oral dose toxicity study of fucoidan from the Sporophyll of Undaria pinnatifida in Sprague–Dawley rats. *Toxicology* **2010**, *267*, 154–158. [CrossRef]

10. Van Weelden, G.; Bobiński, M.; Okła, K.; Van Weelden, W.J.; Romano, A.; Pijnenborg, J.M.A. Fucoidan Structure and Activity in Relation to Anti-Cancer Mechanisms. *Mar. Drugs* **2019**, *17*, 32. [CrossRef]

11. Pan, T.J.; Li, L.X.; Zhang, J.W.; Yang, Z.S.; Shi, D.M.; Yang, Y.K.; Wu, W.Z. Antimetastatic Effect of Fucoidan-Sargassum against Liver Cancer Cell Invadopodia Formation via Targeting Integrin αVβ3 and Mediating αVβ3/Src/E2F1 Signaling. *J. Cancer* **2019**, *10*, 4777–4792. [CrossRef]

12. Chen, L.-M.; Tseng, H.-Y.; Chen, Y.-A.; Al Haq, A.T.; Hwang, P.-A.; Hsu, H.-L. Oligo-Fucoidan Prevents M2 Macrophage Differentiation and HCT116 Tumor Progression. *Cancers* **2020**, *12*, 421. [CrossRef] [PubMed]

13. Hsu, W.-J.; Lin, M.-H.; Kuo, T.-C.; Chou, C.-M.; Mi, F.-L.; Cheng, C.-H.; Lin, C.-W. Fucoidan from Laminaria japonica exerts antitumor effects on angiogenesis and micrometastasis in triple-negative breast cancer cells. *Int. J. Biol. Macromol.* **2020**, *149*, 600–608. [CrossRef] [PubMed]

14. Li, B.; Lu, F.; Wei, X.; Zhao, R. Fucoidan: Structure and Bioactivity. *Molecules* **2008**, *13*, 1671–1695. [CrossRef] [PubMed]

15. Lin, Y.; Qi, X.; Liu, H.; Xue, K.; Xu, S.; Tian, Z. The anti-cancer effects of fucoidan: A review of both in vivo and in vitro investigations. *Cancer Cell Int.* **2020**, *20*, 1–14. [CrossRef] [PubMed]

16. Kim, I.-H.; Nam, T.-J. Fucoidan downregulates insulin-like growth factor-I receptor levels in HT-29 human colon cancer cells. *Oncol. Rep.* **2018**, *39*, 1516–1522. [CrossRef]

17. Duan, Y.; Li, J.; Jing, X.; Ding, X.; Yu, Y.; Zhao, Q. Fucoidan Induces Apoptosis and Inhibits Proliferation of Hepatocellular Carcinoma via the p38 MAPK/ERK and PI3K/Akt Signal Pathways. *Cancer Manag. Res.* **2020**, *12*, 1713–1723. [CrossRef]

18. Wu, T.C.; Hong, Y.H.; Tsai, Y.H.; Hsieh, S.L.; Huang, R.H.; Kuo, C.H.; Huang, C.Y. Degradation of Sargassum crassifolium Fucoidan by Ascorbic Acid and Hydrogen Peroxide, and Compositional, Structural, and In vitro Anti-Lung Cancer Analyses of the Degradation Products. *Mar. Drugs* **2020**, *18*, 334. [CrossRef]

19. Xue, M.; Ji, X.; Xue, C.; Liang, H.; Ge, Y.; He, X.; Zhang, L.; Bian, K.; Zhang, L. Caspase-dependent and caspase-independent induction of apoptosis in breast cancer by fucoidan via the PI3K/AKT/GSK3β pathway in vivo and in vitro. *Biomed. Pharmacother.* **2017**, *94*, 898–908. [CrossRef]

20. Niyonizigiye, I.; Ngabire, D.; Patil, M.P.; Singh, A.A.; Kim, G.-D. In vitro induction of endoplasmic reticulum stress in human cervical adenocarcinoma HeLa cells by fucoidan. *Int. J. Biol. Macromol.* **2019**, *137*, 844–852. [CrossRef]

21. Gupta, D.; Silva, M.; Radziun, K.; Martinez, D.C.; Hill, C.J.; Marshall, J.; Hearnden, V.; Puertas-Mejía, M.A.; Reilly, G.C. Fucoidan Inhibition of Osteosarcoma Cells is Species and Molecular Weight Dependent. *Mar. Drugs* **2020**, *18*, 104. [CrossRef] [PubMed]

22. Sagara, Y.; Miyata, Y.; Nomata, K.; Hayashi, T.; Kanetake, H. Green tea polyphenol suppresses tumor invasion and angiogenesis in N-butyl-(-4-hydroxybutyl) nitrosamine-induced bladder cancer. *Cancer Epidemiol.* **2010**, *34*, 350–354. [CrossRef]

23. Matsuo, T.; Miyata, Y.; Asai, A.; Sagara, Y.; Furusato, B.; Fukuoka, J.; Sakai, H. Green Tea Polyphenol Induces Changes in Cancer-Related Factors in an Animal Model of Bladder Cancer. *PLoS ONE* **2017**, *12*, e0171091. [CrossRef] [PubMed]

24. Wu, P.; Meng, X.; Zheng, H.-D.; Zeng, Q.; Chen, T.; Wang, W.; Zhang, X.; Su, J. Kaempferol Attenuates ROS-Induced Hemolysis and the Molecular Mechanism of Its Induction of Apoptosis on Bladder Cancer. *Molecules* **2018**, *23*, 2592. [CrossRef] [PubMed]

25. Ramchandani, S.; Naz, I.; Lee, J.H.; Khan, R.A.; Ahn, K.S. An Overview of the Potential Antineoplastic Effects of Casticin. *Molecules* **2020**, *25*, 1287. [CrossRef] [PubMed]

26. Cho, T.-M.; Kim, W.-J.; Moon, S.-K. AKT signaling is involved in fucoidan-induced inhibition of growth and migration of human bladder cancer cells. *Food Chem. Toxicol.* **2014**, *64*, 344–352. [CrossRef]

27. Park, H.Y.; Kim, G.-Y.; Moon, S.-K.; Kim, W.-J.; Yoo, Y.H.; Choi, Y.H. Fucoidan Inhibits the Proliferation of Human Urinary Bladder Cancer T24 Cells by Blocking Cell Cycle Progression and Inducing Apoptosis. *Molecules* **2014**, *19*, 5981–5998. [CrossRef]

28. Chen, M.-C.; Hsu, W.-L.; Hwang, P.-A.; Chou, T.-C. Low Molecular Weight Fucoidan Inhibits Tumor Angiogenesis through Downregulation of HIF-1/VEGF Signaling under Hypoxia. *Mar. Drugs* **2015**, *13*, 4436–4451. [CrossRef]

29. Park, H.Y.; Choi, I.W.; Kim, G.Y.; Kim, B.W.; Kim, W.J.; Choi, Y.H. Fucoidan Induces G1 Arrest of the Cell Cycle in EJ Human Bladder Cancer Cells Trough Down-regulation of pRB Phosphorylation. *Rev. Bras. Farmacogn.* **2015**, *25*, 246–251. [CrossRef]

30. Han, M.H.; Lee, D.-S.; Jeong, J.-W.; Hong, S.H.; Choi, I.-W.; Cha, H.-J.; Kim, S.; Kim, A.H.-S.; Park, C.; Kim, G.-Y.; et al. Fucoidan Induces ROS-Dependent Apoptosis in 5637 Human Bladder Cancer Cells by Downregulating Telomerase Activity via Inactivation of the PI3K/Akt Signaling Pathway. *Drug Dev. Res.* **2017**, *78*, 37–48. [CrossRef]

31. Ye, J.; Li, Y.; Teruya, K.; Katakura, Y.; Ichikawa, A.; Eto, H.; Hosoi, M.; Hosoi, M.; Nishimoto, S.; Shirahata, S. Enzyme-digested Fucoidan Extracts Derived from Seaweed Mozuku of Cladosiphon novae-caledoniaekylin Inhibit Invasion and Angiogenesis of Tumor Cells. *Cytotechnology* **2005**, *47*, 117–126. [CrossRef] [PubMed]

32. Oliveira, C.; Granja, S.; Neves, N.M.; Reis, R.L.; Baltazar, F.; Silva, T.H.; Martins, A. Fucoidan from FucusVesiculosus Inhibits New Blood Vessel Formation and Breast Tumor Growth In vivo. *Carbohydr. Polym.* **2019**, *223*, 115034. [CrossRef] [PubMed]

33. Mudassar, F.; Shen, H.; O'Neill, G.; Hau, E. Targeting tumor hypoxia and mitochondrial metabolism with anti-parasitic drugs to improve radiation response in high-grade gliomas. *J. Exp. Clin. Cancer Res.* **2020**, *39*, 1–17. [CrossRef] [PubMed]

34. Shah, V.M.; Sheppard, B.C.; Sears, R.C.; Alani, A.W. Hypoxia: Friend or Foe for drug delivery in Pancreatic Cancer. *Cancer Lett.* **2020**, *492*, 63–70. [CrossRef] [PubMed]

35. Torrisi, F.; Vicario, N.; Spitale, F.M.; Cammarata, F.P.; Minafra, L.; Salvatorelli, L.; Russo, G.; Cuttone, G.; Valable, S.; Gulino, R.; et al. The Role of Hypoxia and SRC Tyrosine Kinase in Glioblastoma Invasiveness and Radioresistance. *Cancers* **2020**, *12*, 2860. [CrossRef] [PubMed]

36. Paternot, S.; Bockstaele, L.; Bisteau, X.; Kooken, H.; Coulonval, K.; Roger, P.P. Rb inactivation in cell cycle and cancer: The puzzle of highly regulated activating phosphorylation of CDK4 versus constitutively active CDK-activating kinase. *Cell Cycle* **2010**, *9*, 689–699. [CrossRef]

37. Asai, A.; Miyata, Y.; Takehara, K.; Kanda, S.; Watanabe, S.-I.; Greer, P.A.; Sakai, H. Pathological significance and prognostic significance of FES expression in bladder cancer vary according to tumor grade. *J. Cancer Res. Clin. Oncol.* **2017**, *144*, 21–31. [CrossRef]

38. Flaig, T.W. NCCN Guidelines Updates: Management of Muscle-Invasive Bladder Cancer. *J. Natl. Compr. Cancer Netw.* **2019**, *17*, 591–593.

39. Kanayama, H. Matrix metalloproteinases and bladder cancer. *J. Med. Investig.* **2001**, *48*, 31–43.

40. Wieczorek, E.; Wasowicz, W.; Gromadzinska, J.; Reszka, E. Functional polymorphisms in the matrix metalloproteinase genes and their association with bladder cancer risk and recurrence: A mini-review. *Int. J. Urol.* **2014**, *21*, 744–752. [CrossRef]

41. Nakamura, Y.; Miyata, Y.; Takehara, K.; Asai, A.; Mitsunari, K.; Araki, K.; Matsuo, T.; Ohba, K.; Sakai, H. The Pathological Significance and Prognostic Roles of Thrombospondin-1, and -2, and 4N1K-peptide in Bladder Cancer. *Anticancer Res.* **2019**, *39*, 2317–2324. [CrossRef]

42. Ohba, K.; Miyata, Y.; Matsuo, T.; Asai, A.; Mitsunari, K.; Shida, Y.; Kanda, S.; Sakai, H. High expression of Twist is associated with tumor aggressiveness and poor prognosis in patients with renal cell carcinoma. *Int. J. Clin. Exp. Pathol.* **2014**, *7*, 3158–3165. [PubMed]

43. Miyata, Y.; Kanda, S.; Mitsunari, K.; Asai, A.; Sakai, H. Heme oxygenase-1 expression is associated with tumor aggressiveness and outcomes in patients with bladder cancer: A correlation with smoking intensity. *Transl. Res.* **2014**, *164*, 468–476. [CrossRef] [PubMed]

44. Dofara, S.G.; Chang, S.-L.; Diorio, C. Gene Polymorphisms and Circulating Levels of MMP-2 and MMP-9: A Review of Their Role in Breast Cancer Risk. *Anticancer Res.* **2020**, *40*, 3619–3631. [CrossRef] [PubMed]

45. Nagai, Y.; Saitoh, Y.; Miwa, N. Fucoidan-Vitamin C complex suppresses tumor invasion through the basement membrane, with scarce injuries to normal or tumor cells, via decreases in oxidative stress and matrix metalloproteinases. *Int. J. Oncol.* **2009**, *35*, 1183–1189. [CrossRef]

46. Lee, H.; Kim, J.S.; Kim, E. Fucoidan from seaweed Fucusvesiculosus inhibits migration and invasion of human lung cancer cell via PI3K-Akt-mTOR pathways. *PLoS ONE* **2012**, *7*, e50624. [CrossRef]

47. Seargent, J.M.; Loadman, P.M.; Martin, S.W.; Naylor, B.; Bibby, M.C.; Gill, J.H. Expression of matrix metalloproteinase-10 in human bladder transitional cell carcinoma. *Urology* **2005**, *65*, 815–820. [CrossRef]

48. Miyata, Y.; Iwata, T.; Maruta, S.; Kanda, S.; Nishikido, M.; Koga, S.; Kanetake, H. Expression of Matrix Metalloproteinase-10 in Renal Cell Carcinoma and Its Prognostic Role. *Eur. Urol.* **2007**, *52*, 791–797. [CrossRef]

49. Maruta, S.; Miyata, Y.; Sagara, Y.; Kanda, S.; Iwata, T.; Watanabe, S.-I.; Sakai, H.; Hayashi, T.; Kanetake, H. Expression of matrix metalloproteinase-10 in non-metastatic prostate cancer: Correlation with an imbalance in cell proliferation and apoptosis. *Oncol. Lett.* **2010**, *1*, 417–421. [CrossRef]

50. Liao, C.-H.; Chang, W.-S.; Tsai, C.-W.; Hu, P.-S.; Wu, H.-C.; Hsu, S.-W.; Chen, G.-L.; Yueh, T.-C.; Shen, T.-C.; Hsia, T.-C.; et al. Association of Matrix Metalloproteinase-7 Genotypes with the Risk of Bladder Cancer. *In Vivo* **2018**, *32*, 1045–1050. [CrossRef]

51. Sagara, Y.; Miyata, Y.; Iwata, T.; Kanda, S.; Hayashi, T.; Sakai, H.; Kanetake, H. Clinical significance and prognostic value of S100A4 and matrix metalloproteinase-14 in patients with organ-confined bladder cancer. *Exp. Ther. Med.* **2010**, *1*, 27–31. [PubMed]

52. Miyata, Y.; Matsuo, T.; Sagara, Y.; Ohba, K.; Ohyama, K.; Sakai, H. A Mini-Review of Reactive Oxygen Species in Urological Cancer: Correlation with NADPH Oxidases, Angiogenesis, and Apoptosis. *Int. J. Mol. Sci.* **2017**, *18*, 2214. [CrossRef] [PubMed]

53. Xiao, W.; Wang, R.-S.; Handy, D.E.; Loscalzo, J. NAD(H) and NADP(H) Redox Couples and Cellular Energy Metabolism. *Antioxid. Redox Signal.* **2018**, *28*, 251–272. [CrossRef] [PubMed]

54. Schieber, M.; Chandel, N.S. ROS Function in Redox Signaling and Oxidative Stress. *Curr. Biol.* **2014**, *24*, R453–R462. [CrossRef]

55. Moloney, J.N.; Cotter, T.G. ROS signalling in the biology of cancer. *Semin. Cell Dev. Biol.* **2018**, *80*, 50–64. [CrossRef]

56. Chen, Y.-C.; Wang, P.-Y.; Huang, B.-M.; Chen, Y.-J.; Lee, W.C.; Chen, Y.-C. 16-Hydroxycleroda-3,13-dien-15,16-olide Induces Apoptosis in Human Bladder Cancer Cells through Cell Cycle Arrest, Mitochondria ROS Overproduction, and Inactivation of EGFR-Related Signalling Pathways. *Molecules* **2020**, *25*, 3958. [CrossRef]

57. Liu, D.; Qiu, X.; Xiong, X.; Chen, X.Q.; Pan, F. Current updates on the role of reactive oxygen species in bladder cancer pathogenesis and therapeutics. *Clin. Transl. Oncol.* **2020**, *22*, 1687–1697. [CrossRef]

58. Witjes, J.A.; Bruins, H.M.; Cathomas, R.; Compérat, E.M.; Cowan, N.C.; Gakis, G.; Hernández, V.; Linares Espinós, E.; Lorch, A.; Neuzillet, Y.; et al. European Association of Urology Guidelines on Muscle-invasive and Metastatic Bladder Cancer: Summary of the 2020 Guidelines. *Eur. Urol.* **2020**, in press. [CrossRef]

59. Albany, C.; Sonpavde, G. Docetaxel for the treatment of bladder cancer. *Expert Opin. Investig. Drugs* **2015**, *24*, 1657–1664. [CrossRef]

60. Miyata, Y.; Matsuo, T.; Nakamura, Y.; Yasuda, T.; Ohba, K.; Takehara, K.; Sakai, H. Expression of Class III Beta-tubulin Predicts Prognosis in Patients with Cisplatin-resistant Bladder Cancer Receiving Paclitaxel-based Second-line Chemotherapy. *Anticancer Res.* **2018**, *38*, 1629–1635. [CrossRef]

61. Blaszczak, W.; Lach, M.S.; Barczak, W.; Suchorska, W.M. Fucoidan Exerts Anticancer Effects Against Head and Neck Squamous Cell Carcinoma In Vitro. *Molecules* **2018**, *23*, 3302. [CrossRef] [PubMed]

62. Abudabbus, A.; Badmus, J.A.; Shalaweh, S.; Bauer, R.; Hiss, D. Effects of Fucoidan and Chemotherapeutic Agent Combinations on Malignant and Non-malignant Breast Cell Lines. *Curr. Pharm. Biotechnol.* **2017**, *18*, 748–757. [CrossRef] [PubMed]

63. Hsu, H.-Y.; Lin, T.-Y.; Hu, C.-H.; Shu, D.T.F.; Lu, M.-K. Fucoidan upregulates TLR4/CHOP-mediated caspase-3 and PARP activation to enhance cisplatin-induced cytotoxicity in human lung cancer cells. *Cancer Lett.* **2018**, *432*, 112–120. [CrossRef]

64. Zhang, Z.; Teruya, K.; Yoshida, T.; Eto, H.; Shirahata, S. Fucoidan Extract Enhances the Anti-Cancer Activity of Chemotherapeutic Agents in MDA-MB-231 and MCF-7 Breast Cancer Cells. *Mar. Drugs* **2013**, *11*, 81–98. [CrossRef]

65. Mathew, L.; Burney, M.; Gaikwad, A.; Nyshadham, P.; Nugent, E.K.; Gonzalez, A.; Smith, J.A. Preclinical Evaluation of Safety of Fucoidan Extracts from Undaria pinnatifida and Fucusvesiculosus for Use in Cancer Treatment. *Integr. Cancer Ther.* **2017**, *16*, 572–584. [CrossRef]

66. Burney, M.; Mathew, L.; Gaikwad, A.; Nugent, E.K.; Gonzalez, A.O.; Smith, J.A. Evaluation Fucoidan Extracts from Undaria pinnatifida and Fucusvesiculosus in Combination with Anticancer Drugs in Human Cancer Orthotopic Mouse Models. *Integr. Cancer Ther.* **2018**, *17*, 755–761. [CrossRef]

67. Zhang, Z.; Teruya, K.; Eto, H.; Shirahata, S. Induction of Apoptosis by Low-Molecular-Weight Fucoidan through Calcium- and Caspase-Dependent Mitochondrial Pathways in MDA-MB-231 Breast Cancer Cells. *Biosci. Biotechnol. Biochem.* **2013**, *77*, 235–242. [CrossRef] [PubMed]

68. Hwang, P.-A.; Lin, X.-Z.; Kuo, K.-L.; Hsu, F.-Y. Fabrication and Cytotoxicity of Fucoidan-Cisplatin Nanoparticles for Macrophage and Tumor Cells. *Materials* **2017**, *10*, 291. [CrossRef] [PubMed]

69. Choi, D.G.; Venkatesan, J.; Shim, M.S. Selective Anticancer Therapy Using Pro-Oxidant Drug-Loaded Chitosan–Fucoidan Nanoparticles. *Int. J. Mol. Sci.* **2019**, *20*, 3220. [CrossRef] [PubMed]

70. Chen, X.; Zhao, X.; Wang, G. Review on marine carbohydrate-based gold nanoparticles represented by alginate and chitosan for biomedical application. *Carbohydr. Polym.* **2020**, *244*, 116311. [CrossRef] [PubMed]

71. Coutinho, A.J.; Lima, S.A.C.; Afonso, C.M.; Reis, S. Mucoadhesive and pH responsive fucoidan-chitosan nanoparticles for the oral delivery of methotrexate. *Int. J. Biol. Macromol.* **2020**, *158*, 180–188. [CrossRef] [PubMed]

72. Oliveira, C.; Neves, N.M.; Reis, R.L.; Martins, A.; Silva, T.H. Gemcitabine delivered by fucoidan/chitosan nanoparticles presents increased toxicity over human breast cancer cells. *Nanomedicine* **2018**, *13*, 2037–2050. [CrossRef] [PubMed]

73. Lai, Y.-H.; Chiang, C.; Hsu, C.-H.; Cheng, H.-W.; Chen, S.-Y. Development and Characterization of a Fucoidan-Based Drug Delivery System by Using Hydrophilic Anticancer Polysaccharides to Simultaneously Deliver Hydrophobic Anticancer Drugs. *Biomolecules* **2020**, *10*, 970. [CrossRef] [PubMed]

74. Chen, M.-L.; Lai, C.-J.; Lin, Y.-N.; Huang, C.-M.; Lin, Y.-H. Multifunctional nanoparticles for targeting the tumor microenvironment to improve synergistic drug combinations and cancer treatment effects. *J. Mater. Chem. B* **2020**. [CrossRef]

75. Miyata, Y.; Nomata, K.; Ohba, K.; Matsuo, T.; Sagara, Y.; Kanetake, H.; Sakai, H. Use of low-dose combined therapy with gemcitabine and paclitaxel for advanced urothelial cancer patients with resistance to cisplatin-containing therapy: A retrospective analysis. *Cancer Chemother. Pharmacol.* **2012**, *70*, 451–459. [CrossRef]

76. Miyata, Y.; Asai, A.; Mitsunari, K.; Matsuo, T.; Ohba, K.; Sakai, H. Safety and efficacy of combination therapy with low-dose gemcitabine, paclitaxel, and sorafenib in patients with cisplatin-resistant urothelial cancer. *Med Oncol.* **2015**, *32*, 235. [CrossRef]

77. Phan, U.T.; Nguyen, K.T.; Van Vo, T.; Duan, W.; Tran, P.H.; Tran, T.T.-D. Investigation of fucoidan-oleic acid conjugate for delivery of curcumin and paclitaxel. *Anti-Cancer Agents Med. Chem.* **2013**, *16*, 1281–1287. [CrossRef]

78. Phan, N.H.; Ly, T.T.; Pham, M.N.; Luu, T.D.; Vo, T.V.; Tran, P.H.; Tran, T.T. A Comparison of Fucoidan Conjugated to Paclitaxel and Curcumin for the Dual Delivery of Cancer Therapeutic Agents. *Anti-Cancer Agents Med. Chem.* **2019**, *18*, 1349–1355. [CrossRef]

79. Miyata, Y.; Matsuo, T.; Araki, K.; Nakamura, Y.; Sagara, Y.; Ohba, K.; Sakai, H. Anticancer Effects of Green Tea and the Underlying Molecular Mechanisms in Bladder Cancer. *Medicines* **2018**, *5*, 87. [CrossRef]

80. Sun, X.; Song, J.; Li, E.; Geng, H.; Li, Y.; Yu, D.; Zhong, C. (-)-Epigallocatechin 3 gallate inhibits bladder cancer stem cells via suppression of sonic hedgehog pathway. *Oncol. Rep.* **2019**, *42*, 425–435. [CrossRef]

81. Piwowarczyk, L.; Stawny, M.; Mlynarczyk, D.T.; Muszalska, I.; Goslinski, T.; Jelińska, A. Role of Curcumin and (−)-Epigallocatechin-3-O-Gallate in Bladder Cancer Treatment: A Review. *Cancers* **2020**, *12*, 1801. [CrossRef] [PubMed]

82. Ikeguchi, M.; Yamamoto, M.; Arai, Y.; Maeta, Y.; Ashida, K.; Katano, K.; Miki, Y.; Kimura, T. Fucoidan reduces the toxicities of chemotherapy for patients with unresectable advanced or recurrent colorectal cancer. *Oncol. Lett.* **2011**, *2*, 319–322. [CrossRef] [PubMed]

83. Fearon, K.C.; Strasser, F.; Anker, S.D.; Bosaeus, I.; Bruera, E.; Fainsinger, R.L.; Jatoi, A.; Loprinzi, C.; Macdonald, N.; Mantovani, G.; et al. Definition and classification of cancer cachexia: An international consensus. *Lancet Oncol.* **2011**, *12*, 489–495. [CrossRef]

84. Schmidt, S.F.; Rohm, M.; Herzig, S.; Diaz, M.B. Cancer Cachexia: More Than Skeletal Muscle Wasting. *Trends Cancer* **2018**, *4*, 849–860. [CrossRef]

85. Donohoe, C.L.; Ryan, A.M.; Reynolds, J.V. Cancer Cachexia: Mechanisms and Clinical Implications. *Gastroenterol. Res. Pract.* **2011**, *2011*, 1–13. [CrossRef]

86. Chen, M.-C.; Hsu, W.-L.; Hwang, P.-A.; Chen, Y.-L.; Chou, T.-C. Combined administration of fucoidan ameliorates tumor and chemotherapy-induced skeletal muscle atrophy in bladder cancer-bearing mice. *Oncotarget* **2016**, *7*, 51608–51618. [CrossRef]

87. Solheim, T.S.; Laird, B.J.A.; Balstad, T.R.; Bye, A.; Stene, G.; Baracos, V.; Strasser, F.; Griffiths, G.; Maddocks, M.; Fallon, M.; et al. Cancer cachexia: Rationale for the MENAC (Multimodal—Exercise, Nutrition and Anti-inflammatory medication for Cachexia) trial. *BMJ Support. Palliat. Care* **2018**, *8*, 258–265. [CrossRef]

88. Cruz, B.L.G.; Oliveira, A.G.; Viana, L.R.; Lopes-Aguiar, L.; Canevarolo, R.; Colombera, M.C.; Valentim, R.R.; Garcia-Fóssa, F.; De Sousa, L.M.; Castelucci, B.G.; et al. Leucine-Rich Diet Modulates the Metabolomic and Proteomic Profile of Skeletal Muscle during Cancer Cachexia. *Cancers* **2020**, *12*, 1880. [CrossRef]

89. Fukushima, H.; Takemura, K.; Suzuki, H.; Koga, F. Impact of Sarcopenia as a Prognostic Biomarker of Bladder Cancer. *Int. J. Mol. Sci.* **2018**, *19*, 2999. [CrossRef]

90. Mayr, R.; Gierth, M.; Zeman, F.; Reiffen, M.; Seeger, P.; Wezel, F.; Pycha, A.; Comploj, E.; Bonatti, M.; Ritter, M.; et al. Sarcopenia as a comorbidity-independent predictor of survival following radical cystectomy for bladder cancer. *J. Cachex. Sarcopenia Muscle* **2018**, *9*, 505–513. [CrossRef]

91. Stangl-Kremser, J.; D'Andrea, D.; Vartolomei, M.; Abufaraj, M.M.; Goldner, G.; Baltzer, P.A.; Shariat, S.F.; Tamandl, D. Prognostic value of nutritional indices and body composition parameters including sarcopenia in patients treated with radiotherapy for urothelial carcinoma of the bladder. *Urol. Oncol. Semin. Orig. Investig.* **2019**, *37*, 372–379. [CrossRef] [PubMed]

92. Chen, M.-C.; Chen, Y.-L.; Lee, C.-F.; Hung, C.-H.; Chou, T.-C. Supplementation of Magnolol Attenuates Skeletal Muscle Atrophy in Bladder Cancer-Bearing Mice Undergoing Chemotherapy via Suppression of FoxO3 Activation and Induction of IGF-1. *PLoS ONE* **2015**, *10*, e0143594. [CrossRef] [PubMed]

93. Miyake, M.; Hori, S.; Itami, Y.; Oda, Y.; Owari, T.; Fujii, T.; Ohnishi, S.; Morizawa, Y.; Gotoh, D.; Nakai, Y.; et al. Supplementary Oral Anamorelin Mitigates Anorexia and Skeletal Muscle Atrophy Induced by Gemcitabine Plus Cisplatin Systemic Chemotherapy in a Mouse Model. *Cancers* **2020**, *12*, 1942. [CrossRef]

94. Song, M.Y.; Ku, S.K.; Kim, H.J.; Han, J.S. Low molecular weight fucoidan ameliorating the chronic cisplatin-induced delayed gastrointestinal motility in rats. *Food Chem. Toxicol.* **2012**, *50*, 4468–4478. [CrossRef]

95. Kim, H.J.; Yoon, Y.M.; Lee, J.H.; Lee, S.H. Protective Role of Fucoidan on Cisplatin-mediated ER Stress in Renal Proximal Tubule Epithelial Cells. *Anticancer Res.* **2019**, *39*, 5515–5524. [CrossRef] [PubMed]

96. Mak, W.; Hamid, N.; Liu, T.; Lu, J.; White, W. Fucoidan from New Zealand Undaria pinnatifida: Monthly variations and determination of antioxidant activities. *Carbohydr. Polym.* **2013**, *95*, 606–614. [CrossRef]

97. Mak, W.; Wang, S.K.; Liu, T.; Hamid, N.; Li, Y.; Lu, J.; White, W.L. Anti-Proliferation Potential and Content of Fucoidan Extracted from Sporophyll of New Zealand Undaria pinnatifida. *Front. Nutr.* **2014**, *1*, 9. [CrossRef] [PubMed]

98. Skriptsova, A.V. Seasonal variations in the fucoidan content of brown algae from Peter the Great Bay, Sea of Japan. *Russ. J. Mar. Biol.* **2016**, *42*, 351–356. [CrossRef]

99. Zhang, W.; Oda, T.; Yu, Q.; Jin, J.O. Fucoidan from Macrocystispyrifera has powerful immune-modulatory effects compared to three other fucoidans. *Mar. Drugs* **2015**, *13*, 1084–1104. [CrossRef]

100. Kalimuthu, S.; Manivasagan, P.; Venkatesan, J.; Kim, S.-K. Brown seaweed fucoidan: Biological activity and apoptosis, growth signaling mechanism in cancer. *Int. J. Biol. Macromol.* **2013**, *60*, 366–374. [CrossRef]

101. Cumashi, A.; Ushakova, N.A.; Preobrazhenskaya, M.E.; D'Incecco, A.; Piccoli, A.; Totani, L.; Tinari, N.; Morozevich, G.E.; Berman, A.E.; Bilan, M.I.; et al. A comparative study of the anti-inflammatory, anticoagulant, antiangiogenic, and antiadhesive activities of nine different fucoidans from brown seaweeds. *Glycobiology* **2007**, *17*, 541–552. [CrossRef] [PubMed]

102. Tokita, Y.; Nakajima, K.; Mochida, H.; Iha, M.; Nagamine, T. Development of a Fucoidan-Specific Antibody and Measurement of Fucoidan in Serum and Urine by Sandwich ELISA. *Biosci. Biotechnol. Biochem.* **2010**, *74*, 350–357. [CrossRef] [PubMed]

103. Irhimeh, M.R.; Fitton, J.H.; Lowenthal, R.M.; Kongtawelert, P. A quantitative method to detect fucoidan in human plasma using a novel antibody. *Methods Find. Exp. Clin. Pharmacol.* **2005**, *27*, 705–710. [CrossRef] [PubMed]

104. Matsubara, K.; Xue, C.; Zhao, X.; Mori, M.; Sugawara, T.; Hirata, T. Effects of middle molecular weight fucoidans on in vitro and ex vivo angiogenesis of endothelial cells. *Int. J. Mol. Med.* **2005**, *15*, 695–699. [CrossRef] [PubMed]

105. Nguyen, M.; Smith, S.T.; Lam, M.; Liow, E.; Davies, A.; Prenen, H.; Segelov, E. An update on the use of immunotherapy in patients with colorectal cancer. *Expert Rev. Gastroenterol. Hepatol.* **2020**, 1–14. [CrossRef] [PubMed]

106. Roviello, G.; Catalano, M.; Nobili, S.; Santi, R.; Mini, E.; Nesi, G. Focus on Biochemical and Clinical Predictors of Response to Immune Checkpoint Inhibitors in Metastatic Urothelial Carcinoma: Where Do We Stand? *Int. J. Mol. Sci.* **2020**, *21*, 7935. [CrossRef]

107. Zhu, M.M.; Shenasa, E.; Nielsen, T.O. Sarcomas: Immune biomarker expression and checkpoint inhibitor trials. *Cancer Treat. Rev.* **2020**, *91*, 102115. [CrossRef]

108. Hayashi, K.; Nakano, T.; Hashimoto, M.; Kanekiyo, K.; Hayashi, T. Defensive effects of a fucoidan from brown alga Undaria pinnatifida against herpes simplex virus infection. *Int. Immunopharmacol.* **2008**, *8*, 109–116. [CrossRef]

109. Chen, L.-M.; Liu, P.-Y.; Chen, Y.-A.; Tseng, H.-Y.; Shen, P.-C.; Hwang, P.-A.; Hsu, H.-L. Oligo-Fucoidan prevents IL-6 and CCL2 production and cooperates with p53 to suppress ATM signaling and tumor progression. *Sci. Rep.* **2017**, *7*, 1–12. [CrossRef]

110. Vetvicka, V.; Vetvickova, J. Fucoidans Stimulate Immune Reaction and Suppress Cancer Growth. *Anticancer Res.* **2017**, *37*, 6041–6046. [CrossRef]

111. Antonelli, A.C.; Binyamin, A.; Hohl, T.M.; Glickman, M.S.; Redelman-Sidi, G. Bacterial immunotherapy for cancer induces CD4-dependent tumor-specific immunity through tumor-intrinsic interferon-γ signaling. *Proc. Natl. Acad. Sci. USA* **2020**, *117*, 18627–18637. [CrossRef] [PubMed]

112. Das, S.; Camphausen, K.; Shankavaram, U. Cancer-Specific Immune Prognostic Signature in Solid Tumors and Its Relation to Immune Checkpoint Therapies. *Cancers* **2020**, *12*, 2476. [CrossRef] [PubMed]

113. Vallo, S.; Stege, H.; Berg, M.; Michaelis, M.; Winkelmann, R.; Rothweiler, F.; Cinatl, J. Tumor necrosis factor-related apoptosis-inducing ligand as a therapeutic option in urothelial cancer cells with acquired resistance against first-line chemotherapy. *Oncol. Rep.* **2020**, *43*, 1331–1337. [CrossRef] [PubMed]

114. Zirakhzadeh, A.A.; Sherif, A.; Rosenblatt, R.; Bergman, E.A.; Winerdal, M.; Yang, D.; Cederwall, J.; Jakobsson, V.; Hyllienmark, M.; Winqvist, O.; et al. Tumour-associated B cells in urothelial urinary bladder cancer. *Scand. J. Immunol.* **2019**, *91*, e12830. [CrossRef]

115. Patel, V.; Oh, W.K.; Galsky, M. Treatment of muscle-invasive and advanced bladder cancer in 2020. *CA A Cancer J. Clin.* **2020**. [CrossRef]

116. Poon, D.M.-C. Immunotherapy for urothelial carcinoma: Metastatic disease and beyond. *Asia-Pac. J. Clin. Oncol.* **2020**, *16*, 18–23. [CrossRef]

117. Luo, D.; Carter, K.A.; Miranda, D.; Lovell, J.F. Chemophototherapy: An Emerging Treatment Option for Solid Tumors. *Adv. Sci.* **2017**, *4*, 1600106. [CrossRef]

118. Li, X.; Lovell, J.F.; Yoon, J.; Chen, X. Clinical development and potential of photothermal and photodynamic therapies for cancer. *Nat. Rev. Clin. Oncol.* **2020**, *17*, 657–674. [CrossRef]

119. Hou, Y.-J.; Yang, X.-X.; Liu, R.-Q.; Zhao, D.; Guo, C.-N.; Zhu, A.-C.; Wen, M.-N.; Liu, Z.; Qu, G.-F.; Meng, H. Pathological Mechanism of Photodynamic Therapy and Photothermal Therapy Based on Nanoparticles. *Int. J. Nanomed.* **2020**, *15*, 6827–6838. [CrossRef]

120. Sundaram, P.; Abrahamse, H. Phototherapy Combined with Carbon Nanomaterials (1D and 2D) and their Applications in Cancer Therapy. *Materials* **2020**, *13*, 4830. [CrossRef]

121. Lu, K.-Y.; Jheng, P.-R.; Lu, L.-S.; Rethi, L.; Mi, F.-L.; Chuang, E.-Y. Enhanced anticancer effect of ROS-boosted photothermal therapy by using fucoidan-coated polypyrrole nanoparticles. *Int. J. Biol. Macromol.* **2020**. [CrossRef] [PubMed]

122. Mitsunari, K.; Miyata, Y.; Asai, A.; Matsuo, T.; Shida, Y.; Hakariya, T.; Sakai, H. Human antigen R is positively associated with malignant aggressiveness via upregulation of cell proliferation, migration, and vascular endothelial growth factors and cyclooxygenase-2 in prostate cancer. *Transl. Res.* **2016**, *175*, 116–128. [CrossRef] [PubMed]

123. Ismail, T.; Kim, Y.; Lee, H.; Lee, D.-S.; Lee, H.-S. Interplay Between Mitochondrial Peroxiredoxins and ROS in Cancer Development and Progression. *Int. J. Mol. Sci.* **2019**, *20*, 4407. [CrossRef] [PubMed]

124. Ntellas, P.; Mavroeidis, L.; Gkoura, S.; Gazouli, I.; Amylidi, A.-L.; Papadaki, A.; Zarkavelis, G.; Mauri, D.; Karpathiou, G.; Kolettas, E.; et al. Old Player-New Tricks: Non Angiogenic Effects of the VEGF/VEGFR Pathway in Cancer. *Cancers* **2020**, *12*, 3145. [CrossRef] [PubMed]

125. Nagamine, T.; Kadena, K.; Tomori, M.; Nakajima, K.; Iha, M. Activation of NK cells in male cancer survivors by fucoidan extracted from Cladosiphonokamuranus. *Mol. Clin. Oncol.* **2020**, *12*, 81–88. [PubMed]

126. Gueven, N.; Spring, K.J.; Holmes, S.; Ahuja, K.D.K.; Eri, R.; Park, A.Y.; Fitton, J.H. Micro RNA Expression after Ingestion of Fucoidan; A Clinical Study. *Mar. Drugs* **2020**, *18*, 143. [CrossRef]

127. Zheng, K.H.; Kaiser, Y.; Poel, E.; Verberne, H.; Aerts, J.; Rouzet, F.; Stroes, E.; Letourneur, D.; Chauvierre, C. 99mTc-Fucoidn as diagnostic agent for P-selectin imaging: First-in-human evaluation (phase I). *Atherosclerosis* **2019**, *287*, e143. [CrossRef]

128. Rui, X.; Pan, H.-F.; Shao, S.-L.; Xu, X.-M. Anti-tumor and anti-angiogenic effects of Fucoidan on prostate cancer: Possible JAK-STAT3 pathway. *BMC Complement. Altern. Med.* **2017**, *17*, 1–8. [CrossRef]

2

Profiling and Targeting of Energy and Redox Metabolism in Grade 2 Bladder Cancer Cells with Different Invasiveness Properties

Valentina Pasquale [1,2,†]🆔, Giacomo Ducci [1,2,†], Gloria Campioni [1,2]🆔, Adria Ventrici [1], Chiara Assalini [3], Stefano Busti [1,2], Marco Vanoni [1,2,*]🆔, Riccardo Vago [3,4,*]🆔 and Elena Sacco [1,2,*]🆔

[1] Department of Biotechnology and Biosciences, University of Milano-Bicocca, Piazza della Scienza 2, 20126 Milan, Italy; valentina.pasquale@unimib.it (V.P.); g.ducci@campus.unimib.it (G.D.); g.campioni@campus.unimib.it (G.C.); a.ventrici@campus.unimib.it (A.V.); stefano.busti1@unimib.it (S.B.)

[2] SYSBIO-ISBE-IT-Candidate National Node of Italy for ISBE, Research Infrastructure for Systems Biology Europe, 20126 Milan, Italy

[3] Urological Research Institute, Division of Experimental Oncology, IRCCS San Raffaele Hospital, 20132 Milan, Italy; assalini.chiara@hsr.it

[4] Università Vita-Salute San Raffaele, 20132 Milan, Italy

[*] Correspondence: marco.vanoni@unimib.it (M.V.); vago.riccardo@hsr.it (R.V.); elena.sacco@unimib.it (E.S.)

[†] These authors equally contributed to this work.

Abstract: Bladder cancer is one of the most prevalent deadly diseases worldwide. Grade 2 tumors represent a good window of therapeutic intervention, whose optimization requires high resolution biomarker identification. Here we characterize energy metabolism and cellular properties associated with spreading and tumor progression of RT112 and 5637, two Grade 2 cancer cell lines derived from human bladder, representative of luminal-like and basal-like tumors, respectively. The two cell lines have similar proliferation rates, but only 5637 cells show efficient lateral migration. In contrast, RT112 cells are more prone to form spheroids. RT112 cells produce more ATP by glycolysis and OXPHOS, present overall higher metabolic plasticity and are less sensitive than 5637 to nutritional perturbation of cell proliferation and migration induced by treatment with 2-deoxyglucose and metformin. On the contrary, spheroid formation is less sensitive to metabolic perturbations in 5637 than RT112 cells. The ability of metformin to reduce, although with different efficiency, cell proliferation, sphere formation and migration in both cell lines, suggests that OXPHOS targeting could be an effective strategy to reduce the invasiveness of Grade 2 bladder cancer cells.

Keywords: bladder cancer; energy and redox metabolism; cellular bioenergetics; mitochondrial function; glycolysis; fatty acids oxidation; oxidative stress; 2D and 3D cultures; Seahorse Extracellular Flux Analyzer; quantitative imaging; Operetta CLS™

1. Introduction

Bladder cancer (BC) is among the most common malignancies worldwide and one of the most expensive cancers to manage [1]. Most BC patients (75–80%) are diagnosed with non-muscle invasive BC (NMIBC). Recurrences are frequent (50–70%), sometimes including progression to invasive tumors (Muscle invasive BC, MIBC), which drastically reduce survival expectations. NMIBC is usually treated by transurethral resection (TUR) to remove the tumor and obtain histological examination material. After resection, patients are introduced to a treatment regimen, which reflects the disease's nature and potential, based on histological grade and tumor-node-metastasis stage. Therefore, a proper definition of urothelial neoplasms grading is a crucial driver to stratify tumor behavior, including progression and recurrence for optimal patient management and surveillance follow-up [2,3]. In 2004, the World Health Organization (WHO) introduced a classification, confirmed in 2016, including the concept of Low-Grade (LG) and High-Grade (HG) tumors, as well as the papillary urothelial neoplasm of low malignant potential category [4]. One critical issue in this categorization is grade heterogeneity in papillary neoplasms, a mixture of non-invasive HG and LG features that can be observed in around 25% of cases [5]. So far, molecular markers are not part of standard clinical practice, even if molecular changes in HG tumors occur at early stages before developing the corresponding morphological features [6]. In the case of borderline histology, to distinguish LG and HG tumors, other parameters such as urinary cytology, multifocality, size of the lesion, prior history, and recurrence can be considered for grading determination, but they are often not consistent. Mixed lesions represent a challenging topic and no authoritative recommendations on reporting them are available from the WHO 2016 [3].

In this context, it is crucial to identify new markers that can contribute to patients' stratification to direct them to more effective and less toxic targeted treatments, even to be combined with conventional therapies, to improve prognosis, avoid relapses, or to promote the overcoming of chemoresistance. Reprogramming of energy metabolism has emerged as a hallmark of cancer, and altered metabolic pathways can represent attractive clinical targets exploitable in new therapeutic strategies [7,8]. Cancer cells exhibit profound metabolic rearrangements, which support their enhanced growth, allowing them to proliferate and survive in conditions where normal cells do not [9,10]. Among the most common rearrangements there is the well-known Warburg effect, which consists of enhancing aerobic glycolysis at the expense of mitochondrial respiration, which leads to ferment the glycolysis-derived pyruvate to lactic acid, even under normoxic condition [11]. This metabolic rewiring allows obtaining energy, reducing power and building blocks for biosynthetic processes, faster than through alternative metabolic pathways. This type of metabolism is usually exploited by actively proliferating cells [12,13] and maximally contracted skeletal muscle cells, which must reach short-term high energy goals [14]. Although initially associated with mitochondrial defects, it is clear by now that the Warburg effect also occurs in the presence of functional mitochondria. The activation of specific signaling pathways (i.e., Hypoxia-induced HIF-1α, PI3K-Akt-mTOR, RAS/MEK/MAPK), of specific oncogenes (i.e., RAS [15–17], Myc [18]), the inactivation of tumor suppressors (i.e., p53 [19,20]), and/or the selective pressure exerted by the microenvironment [21–24] all contribute to driving the Warburg effect. The hyperglycolytic phenotype, characterized by increased glucose uptake and glycolysis, is associated with further metabolic changes that include the extensive anaplerotic use of other nutrients, such as glutamine, for the replenishment of the TCA cycle intermediates [25–27]. Although these rearrangements can provide selective advantages to cancer cells, they also confer dependence on specific enzymatic activities and specific nutrients and open to novel therapeutic opportunities [28–30]. For example, glutamine addicted cancer cells need glutamine to survive because they depend on glutaminolysis for anaplerosis and their biosynthetic needs [27,31]. Many other metabolic targets have been identified in cancers, including urothelial bladder cancers [32,33], and are also evaluated as prognostic markers [34]. Several drugs that affect the altered metabolism are under clinical trial in the perspective of precision medicine [35–37]. Deregulations of energy metabolism can also affect reducing equivalents and impact on redox homeostasis by making cancer cells more sensitive to oxidative stress [38–40].

In this work we present a characterization of the energy and redox metabolism of two bladder cancer cell lines with a low histological grade of tumor progression (Grade 2), RT112, and 5637. Grade 2 represents a therapeutic window that strongly requires post-surgical resection pharmacological treatments that help to eliminate residual tumor cells and prevent the formation of tumor relapses. Based on gene mutation patterns and genomic changes, the two cell lines are representative of luminal like FGFR3-driven cancer (RT112), and of the basal-like TP53/RB tumor suppressor-driven cancer (5736), often used as models of non-aggressive and aggressive BCs, respectively [41,42]. Here we show that the RT112 cell line is largely less efficient in migration, but forms spheroids more efficiently. Both cell lines produce ATP by both OXPHOS and glycolysis. However, RT112 cells are more energetic, have higher metabolic plasticity and are less sensitive than 5637 to nutritional perturbation of cell proliferation and migration. Although both cell lines, when grown under adhesion are sensitive to targeting of both OXPHOS and glycolysis, although with different efficiency, only targeting of OXPHOS significantly affects spheroid formation of both cell lines.

2. Materials and Methods

2.1. Materials and Cell Cultures

Grade 2 bladder cancer cell lines RT112 and 5637, originally established from primary urinary bladder carcinoma [43,44], were purchased from American Collection of Cell Cultures (ATCC, Manassas, VA, USA). Cell lines were routinely grown in RPMI-1640 medium (R0883-Merck Life Science, Darmstadt, Germany) supplemented with 10% fetal bovine serum (FBS, Gibco-ThermoFisher, Waltham, MA, USA), 4 mM glutamine, 100 U/mL penicillin and 100 mg/mL streptomycin, at 37 °C in a humidified atmosphere of 5% CO_2. Cells were passaged using trypsin-ethylenediaminetetraacetic acid (EDTA). Assays on adherent cells were performed in experimental medium: DMEM w/o phenol red (Gibco™-Thermo Fisher Scientific), FBS 10%, 10 mM glucose, 2 mM glutamine, 100 U/mL penicillin and 100 mg/mL streptomycin. Sphere formation was performed in 3D experimental medium DMEM w/o phenol red (Gibco™-Thermo Fisher Scientific), 1% BSA, 10 mM glucose, 2 mM glutamine, 10 µg/mL Insulin (I9278, Merck Life Science), 0.5 µg/mL Hydrocortisone (H0888-1G, Merck Life Science), 20 ng/mL EGF (EGF Human Recombinant, Peprotech, London, UK) 100 ng/mL Cholera Toxin (C8052, Merck Life Science), 100 U/mL penicillin and 100 mg/mL streptomycin).

Anti-β-Actin mouse monoclonal antibody (Catalog number A5441, Sigma-Aldrich, St. Louis, MO, USA), dilution 1:10,000; anti-vimentin mouse monoclonal antibody (Catalog number sc-32322, Santa Cruz Biotechnology, Dallas, TX, USA), dilution 1:2000; Anti-PSrc (Tyr416) rabbit polyclonal antibody (Catalog number 2101, Cell Signaling Technology®, Danvers, MA, USA), dilution 1:1000; Anti-Src rabbit polyclonal antibody (Catalog number 2109, Cell Signaling Technology®), dilution 1:1000. Unless specified, all reagents were from Merck Life Science. Stocks used: 0.9 M 2-Deoxy-D-glucose (2-DG) in assay medium; 2.5 mM antimycin A in DMSO; 10 mM etomoxir in sterile water; 25 mM carbonyl cyanide p-triflouromethoxyphenylhydrazone (FCCP) in DMSO; 1 M H_2O_2; 1 M metformin in assay medium; 2.5 mM oligomycin A in DMSO; 2.5 mM rotenone in DMSO; 20 mM UK5099 in DMSO.

2.2. Cell Proliferation and Viability Assays

Cell proliferation under H_2O_2 treatment was analyzed by growth kinetics: 3.8×10^5 cells were plated in 6-well plates with 2 mL of standard medium and incubated at 37 °C and 5% CO_2. After 18 h medium was changed and cells were exposed to different perturbed conditions (medium containing different concentrations of H_2O_2; 0–50 mM). At different time points the viable cell number was counted using Trypan-Blue exclusion method.

Cell viability under etomoxir treatment was analyzed by an MTT assay: 5×10^3 cells were plated in 96-well plates in 50 µL of standard medium and incubated at 37 °C and 5% CO_2. The day after 50 µL of medium supplemented with 2× serial dilutions of etomoxir or vehicle was added to the wells. 72 h after treatment, 20 µL of MTT formazan (20 mg/mL in isopropanol) was added to the culture media. After 1 h of incubation at 37 °C, the medium was gently removed and cells were suspended in 100 µL DMSO and then absorbance at 570 nm was recorded by using a Victor Multilabel Plate Reader (Perkin–Elmer, Waltham, MA, USA). The viability of cells treated with increasing concentrations of drugs was tested relative to the viability of the same cells treated with vehicle.

Cell proliferation in response to metabolic targeting was analyzed by growth kinetics: 2.1×10^4 cells were plated in Cell Imaging 24-well Plates in 500 µL of experimental medium at 37 °C and 5% CO_2. After 24 h medium was changed, and cells were exposed to experimental medium containing dose-response concentrations of selected drugs (2DG 0-0.5-5-15 mM, metformin 0-1-5-10-20 mM). Cell growth was monitored through imaging acquisitions every 24 h using Operetta CLS™ high-content analysis system in brightfield using 10× magnification. After 72 h cells were stained with Hoechst 33342 (working concentration 1 ug/mL incubated for 15 min at 37 °C and 5% CO_2) and imaging acquisitions were made using Operetta CLS™ with 10× magnification in brightfield and widefield fluorescence microscopy. Total cell count (nuclei positive for Hoechst 33342) was obtained using the Harmony software.

2.3. Wound Healing Assay

Cell migratory capacity was evaluated with wound healing assay. 10^5 cells were plated in Cell Imaging 24-well Plates in 500 μL of experimental medium at 37 °C and 5% CO_2. As an adherent confluent monolayer formed, cells were stained using CellTracker™ Red CMTPX Dye 5 μM (C34552, stock 10 mM in DMSO, Invitrogen™-Thermo Fisher Scientific), according to the supplier's instructions, to track cell movements. Cell starvation lasting 8 h, with FBS-free experimental medium, was performed to stop cell proliferation. At the end of starvation protocol, pre-wound images of the entire well were acquired using Operetta CLS™ using 10× magnification in brightfield and widefield fluorescence microscopy to detect CellTracker. Next, a wound was made by scratching the monolayer cells with a sterile 10 μL pipette tip, and, after washing, the medium was changed to 0.1% FBS experimental medium containing dose-response concentrations of selected drugs (2DG 0-0.5-5-15 mM, metformin 0-1-5-10 mM). Wound coverage was monitored with automatized time-lapse imaging acquisition using Operetta CLS™, acquiring every entire well of the 24-well plate, both in brightfield and widefield fluorescence microscopy, using 10× magnification, every 35 min (time of acquisition of the entire plate) for 40 h with monitored temperature (37 °C) and atmosphere (5% CO_2). Evaluation of drug-dependent wound coverage was obtained using the Harmony software.

2.4. Sphere Formation Assays

Sphere formation was evaluated using different cell growth supports: 6-well plates not treated for cell adhesion, 6-well cell-repellent plates and Cell Imaging 24-well Plates coated with Poly(2-hydroxyethyl methacrylate) (Poly-HEMA, Merck Life Science). 4×10^5 cells in 6-well and 1.5×10^5 cells in 24-well were seeded in 3D experimental medium and sphere formation was monitored every 24 h with phase contrast microscopy and with Operetta CLS™, respectively, until the endpoint (72 h). We monitored sphere formation with imaging analysis. 4×10^4 cells were seeded on CellCarrier-96 ULA Ultra Microplates 96-well (PerkinElmer) pre-stained with CellTracker™ Red CMTPX Dye 5 μM (Invitrogen™-Thermo Fisher Scientific). Assay was performed in 200 μL 3D experimental medium containing dose-response concentrations of selected drugs (2DG 0-0.5-5-15 mM, metformin 0-1-5-10-20 mM). Sphere morphology was monitored through imaging acquisitions of every complete well every 24 h, for 72 h, using Operetta CLS™, both in brightfield and widefield fluorescence microscopy with 10× magnification. We analyzed sphere formation using the Harmony software.

2.5. Metabolic Profiling by Seahorse Assays

Bioenergetic parameters of RT112 and 5637 cells under standard and nutritionally perturbed growth conditions were measured with the Seahorse Extracellular Flux XF24 and XFe96 analyzers (Agilent, Santa Clara, CA, USA; https://www.agilent.com/en/products/cell-analysis/how-seahorse-xf-analyzers-work). XF Glycolysis stress test, Mitochondrial stress test, and Palmitate-BSA Fatty Acid Oxidation assay kit protocols (Agilent) were performed using the XF24 analyzer, while ATP rate assay and Mitochondrial Fuel Flex test kit protocols (Agilent) were performed with the XFe96 analyzer, according to the manufacturer's instructions. Briefly cells were seeded in Seahorse XF plates at a density of 5×10^4 (XF24) or 4×10^4 (XFe96) cells per well and cultured for 24 h. The next day medium was replaced with low buffered XF assay medium (103575-100 Agilent), supplemented with 10 mM glucose, unless otherwise specified, and 2 mM glutamine and cell cultures were allowed to equilibrate for 1 h at

37 °C in a no-CO_2 incubator. Seahorse XF analysis was performed at 37 °C simultaneously measuring Oxygen Consumption Rate (OCR = pmole O_2/min) and ExtraCellular Acidification Rate (ECAR = mpH/min). The XFe96 analyzer allows also measuring the Proton Efflux Rate (PER = pmolesH$^+$/min). At the end of the analysis performed in XF24 plates, the medium was removed, cells were gently washed with PBS, suspended in JS lysis buffer and scraped after two freezing and thawing cycles. The protein content of cell lysates was measured by Bradford assay and used to normalize respiratory and glycolytic parameters. Subsequently these parameters were normalized on cell number, taking into consideration the protein content per cell. For the assays in XFe96 format, at the end of the Seahorse measurements, Hoechst 33342 was added to each well at the final working concentration of 1 ug/mL and after 15 min incubation nuclei/well were imaged and counted by Operetta CLS™ software Harmony, and directly used to normalize the Seahorse parameters per cell number. Samples were analyzed with at least 10 technical replicates. Data derive from two independent experiments.

2.5.1. XF Cell Mitochondrial Stress Test

This assay was performed to determine the mitochondrial bioenergetics. Oxygen Consumption Rate was analyzed under basal condition and after the treatment with different drugs including the ATP synthase inhibitor oligomycin A (optimal dose chosen after dose-response optimization assay: 0.125–2 μM oligomycin A), an ETC accelerator ionophore (optimal dose chosen after dose-response optimization assay: 0.25–4 μM FCCP), and an ETC inhibitors mixture (1 μM rotenone and 1 μM antimycin A). The response to the minimal dose of oligomycin A and FCCP, generating the maximal effect, accounts for non-phosphorylating mitochondrial respiration and maximal FCCP-uncoupled respiration, respectively. The response to the rotenone and antimycin A mixture accounts for non-mitochondrial oxygen consumption. Respiratory parameters were elaborated using the following formulas:

$$\text{Basal Mitochondrial Respiration (Basal-MR)} = OCR_{basal} - OCR_{rot/ant}$$

$$\text{Non-Phosphorylating Mitochondrial Respiration (oligo-NPMR)} = OCR_{oligo} - OCR_{rot/ant}$$

$$\text{FCCP-uncoupled Mitochondrial Respiration (FCCP-MR)} = OCR_{FCCP} - OCR_{rot/ant}$$

$$\text{Sare respiratory capacity} = OCR_{FCCP} - OCR_{rot/ant}/OCR_{basal} - OCR_{rot/ant}$$

$$\text{Coupling efficiency} = 1 - (OCR_{oligo} - OCR_{rot/ant}/OCR_{basal} - OCR_{rot/ant})$$

2.5.2. XF Glycolysis Stress Test

This assay was performed to determine the glycolytic bioenergetics. Extracellular acidification was analyzed in glucose-free-medium before and after the sequential injections of 10 mM glucose, oligomycin A (optimal dose chosen after dose-response optimization assay: 0.125–2 μM oligomycin A), and 50 mM 2-Deoxy-D-glucose (2-DG), a glycolysis inhibitor. The response to the minimum dose generating the maximal effect of oligomycin A accounts for glycolytic capacity. The response to 2-DG accounts for non-glycolytic extracellular acidification. Data were elaborated using the following formulas:

$$\text{Basal glycolysis} = ECAR_{glc} - ECAR_{2\text{-DG}}$$

$$\text{Glycolytic capacity} = ECAR_{oligo} - ECAR_{2\text{-DG}}$$

$$\text{Glycolytic reserve} = ECAR_{oligo} - ECAR_{glc}$$

2.5.3. XF ATP Rate Assay

This assay measures OXPHOS and glycolysis's contribution to ATP production. This assay was performed under standard and 2 h glucose deprivation. OCR and acidification were measured before and after sequential injection of 1.5 μM oligomycin A and 0.5 μM rotenone/antimycin A. Data were assessed with XF Wave Software (Seahorse Bioscience, Agilent).

2.5.4. XF Palmitate-BSA FAO Assay

Fatty Acid Oxidation (FAO) of RT112 and 5637 cells were analyzed using the XF Palmitate-BSA FAO Substrate, namely 1 mM palmitate, a long chain fatty acid, conjugated to 0.17 mM BSA (6:1 palmitate:BSA ratio). For the FAO assay 3.5×10^5 cells were seeded in 100 μL of the standard medium onto Seahorse XF24-well plates and incubated at 37 °C and 5% CO_2. After 24 h, medium was replaced with substrate-limited medium (DMEM medium supplemented with 0.5 mM glucose, 1 mM glutamine, 0.5 mM carnitine and 1% FBS, 5 mM Hepes pH 7.4) and cells were incubated at 37 °C, and 5% CO_2. After 24 h (45 min before XF analysis), the medium was replaced with FAO-assay medium (KHB supplemented with 5 mM glucose, 0.5 mM glutamine, 0.5 mM carnitine and 5 mM Hepes pH 7.4) and cell cultures were allowed to equilibrate for 1 h at 37 °C in a no-CO_2 incubator. After 30 min (15 min before XF analysis) 40 μM etomoxir or vehicle was added to appropriate wells on the microplate, and just before initiating XF analysis 220 μM palmitate-BSA or BSA was added to appropriate wells on the microplate. In summary we tested four different conditions for each XF FAO assay:

(1) BSA-Eto (BSA control without etomoxir) accounting for total respiration, including that one deriving from endogenous fatty acids oxidation;

(2) BSA+Eto (BSA control with etomoxir) accounting for respiration not depending on endogenous fatty acids oxidation;

(3) Palm:BSA-Eto (palmitate-BSA without etomoxir) accounting for total respiration, including that one deriving from exogenous fatty acids oxidation;

(4) Palm:BSA+Eto (palmitate-BSA with etomoxir) accounting for respiration not depending on exogenous fatty acids oxidation.

2.5.5. XF Mitochondrial Fuel Flex Test

This assay was performed to measure the dependency, capacity and flexibility of cells to oxidize three critical mitochondrial fuels—glucose, glutamine and fatty acids. The assay was performed in an XF assay medium containing 10 mM glucose, 2 mM glutamine and 1 mM Na-pyruvate. Cells were exposed to BPTES (3 μM), etomoxir (4 μM) or UK5099 (2 μM) in succession and OCR was measured before and after injection of each compound. Data were assessed with XF Wave Software (Seahorse Bioscience, Agilent).

2.6. Flow Cytometry

For FACS analysis 1×10^6 cells were plated in 6-well plates with 2 mL of experimental medium and incubated overnight at 37 °C and 5% CO_2. Cells were then stained with different dyes, as described below, before or after treatment with trypsin-EDTA following dye and antibody protocols and the supplier's recommendations, suspended in PBS supplemented with 0.2% BSA and acquired by CytoFlex S (Beckman Coulter, Brea, CA, USA). Data were elaborated using CytExpert 2.0 software (Beckman Coulter).

To evaluate mitochondrial membrane potential and mass cells were stained with 100 nM MitoTracker™ Red CMXRos (Invitrogen™ Thermo Fisher Scientific, 1 mM stock in DMSO) and 25 nM MitoTracker™ Green FM (Invitrogen™ Thermo Fisher Scientific, 1 mM stock in DMSO), respectively, in FBS-free medium for 20 min at 37 °C and 5% CO_2.

To evaluate mitochondrial and intracellular ROS, cells were stained with 5 μM MitoSOX™ Red Mitochondrial Superoxide Indicator (MitoSOX, Invitrogen™ Thermo Fisher Scientific, 5 mM stock in DMSO), and 10 mM 2′,7′-dichlorodihydrofluoresceine diacetate (H2DCFDA Merck Life Science, 5 mM stock in ethanol), respectively, in FBS-free medium for 30 min at 37 °C and 5% CO_2. According to fluorescence panel necessity, dead cells were excluded from analysis using viability dyes

7-aminoactinomycin D (Thermo Fisher Scientific) or LIVE/DEAD™ Fixable Green Dead Cell Stain (Thermo Fisher Scientific). Cell staining was performed according to supplier's instruction.

To evaluate stemness, cells were stained as single cell suspension with conjugated antibody CD44-APC (cod. 17-0441-82 eBioscience™, San Diego, CA, USA), CD133-PE (cod. 12-1338-42 eBioscience™), and Aldefluor, Stem Cell Identification Kit (STEMCELL Technologies™, Vancouver, BC, Canada) according to supplier's protocol. Dead cells were excluded from analysis using viability dyes 7-aminoactinomycin D.

Data were expressed as Median Fluorescence Intensity (MFI) of labeled living cells corrected for MFI of unlabeled living cells' autofluorescence.

2.7. Imaging

Analysis of mitochondrial machinery and redox status was performed by high-resolution imaging.

2.7.1. High-Resolution Imaging for Quantitative Analysis

Cells (6.5×10^4) were seeded per well on Cell Imaging 24-well Plates, incubated overnight at 37 °C and 5% CO_2. The day after cells were stained with selected dye, then gently washed with phenol red-free medium and promptly analyzed in the experimental medium using Operetta CLS™, with confocal imaging set-up and 63× magnification. To evaluate mitochondrial membrane potential and mass, cells were stained with 100 nM MitoTracker™ Red CMXRos and 25 nM MitoTracker™ Green FM, respectively, for 20 min at 37 °C and 5% CO_2.

To evaluate mitochondrial ROS, intracellular ROS and lipid oxidation status, cells were stained with 3 μM MitoSOX (5 mM stock in DMSO), 10 μM H2DCFDA (20 mM stock in DMSO) and 10 μmM BODIPY™ 581/591 C11 (Lipid Peroxidation Sensor, Invitrogen™ Thermo Fisher Scientific, 20 mM stock in DMSO), respectively, for 25, 10, and 30 min at 37 °C and 5% CO_2. Following imaging acquisition of selected dye, cells were stained with Hoechst 33342 (1 μg/mL incubated for 15 min at 37 °C and 5% CO_2) and further imaging acquisitions were made using Operetta CLS™ with 63× magnification with the confocal set-up. Dye quantitative analysis and total cell count (nuclei positive for Hoechst 33342) were obtained using Harmony software (as schematized in Supplementary Figure S1D–F).

To analyze mitochondrial mass, we plated 1.2×10^4 cells in CellCarrier-96 Ultra Microplates 96-well (PerkinElmer) and incubated at 37 °C and 5% CO_2 overnight. The day after, cells were transiently transfected using Lipofectamine reagent (Invitrogen, Carlsbad, CA, USA), according to the manufacturer's instruction, with 1.0 μg of pEYFP-mito vector expressing the mitochondrially targeted yellow fluorescent protein MitoYFP (Clontech, Mountain View, CA, USA). After 48 h, cells were stained with Hoechst 33342 (working concentration 1 ug/mL incubated for 15 min at 37 °C and 5% CO_2) and imaging acquisitions were made using Operetta CLS™ with 63× magnification with the confocal set-up. Quantitative analysis and total cell count (nuclei positive for Hoechst 33342) were obtained using the Harmony software.

For cell area measurements, 6.5×10^4 cells were seeded per well on Cell Imaging 24-well Plates, incubated overnight at 37 °C and 5% CO_2. The day after cells were stained using Vybrant™ DiI Cell-Labeling Solution 5 μM (V22885, stock solution 1 mM, Invitrogen™-Thermo Fisher Scientific) according to supplier's instruction, then analyzed in the experimental medium using Operetta CLS™ with confocal imaging set-up and 63× magnification. Cell area was obtained using the Harmony software.

2.7.2. High-Resolution Imaging with Manually Operated Confocal Microscopy

To analyze SOX2 expression in cells grown as monolayers or spheroids, cells were seeded in different 6-well plates: 1×10^5 cells for RT112 cells and 1.2×10^5 cells for 5637 cells in tissue culture-treated plates in 2 mL 2D experimental medium and 4×10^5 cells for both RT112 and 5637 cells in not-treated and cell repellent plates in 2 mL 3D experimental medium and incubated at 37 °C and 5% CO_2. Sphere formation was monitored every 24 h with phase contrast microscopy until endpoint

(72 h). Adherent cells were harvested by trypsinization and spheres were dissociated. Cells were seeded at subconfluent concentration on 13 mm microscopy slides and incubated at 37 °C, 5% CO_2 for 24 h. Cells were fixed in two passages with progressive higher concentration of paraformaldehyde at room temperature. After washing with PBS, blocking solution (PBS 1×, 10% normal goat serum (NGS), 0.2% Triton X) was added, incubation lasted for 1 h and 30 min at room temperature. Incubation with primary antibody 1:100 in PBS 1×, NGS 10% was performed overnight at 4 °C (anti-h/mSOX2 MAB2018 Clone 245610 R&D Systems, Minneapolis, MN, USA). After washing with PBS, each slide was incubated with secondary antibody 1:1000 (anti-mouse IgG2a conjugated PE) in the same buffer for 45 min at room temperature in an obscured chamber. Cells were stained with Hoechst 33342 (0.5 ug/mL incubated for 15 min at RT and 5% CO_2) and image acquisitions were made using an A1R confocal microscope (Nikon, Tokio, Japan) with 40× magnification.

For high resolution imaging of mitochondrial machinery, 2×10^4 cells were plated in 10 compartment CellView culture slide with glass bottom (GreinerBioOne, Kremsmünster, Austria) and incubated overnight at 37 °C and 5% CO_2. Afterward, cells were stained as previously described with MitoTracker™ Green FM and MitoTracker™ Red CMXRos and analyzed by live imaging confocal microscopy with a Nikon A1R confocal microscope for 48 h with 63× magnification.

For analysis of mitochondrial network morphology, 2.5×10^5 cells were plated in Cellview cell culture dishes with glass bottom (Greiner BioOne) and incubated at 37 °C and 5% CO_2 overnight. The day after, cells were transiently transfected using Lipofectamine reagent (Invitrogen), according to the manufacturer's instruction, with 1 μg of pEYFP-Mito vector. Forty-eight h after transfection cells were stained with Hoechst 33342 (1 μg/mL incubated for 15 min at 37 °C and 5% CO_2) and analyzed by live imaging with a Nikon A1R confocal microscope with 100× magnification.

2.8. RNA Extraction and qRT-PCR

Total RNA from bladder cancer cells was extracted using TRIzol LS Reagent (Invitrogen) according to the manufacturer's recommended protocols. The total RNA quantity was assessed using a Nanodrop spectrophotometer (ND-1000, Nanodrop, Labtech International, Uckfield, UK). Each RNA sample was then retrotranscribed with High Capacity cDNA Reverse Transcription Kit (Applied Biosystems, Foster City, CA, USA). A calibration curve was performed for each gene of interest to test primers and to determine the correct concentration of cDNA to be used for quantitative real time PCR. Reactions were run on an ABI 7000 Real Time PCR system (Applied Biosystems). Primers were purchased from Eurofins (Luxembourg). ATP5A1, ATP5B1, ALDH3A1, GAPDH, LDHA, PKM1 and PKM2 expression levels (indicated as "fold change") were analyzed in triplicate, normalized to HPRT1 and calculated according to the CT method. Primers used: ATP5A1F 5'-CATTGGTGATGGTATTGCGC-3'; ATP5A1R 5'-TCCCAAACA CGACAACTCC-3'; ATP5B1F 5'-CCGTGAGGGCAATGATTTATAC-3'; ATP5B1R 5'-GTCAAAC CAGTCAGAGCTACC-3'; ALDH3A1-F 5'-GCAGACCTGCACAAGAATGA-3' ALDH3A1-R 5'-TGTA GAGCTCGTCCTGCTGA-3'; GAPDH-F 5'-GGACTCATGACCACAGTCCA-3', GAPDH-R 5'-CCA GTAGAGGCAGGGATGAT-3'; LDHA-F5'-AGCCCGATTCCGTTACCT-3', LDHA-R 5'-CA CCAGCAACATTCATTCCA-3'; PKM1-F5'-ACCGCAAGCTGTTTGAAGAA-3', PKM1-R 5'-TCCA TGAGGTCTGTGGAGTG-3'; PKM2-F 5'-ATCGTCCTCACCAAGTCTGG-3', PKM2-F 5'-GAAG ATGCCACGGTACAGGT-3'; HPRT1-F 5'-TGCAGACTTTGCTTTCCTTG-3', HPRT1-R 5'- CTGGCT TATATCCAACACTTCG-3'.

2.9. Protein Content, Western Blotting

To determine the cell size of RT112 and 5637 cells, we measured the protein content by Bradford assay (Bio-Rad, Hercules, CA, USA) on cell lysates obtained from 1×10^6 cells harvested by trypsinization, gently washed in PBS, suspended in lysis buffer (50 mM Tris-HCl pH 7.4, 5 mM EDTA, 1 mM EGTA, 10 mM 2-mercaptoethanol), and subjected to three freeze and thaw cycles. For western blotting analysis, 1×10^6 cells were seeded in p100 plates in complete medium and incubated overnight for the attachment. After 24h cells were washed with phosphate buffer saline without calcium and magnesium (PBS), scraped and lysed in lysis buffer supplemented with protease and phosphatase inhibitors. Proteins quantification was performed using BIO-RAD BCA Protein Assay Kit. Cellular lysates (10–30 μg proteins) were resuspended in Sample Buffer with β-mercaptoethanol (312.5 mM Tris-HCl pH 6.8, 10% SDS, 50% glycerol, 25% β-mercaptoethanol and 0.01% bromophenol blue) and analyzed by SDS-PAGE. After electrophoresis, proteins were transferred to nitrocellulose membrane by electroblotting. The membrane was incubated 1 h or overnight with 5% nonfat milk in Tris Buffered Saline supplemented with Tween 20 (TBS-T): 10 mM Tris, pH 8.0, 150 mM NaCl, 0.1% Tween 20. Membranes were probed with specific antibodies for 1 h or overnight. Blots were washed with TBS-T for three times and incubated with ECL (Amersham ECL Prime Western Blotting Detection Reagent, GE Healthcare UK, Little Chalfont, UK) according to the manufacturer's protocols. Bands were analyzed with the ImageJ software.

2.10. Statistical Analysis

Unless specified otherwise, all experiments were carried out at least in triplicate. The number of technical replicates within each experiment is reported in the Results section. Results were expressed as means ± standard deviation and variables were compared using unpaired Student's t-test or general linear model according to their distribution. A p-value < 0.05 was considered statistically significant. All statistical analyses were performed using GraphPad version 6 (GraphPad Software, Inc., San Diego, CA, USA) software.

3. Results

3.1. Morpho/Functional Features of RT112 and 5637 Grade 2 Bladder Cancer Cells

RT112 and 5637 (Figure 1a) are bladder cancer cell lines, of the same histological Low Grade (G2). The two cell lines have a similar proliferation rate (Figure 1b), but RT112 cells are significantly larger, as shown by imaging data (average area in square micrometers, Figure 1c) and biochemical determination of the protein content/cell (Figure 1d).

A wound healing assay (Figure 1e,f, Supplementary Video S1) shows that 5637 cells present a significantly higher migration rate than RT112. Consistently, 5637—but not RT112—cells show a significant level of vimentin (Figure 1g), the main protein of intermediate filaments, a canonical marker of epithelial-mesenchymal transition (EMT) reprogramming, associated with the acquisition of migratory and invasive phenotype [45,46]. The increase in the migratory capacity of 5637 is also associated with a reduction in the Src kinase specific activity (here measured as the ratio between Y416-phosphorylated form and the total protein) (Figure 1h,i). This protein plays a key role in the process called "adhesion turnover", consisting of the continuous formation of cellular matrix at the front pole of the cell and continue old cellular matrix disassembly at the rear [47]. The expression and activity of Src are inversely related to the migratory and metastatic capacity also in other bladder cancer cell lines [48].

A significant difference in the RT112 and 5637 cell lines' adhesive properties is highlighted by the cells' different behavior when seeded on polystyrene plates not subjected to the tissue culture treatment, which makes them more hydrophilic, that we refer to as "not treated". On these plates in serum-free medium, only RT112 cells form spheroids, while the 5637 cell line grows as a monolayer (Figure 1j). On cell repellent plates (in serum-free medium) both cell lines form spheroids. Compared to 5637, RT112 cells form a significantly higher number of spheroids (Supplementary Figure S2a,b), characterized by a significantly larger area (Supplementary Figure S2c).

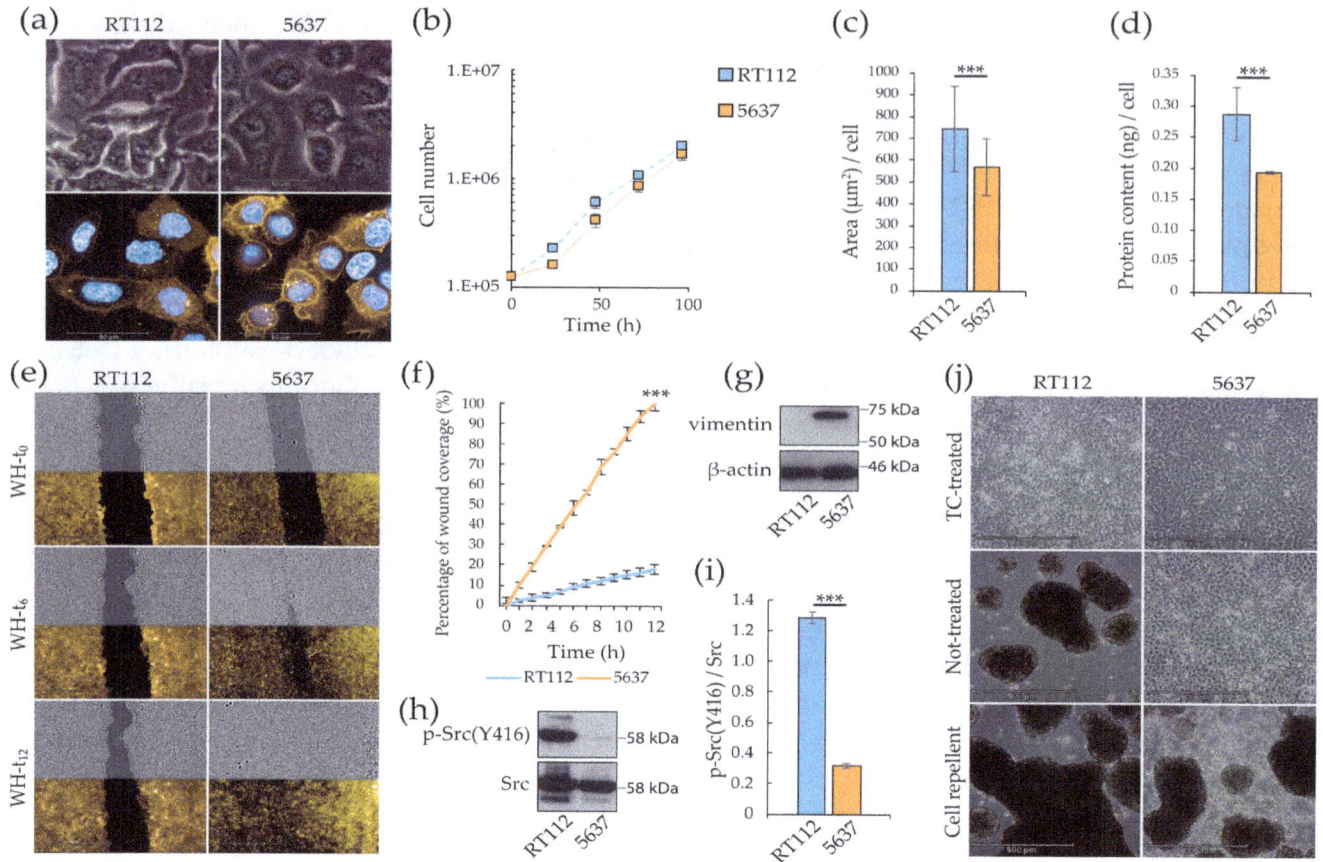

Figure 1. Morpho/functional readouts of RT112 and 5637 cells: proliferation rate, migration and spheroids formation capacity. (**a**) RT112 and 5637 cell morphology by phase contrast and confocal microscopy. For confocal microscopy cell membranes and nuclei were stained with fluorescent Vybrant™ DiI Cell-Labeling Solution (orange) and Hoechst 33342 (blue) dye respectively. (**b**) RT112 and 5637 cell growth curves in standard medium. Viable cells were counted by the Trypan-Blue exclusion method. (**c**) RT112 and 5637 average cell surface area measured as Vybrant™ fluorescent area using Harmony software. (**d**) RT112 and 5637 average protein content per cell measured by Bradford assay. (**e**) Representative wound healing assay images acquired by brightfield and fluorescence microscopy with Operetta CLS™ at 0 h, 6 h and 12 h after scratch (orange: CellTracker™ Red CMTPX Dye). (**f**) Percentage of wound coverage in wound healing assay through time (0–12 h), measured using Harmony software. (**g,h**) Western blot analysis for vimentin (**g**) and for Src and p-Src(Y416) (**h**) proteins in RT112 and 5637 cells. (**i**) p-Src(Y416)/Src ratio in RT112 and 5637 cells measured after densitometric analysis of Western Blot bands with ImageJ. (**j**) Spheroids formation assay in different supports: tissue culture treated (upper panels), not-treated (middle panels) and cell repellent supports (lower panels). Images were acquired in phase contrast light microscopy. Results are the mean of two (**f**) or three (**b**–**d**,**i**) experimental replicates. Statistical test: *t*-test and linear regression, *** for $p < 0.001$.

Compared to RT112, monolayers of 5637 cells show higher levels of some markers of stemness, and invasiveness, typically linked to tumor malignancy [49,50], namely a higher positivity to the fluorescent dye Aldefluor™ (Figure 2a), a readout of the expression of ALDH1A1 [51,52], and in expression level of the transmembrane glycoprotein CD44 [53,54] (Figure 2b), but not of CD133 [55,56] (Figure 2c). In agreement with previous studies [57], spheroid growth in both lines is associated with increased expression and nuclear localization (activation) of the transcription factor SOX2 (Figure 2d), a member of the SRY-related HMG-box (SOX) family. SOX2 is a known marker of stemness not expressed in healthy urothelial cells and related to the presence of cancer stem cells (CSCs), also in bladder cancer [49].

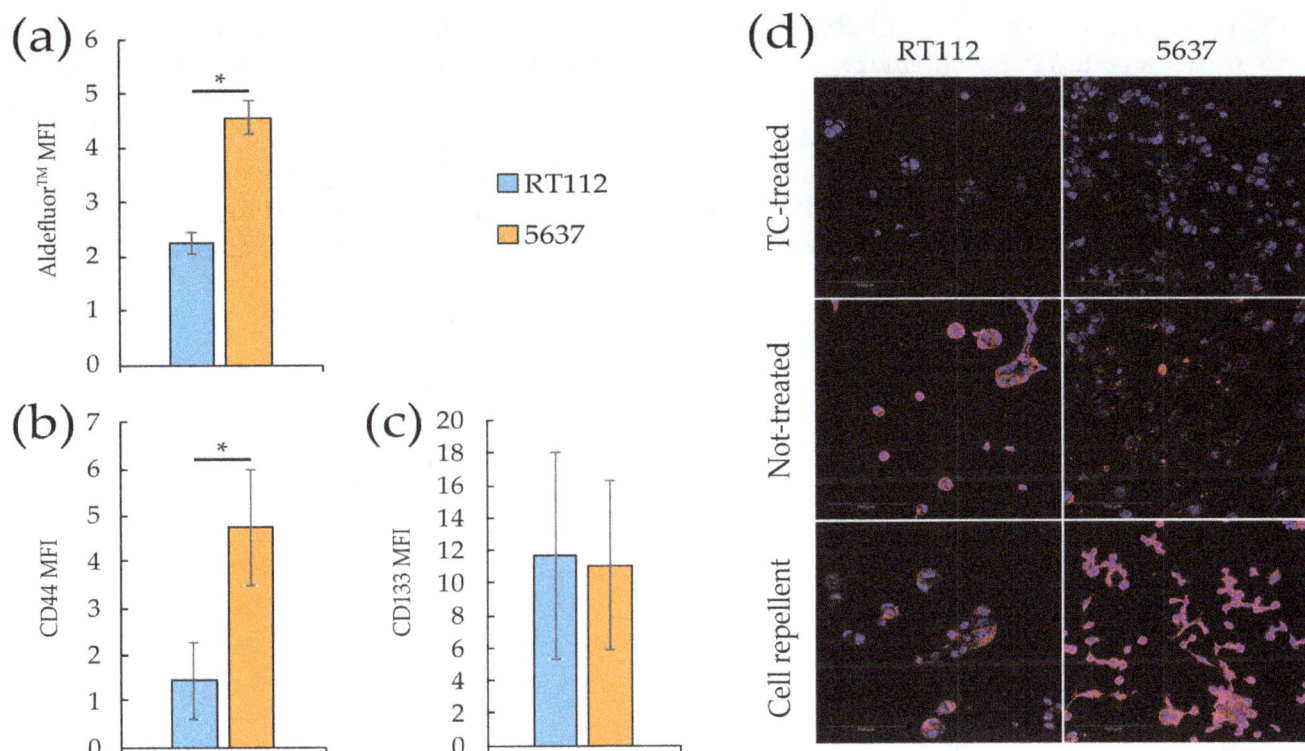

Figure 2. Stemness markers of monolayers and spheroids from RT112 and 5637 cells. (**a**–**c**) Median fluorescence intensity of Aldefluor^TM (**a**), CD44 (**b**) and CD133 (**c**) by flow cytometry analysis on RT112 and 5637 cells grown as monolayers. Results are the mean of two (**a**) and three (**b**,**c**) experimental replicates. Statistical test: t-test, * for $p < 0.05$. (**d**) Representative images from confocal immunofluorescence (IF) microscopy of RT112 and 5637 cells using SOX2 Antibody (red) and Hoechst 33342 (blue) for nuclei. Cells were grown as monolayer or spheroids on different (Tissue culture-treated, Not-treated or Cell repellent) supports, before being seeded in adherent condition on chamber slides for IF.

3.2. Glycolytic and Mitochondrial Bioenergetics of RT112 and 5637 Grade 2 Bladder Cancer Cells

Metabolic rewiring is a hallmark of cancer [7,58], allowing cancer cells to meet their energy and biosynthetic needs to support enhanced cell growth and survival under nutrient-poor environmental conditions, not allowing survival or proliferation of normal cells.

The main metabolic routes contributing to the energy homeostasis are glycolysis and oxidative phosphorylation (OXPHOS), which couple the breakdown of nutrients as glucose, amino acids and fatty acids to ATP production. These two pathways also play a pivotal role in redox homeostasis since they contribute to producing the reducing power required for anabolic processes and for counteracting oxidative stress. The Seahorse Extracellular Flux Analyzer (Agilent) measures in real time the ExtraCellular Acidification Rate (ECAR) related to the excretion of lactate that in turn is strictly related to the glycolytic flux, and the Oxygen Consumption Rate (OCR), that is primarily due to mitochondrial respiration, in living cells [59]. The Seahorse XF Glycolysis Stress Test and Mitochondrial Stress Test protocols dissect the glycolytic and respiratory fluxes components into basal, maximal and reserve (spare) glycolytic or respiratory capacity through the consecutive addition of specific drugs, whose optimization is reported in Supplementary Figure S3a–c.

Seahorse analysis demonstrated that, compared to RT112, 5637 cells show a significant reduction in basal and maximal (i.e., oligomycin induced) glycolytic capacity as well as in glycolytic reserve (Figure 3a,c). Consistently, the levels of mRNAs encoding two key glycolytic enzymes are down-regulated in 5637 cells compared RT112: glyceraldehyde 3-phosphate dehydrogenase (GAPDH), responsible of the conversion of glyceraldehyde-3-phosphate to 1,3-biphosphoglycerate with the production of NADH and H+, and lactate dehydrogenase A (LDHA), that catalyzes fermentation of pyruvate to lactate (Supplementary Figure S3d,e). The level of mRNAs encoding the M1 and M2 isoforms of pyruvate kinase M (PKM), that catalyzes the transfer of a phosphoryl group from phosphoenolpyruvate (PEP) to ADP generating ATP, are instead similar in both cell lines (isoform M2, associated with cancer) or higher in 5637 (isoform M1) (Supplementary Figure S3f,g). The physio-pathological consequence of the PKM expression pattern is difficult to predict, since the sugar kinase activity of the enzyme is regulated by a complex interplay between allosteric activators and inhibitors [60,61].

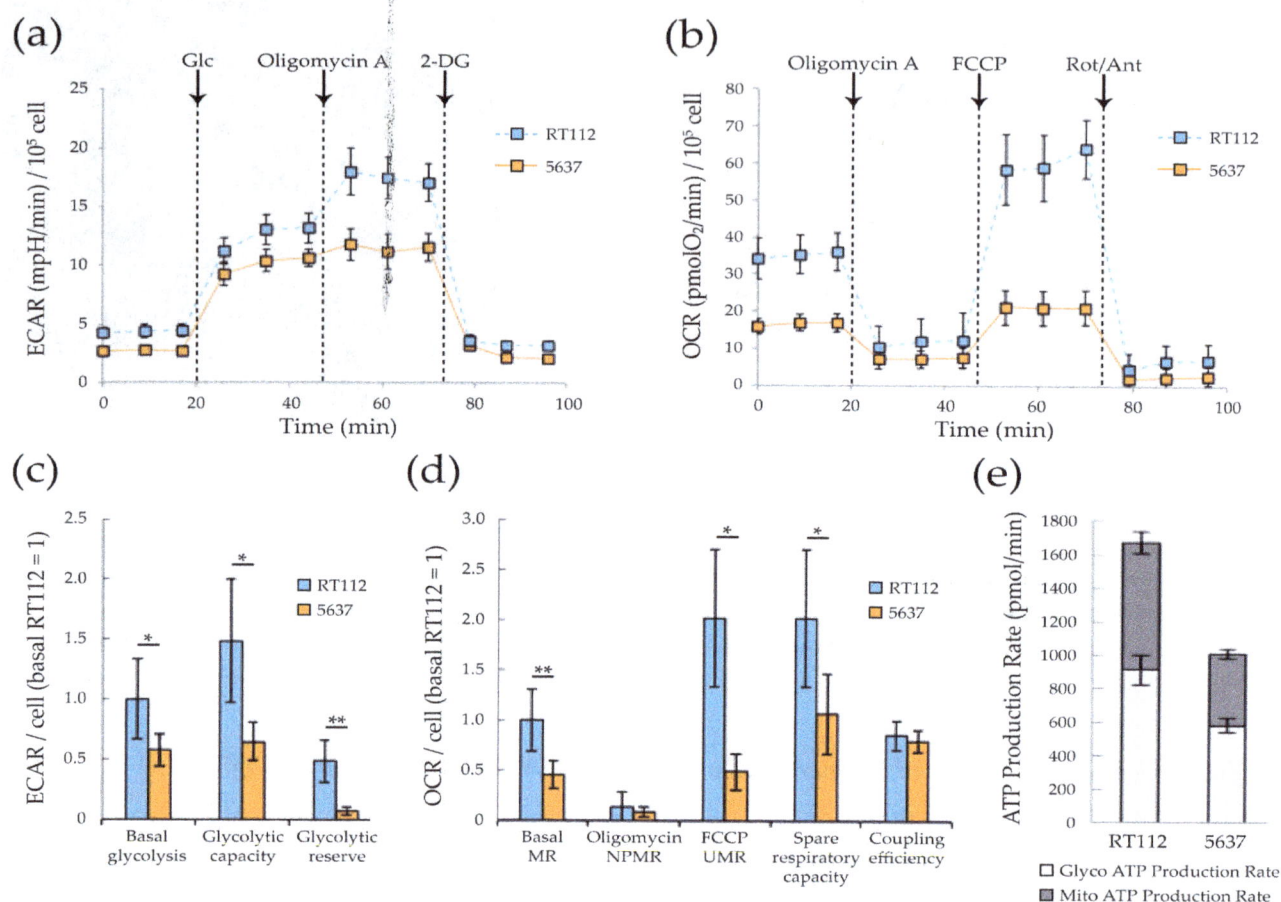

Figure 3. Glycolysis and respiratory bioenergetics of RT112 and 5637 cells. (**a**) Representative ExtraCellular Acidification Rate (ECAR) profile of monolayer cells subjected to XF Glycolysis Stress Test with XF24 Agilent Seahorse under sequential injections of 10 mM glucose, 0.25 μM oligomycin A and 50 mM 2-deoxy-glucose (**b**) Representative Oxygen Consumption Rate (OCR) profile of monolayer cells subjected to XF Mito Stress Test with XF24 Agilent Seahorse under sequential injections of 0.25 μM oligomycin A, 2 μM FCCP and 1 μM Rotenone + 1 μM Antimycin A. ECAR and OCR values measured using XF24 Agilent Seahorse were normalized on protein content measured by Bradford assay. Data were further normalized per cell number, taking into consideration the protein content per cell (Figure 1d) (**c**) Glycolytic bioenergetic parameters measured from Seahorse results: basal glycolysis, glycolytic capacity and glycolytic reserve (**d**). Respiratory bioenergetics parameter measured from Seahorse results: basal mitochondrial respiration (MR), non-phosphorylating mitochondrial respiration (NPMR) and FCCP-uncoupled respiration (UMR), spare respiratory capacity and coupling efficiency. (**e**) ATP production rates due to glycolysis or mitochondrial respiration as measured with XF Real-Time ATP rate assay using XFe96 Agilent Seahorse. Proton Efflux Rate (PER) and OCR values were normalized on cell number measured by counting Hoechst-positive nuclei with Operetta CLS™ and Harmony software. Statistical test: *t*-test, * for $p < 0.05$; ** for $p < 0.01$.

Compared to RT112, 5637 cells show a significantly reduced basal mitochondrial (MR, 2-fold reduction) and FCCP-uncoupled (UMR, 4-fold reduction) respiration (Figure 3b,d). Non-phosphorylating mitochondrial respiration (NPMR) is low and very similar in both cell lines, indicating that the enhanced basal mitochondrial respiration in RT112 is essentially devoted to ATP production. As expected, 5637 cells produce significantly less ATP than RT112 by mitochondrial respiration, and by glycolysis as well (Figure 3e).

We further analyzed mitochondrial morphology and function by confocal microscopy and high content analysis performed with Operetta CLS™. We first determined mitochondrial mass using either quantification of a transiently expressed mitochondrial-specific YFP protein (MitoYFP, Figure 4a,b) or staining with MitoTracker Green, a dye which localizes into mitochondria regardless of mitochondrial membrane potential [62] (Figure 4c,d). Quantification of both the MitoYFP- positive area/cell (Supplementary Figure S1a) and of the intensity of the MitoTracker Green signal/cell (Supplementary Figure S1b), suggests that 5637 cells have a higher mitochondrial mass compared to RT112.

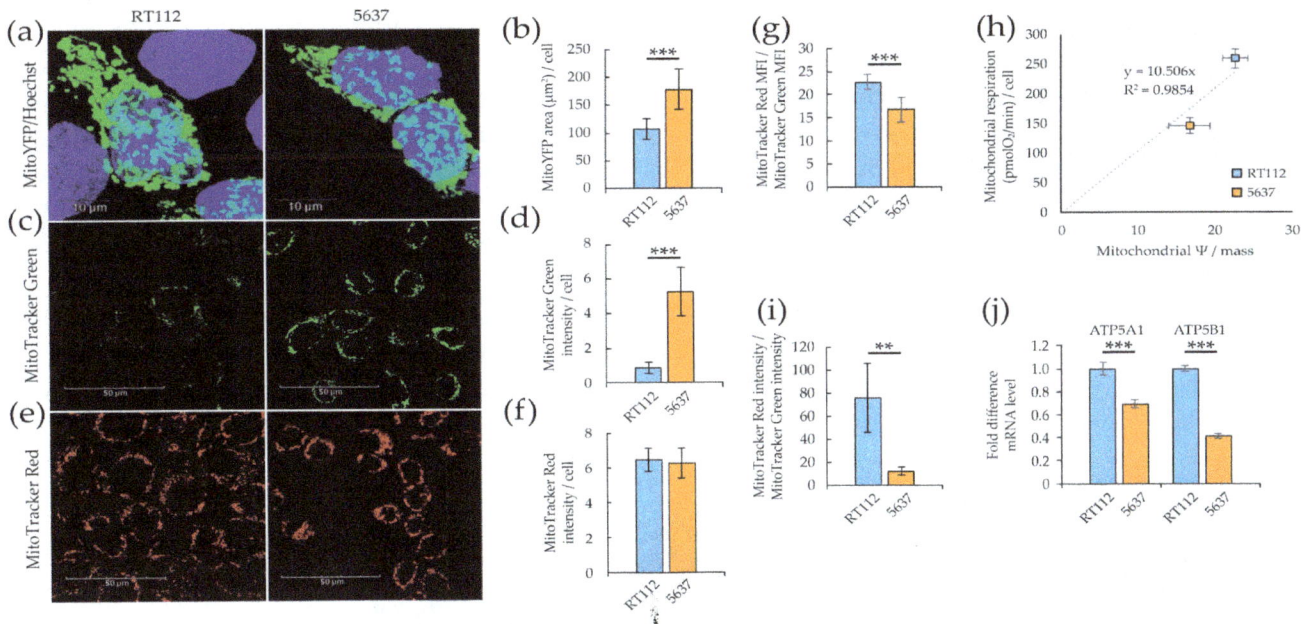

Figure 4. Mitochondrial efficiency of RT112 and 5637 cells. (**a**) Confocal imaging of fixed cells transiently transfected for the expression of the mitochondrial-specific MitoYFP protein (green), stained with Hoechst 33342 dye labeling nuclei (blue). (**b**) Mitochondrial area per cell quantified as the ratio of green (MitoYFP) fluorescent area to blue Hoechst-positive objects (nuclei) in manually selected 30-40 ROIs containing green positive cells. (**c**) Confocal imaging of living cells stained with mitochondrion-selective MitoTracker™ Green FM (green). (**d**) Mitochondrial mass per cell calculated as the ratio of MitoTracker™ green fluorescence intensity to blue Hoechst-positive objects (nuclei). (**e**) Confocal imaging of living cells stained with the potentiometric mitochondrion-selective MitoTracker™ Red CMXRos dye (red). (**f**) Mitochondrial membrane potential per cell calculated as the ratio of MitoTracker™ Red CMXRos fluorescence intensity to blue Hoechst-positive objects (nuclei). (**g**) Mitochondrial membrane potential per mitochondrial mass unit calculated as the ratio of the median fluorescence intensity of MitoTracker Red CMXRos per cell and the median fluorescence intensity of MitoTracker Green per cell by flow cytometry analysis. (**h**) Correlation between basal respiration OCR and mitochondrial membrane potential per mitochondrial mass unit measured by flow cytometry. (**i**) Mitochondrial membrane potential per mitochondrial mass unit calculated by quantitative imaging as the ratio of the Mitotracker Red and Green's fluorescence intensity per cell. (**j**) mRNA level by qRT-PCR of ATP5A1 and ATP5B1 genes normalized to the house-keeping HPRT-1 gene level. Quantitative imaging analysis was performed with Harmony software (**b,d,f,i**). All results are the mean of at least three experimental replicates. Statistical test: t-test, ** for $p < 0.01$; *** for $p < 0.001$.

We then investigated the mitochondrial membrane potential with MitoTracker Red, a potentiometric fluorescent red dye that accumulates into mitochondria depending on membrane potential, and mitochondrial activity [63]. MitoTracker Red intensity/cell is similar in the two cell lines (Figure 4e,f and Figure S1c). The ratio between the MitoTracker Red and MitoTracker Green intensities determined by imaging (Figure 4i), or the ratio between the median fluorescence intensities determined by FACS (Figure 4g) defines mitochondrial activity per unit of mitochondrial mass (*i.e.*, mitochondrial specific activity). Both measurements indicate that mitochondrial specific activity is higher in RT112 than in 5637 cells and well correlates with enhanced mitochondrial respiration measured by Seahorse flux analysis (basal OCR, Figure 3d), as reported in Figure 4h. In keeping with these data RT112 cells have higher expression level of two ATP synthase subunits, ATP5A1 and ATP5B1 (Figure 4j), and produce more ATP by mitochondrial respiration (Figure 3e).

3.3. Redox Homeostasis in RT112 and 5637 Cell Lines

Mitochondrial respiration is the primary source of cellular ROS and both cell lines under investigation are oxidative. Therefore, we analyzed mitochondrial and cytoplasmatic ROS levels by flow cytometry, and quantitative imaging (Operetta CLS™) on living cells stained with MitoSOX and 2′,7′-dichlorofluorescein diacetate (H2DCFDA), respectively [64]. MitoSOX is a mitochondrion selective dye which is oxidized by superoxide but not by other reactive oxygen species (ROS) and reactive nitrogen species (RNS), while H2DCFDA is a fluorogenic dye that allow measuring hydroxyl, peroxyl and other ROS species within the cell. After passive diffusion into cells, H2DCFDA is deacetylated by cellular esterases to the corresponding dichlorodihydrofluorescein derivative, whose ROS oxidization originates a fluorescent adduct, 2′,7′-dichlorofluorescin (DCF), that remains trapped inside the cells. Quantitative imaging results, confirmed by flow cytometry analysis (Figure 5a–f), showed that although RT112 cells have a higher (30% more) content of mitochondrial superoxide than 5637, in keeping with their higher respiratory rate, they are characterized by a significantly lower total intracellular ROS level.

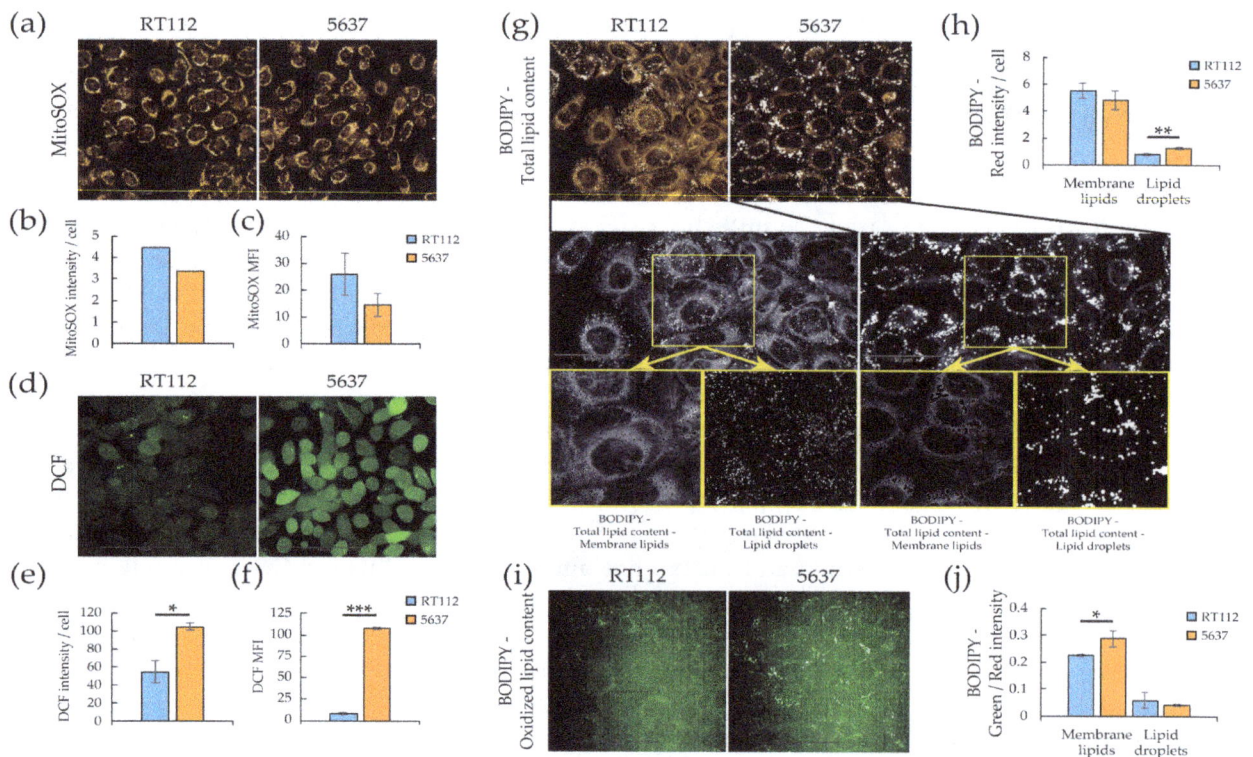

Figure 5. Redox homeostasis and lipid peroxidation in RT112 and 5637 cells. Quantitative imaging was performed with Operetta CLS™ and Harmony software (**a**) Confocal imaging of living cells stained

with MitoSOX (orange). (**b**) Mitochondrial ROS level per cell calculated as the ratio of MitoSOX red fluorescence intensity to blue Hoechst-positive objects (nuclei) (**c**) MitoSOX median fluorescence intensity obtained by flow cytometry. (**d**) Confocal imaging of living cells stained with 2′,7′-Dichlorofluorescin diacetate (green). (**e**) Total ROS level per cell calculated as the ratio of DCF green fluorescence intensity to blue Hoechst-positive objects (nuclei). (**f**) Total ROS level per cell obtained from DCF median fluorescence intensity obtained from flow cytometry. (**g**) Confocal imaging of red fluorescence of living cells stained with the Lipid Peroxidation Sensor BODIPY™ 581/591 C11 (orange, total lipid content, upper panels) and grayscale representative image as used for quantitative analysis of total lipid content (middle panels), membrane lipids and lipid droplets (lower panels). (**h**) Lipids per cell quantified as membrane lipids and lipid droplets measured using Harmony software. (**i**) Confocal imaging of green fluorescence of living cells stained with the Lipid Peroxidation Sensor BODIPY™ 581/591 C11 (green, oxidized lipid content). (**j**) Oxidized/total membrane lipids and lipid droplets ratio, calculated as the ratio of green to red fluorescence intensity. All results are the mean of at least three experimental replicates. Statistical test: t-test, * for $p < 0.05$; ** for $p < 0.01$; *** for $p < 0.001$.

Since high ROS concentrations lead to free radical mediated chain reactions that indiscriminately target intracellular molecules, including polyunsaturated fatty acids of lipid membranes [65], we analyzed by confocal microscopy (Operetta CLS™) lipid peroxidation using a ratio-fluorescence assay on living cells stained with the oxidative sensitive C11-BODIPY581-591 dye [66]. This probe incorporates readily into cellular membranes and its fluorescence shifts from red to green upon oxidation. Figure 5g,i report confocal images of red and green fluorescence of RT112 and 5637 cells stained with C11-BODIPY581-591. It is possible to distinguish bright fluorescent spots corresponding to lipid droplets, and a diffuse fluorescence corresponding to membrane lipid content. The bottom part of the same panel reports an enlarged, grayscale version of the images to highlight the quantification procedure. Although 5637 and RT112 have a similar total lipid content, quantitative imaging shows that 5463 have a slightly lower membrane lipid content and a lower number of significantly larger and denser lipid droplets on a cellular basis (Figure 5h and Figure S4a,b). In contrast, 5637 show higher oxidation of membrane lipids (diffuse green fluorescence). The two cell lines show no significant difference in lipid droplets' oxidation (Figure 5j and Figure S4c,d). In keeping with the higher ROS and peroxidized lipids levels, 5637 cells are more sensitive to oxidative stress, namely H_2O_2 treatment (Supplementary Figure S4g).

3.4. Metabolic Plasticity in RT112 and 5637 Cell Lines

As highlighted by the Seahorse experiments described above (Figure 3b,d), RT112 cells are more energetic than 5637, having a more efficient glycolytic and mitochondrial apparatus both for the production of energy in basal conditions, and for responding to eventual energy stress (greater glycolytic reserve, and spare respiratory capacity, or nutrient perturbation). Consistently, when exposed to glucose deprivation (blocking glycolysis) the RT112 cells increase the mitochondrial respiration more effectively compared to 5637. The reduced plasticity of 5637 is appreciable in Figure 6a which reports the two lines' energy phenotype under basal (in presence or absence of glucose) and maximal conditions (oligomycin-induced glycolysis, and FCCP-uncoupled respiration).

To understand the two cell lines' ability and flexibility to oxidize different nutrients, we performed the Seahorse XF Mitochondrial Fuel Flex test (Figure 6b). The test showed that both cell lines strongly depend on glucose as a fuel for mitochondrial respiration, make limited use of fatty acids and no use of glutamine at all (dependency, gray bars). Both cell lines are flexible enough to increase allocation of glucose, glutamine and fatty acids for mitochondrial respiration (Flexibility, white bars).

Fatty acid oxidation into mitochondria provides twice as much ATP as carbohydrates on a dry mass basis. Indeed, energy-demanding tissues generally carried out fatty acid β-oxidation (FAO). Furthermore, several cancer cells are dependent on FAO for survival and growth, since it can eliminate potentially toxic lipids, inhibit pro-apoptotic pathways and provide metabolic intermediates for anaplerosis, besides providing ATP and NADPH, counteracting energy and oxidative stress [67].

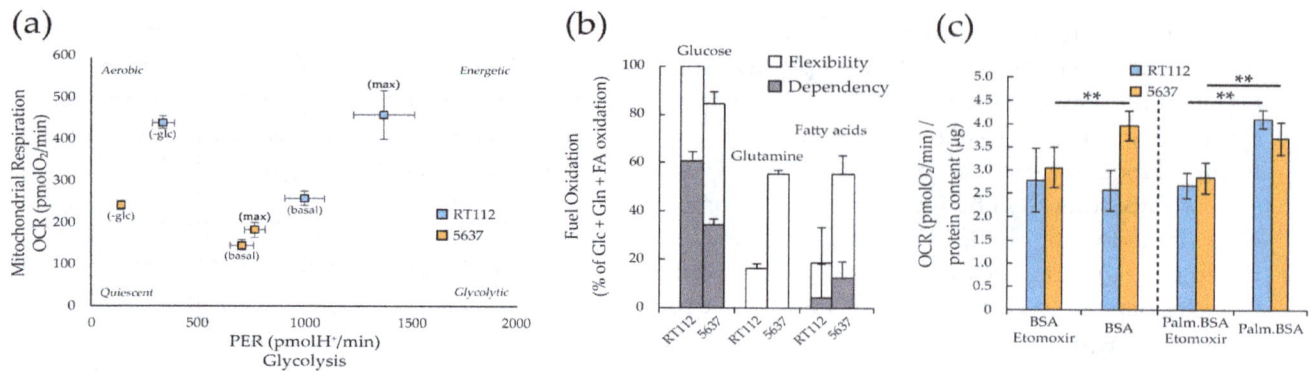

Figure 6. Glycolytic and respiratory capacity and nutrient usage in RT112 and 5637 cells. (**a**) PER and OCR values (attributable to glycolysis and oxidative phosphorylation respectively) in basal condition, maximal capacity (reached with treatment with optimized concentration of oligomycin A for maximal glycolytic capacity or FCCP for maximal respiratory capacity) and under 5 h-glucose deprivation. Seahorse data were normalized on cell number measured after Hoechst 33342 staining as blue-positive objects acquired by Operetta CLS™ and counted using Harmony software. (**b**) The ability to oxidize three different nutrients (glucose, glutamine and fatty acids) reported as dependency and flexibility from XF Mito Fuel Flex Test performed using Agilent Seahorse XFe96 Analyzer. (**c**) OCR values measured in presence/absence of 5 µM Etomoxir from XF Palmitate-BSA FAO Substrate assay using Agilent Seahorse XF24 Analyzer. OCR values were normalized on protein content measured by Bradford assay. All results are the mean of at least three experimental replicates. Statistical test: t-test, ** for $p < 0.01$.

We extended our studies dealing with energy homeostasis of RT112 and 5637 cells to FAO for these reasons. The Seahorse XF fatty acid β-oxidation (FAO) test assays the cells' capability to oxidize endogenous fatty acids and/or the long chain fatty acid palmitate, exogenously added in the culture medium. The share of respiration devoted to FAO can be calculated as the difference between the basal respiration and the residual respiration obtained after treatment with 40 µM etomoxir, an irreversible inhibitor of carnitine palmitoyltransferase-1 (CPT1), which is a mitochondrial transporter required for FAO [68]. The FAO assay (Figure 6c) demonstrates that both cell lines can oxidize the exogenous palmitate, while only 5637 cells can also oxidize also the endogenous fatty acids.

3.5. Targeting Metabolism in RT112 and 5637 Cell Lines

The different assays reported above (Figure 5; Figure 6) indicate that both cell lines present, albeit with some differences, some kind of metabolic flexibility. Here we tested the pharmacological effect of the inhibition of glycolysis and OXPHOS on cell proliferation, migration and propensity to form spheroids. We used the non-hydrolyzable glucose analog 2-Deoxy-D-glucose (2-DG), to inhibit glycolysis, and metformin to inhibit, possibly indirectly, mitochondrial respiration [69–71].

Treatment with both 2-DG and metformin inhibits cell proliferation of both bladder cancer cell lines (Figure 7a,b). Compared to RT112, the 5637 cell line's proliferation was more sensitive to both 2-DG and metformin. This behavior could be due to the more remarkable metabolic plasticity of RT112 cells, which would improve resistance to the inhibition of any of the two energy pathways.

While metformin inhibits in a dose–dependent manner the already limited lateral migration of RT112, 2-DG does not inhibit migration of this cell line (Figure 7c). Indeed, 2-DG seems to paradoxically stimulate cell migration. Whether this is caused by the enhanced metabolic flexibility of RT112 cells or by the short timeframe of this experiment (12 h compared to the 72 h used in the cell proliferation and spheroid formation assays), remains to be seen. Treatments with both metformin and 2DG significantly reduce the migratory capacity of 5637 (Figure 7d).

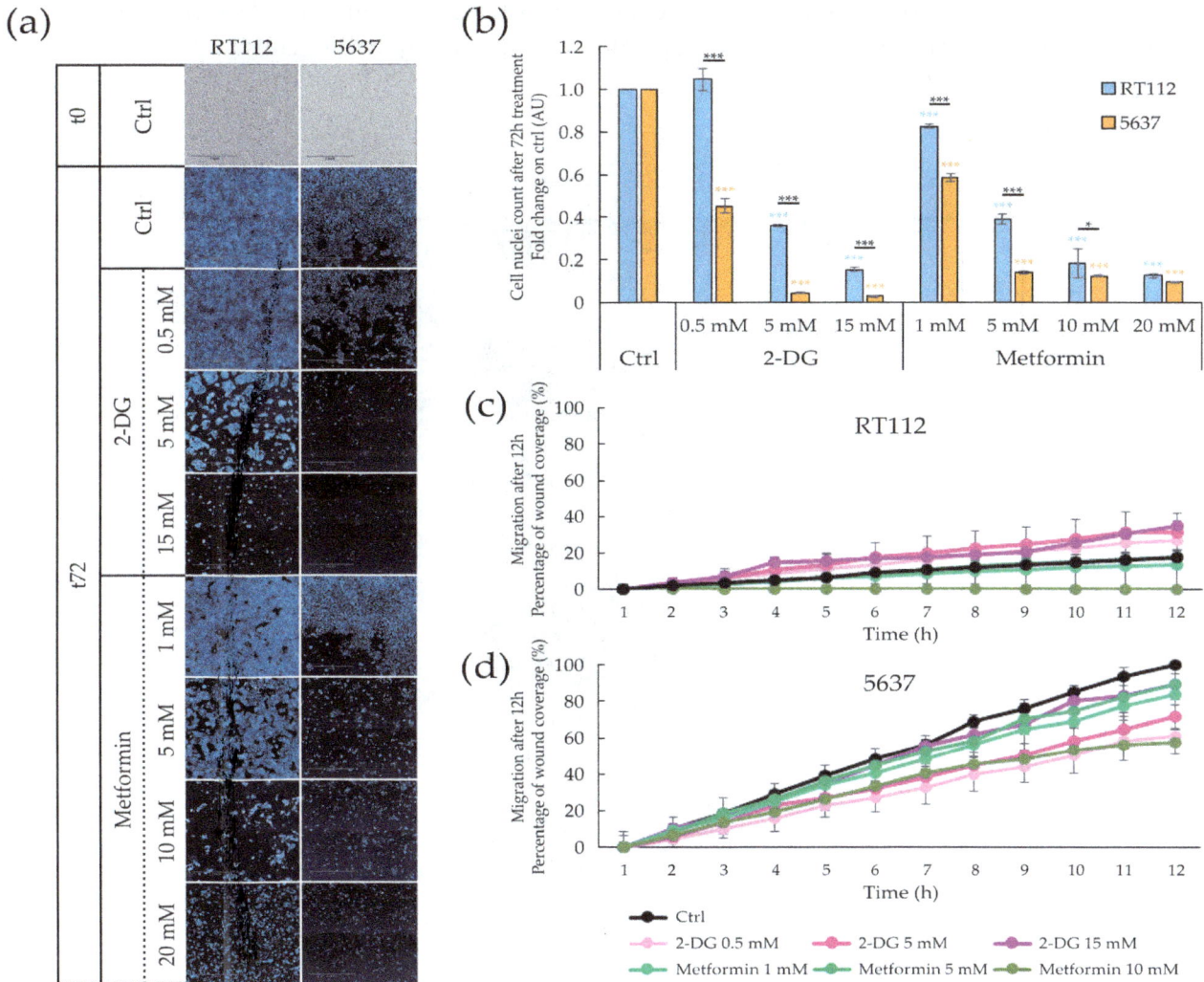

Figure 7. Effect of pharmacological treatment on proliferation and migratory capacity of RT112 and 5637 cells grown as adherent cells. (**a**) Representative images of brightfield (T0) and Hoechst 33342 stained nuclei acquired with Operetta CLS™ of adherent cells after 72 h-treatment with increasing concentration of 2-Deoxy-D-glucose (2-DG) (0, 0.5, 5, 15 mM) and metformin (0, 1, 5, 10, 20 mM). (**b**) Fold change relative to the control condition of nuclei count of cells treated for 72 h grown with 2-Deoxy-D-glucose (2-DG) and metformin treatment. Results are the mean of three experimental replicates. (**c,d**) Percentage of wound coverage in wound healing assay after 12 h-treatment condition of increasing concentration of 2-Deoxy-D-glucose (2-DG) (0, 0.5, 5, 15 mM) and metformin (0, 1, 5, 10 mM) of RT112 cells (**c**) and 5637 cells Results are the mean of two experimental replicates, except for 15 mM 2-DG and 10 mM metformin conditions performed in single replicate. Statistical test: t-test, * for $p < 0.05$; *** for $p < 0.001$.

Then we tested the effect of 2-DG and metformin on the ability of RT112 and 5637 to form spheroids from single cells in non-adherent conditions. Spheroid formation exploits features of cell progenitors or cancer stem cells (CSC), such as anchorage-independent growth, anoikis resistance and self-renewal [72,73]. Figure 8 and Supplementary Figure S5 show cell tracker-labeled spheroids at 0 and 72 h after seeding and during time course (24-48-72 h) respectively. Untreated spheroids (upper line) have a compact, regular, bright shape and may be surrounded by some cells, especially in the case of the 5637 cell line. The 2-DG treatment has little effect at the lowest tested concentration, while higher concentrations inhibit the development of a properly formed spheroid, originating less bright and more spread aggregates. The effect appears more potent in 5637 cells. A more substantial disruptive effect on the proper formation of spheroids is elicited by treatment with metformin, in keeping with literature data suggesting that spheroid formation is exquisitely dependent on mitochondrial respiration [74–77]. The aggregates formed after both pharmacological perturbations by RT112 cells appear irregular than those formed by 5637 cells.

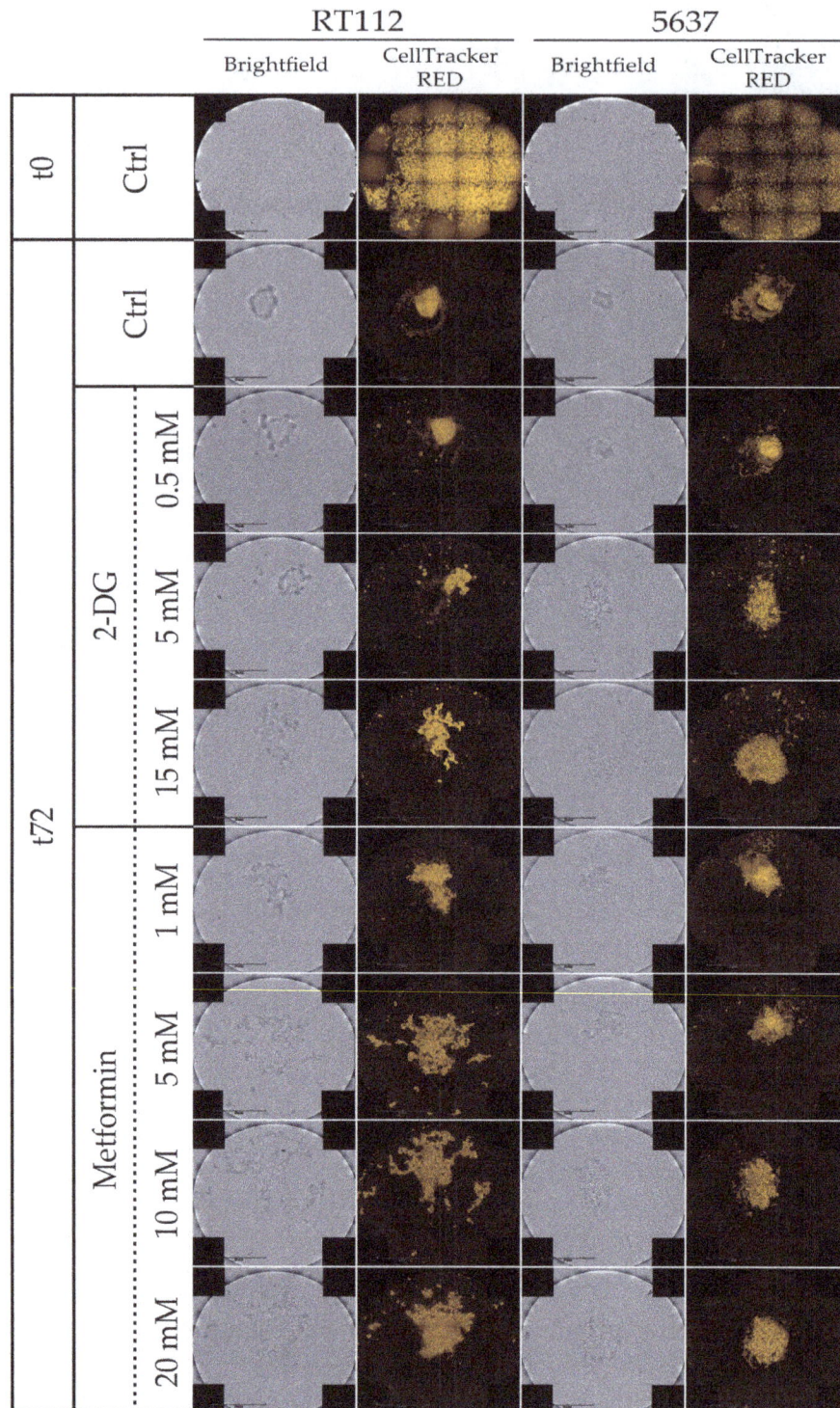

Figure 8. Spheroid formation under pharmacological treatment of RT112 and 5637 cells. Representative images from brightfield and fluorescence microscopy (orange: CellTracker™ Red CMTPX Dye) acquired with Operetta CLS™ at 0 h and 72 h of cells grown in cell repellent 96-well plate under treatment with increasing concentration of 2-Deoxy-D-glucose (2-DG) (0, 0.5, 5, 15 mM) and metformin (0, 1, 5, 10, 20 mM).

4. Discussion

Bladder cancer ranks eleventh among the most diagnosed cancer globally. Nearly 90% of these cancers are urothelial carcinomas [78]. Early and accurate diagnostic staging and development of sensitive biomarkers are crucial for identifying the most aggressive cancers and developing appropriate therapeutic interventions. Metabolism is increasing recognized as a driver in the development and maintenance of multifactorial diseases such as cancer [79,80]. Accordingly, detection and characterization of the metabolic footprint of bladder cancers [81,82] could be instrumental for both early diagnosis and therapy monitoring.

Fast cell growth, ability to move and to form 3D structures contribute to defining a cancer cell's aggressiveness. RT112 and 5637 cells are classified at the same histological low grade, but express molecular markers related to different aggressiveness. The two cell lines present a similar growth rate, but RT112 cells are significantly larger. RT112 form spheroids more efficiently, even on surfaces where 5637 do not form spheroids at all. Even on cell repellent plates, where both cell lines generate spheroids, RT112 form more spheroids with a larger size. In contrast, the 5637 cells migrate much faster (Figure 1 and Video S1). This phenotypic trait is consistent with data that classify RT112 as luminal-like cells enriched in papillary architecture, [43,83,84], and 5637 as basal-like cells enriched for squamous differentiation, considered as models of non-aggressive and aggressive BCs, respectively [44,84,85].

Once characterized the cellular properties associated with spreading and tumor progression of RT112 and 5637, we analyzed their cellular bioenergetics, and nutrient usage in order to identify a potential fragility or dependency to be targeted with a pharmacological treatment.

Seahorse analysis showed that both cell lines can use glycolysis and respiration to produce ATP. However, the RT112 cell line is more energetic than 5637 with a higher basal respiration and glycolytic flux (Figure 6a), essentially due to a potentiated respiratory and glycolytic machinery.

Most cells exploit only a part of their total bioenergetic capacity, operating at a basal level and maintaining a reserve capacity for sudden surges in energy requirements due to stress or increased workload. Under standard growth conditions, 5637 cells use most of their glycolytic and respiratory potential, while RT112 cells have a large, unused glycolytic and respiratory reserve. Both cell lines respond to glucose deprivation by increasing respiration, possibly because glucose starvation unlocks the respiratory machinery. The increase in respiration is less striking in 5637 cells.

Mitochondria are both the source and target of reactive oxygen species (ROS), and damaged mitochondria can release more ROS [86,87]. In detail, about 1–2% O_2 uptaken by the mitochondria is reduced to superoxide anion radical and ROS as a byproduct of electron transport during oxidative phosphorylation, in particular through the activity of complex I (NADH dehydrogenase ubiquinone-ubiquinol reductase) [88] and complex III (ubiquinol cytochrome c reductase) [89]. Electron transport chain (ETC) generates ROS particularly when is slowed down by high mitochondrial membrane potential ($\Delta\psi m$), or functions in reverse from complex II to complex I, as for ubiquinol excess produced in several mitochondrial metabolic pathways such as fatty acid β-oxidation or oxidation of α-glycerophosphate. ROS generation can also be attributed to the TCA cycle's specific dehydrogenases due to an increased NADH/NAD+ ratio.

Consistently with their higher respiratory rate, RT112 cells have higher levels of mitochondrial ROS. However, the total level of ROS is higher in 5637 cells. This can be due to a less efficient detoxification system, or poor supply of reducing equivalents required to maintain the antioxidant capacity of the glutathione system. The increased intracellular ROS level in 5637 cells correlates with increased lipid peroxidation. Lipid peroxidation produces highly-reactive aldehyde species, including 4-hydroxy 2-nonenal (4-HNE), considered second messengers of oxidative stress and playing a critical role in cell proliferation and survival, and thereby in cancer progression as reviewed in [90–92]. The aldehyde dehydrogenase ALDH3A1 acts as a specific scavenger for these fatty aldehydes [93,94]. RT-PCR analysis (Figure S4h) demonstrates that ALDH3A1 is not expressed in 5637, unlike RT112, indicating that the accumulation of peroxidized lipids could be associated with an ineffective detoxification system. 5637 cells are also more sensitive to H_2O_2-induced oxidative stress, suggesting a differential balance between ROS production and detoxification mechanisms in the two bladder cancer cell lines.

Metabolic plasticity is the ability to modulate the use of glycolysis and OXPHOS, to meet the energy and biosynthetic needs depending on the nutritional/environmental conditions, enabling the cancer cells to adapt to various microenvironmental conditions including hypoxia and acidosis. Although most cancer cells, according to the Warburg paradigm, internalize glucose faster and metabolize it via aerobic glycolysis to sustain active proliferation, they remain able to completely oxidize glucose, unless they display significant mitochondrial defects [95]. Indeed both glycolysis and respiration can be simultaneously turned on [9].

In addition to glucose-derived pyruvate, other nutrients provide substrates to the TCA cycle to support mitochondrial metabolism, including lactate and amino acids, i.e., glutamine, and fatty acids. Glucose appears the favorite respiratory substrate for both cell lines, although they can use glutamine and fatty acids when required. Contrary to RT112, the 5637 cell line appears able to use endogenous fatty acids. However, in keeping with the negligible contribution of fatty acids to mitochondria respiration in both cell lines (Figure 6b), in vivo administration of low concentrations of etomoxir [68,96,97]—that guarantee to avoid off-target effects reported at higher dosage [98] and that led to the stoppage of etomoxir clinical trials—does not significantly affect the viability of RT112 and 5637 monolayers (Supplementary Figure S4e,f).

While inhibition of either glycolysis (through treatment with the glucose analog 2-deoxyglucose (2-DG) or respiration (through metformin) results in general down-regulation of cell proliferation, cell migration and spheroid formation in both RT112 and 5637 cells, some difference is worth noting. RT112 cells are less sensitive than 5637 to the inhibitory effect of both drugs on proliferation and cell migration. 2-DG does not inhibit migration in RT112 cells. Migration results with this cell line should be taken cautiously, because of the extremely low migration rate. This overall lower sensitivity to metabolic perturbations is consistent with the more energetic phenotype of the RT112 cell line and its higher ability to cope with metabolic stress, as shown by Seahorse analysis (Figure 3). Metformin appears to inhibit spheroid formation more than 2-DG, in both cell lines. Consistently, recent data indicate that mitochondrial respiration is particularly important in metastatic/circulating cancer cells [99,100], in the development and maintenance of chemoresistance mechanisms [77], and in cancer stem cells [74,101,102], which are particularly enriched in 3D cellular structures, as spheroids.

5. Conclusions

In conclusion, our study highlights that two bladder cancer cell lines, established from primary urinary bladder carcinoma of the same histological grade, associated with different aggressiveness and prognoses, present distinct metabolic and invasive properties. Although both cell lines use both glycolysis and respiration to support energy production, RT112 cells present overall higher metabolic plasticity and a higher propensity to form 3D structures while being vastly less efficient in migration. Despite these differences, both cell lines have sizable respiration, and the metformin treatment gives a global down-regulation of the proliferation, migration, and the ability to form spheroids. This suggests that the targeted inhibition of energy metabolism may also be effective in a heterogeneous tumor context. Intriguingly, while RT112 are less sensitive than 5637 to pharmacological perturbation of cell proliferation and migration by 2-DG and metformin, they are more sensitive in the spheroid formation assay. These differences may be partially due to transcriptional rewiring and altered signaling and communication within the forming spheroid architecture. As the molecular and metabolic characterization of these cancers and derived cellular and animal [103] models increase, we will be able to design ever more effective single and combinatorial [104,105] anti-cancer regimens based on the detected metabolic fragilities. This ability appears particularly important for cancers of low histological grade, such as the Grade 2 bladder tumors, representing a critical therapeutic window for adjuvant or post-operative treatments to reduce the tumor mass or avoid the formation of relapses.

Supplementary Materials:
Figure S1: Quantitative imaging by Operetta CLS™ high-content analysis and the Harmony software. Figure S2: RT112 and 5637 cells spheroids formation capacity. Figure S3: Figure S3 Oligomycin and FCCP optimization for the measurement of glycolytic and respiratory bioenergetics, and mRNA levels of selected glycolytic enzymes differentially expressed in RT112 and 5637 cells. Figure S4: Figure S4. Lipid content, lipid peroxidation and redox homeostasis in RT112 and 5637 cells. Figure S5: Spheroid formation capacity of RT112 and 5637 cells under pharmacological treatment; Video S1: RT112 and 5637 cells migration time-lapse.

Author Contributions: Conceptualization, M.V. and E.S.; Data curation, V.P., G.D., G.C., A.V., C.A., R.V. and E.S.; Funding acquisition, M.V., R.V. and E.S.; Investigation, V.P., G.D., G.C., A.V., C.A., S.B. and E.S.; Writing—original draft, V.P., G.D. and E.S.; Writing—review & editing, M.V., R.V. and E.S. All authors have read and agreed to the published version of the manuscript.

Acknowledgments: The authors would like to thank SYSBIO/ISBE.IT Center of Systems Biology and the Project of Excellence CHRONOS (CHRonical multifactorial disorders explored by NOvel integrated Strategies) for providing advanced technologies used in this study. The authors also warmly thank Silvia Nicolis for the kind gift of anti-SOX2 antibodies.

References

1. Yeung, C.; Dinh, T.; Lee, J. The Health Economics of Bladder Cancer: An Updated Review of the Published Literature. *Pharm. Econ.* **2014**, *32*, 1093–1104. [CrossRef] [PubMed]

2. Babjuk, M.; Böhle, A.; Burger, M.; Capoun, O.; Cohen, D.; Compérat, E.; Hernández, V.; Kaasinen, E.; Palou, J.; Rouprêt, M.; et al. EAU Guidelines on Non–Muscle-invasive Urothelial Carcinoma of the Bladder: Update 2016. *Eur. Urol.* **2017**, *71*, 447–461. [CrossRef] [PubMed]

3. Witjes, F.; Lebret, T.; Compérat, E.; Cowan, N.C.; De Santis, M.; Bruins, H.M.; Hernández, V.; Espinós, E.L.; Dunn, J.; Rouanne, M.; et al. Updated 2016 EAU Guidelines on Muscle-invasive and Metastatic Bladder Cancer. *Eur. Urol.* **2017**, *71*, 462–475. [CrossRef]

4. Compérat, E.M.; Burger, M.; Gontero, P.; Mostafid, H.; Palou, J.; Rouprêt, M.; Van Rhijn, B.W.; Shariat, S.F.; Sylvester, R.J.; Zigeuner, R.; et al. Grading of Urothelial Carcinoma and The New "World Health Organisation Classification of Tumours of the Urinary System and Male Genital Organs 2016". *Eur. Urol. Focus* **2019**, *5*, 457–466. [CrossRef]

5. Cheng, L.; Neumann, R.M.; Nehra, A.; Spotts, B.E.; Weaver, A.L.; Bostwick, D.G. Cancer heterogeneity and its biologic implications in the grading of urothelial carcinoma. *Cancer* **2000**, *88*, 1663–1670. [CrossRef]

6. Downes, M.R.; Weening, B.; Van Rhijn, B.W.G.; Have, C.L.; Treurniet, K.M.; Van Der Kwast, T.H. Analysis of papillary urothelial carcinomas of the bladder with grade heterogeneity: Supportive evidence for an early role ofCDKN2Adeletions in theFGFR3pathway. *Histopathology* **2016**, *70*, 281–289. [CrossRef] [PubMed]

7. Hanahan, D.; Weinberg, R.A. Hallmarks of cancer: The next generation. *Cell* **2011**, *144*, 646–674. [CrossRef]

8. Warburg, O. On the Origin of Cancer Cells. *Science* **1956**, *123*, 309–314. [CrossRef]

9. DeBerardinis, R.J.; Chandel, N.S. Fundamentals of cancer metabolism. *Sci. Adv.* **2016**, *2*, e1600200. [CrossRef]

10. Zhu, J.; Thompson, C.B. Metabolic regulation of cell growth and proliferation. *Nat. Rev. Mol. Cell Biol.* **2019**, *20*, 436–450. [CrossRef]

11. DeBerardinis, R.J.; Chandel, N.S. We need to talk about the Warburg effect. *Nat. Metab.* **2020**, *2*, 127–129. [CrossRef] [PubMed]

12. Wang, T.; Marquardt, C.; Foker, J. Aerobic glycolysis during lymphocyte proliferation. *Nat. Cell Biol.* **1976**, *261*, 702–705. [CrossRef] [PubMed]

13. Bauer, D.E.; Harris, M.H.; Plas, D.R.; Lum, J.J.; Hammerman, P.S.; Rathmell, J.C.; Riley, J.L.; Thompson, C.B. Cytokine stimulation of aerobic glycolysis in hematopoietic cells exceeds proliferative demand. *FASEB J.* **2004**, *18*, 1303–1305. [CrossRef] [PubMed]

14. Peek, C.B.; Levine, D.C.; Cedernaes, J.; Taguchi, A.; Kobayashi, Y.; Tsai, S.J.; Bonar, N.A.; McNulty, M.R.; Ramsey, K.M.; Bass, J. Circadian Clock Interaction with HIF1α Mediates Oxygenic Metabolism and Anaerobic Glycolysis in Skeletal Muscle. *Cell Metab.* **2017**, *25*, 86–92. [CrossRef]

15. Chiaradonna, F.; Sacco, E.; Manzoni, R.; Giorgio, M.; Vanoni, M.; Alberghina, L. Ras-dependent carbon metabolism and transformation in mouse fibroblasts. *Oncogene* **2006**, *25*, 5391–5404. [CrossRef]

16. Ying, H.; Kimmelman, A.C.; Lyssiotis, C.A.; Hua, S.; Chu, G.C.; Fletcher-Sananikone, E.; Locasale, J.W.; Son, J.; Zhang, H.; Coloff, J.L.; et al. Oncogenic Kras Maintains Pancreatic Tumors through Regulation of Anabolic Glucose Metabolism. *Cell* **2012**, *149*, 656–670. [CrossRef]

17. Damiani, C.; Colombo, R.; Gaglio, D.; Mastroianni, F.; Pescini, D.; Westerhoff, H.V.; Mauri, G.; Vanoni, M.; Alberghina, L. A metabolic core model elucidates how enhanced utilization of glucose and glutamine, with enhanced glutamine-dependent lactate production, promotes cancer cell growth: The WarburQ effect. *PLoS Comput. Biol.* **2017**, *13*, e1005758. [CrossRef]

18. Pupo, E.; Avanzato, D.; Middonti, E.; Bussolino, F.; Lanzetti, L. KRAS-Driven Metabolic Rewiring Reveals Novel Actionable Targets in Cancer. *Front. Oncol.* **2019**, *9*, 848. [CrossRef]

19. Matoba, S.; Kang, J.-G.; Patino, W.D.; Wragg, A.; Boehm, M.; Gavrilova, O.; Hurley, P.J.; Bunz, F.; Hwang, P.M. p53 Regulates Mitochondrial Respiration. *Science* **2006**, *312*, 1650–1653. [CrossRef]

20. Lago, C.U.; Sung, H.J.; Ma, W.; Wang, P.Y.; Hwang, P.M. P53, aerobic metabolism, and cancer. *Antioxid. Redox Signal.* **2011**, *15*, 1739–1748. [CrossRef]

21. Hoxhaj, G.; Manning, B.D. The PI3K–AKT network at the interface of oncogenic signalling and cancer metabolism. *Nat. Rev. Cancer* **2019**, *20*, 74–88. [CrossRef] [PubMed]

22. Sciacovelli, M.; Frezza, C. Oncometabolites: Unconventional triggers of oncogenic signalling cascades. *Free Radic. Biol. Med.* **2016**, *100*, 175–181. [CrossRef] [PubMed]

23. Tommasini-Ghelfi, S.; Murnan, K.; Kouri, F.M.; Mahajan, A.S.; May, J.L.; Stegh, A.H. Cancer-associated mutation and beyond: The emerging biology of isocitrate dehydrogenases in human disease. *Sci. Adv.* **2019**, *5*, eaaw4543. [CrossRef] [PubMed]

24. Dang, C.V.; Lewis, B.C.; Dolde, C.; Dang, G.; Shim, H. Oncogenes in tumor metabolism, tumorigenesis, and apoptosis. *J. Bioenerg. Biomembr.* **1997**, *29*, 345–354. [CrossRef]

25. DeBerardinis, R.J.; Mancuso, A.; Daikhin, E.; Nissim, I.; Yudkoff, M.; Wehrli, S.; Thompson, C.B. Beyond aerobic glycolysis: Transformed cells can engage in glutamine metabolism that exceeds the requirement for protein and nucleotide synthesis. *Proc. Natl. Acad. Sci. USA* **2007**, *104*, 19345–19350. [CrossRef]

26. Gaglio, D.; Metallo, C.M.; A Gameiro, P.; Hiller, K.; Danna, L.S.; Balestrieri, C.; Alberghina, L.; Stephanopoulos, G.; Chiaradonna, F. Oncogenic K-Ras decouples glucose and glutamine metabolism to support cancer cell growth. *Mol. Syst. Biol.* **2011**, *7*, 523. [CrossRef]

27. Son, J.; Lyssiotis, C.A.; Ying, H.; Wang, X.; Hua, S.; Ligorio, M.; Perera, R.M.; Ferrone, C.R.; Mullarky, E.; Shyh-Chang, N.; et al. Glutamine supports pancreatic cancer growth through a KRAS-regulated metabolic pathway. *Nat. Cell Biol.* **2013**, *496*, 101–105. [CrossRef]

28. Rashkovan, M.; Ferrando, A. Metabolic dependencies and vulnerabilities in leukemia. *Genes Dev.* **2019**, *33*, 1460–1474. [CrossRef]

29. Chajès, V.; Cambot, M.; Moreau, K.; Lenoir, G.M.; Joulin, V. Acetyl-CoA Carboxylase α Is Essential to Breast Cancer Cell Survival. *Cancer Res.* **2006**, *66*, 5287–5294. [CrossRef]

30. Wang, Z.; Liu, F.; Fan, N.; Zhou, C.; Li, D.; MacVicar, T.; Dong, Q.; Bruns, C.J.; Zhao, Y. Targeting Glutaminolysis: New Perspectives to Understand Cancer Development and Novel Strategies for Potential Target Therapies. *Front. Oncol.* **2020**, *10*, 589508. [CrossRef]

31. Gaglio, D.; Soldati, C.; Vanoni, M.; Alberghina, L.; Chiaradonna, F. Glutamine Deprivation Induces Abortive S-Phase Rescued by Deoxyribonucleotides in K-Ras Transformed Fibroblasts. *PLoS ONE* **2009**, *4*, e4715. [CrossRef] [PubMed]

32. Massari, F.; Ciccarese, C.; Santoni, M.; Iacovelli, R.; Mazzucchelli, R.; Piva, F.; Scarpelli, M.; Berardi, R.; Tortora, G.; Lopez-Beltran, A.; et al. Metabolic phenotype of bladder cancer. *Cancer Treat. Rev.* **2016**, *45*, 46–57. [CrossRef] [PubMed]

33. Petrella, G.; Ciufolini, G.; Vago, R.; Cicero, D.O. The Interplay between Oxidative Phosphorylation and Glycolysis as a Potential Marker of Bladder Cancer Progression. *Int. J. Mol. Sci.* **2020**, *21*, 8107. [CrossRef] [PubMed]

34. Loras, A.; Trassierra, M.; Sanjuan-Herráez, D.; Martínez-Bisbal, M.C.; Castell, J.V.; Quintás, G.; Ruiz-Cerdá, J.L. Bladder cancer recurrence surveillance by urine metabolomics analysis. *Sci. Rep.* **2018**, *8*, 1–10. [CrossRef] [PubMed]

35. Sborov, D.W.; Haverkos, B.M.; Harris, P.J. Investigational cancer drugs targeting cell metabolism in clinical development. *Expert Opin. Investig. Drugs* **2015**, *24*, 79–94. [CrossRef] [PubMed]

36. A Pierotti, M.; Berrino, F.; Gariboldi, M.B.; Melani, C.; Mogavero, A.; Negri, T.; Pasanisi, P.; Pilotti, S. Targeting metabolism for cancer treatment and prevention: Metformin, an old drug with multi-faceted effects. *Oncogene* **2013**, *32*, 1475–1487. [CrossRef]

37. Luengo, A.; Gui, D.Y.; Vander Heiden, M.G. Targeting Metabolism for Cancer Therapy. *Cell Chem. Biol.* **2017**, *24*, 1161–1180. [CrossRef]

38. De Sanctis, G.; Spinelli, M.; Vanoni, M.; Sacco, E. K-Ras Activation Induces Differential Sensitivity to Sulfur Amino Acid Limitation and Deprivation and to Oxidative and Anti-Oxidative Stress in Mouse Fibroblasts. *PLoS ONE* **2016**, *11*, e0163790. [CrossRef]

39. Baracca, A.; Chiaradonna, F.; Sgarbi, G.; Solaini, G.; Alberghina, L.; Lenaz, G. Mitochondrial Complex I decrease is responsible for bioenergetic dysfunction in K-ras transformed cells. *Biochim. Biophys. Acta (BBA) Bioenerg.* **2010**, *1797*, 314–323. [CrossRef]

40. Weinberg, F.; Hamanaka, R.; Wheaton, W.W.; Weinberg, S.; Joseph, J.; Lopez, M.; Kalyanaraman, B.; Mutlu, G.M.; Budinger, G.R.S.; Chandel, N.S. Mitochondrial metabolism and ROS generation are essential for Kras-mediated tumorigenicity. *Proc. Natl. Acad. Sci. USA* **2010**, *107*, 8788–8793. [CrossRef]

41. Earl, J.; Rico, D.; De Pau, E.C.S.; Rodríguez-Santiago, B.; Méndez-Pertuz, M.; Auer, H.; Gómez-López, G.; Grossman, H.B.; Pisano, D.G.; Schulz, W.A.; et al. The UBC-40 Urothelial Bladder Cancer cell line index: A genomic resource for functional studies. *BMC Genom.* **2015**, *16*, 1–16. [CrossRef]

42. Sjödahl, G.; Eriksson, P.; Patschan, O.; Marzouka, N.; Jakobsson, L.; Bernardo, C.; Lövgren, K.; Chebil, G.; Zwarthoff, E.; Liedberg, F.; et al. Molecular changes during progression from nonmuscle invasive to advanced urothelial carcinoma. *Int. J. Cancer* **2019**, *146*, 2636–2647. [CrossRef] [PubMed]

43. Marshall, C.J.; Franks, L.M.; Carbonell, A.W. Markers of Neoplastic Transformation in Epithelial Cell Lines Derived From Human Carcinomas. *J. Natl. Cancer Inst.* **1977**, *58*, 1743–1751. [CrossRef] [PubMed]

44. Fogh, J.; Fogh, J.M.; Orfeo, T. One Hundred and Twenty-Seven Cultured Human Tumor Cell Lines Producing Tumors in Nude Mice23. *J. Natl. Cancer Inst.* **1977**, *59*, 221–226. [CrossRef] [PubMed]

45. Chung, B.-M.; Rotty, J.D.; A Coulombe, P. Networking galore: Intermediate filaments and cell migration. *Curr. Opin. Cell Biol.* **2013**, *25*, 600–612. [CrossRef] [PubMed]

46. Strouhalova, K.; Přechová, M.; Gandalovičová, A.; Brábek, J.; Gregor, M.; Rösel, D. Vimentin Intermediate Filaments as Potential Target for Cancer Treatment. *Cancers* **2020**, *12*, 184. [CrossRef]

47. Webb, D.J.; Donais, K.; Whitmore, L.A.; Thomas, S.M.; Turner, C.E.; Parsons, J.T.; Horwitz, A.F. FAK–Src signalling through paxillin, ERK and MLCK regulates adhesion disassembly. *Nat. Cell Biol.* **2004**, *6*, 154–161. [CrossRef]

48. Thomas, S.; Overdevest, J.B.; Nitz, M.D.; Williams, P.D.; Owens, C.R.; Sanchez-Carbayo, M.; Frierson, H.F.; Schwartz, M.A.; Theodorescu, D. Src and Caveolin-1 Reciprocally Regulate Metastasis via a Common Downstream Signaling Pathway in Bladder Cancer. *Cancer Res.* **2010**, *71*, 832–841. [CrossRef]

49. Zhang, X.; Zhao, W.; Li, Y. Stemness-related markers in cancer. *Cancer Transl. Med.* **2017**, *3*, 87–95. [CrossRef]

50. Reya, T.; Morrison, S.J.; Clarke, M.F.; Weissman, I.L. Stem cells, cancer, and cancer stem cells. *Nature* **2001**, *414*, 105–111. [CrossRef]

51. Toledo-Guzmán, M.E.; Hernández, M.I.; Gómez-Gallegos, Á.A.; Ortiz-Sánchez, E. ALDH as a Stem Cell Marker in Solid Tumors. *Curr. Stem Cell Res. Ther.* **2019**, *14*. [CrossRef] [PubMed]

52. Rodriguez-Torres, M.; Allan, A.L. Aldehyde dehydrogenase as a marker and functional mediator of metastasis in solid tumors. *Clin. Exp. Metastasis* **2016**, *33*, 97–113. [CrossRef] [PubMed]

53. Farid, R.M.; Sammour, S.A.E.-M.; El-Din, Z.A.E.-K.S.; Salman, M.I.; Omran, T.I. Expression of CD133 and CD24 and their different phenotypes in urinary bladder carcinoma. *Cancer Manag. Res.* **2019**, *11*, 4677–4690. [CrossRef] [PubMed]

54. Shmelkov, S.V.; Butler, J.M.; Hooper, A.T.; Hormigo, A.; Kushner, J.; Milde, T.; Clair, R.S.; Baljevic, M.; White, I.; Jin, D.K.; et al. CD133 expression is not restricted to stem cells, and both CD133+ and CD133– metastatic colon cancer cells initiate tumors. *J. Clin. Investig.* **2008**, *118*, 2111–2120. [CrossRef]

55. Höfner, T.; Macher-Goeppinger, S.; Klein, C.; Schillert, A.; Eisen, C.; Wagner, S.; Rigo-Watermeier, T.; Baccelli, I.; Vogel, V.; Trumpp, A.; et al. Expression and prognostic significance of cancer stem cell markers CD24 and CD44 in urothelial bladder cancer xenografts and patients undergoing radical cystectomy. *Urol. Oncol. Semin. Orig. Investig.* **2014**, *32*, 678–686. [CrossRef]

56. Chan, K.S.; Espinosa, I.; Chao, M.; Wong, D.; Ailles, L.; Diehn, M.; Gill, H.; Presti, J.; Chang, H.Y.; Van De Rijn, M.; et al. Identification, molecular characterization, clinical prognosis, and therapeutic targeting of human bladder tumor-initiating cells. *Proc. Natl. Acad. Sci. USA* **2009**, *106*, 14016–14021. [CrossRef]

57. Wen, Y.; Hou, Y.; Huang, Z.; Cai, J.; Wang, Z. SOX2 is required to maintain cancer stem cells in ovarian cancer. *Cancer Sci.* **2017**, *108*, 719–731. [CrossRef]

58. Pavlova, N.N.; Thompson, C.B. The Emerging Hallmarks of Cancer Metabolism. *Cell Metab.* **2016**, *23*, 27–47. [CrossRef]

59. Ferrick, D.A.; Neilson, A.; Beeson, C. Advances in measuring cellular bioenergetics using extracellular flux. *Drug Discov. Today* **2008**, *13*, 268–274. [CrossRef]

60. Dombrauckas, J.D.; Santarsiero, B.D.; Mesecar, A.D. Structural Basis for Tumor Pyruvate Kinase M2 Allosteric Regulation and Catalysis. *Biochemistry* **2005**, *44*, 9417–9429. [CrossRef]

61. Yuan, M.; McNae, I.; Chen, Y.; Blackburn, E.A.; Wear, M.A.; Michels, P.A.; Gilmore, L.; Hupp, T.; Walkinshaw, M.D. An allostatic mechanism for M2 pyruvate kinase as an amino-acid sensor. *Biochem. J.* **2018**, *475*, 1821–1837. [CrossRef] [PubMed]

62. Poot, M.; Zhang, Y.Z.; Krämer, J.A.; Wells, K.S.; Jones, L.J.; Hanzel, D.K.; Lugade, A.G.; Singer, V.L.; Haugland, R.P. Analysis of mitochondrial morphology and function with novel fixable fluorescent stains. *J. Histochem. Cytochem.* **1996**, *44*, 1363–1372. [CrossRef] [PubMed]

63. Mitra, K.; Lippincott-Schwartz, J. Analysis of Mitochondrial Dynamics and Functions Using Imaging Approaches. *Curr. Protoc. Cell Biol.* **2010**, *46*, 4–25. [CrossRef] [PubMed]

64. Iannetti, E.F.; Prigione, A.; Smeitink, J.A.M.; Koopman, W.J.H.; Beyrath, J.; Renkema, H. Live-Imaging Readouts and Cell Models for Phenotypic Profiling of Mitochondrial Function. *Front. Genet.* **2019**, *10*, 131. [CrossRef] [PubMed]

65. Halliwell, B.; Chirico, S. Lipid peroxidation: Its mechanism, measurement, and significance. *Am. J. Clin. Nutr.* **1993**, *57*, 715S–725S. [CrossRef] [PubMed]

66. Pap, E.; Drummen, G.; Winter, V.; Kooij, T.; Rijken, P.; Wirtz, K.; Kamp, J.O.D.; Hage, W.; Post, J. Ratio-fluorescence microscopy of lipid oxidation in living cells using C11-BODIPY581/591. *FEBS Lett.* **1999**, *453*, 278–282. [CrossRef]

67. Carracedo, A.; Cantley, L.C.; Pandolfi, P.P. Cancer metabolism: Fatty acid oxidation in the limelight. *Nat. Rev. Cancer* **2013**, *13*, 227–232. [CrossRef]

68. Ceccarelli, S.M.; Chomienne, O.; Gubler, M.; Arduini, A. Carnitine Palmitoyltransferase (CPT) Modulators: A Medicinal Chemistry Perspective on 35 Years of Research. *J. Med. Chem.* **2011**, *54*, 3109–3152. [CrossRef]

69. El-Mir, M.-Y.; Nogueira, V.; Fontaine, E.; Avéret, N.; Rigoulet, M.; Leverve, X. Dimethylbiguanide Inhibits Cell Respiration via an Indirect Effect Targeted on the Respiratory Chain Complex I. *J. Biol. Chem.* **2000**, *275*, 223–228. [CrossRef]

70. Owen, M.R.; Doran, E.; Halestrap, A.P. Evidence that metformin exerts its anti-diabetic effects through inhibition of complex 1 of the mitochondrial respiratory chain. *Biochem. J.* **2000**, *348*, 607–614. [CrossRef]

71. Vial, G.; Detaille, D.; Guigas, B. Role of Mitochondria in the Mechanism(s) of Action of Metformin. *Front. Endocrinol.* **2019**, *10*, 294. [CrossRef] [PubMed]

72. Ishiguro, T.; Ohata, H.; Sato, A.; Yamawaki, K.; Enomoto, T.; Okamoto, K. Tumor-derived spheroids: Relevance to cancer stem cells and clinical applications. *Cancer Sci.* **2017**, *108*, 283–289. [CrossRef] [PubMed]

73. Mehta, P.; Novak, C.; Raghavan, S.; Ward, M.; Mehta, G. Self-Renewal and CSCs In Vitro Enrichment: Growth as Floating Spheres. In *Bioinformatics in MicroRNA Research*; Springer Science and Business Media LLC: Berlin, Germany, 2018; Volume 1692, pp. 61–75.

74. Sancho, P.; Barneda, D.; Heeschen, C. Hallmarks of cancer stem cell metabolism. *Br. J. Cancer* **2016**, *114*, 1305–1312. [CrossRef] [PubMed]

75. Sotgia, F.; Fiorillo, M.; Lisanti, M.P. Hallmarks of the cancer cell of origin: Comparisons with "energetic" cancer stem cells (e-CSCs). *Aging* **2019**, *11*, 1065–1068. [CrossRef]

76. Fiorillo, M.; Lamb, R.; Tanowitz, H.B.; Mutti, L.; Krstic-Demonacos, M.; Cappello, A.R.; Martinez-Outschoorn, U.E.; Sotgia, F.; Lisanti, M.P. Repurposing atovaquone: Targeting mitochondrial complex III and OXPHOS to eradicate cancer stem cells. *Oncotarget* **2016**, *7*, 34084–34099. [CrossRef]

77. Denise, C.; Paoli, P.; Calvani, M.; Taddei, M.L.; Giannoni, E.; Kopetz, S.; Kazmi, S.M.A.; Pia, M.M.; Pettazzoni, P.; Sacco, E.; et al. 5-Fluorouracil resistant colon cancer cells are addicted to OXPHOS to survive and enhance stem-like traits. *Oncotarget* **2015**, *6*, 41706–41721. [CrossRef]

78. Ferlay, J.; Steliarova-Foucher, E.; Lortet-Tieulent, J.; Rosso, S.; Coebergh, J.; Comber, H.; Forman, D.; Bray, F. Cancer incidence and mortality patterns in Europe: Estimates for 40 countries in 2012. *Eur. J. Cancer* **2013**, *49*, 1374–1403. [CrossRef]

79. Nielsen, J. Systems Biology of Metabolism: A Driver for Developing Personalized and Precision Medicine. *Cell Metab.* **2017**, *25*, 572–579. [CrossRef]

80. Damiani, C.; Gaglio, D.; Sacco, E.; Alberghina, L.; Vanoni, M. Systems metabolomics: From metabolomic snapshots to design principles. *Curr. Opin. Biotechnol.* **2020**, *63*, 190–199. [CrossRef]

81. Tan, G.; Wang, H.; Yuan, J.; Qin, W.; Dong, X.; Wu, H.; Meng, P. Three serum metabolite signatures for diagnosing low-grade and high-grade bladder cancer. *Sci. Rep.* **2017**, *7*, srep46176. [CrossRef]

82. Mpanga, A.Y.; Siluk, D.; Jacyna, J.; Szerkus, O.; Wawrzyniak, R.; Markuszewski, M.; Kaliszan, R.; Markuszewski, M.J. Targeted metabolomics in bladder cancer: From analytical methods development and validation towards application to clinical samples. *Anal. Chim. Acta* **2018**, *1037*, 188–199. [CrossRef] [PubMed]

83. Zuiverloon, T.C.; De Jong, F.C.; Costello, J.C.; Theodorescu, D. Systematic Review: Characteristics and Preclinical Uses of Bladder Cancer Cell Lines. *Bladder Cancer* **2018**, *4*, 169–183. [CrossRef] [PubMed]

84. Warrick, J.I.; Walter, V.; Yamashita, H.; Chung, E.; Shuman, L.; Amponsa, V.O.; Zheng, Z.; Chan, W.; Whitcomb, T.L.; Yue, F.; et al. FOXA1, GATA3 and PPARγ Cooperate to Drive Luminal Subtype in Bladder Cancer: A Molecular Analysis of Established Human Cell Lines. *Sci. Rep.* **2016**, *6*, 38531. [CrossRef] [PubMed]

85. Rebouissou, S.; Bernard-Pierrot, I.; De Reyniès, A.; Lepage, M.-L.; Krucker, C.; Chapeaublanc, E.; Hérault, A.; Kamoun, A.; Caillault, A.; Letouzé, E.; et al. EGFR as a potential therapeutic target for a subset of muscle-invasive bladder cancers presenting a basal-like phenotype. *Sci. Transl. Med.* **2014**, *6*, 244ra91. [CrossRef] [PubMed]

86. Turrens, J.F. Mitochondrial formation of reactive oxygen species. *J. Physiol.* **2003**, *552*, 335–344. [CrossRef]

87. Zorov, D.B.; Juhaszova, M.; Sollott, S.J. Mitochondrial Reactive Oxygen Species (ROS) and ROS-Induced ROS Release. *Physiol. Rev.* **2014**, *94*, 909–950. [CrossRef]

88. Vinogradov, A.; Grivennikova, V.G. Oxidation of NADH and ROS production by respiratory complex I. *Biochim. Biophys. Acta (BBA) Bioenerg.* **2016**, *1857*, 863–871. [CrossRef]

89. Bleier, L.; Dröse, S. Superoxide generation by complex III: From mechanistic rationales to functional consequences. *Biochim. Biophys. Acta (BBA) Bioenerg.* **2013**, *1827*, 1320–1331. [CrossRef]

90. Barrera, G.; Pizzimenti, S.; Dianzani, M.U. Lipid peroxidation: Control of cell proliferation, cell differentiation and cell death. *Mol. Asp. Med.* **2008**, *29*, 1–8. [CrossRef]

91. Barrera, G. Oxidative Stress and Lipid Peroxidation Products in Cancer Progression and Therapy. *ISRN Oncol.* **2012**, *2012*, 1–21. [CrossRef]

92. Ayala, A.; Muñoz, M.F.; Argüelles, S. Lipid Peroxidation: Production, Metabolism, and Signaling Mechanisms of Malondialdehyde and 4-Hydroxy-2-Nonenal. *Oxidative Med. Cell. Longev.* **2014**, *2014*, 1–31. [CrossRef] [PubMed]

93. Black, W.; Chen, Y.; Matsumoto, A.; Thompson, D.C.; Lassen, N.; Pappa, A.; Vasiliou, V. Molecular mechanisms of ALDH3A1-mediated cellular protection against 4-hydroxy-2-nonenal. *Free Radic. Biol. Med.* **2012**, *52*, 1937–1944. [CrossRef] [PubMed]

94. Singh, S.; Brocker, C.; Koppaka, V.; Chen, Y.; Jackson, B.C.; Matsumoto, A.; Thompson, D.C.; Vasiliou, V. Aldehyde dehydrogenases in cellular responses to oxidative/electrophilicstress. *Free Radic. Biol. Med.* **2013**, *56*, 89–101. [CrossRef] [PubMed]

95. Corbet, C.; Feron, O. Cancer cell metabolism and mitochondria: Nutrient plasticity for TCA cycle fueling. *Biochim. Biophys. Acta (BBA) Bioenerg.* **2017**, *1868*, 7–15. [CrossRef] [PubMed]

96. Bentebibel, A.; Sebastián, D.; Herrero, L.; López-Viñas, E.; Serra, D.; Asins, G.; Gómez-Puertas, P.; Hegardt, F.G. Novel Effect of C75 on Carnitine Palmitoyltransferase I Activity and Palmitate Oxidation. *Biochemistry* **2006**, *45*, 4339–4350. [CrossRef] [PubMed]

97. Declercq, P.E.; Falck, J.R.; Kuwajima, M.; Tyminski, H.; Foster, D.W.; McGarry, J.D. Characterization of the mitochondrial carnitine palmitoyltransferase enzyme system. I. Use of inhibitors. *J. Biol. Chem.* **1987**, *262*, 9812–9821.

98. Raud, B.; Roy, D.G.; Divakaruni, A.S.; Tarasenko, T.N.; Franke, R.; Ma, E.H.; Samborska, B.; Hsieh, W.Y.; Wong, A.H.; Stüve, P.; et al. Etomoxir Actions on Regulatory and Memory T Cells Are Independent of Cpt1a-Mediated Fatty Acid Oxidation. *Cell Metab.* **2018**, *28*, 504–515.e7. [CrossRef]

99. LeBleu, V.S.; O'Connell, J.T.; Herrera, K.N.G.; Wikman-Kocher, H.; Pantel, K.; Haigis, M.C.; De Carvalho, F.M.; Damascena, A.; Chinen, L.T.D.; Rocha, R.M.; et al. PGC-1α mediates mitochondrial biogenesis and oxidative phosphorylation in cancer cells to promote metastasis. *Nat. Cell Biol.* **2014**, *16*, 992–1003. [CrossRef]

100. Sotgia, F.; Whitaker-Menezes, D.; Martinez-Outschoorn, U.E.; Flomenberg, N.; Birbe, R.C.; Witkiewicz, A.K.; Howell, A.; Philp, N.J.; Pestell, R.G.; Lisanti, M.P. Mitochondrial metabolism in cancer metastasis. *Cell Cycle* **2012**, *11*, 1445–1454. [CrossRef]

101. Sancho, P.; Burgos-Ramos, E.; Tavera, A.; Kheir, T.B.; Jagust, P.; Schoenhals, M.; Barneda, D.; Sellers, K.; Campos-Olivas, R.; Graña, O.; et al. MYC/PGC-1α Balance Determines the Metabolic Phenotype and Plasticity of Pancreatic Cancer Stem Cells. *Cell Metab.* **2015**, *22*, 590–605. [CrossRef]

102. Lagadinou, E.D.; Sach, A.; Callahan, K.; Rossi, R.M.; Neering, S.J.; Minhajuddin, M.; Ashton, J.M.; Pei, S.; Grose, V.; O'Dwyer, K.M.; et al. BCL-2 Inhibition Targets Oxidative Phosphorylation and Selectively Eradicates Quiescent Human Leukemia Stem Cells. *Cell Stem Cell* **2013**, *12*, 329–341. [CrossRef] [PubMed]

103. Invrea, F.; Rovito, R.; Torchiaro, E.; Petti, C.; Isella, C.; Medico, E. Patient-derived xenografts (PDXs) as model systems for human cancer. *Curr. Opin. Biotechnol.* **2020**, *63*, 151–156. [CrossRef] [PubMed]

104. Reckzeh, E.S.; Karageorgis, G.; Schwalfenberg, M.; Ceballos, J.; Nowacki, J.; Stroet, M.C.; Binici, A.; Knauer, L.; Brand, S.; Choidas, A.; et al. Inhibition of Glucose Transporters and Glutaminase Synergistically Impairs Tumor Cell Growth. *Cell Chem. Biol.* **2019**, *26*, 1214–1228.e5. [CrossRef] [PubMed]

105. Gaglio, D.; Bonanomi, M.; Valtorta, S.; Bharat, R.; Ripamonti, M.; Conte, F.; Fiscon, G.; Righi, N.; Napodano, E.; Papa, F.; et al. Disruption of redox homeostasis for combinatorial drug efficacy in K-Ras tumors as revealed by metabolic connectivity profiling. *Cancer Metab.* **2020**, *8*, 1–15. [CrossRef]

3

Liquid Biopsy Biomarkers in Bladder Cancer: A Current Need for Patient Diagnosis and Monitoring

Iris Lodewijk [1,2], **Marta Dueñas** [1,2,3], **Carolina Rubio** [1,2,3], **Ester Munera-Maravilla** [1,2], **Cristina Segovia** [1,2,3], **Alejandra Bernardini** [1,2,3], **Alicia Teijeira** [1], **Jesús M. Paramio** [1,2,3] and **Cristian Suárez-Cabrera** [1,2,*]

[1] Molecular Oncology Unit, CIEMAT (Centro de Investigaciones Energéticas, Medioambientales y Tecnológicas), Avenida Complutense nº 40, 28040 Madrid, Spain; IrisAdriana.Lodewijk@externos.ciemat.es (I.L.); marta.duenas@ciemat.es (M.D.); carolina.rubio@externos.ciemat.es (C.R.); ester.munera@ciemat.es (E.M.-M.); cristina.segovia@ciemat.es (C.S.); Alejandra.bernardini@externos.ciemat.es (A.B.); aliciateijeira.merced@gmail.com (A.T.); jesusm.paramio@ciemat.es (J.M.P.)

[2] Biomedical Research Institute I+12, University Hospital "12 de Octubre", Av Córdoba s/n, 28041 Madrid, Spain

[3] Centro de Investigación Biomédica en Red de Cáncer (CIBERONC), 28029 Madrid, Spain

* Correspondence: cristian.suarez@externos.ciemat.es

Abstract: Bladder Cancer (BC) represents a clinical and social challenge due to its high incidence and recurrence rates, as well as the limited advances in effective disease management. Currently, a combination of cytology and cystoscopy is the routinely used methodology for diagnosis, prognosis and disease surveillance. However, both the poor sensitivity of cytology tests as well as the high invasiveness and big variation in tumour stage and grade interpretation using cystoscopy, emphasizes the urgent need for improvements in BC clinical guidance. Liquid biopsy represents a new non-invasive approach that has been extensively studied over the last decade and holds great promise. Even though its clinical use is still compromised, multiple studies have recently focused on the potential application of biomarkers in liquid biopsies for BC, including circulating tumour cells and DNA, RNAs, proteins and peptides, metabolites and extracellular vesicles. In this review, we summarize the present knowledge on the different types of biomarkers, their potential use in liquid biopsy and clinical applications in BC.

Keywords: bladder cancer; liquid biopsy; biomarkers

1. Introduction: Bladder Cancer Issues and Liquid Biopsy

Bladder cancer (BC) is the most common malignancy of the urinary tract, representing a highly prevalent disease which affects primarily elderly people. For both sexes combined, it is the 9th most common cancer diagnosed worldwide and a significant cause of tumour-related death, with an estimated 165,000 deaths per year [1]. BC represents an important health problem with an age-standardized incidence rate (per 100,000 person-years) of 9 in men versus 2.2 in women and an age-standardized mortality rate (per 100,000 person-years) of 3.2 and 0.9, respectively [2–4]. The incidence and mortality rate are stagnant due to the scarcity of newly developed effective treatments and options for prevention [5,6].

BC can be divided in two major classes based on tumour stage, I) non-muscle invasive bladder cancer (NMIBC), which is either confined to the urothelium (carcinoma in situ (CIS)-or stage Ta, 5-year survival rate of 95.4%) or the lamina propia (stage T1, 5-year survival rate of approximately 88%) and II) muscle-invasive bladder cancer (MIBC) (stage T2, T3 and T4, representing 5-year survival rates of 69.4%, 34.9% and 4.8%, respectively) [7,8]. NMIBC represents the most frequent form of BC, presented by approximately 70–80% of patients at diagnosis and is primarily treated by transurethral resection of the bladder tumour (TURBT), which is considered fundamental for the diagnosis and prognosis of the disease [9,10]. Dependent upon certain pathological characteristics (e.g., size and number of implants), TURBT is followed by intravesical instillation with chemotherapeutics, such as mitomycin, or the immunotherapeutic Bacillus Calmette-Guérin (BCG) [11,12]. However, despite TURBT and chemo/immunotherapy as first-line treatment, NMIBC displays a high recurrence incidence (50–70%) with tumour progression towards invasive tumours in at least 10–15% of the cases, due to minimal residual disease (MRD) which remained undetected [9,10]. The extraordinary rates of recurrence and the likelihood to progress require continuous follow-up of NMIBC patients by cystoscopy (every 3–6 months during the next 5 years) and urine cytology, making NMIBC one of the most costly malignancies for the National Health systems of developed countries [11,13]. Accordingly, BC represents the most expensive human cancer from diagnosis to death, with an estimated cost of $187,000 per patient in the United States [14]. In 2010, its total annual cost was estimated at $4 billion, which is expected to rise to approximately $5 billion by 2020 [14,15]. In the European Union, in 2012, the total BC expenditure has been determined at €4.9 billion, with health care accounting for €2.9 billion (59%) [16].

The remaining 20–30% of BC patients presents MIBC at diagnosis. Once tumour progression is observed the prognosis declines [17,18]. Treatment of invasive BC currently consists of radical cystectomy followed by platin-based chemotherapy. Nevertheless, clinical benefit of the addition of neoadjuvant chemotherapy (NAC) (like cisplatin, methotrexate, vinblastine and gemcitabine) has been evaluated by several studies [19–21]. NAC is presumed to diminish the burden of micrometastatic disease and can be used to predict chemosensitivity of the tumour [2]. Despite conflicting results shown by multiple randomized phase III trials (due to differences in for example, chemotherapy used, number of cycles and trial design), a significant survival benefit in favour of NAC has been indicated by various meta-analyses [19,20]. Unfortunately, metastatic spreading remains an important problem in a high fraction of the cases (50–70%), resulting in very low survival rates (5-year survival rate of 4.8%) [2,8,22].

Despite multiple trials, no new effective therapeutic options have been developed throughout the last decades [23], with the exception of immunotherapy based on checkpoint inhibitors. Even though these checkpoint inhibitors have shown promising results in patients with advanced or recurrent BC, only 20–35% of the BC patients benefit from this therapy and overall survival is still limited [24,25].

The typical and most important clinical indication for BC is haematuria. Nowadays, a combination of urine cytology and cystoscopy is still the routinely used methodology by excellence for detection, diagnosis and surveillance of this disease. Cytology remains the gold standard for detection of urothelial carcinoma. BC urinary cytology shows a specificity of approximately 98% and a sensitivity of 38% [26] (Table 1). However, the sensitivity of this test significantly increases with malignancy grade, reaching a reasonable sensitivity of >60% for CIS and high-grade lesions [26,27]. In 1997, in order to improve cytology predictive values, Fradet and Lockhard developed an immunofluorescence test (uCyt+) which was based on detection of three BC antigens (M344, LDQ10 and 19A11) in exfoliated cells [28], improving the sensitivity of cytology to approximately 73% but decreasing the specificity to 66% due to the requirement of a large number of exfoliated cells [29] (Table 1). Cystoscopy is currently the gold standard technique in clinical practice for detection and follow-up of BC, achieving a sensitivity of approximately 85–90% and 65–70% to detect exophytic tumours and CIS, respectively [27,30–33]. Nevertheless, this procedure is highly invasive, showing a big inter-observer and intra-observer variation in the tumour stage and grade interpretation [27,30–33].

Therefore, it is clear that there is an urgent need for improvements in diagnosis, prognosis and follow-up of BC patients. Over the last decades, tumour biopsies have revealed details with regard to the genetic profile of tumours, allowing the prediction of prognosis, tumour progression as well as therapy response and resistance [34]. Recently, the potential use of liquid biopsy as a new non-invasive way to determine the genomic landscape of cancer patients, screen treatment response, quantify MRD and assess therapy resistance is gaining significant attention [34–40]. The term "liquid biopsy" means the sampling and analysis of biological fluids, including blood, plasma, urine, pleural liquid, cerebrospinal fluid and saliva (Figure 1) [36,39]. The analysis is based on different cells and molecules which can be obtained from liquid biopsies: circulating tumour cells (CTCs), circulating cell-free tumour DNA (ctDNA), messenger RNAs (mRNAs), micro-RNAs (miRNAs), long non-coding RNAs (lncRNAs), proteins and peptides, metabolites and vesicles (exosomes and endosomes) (Figure 1). Even though the presence of circulating free DNA and RNA in human blood was first demonstrated in 1948 [41], only a few liquid biopsies are currently approved for clinical use. In recent years, cancer research has been mainly focused on the introduction of suitable biomarkers, indicating the presence, recurrence and progression of a disease, as well as the appropriated treatment for a specific type of cancer. Taken together, biomarkers present in liquid biopsies hold great promise, as they are able to record and monitor the disease stage at real time and predict prognosis, recurrence, therapy response and resistance, without invasive intervention.

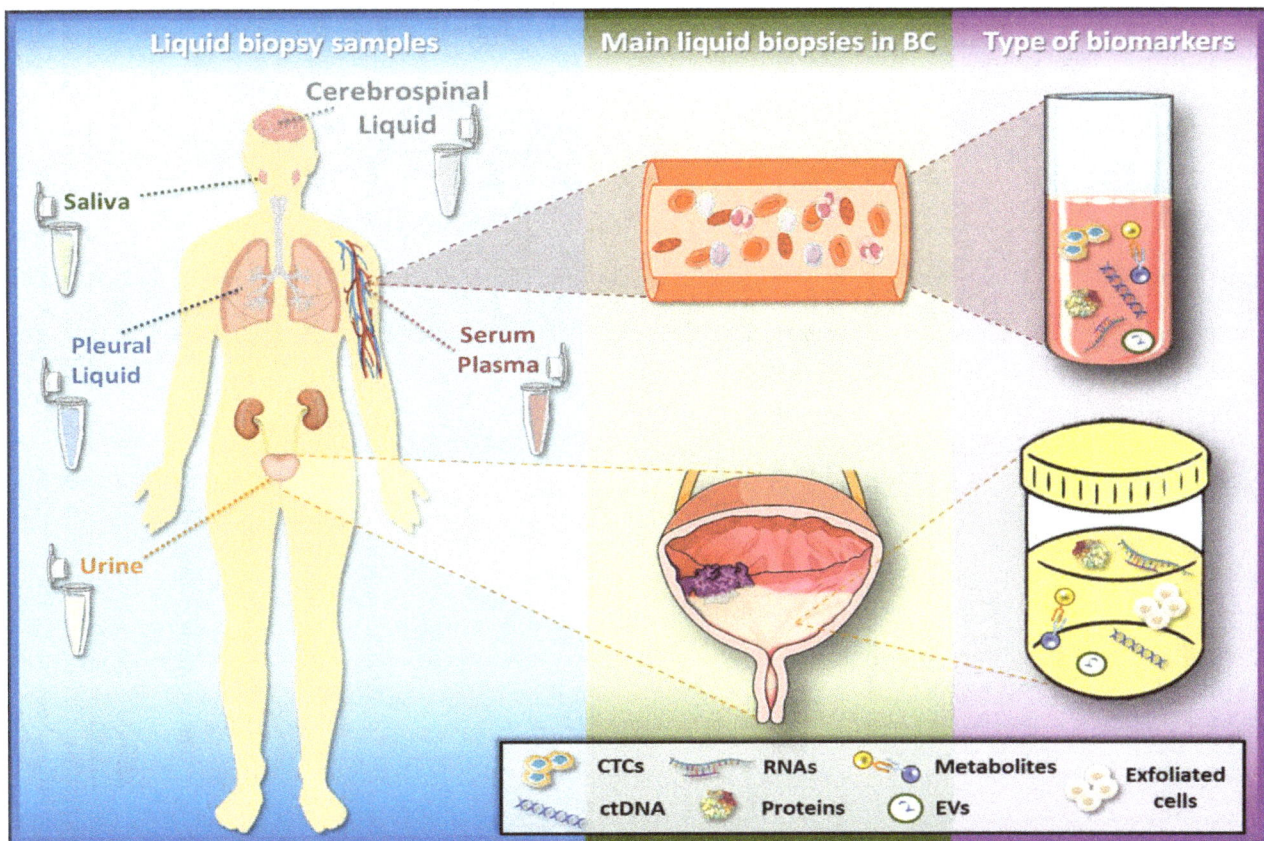

Figure 1. Liquid biopsy samples and biomarkers. Liquid biopsy samples include urine, serum, plasma, saliva, cerebrospinal and pleural fluid, among others. In BC, the liquid biopsies more widely used as detection and surveillance systems are urine (by its intimate contact with the tumour), as well as serum and plasma, which allow the follow-up of advanced disease. These liquid biopsies present several biomarkers, such as circulating tumour cells (CTCs), circulating cell-free tumour DNA (ctDNA), RNAs, proteins, metabolites and extracellular vesicles (EVs). Additionally, exfoliated cells derived from a tumour can be found in urine.

Table 1. Commercial kits to detect and follow-up bladder cancer (BC) using liquid biopsy biomarkers.

Commercial Kits	Biomarker	Assay Type	Sample Type	FDA Approved	Purpose	Predictive Capacity	Source	Refs.
Cytology	Sediment cells	Giemsa and HE staining	Urine	Yes	Diagnostic and surveillance (1)	Sensitivity = 38% Specificity = 98%	-	[26]
uCyt+	Sediment cells	Immunofluorescence	Urine	Yes	Surveillance in adjunct to cystoscopy	Sensitivity = 73% Specificity = 66%	DiagnoCure (2)	[29]
UroVysion	Sediment cells	Multi-target FISH	Urine	Yes	Diagnostic	Sensitivity = 72% Specificity = 83%	Abbott	[42]
UroMark(3)	Sediment cells	Bisulfite-based methylation assay	Urine	No	Diagnostic	Sensitivity = 98% Specificity = 97%	Kelly:Feber	[43]
CellSearch	CTCs	Immunomagnetic enrichment	Plasma/serum	Yes	Surveillance	Sensitivity = 48% Specificity = 98%	Menarini-Silicon Biosystems	[44]
CxBladder	mRNA	RT-qPCR	Urine	No	Diagnostic	Sensitivity = 82% Specificity = 85%	Pacific Edge	[32]
CxBladder Monitor	mRNA	RT-qPCR	Urine	No	Surveillance	Sensitivity = 91% NPV = 96%	Pacific Edge	[45]
Xpert BC Detection	mRNA	RT-qPCR	Urine	No	Diagnostic	Sensitivity = 76% Specificity = 85%	Cepheid	[46]
Xpert BC Monitor	mRNA	RT-qPCR	Urine	No	Surveillance	Sensitivity = 84% Specificity = 91%	Cepheid	[47]
PanC-Dx	mRNA	RT-qPCR	Urine	No	Diagnostic	Sensitivity = 90% Specificity = 83%	Oncocyte	[48]
UROBEST (4)	mRNA	RT-qPCR	Urine	No	Diagnostic and surveillance (5)	Sensitivity = 80% Specificity = 94%	Biofina Diagnostics	-
NMP22	Protein	Sandwich ELISA	Urine	Yes	Surveillance	Sensitivity = 40% Specificity = 99%	Abbott	[49]
NMP22 BladderChek	Protein	Dipstick immunoassay	Urine	Yes	Diagnostic and surveillance (1)	Sensitivity = 68% Specificity = 79%	Abbott	[50]
BTA TRAK	Protein	Sandwich ELISA	Urine	Yes	Diagnostic and surveillance (1)	Sensitivity = 66% Specificity = 65%	Polymedco	[51]
BTA stat	Protein	Dipstick immunoassay	Urine	Yes	Diagnostic and surveillance (1)	Sensitivity = 70% Specificity = 75%	Polymedco	[51]
CYFRA 21.1	Protein	Immunoradiometric assay or ELISA	Urine	No	Diagnostic	Sensitivity = 82% Specificity = 80%	CIS Bio International	[52]
UBC test	Protein	Sandwich ELISA or dipstick immunoassay	Urine	No	Diagnostic	Sensitivity = 64% Specificity = 80%	IDL Biotech	[53]

(1) Although these tests have been proposed for diagnosis and follow-up of BC, predictive values correspond to the detection of primary tumour. (2) DiagnoCure company was dissolved in 2016 and the uCyt+ test is not available at present. (3) The performance of the UroMark test is currently evaluated in Phase III studies. (4) UROBEST is not yet commercially available. (5) Biofina Diagnostics provides these predictive values for diagnostic and surveillance purposes together. NPV = Negative predictive value.

Thus, the potential use of liquid biopsy as a new non-invasive approach to improve BC management is far reaching. Even though their extensive applications are only starting to emerge in clinical practice, multiple studies have indicated the potential use of different biomarkers in liquid biopsies for BC. In this review, we provide an overview of the more important studies regarding the different types of biomarkers in liquid biopsy and their clinical applications in BC.

2. Liquid Biopsy Biomarkers and Their Clinical Applications

2.1. Circulating Tumour Cells (CTCs)

CTCs were first discovered in breast cancer patients in 1869 by Ashworth and colleagues [54]. They are tumour cells of approximately 4 to 50 µm, which are being released from the tumour site into the bloodstream, thereby representing the main mechanism for metastasis [54,55]. CTC detection systems emerged from the need to find new methods to detect early metastatic disease in a less invasive way compared to conventional methods currently available, such as radiological evaluation. In recent years, a wide variety of approaches has been developed for the detection of CTCs, some of which have been implemented in clinical practice. These techniques include immunocytochemistry, reverse-transcriptase polymerase chain reaction, flow cytometry and the CellSearch system, which is the only approach approved by the USA Food and Drug Administration (FDA) [56].

In certain types of solid tumours, such as breast, colorectal cancer and gastric tumours, it has been reported that the presence of CTCs is an indicator of poor prognosis [57–60]. In BC, the presence of CTCs has also been proposed to be associated with a bad prognosis and the amount of CTCs found in blood has been indicated to correlate with short disease-free survival in metastatic BC [61]. However, the relevance for NMIBC is still controversial.

2.1.1. CTC Detection Methods

Since CTCs are very rare and the amount of cells available is around 1 to 10 in 10^6–10^8 white blood cells, their detection, enumeration and molecular characterization is a challenge [62]. Accordingly, an efficient and reliable method for both isolation and characterization of these cells is needed [62,63]. Nowadays, different isolation techniques have been developed, all of which have a first enrichment step before the cells can finally be analysed. Enrichment can be carried out by different methods, including techniques based on physical properties such as size (by microfilters that isolate CTCs regarding to their greater size), density or deformability, as well as on biological properties of CTCs (for example, using immunomagnetic assays) (Figure 2) (reviewed in [64]). Immunomagnetic enrichment can be either negative or positive, both of which are available for in vivo assays, enabling a better sample analysis. Whereas negative enrichment does not rely on the biomarker expression of CTCs but on markers of hematopoietic cells (like CD45, a leukocytic antigen) and allows collection of cells in their intact form (depleting most of the leukocytes and erythrocytes), positive enrichment (using specific CTC biomarkers) has its own advantages including a low false-positive CTC detection rate (Figure 2) (reviewed in [64]).

The CellSearch system (Veridex, LLC, Warren, NJ, USA) is one of those technologies developed and, in this case, approved by the FDA for the isolation of CTCs (Table 1). CellSearch CTC Test is based on immunomagnetic enrichment and, initially, permitted enumeration of CTCs of epithelial origin by targeting only EpCAM for capturing CTCs. However, some studies have pointed out the difficulty in obtaining sufficient EpCAM-expressing CTCs from patients with advanced disease to reach statistically significant conclusions from a study or clinical trial [65]. Therefore, the recent versions of this test also select CTCs by other surface proteins, selecting those cells that are CD45−, EpCAM+ and cytokeratin 8/18+ and/or 19+. Though CellSearch is the most frequently used and still the gold standard today, new ways to detect CTCs have come up recently. CytoTrack is a similar method which allows detection and quantification of CTCs using a scanning fluorescence microscope [66]. For this test, a cocktail of a range of cytokeratins (pan-cytokeratin antibody) and CD45 (to deplete blood cells) is used [66].

Given that CytoTrack relies on a cytokeratin signal to detect cells and CellSearch depends on both EpCAM and cytokeratin expression, these two different approaches could give rise to significantly different results with regard to CTC detection. The advantage of Cytotrack is the possibility of staining with different antibodies which allows identification of new CTC biomarkers [67]. For example, HER2, which is considered a breast cancer biomarker, has also been used as target antigen for this technique [68,69]. By performing a comparative analysis between both systems, CellSearch and Cytotrack, Hillig et al. found that the two CTC technologies have similar recovery of cells spiked into blood (69% vs. 71%, $p = 0.58$, respectively) [67]. However, CellSearch shows a lower variability in the analysis [67]. Another promising method is the Epic CTC Platform, whose detection system is based on the use of cytokeratins as CTC biomarkers and CD45 as hematopoietic marker. Even though this approach is similar to CytoTrack, the Epic CTC platform also integrates downstream capabilities for the evaluation of cell morphology characteristics, protein biomarker expression and genomic analyses (Fluorescence In Situ Hybridization (FISH) and Next-Generation Sequencing (NGS)) [70]. In an analytical validation of the Epic CTC Platform capabilities, Werner et al. assayed the performance, including accuracy, linearity, specificity and intra/inter-assay precision, of CTC enumeration in healthy donor blood samples spiked with varying concentrations of cancer cell line controls [71]. They found a high percentage of nucleated cell recovery for all cancer cell concentrations tested and showed excellent assay linearity ($R^2 = 0.999$). Besides, using a small cohort of metastatic castration-resistant prostate cancer patient samples tested with the Epic CTC Platform, detection of ≥ 1 traditional CTC/mL in 89% of patient samples was shown, whereas 100% of the cancer patient samples had ≥ 1 CTC/mL when additionally considering the cytokeratin negative and apoptotic CTC subpopulations, compared to healthy donor samples (in which zero CTCs were enumerated in all 18 samples) (Figure 2) [70].

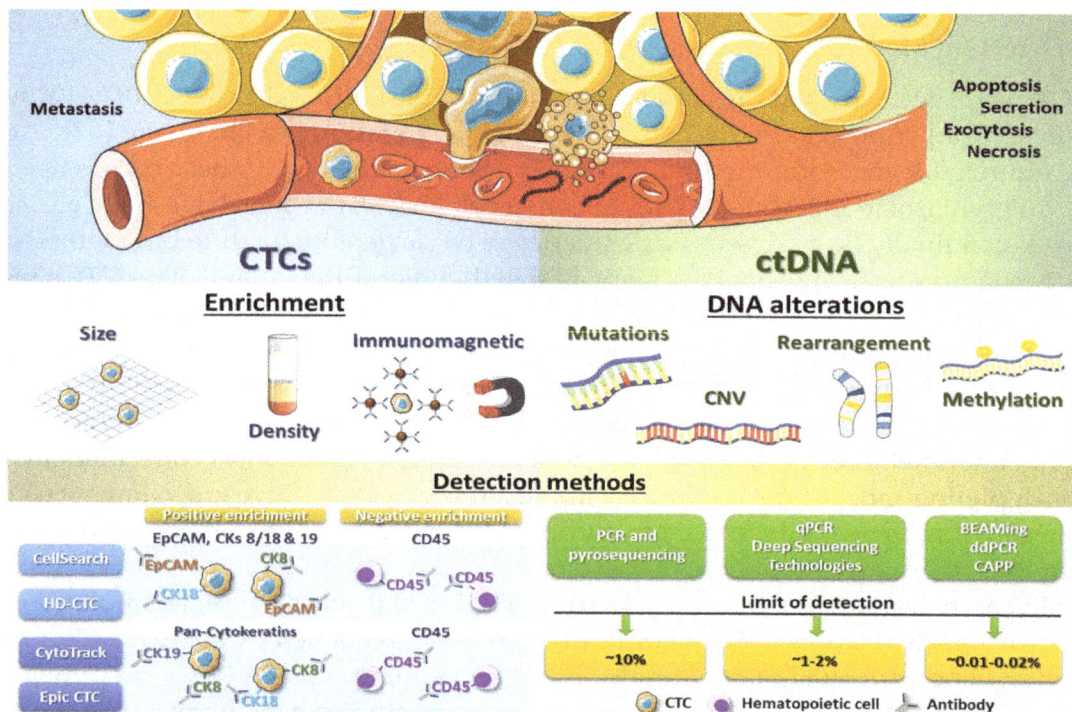

Figure 2. CTC and ctDNA processing methods. Scheme showing some enrichment techniques to isolate CTCs from peripheral blood cells (erythrocytes and leukocytes) and different detection systems based on immunomagnetic assays, using specific antibodies to recognize antigens present in tumour cells (like EpCAM or cytokeratins) as well as to exclude leukocytes (using antibodies against CD45) (left panel). Right panel displays the different DNA alterations (including mutations, copy number variations (CNVs), gene rearrangements or methylation variations) which can be analysed from ctDNA, as well as different detection methods and their correspondent limit of detection.

An improved CellSearch method is HD-CTC (from High Definition CTC; Epic Sciences, Inc., San Diego, CA, USA), which is not only based on EpCAM, cytokeratins and CD45 immunofluorescence staining but also on morphological characterization, size and high throughput counting, allowing the identification of apoptotic cells by DAPI staining and imaging using a high definition scanner (Figure 2). This detection method has been demonstrated to be more sensitive than the original CellSearch [71]. Additional to previously described detection methods, many other approaches have been developed over the last years by multiple commercial laboratories, evidencing the great potential of CTC detection at present and in future clinical procedures (reviewed in [64]).

However, these detection systems usually use small volumes of peripheral blood (<10 mL), showing a yield of 0.1–0.2% with respect to all tumour cells present in whole blood [72]. To overcome this problem in CTC detection and to evaluate large blood volumes, some groups have been exploring the potential of apheresis as CTC isolation method previous to the use of detection systems. In breast and pancreatic cancer patients, apheresis has demonstrated to improve the recovery of CTCs, showing better yield than the CellSearch system [73,74]. Besides, since CTCs probably have representative features of primary tumours, obtaining a sufficient number of CTCs could depict a global view of the tumour alterations and would allow carrying out different genomic analyses in order to define tumour and metastasis features. At present, there is a European Consortium "CTC Therapeutic Apheresis: CTCTrap project" (http://www.utwente.nl/en/tnw/ctctrap/) focused on improving this method in order to characterize all tumour cells circulating in blood and apply it into the clinic in a real-rime liquid biopsy system.

2.1.2. CTCs in Bladder Cancer

CTC detection in BC was first reported in 2000 by Lu et al., when they published a method for CTC detection in peripheral blood of patients with urothelial carcinoma using nested reverse transcription-PCR assay for *UPK2* (Uroplakin II) [75]. Their results were modest, being able to detect 3 out of 29 patients (10.3%) with superficial cancers (pTa-1N0M0), 4 out of 14 patients (28.6%) with MIBC (pT2-4N0M0), 2 out of 5 loco-regional node-positive patients (40.0%) (pN1-2M0) and 6 out of 8 patients (75.0%) with distant metastases [75].

More recently, several studies have evaluated CTCs in BC, mainly using CellSearch Technology, showing an average close to 50% of positive detection for metastatic BC and a low (around 15%) detection level for clinically localized BC [76]. Besides, even though CTC quantification has also been employed for prognosis and patient stratification, the detection of recurrent tumours is approximately 20–44% in patients showing progression upon recurrence. Additionally, Busetto and colleagues found a strong correlation between CTC presence and the time to first recurrence (75%) and they suggested that the time of progression is strongly correlated with CTCs [77].

In 2017, Zhang et al. published a meta-analysis of the impact of CTCs in BC. This study showed that the number of CTCs in peripheral blood is correlated with tumour stage, histological grade, metastasis and regional lymph node metastasis [45]. They also reported that the overall sensitivity and specificity of CTC detection assays are, respectively, 35% (95% CI: 28–43) and 97% (95% CI: 92–99), concluding that the presence of CTCs in peripheral blood is an independent predictive indicator of poor outcomes for urothelial cancer patients [44].

Even though CTC quantitation has to be studied more profoundly, this procedure could be incorporated into risk stratification algorithms and, therefore, aid patient management. In addition, CTC detection may not be accurate to be used as initial screening test but as a method for confirming BC diagnosis, due to the limited diagnostic sensitivity and high overall specificity. With improvements in clinical and laboratory techniques, the detection of CTCs at different time points in the future may allow real-time surveillance of dynamic changes of disease and crucially enhance our understanding of the metastatic cascade, thus facilitating novel targeted therapy approaches.

Regarding BC, the employability of CTCs in diagnosis and prognosis will be determined by the optimal combination of sensitivity, specificity, simplicity and cost of its implementation in the hospital routine. CTC enrichment techniques accompanied by a good cytological characterization may improve the fundamental weakness of cytology in the diagnosis/prognosis of low-grade disease. However, more well-designed, high-quality and large-scale prospective studies, especially including the CTCs and survival, are required to further strengthen current observations and shed more light on the potential of CTCs as a promising biomarker.

2.2. Circulating Cell-Free Tumour DNA (ctDNA)

2.2.1. Detection and Genomic Analysis of ctDNA: First Clinical Approaches

As previously mentioned, the presence of cell-free DNA fragments in human blood was first discovered in 1948 [41]. In 1977, increased total cell-free DNA levels were observed in serum of cancer patients compared to healthy individuals, showing potential for therapeutic evaluation [78]. In blood, fragments of cell-free DNA have a typical size of 160–180 bp and are released from apoptotic as well as necrotic cells and possibly by active secretion, phagocytosis and exocytosis [40,79]. Methylation analysis has been used to trace the tissue of origin of cell-free DNA and showed that the biggest part in plasma is released by blood cells in healthy individuals [80]. At the end of the 1980s, Stroun et al. described that at least part of circulating free DNA in the plasma of cancer patients derived from cancer cells [81]. In 1991, DNA bearing *TP53* mutations were found in urinary sediments from MIBC patients, paving the way for the use of genomics in liquid biopsy [82]. Posteriorly, studies based on mutated *KRAS* sequences in plasma confirmed the tumour origin of mutant cell-free DNA [83]. Mutated genes in plasma were subsequently proposed to represent tumour markers and the term "circulating tumour DNA" was coined. On the other hand, ctDNA levels are very variable between individuals and the presence of metastasis as well as disease burden increase the heterogeneity of ctDNA levels [84]. In fact, the ctDNA fraction in plasma could represent up to 50% of all cell-free DNA in metastatic patients [85], whereas ctDNA may be undetectable in patients with MRD [86].

Despite these findings, poor technological advances have limited progress in this area for decades. For many years, multiple studies have been carried out to improve the detection systems that are used to observe tumour-associated genomic alterations in ctDNA, such as tumour-specific mutations, amplifications, deletions, gene rearrangements or methylation variations (Figure 2). These studies have tried to validate the potential of ctDNA as a diagnostic and prognostic marker in cancer as well as their value in MRD detection and therapeutic monitoring, mainly for patients with advanced malignancies [87–91]. However, the detection and quantification of ctDNA with a sensitivity required for significant clinical practice has not been easy, due to the small number of ctDNA fragments compared to the number of normal circulating DNA fragments.

Initially, allele-specific primers in conventional PCR and Pyrosequencing were used to detect and quantify the percentage of specific mutations in cell-free DNA present in liquid biopsy samples but the restriction to specific mutations as well as a low sensitivity (requiring, at least, a 10% of mutant DNA) has limited the success of these techniques [90,92]. This limitation in detection was improved by using quantitative PCR and different deep sequencing technologies such as NGS, being able to identify a 1–2% of mutations in different types of tumours [92–97]. Nowadays, digital droplet polymerase chain reaction (ddPCR) has improved accuracy and quantification of mutations, enabling more effective extraction and analysis of ctDNA, even in highly diluted cell-free DNA samples [98]. In 2005, Diehl and colleagues described for the first time the quantification of the mutant allele fraction of the *APC* gene in plasma of colorectal cancer patients by means of BEAMing technology, which is an approach based on digital PCR, binding to streptavidin beads, attachment of base pair-specific fluorescent probes and flow cytometry [99,100]. Both ddPCR and BEAMing have allowed the reduction of the detection limit of ctDNA mutations to 0.01–0.02% (Figure 2).

Despite the previously described technological advances, the abovementioned detection systems have some restrictions. Using PCR-based methods, the number of ctDNA alterations detected per assay is limited, only evaluating known and specific mutations. Besides, some techniques (like BEAMing) are laborious processes, keeping off a high productivity. Since the percentage of patients bearing known driver mutations is low, assays based on genome-wide analysis, which detection capacity has increased over the last years, have currently gained much importance. Newman et al. have developed a new system, called "cancer personalized profiling by deep sequencing (CAPP-Seq)" [101]. Here, they designed a multiple panel including somatic alterations from Catalogue Of Somatic Mutations In Cancer (COSMIC) and The Cancer Genome Atlas (TCGA) databases for non-small cell lung cancer, thereby detecting some of these alterations in 100% of high stage patients and in 50% of low stage patients, with a detection limit of approximately 0.02% [101] (Figure 2). Accordingly, these advanced techniques open a wide spectrum of possibilities to increase accuracy of diagnostic and predictive systems in a non-invasive form in cancer patients.

Worthy of note, the exact origin of ctDNA is not completely clear yet. Since ctDNA can be released from apoptotic or necrotic tumour cells which have died, genomic features derived from these cells may not entirely reflect the biology of primary tumours or metastasis at diagnosis, and, consequently, these alterations might not contribute to subsequent tumour progression and/or metastasis. This should also be taken into consideration during the clinical decision-making process.

2.2.2. ctDNA in Bladder Cancer

Regarding ctDNA detection in BC patients, several studies have focused on the detection of different DNA alterations in liquid biopsy samples in order to find predictive biomarkers. In particular, urine has been proposed to be a bona fide liquid biopsy for diagnosis and prognosis of BC, given the proximity of tumours. The presence of ctDNA has been found in urine and plasma of BC patients and multiple studies have shown that high levels of ctDNA could be observed in urine of patients with progressive disease, even if ctDNA was not detected in plasma. These results support the usage of both plasma and urine liquid biopsy to detect BC, as well as to monitor recurrence and progression of the disease (reviewed in [86]).

As previously mentioned, *TP53* mutations in urinary sediments from invasive BC patients were described three decades ago [82]. Ever since, specific mutation hotspots in some genes, such as *PIK3CA*, *TERT*, *FGFR3*, *RAS* and *TP53*, have been targeted to detect mutations in ctDNA from BC patients, which has led to the discovery of associations between the presence of ctDNA mutations in these genes in urine as well as plasma samples and disease recurrence and progression [102–104]. Furthermore, using multiplex ligation-dependent probe amplification and NGS, copy number variations (CNVs) and mutations in tumour-related genes in plasma and urine of non-metastatic BC patients were identified, respectively. In this study, Patel et al. reported that the most common mutated genes were *TP53*, *KRAS*, *PIK3CA*, *BRAF*, *CTNNB1* and *FGFR3* and they found a loss of *CDKN2A* and *CREBBP* and gain of *E2F3*, *SOX4*, *PPARG*, *YWHAZ* and *MYCL1* [102]. The presence of some of these ctDNA mutations in plasma or urine (with a technical threshold of 0.5%) has been associated with early disease recurrence, achieving a sensitivity of 83% and specificity of 100% [102]. In plasma from MIBC patients, who show a high mutation rate, at least one mutation in the *PIK3CA*, *TP53* or *ARDIA1* hotspot regions or promoter region of *TERT* gene has been detected in 90% of the cases, as well as CNVs, observing *TP53* and *RB1* inactivating changes, *MDM2* gain or *CDKN2A* loss [85].

Moreover, loss of heterozygosity (LOH) has been shown by microsatellite-based PCR analysis in serum, plasma and urine of BC patients [69,105,106]. Microsatellite instability and LOH in liquid biopsy samples of BC patients are found relatively frequently using markers to detect alterations on chromosomes 4, 8, 9, 14 and 17 [105,106]. Chromosomal regions 17p and 9p are often affected in BC, disrupting the activity of tumour suppressor genes *TP53* and *CDKN2A*. This LOH seems to be associated with reduced disease-free survival and high risk of disease progression [107,108]. Since mutations and CNVs in ctDNA from plasma and urinary biopsies are detectable in high levels before progression, even in NMIBC patient and especially in urine samples, these biomarkers may be useful for disease monitoring [103]. Besides, some studies have revealed unknown alterations with differential sensitivity to therapeutic agents in metastatic patients, emphasizing the importance of ctDNA analysis as a useful tool for the detection of markers of therapy response and guidance of individualized therapies [86].

On the other hand, epigenetic alterations can be detected in BC patients using methylation -specific PCR (MSP) on ctDNA [69]. The combination of methylation levels of the *POU4F2* and *PCDH17* or *TWIST1* and *NID2* genes in urine samples showed a high capacity to differentiate BC patients from healthy volunteers, with 90% sensitivity and 93–94% specificity in both cases [109,110]. Dulaimi et al. reported the hypermethylation of *APC*, *RASSF1A* or *CDKN2A* (p14ARF) in urine ctDNA from 39 out of 45 BC patients (87% sensitivity and 100% specificity), even detecting 16 cases that showed a negative result in cytology assays [111]. Accordingly, hypermethylated DNA in urine of BC patients seems to be more common than positive cytology [111]. Besides, Hoque and colleagues described the combined methylation analysis of *CDKN2A*, *MGMT* and *GSTP1* using urine, enabling the differentiation between BC patients and control subjects, achieving 69% sensitivity and 100% specificity [112]. Furthermore, promoter methylation of both *CDKN2A* (p14ARF) and *MGMT* has been associated with tumour stage and the addition of *GSTP1* and *TIMP3* promoter methylation allowed to discriminate invasive tumours [112]. In cell-free serum DNA, hypermethylation of *APC*, *GSTP1* or *TIG1* has been shown to allow distinction between BC patients and control subjects with 80% sensitivity and 93% specificity [113]. Thus, the potential importance of methylation markers has been proposed for BC prevention and guidance of individual patient management in unpredictable BCs [114–116].

In addition to the alterations found in ctDNA, some commercial kits are based on DNA modifications present in exfoliated cells of the urine sediment. The UroVysion BC Kit is a multi-target FISH assay using exfoliated cells in urine that identifies aneuploidy of chromosomes 3, 7 and 17, as well as the loss of the 9p21 locus (which harbours tumour suppressor gene *CDKN2A*) [117]. A meta-analysis from 14 studies showed that the UroVysion kit has a diagnostic accuracy of 72% sensitivity and 83% specificity (AUC = 0.87) [42] (Table 1). Furthermore, based on methylation patterns of urine exfoliated cells, the 150 loci UroMark assay allows the detection of primary BC when compared to non-BC urine with a sensitivity of 98% and specificity of 97% (AUC = 0.97) [43] (Table 1).

2.3. Circulating Cell-Free RNAs

The presence of circulating cell-free RNA in liquid biopsy samples of cancer patients was described three decades ago, when alterations in the expression levels of some of them were observed in different types of cancer patients [118–120] and even associations with clinical outcome and disease prognosis were found [121–124]. Ever since, coding (mRNA) and non-coding (miRNA, lncRNA and piwi-interacting RNA) cell-free RNAs have gained much relevance as potential biomarkers in these sample types. Subsequently, principal studies related to each type of cell-free RNA in liquid biopsy in BC are described:

2.3.1. Messenger RNAs

Circulating mRNAs were the first RNA molecules described in liquid biopsy in cancer patients [41]. Due to their intracellular role, cell-free mRNAs could be an important source of information about the status of activated or repressed signalling pathways into the tumour cells. Although a high percentage of these mRNAs are usually degraded by RNases, showing lack of stability and high variability between individuals [125–127], some mRNAs have demonstrated to have potential as biomarkers with diagnostic and predictive capacities.

With respect to total isoforms, the percentage of a full-length splicing variant of the *CA9* gene in urine sediments has shown to have diagnostic value to identify BC patients (AUC = 0.896) and this percentage was further increased in high grade and stage tumours [128]. Expression levels of *UBE2C* and *KRT20* mRNAs were significantly elevated in urine of urothelial cancer patients (sensitivity 82.5% and 85%; specificity 76.2% and 94.3%, respectively), increasing gradually with tumour grade and stage [129,130]. Bacchetti and collaborators observed significant differences in urine *PON2* expression when compared Ta and T1-3 tumours, showing higher expression in tumours confined to the basement membrane than in those invading other histological layers [131].

In order to improve the sensitivity and specificity of diagnostic and prognostic systems based on urine samples, several research groups have investigated different mRNA panels. Urquidi et al. carried out the combination of three different gene signatures [32,132,133] together with 6 other independent genes from different biomarker studies, after which they stablished a new diagnostic gene signature based on detected expression of 18 mRNAs (*ANXA10, BIRC5, CA9, CCL18, CDK1, CTSE, DSC2, IGF2, KFL9, KRT20, MDK, MMP1, MMP9, MMP10, MMP12, RAB1A, SEMA3D* and *SNAI2*) in urine samples from BC patients, achieving 85% sensitivity and 88% specificity (AUC = 0.935) [134]. Recently, the CxBladder Monitor and the Xpert Bladder Cancer Monitor (Table 1), two urine-based tests for BC surveillance which measure the expression levels of different sets of five mRNAs (*CDK1, CXCR2, HOXA13, IGFBP5* and *MDK*; and *ABL1, ANXA10, CRH, IGF2* and *UPK1B*, respectively), have been evaluated as follow-up methods for NMIBC patients after TURBT of primary or recurrent tumours. The CxBladder Monitor test was able to predict new recurrences after surgery with a sensitivity of 91% and a negative predictive value (NPV) of 96% (AUC = 0.73) [45,135], whereas the second test achieved a sensitivity of 84% and a specificity of 91% (AUC = 0.872) [47]. Biofina Diagnostics laboratory has developed a test based on ten differentially-expressed genes for the diagnosis and surveillance of BC from urine (UROBEST), achieving 80% sensitivity and 94% specificity (AUC = 0.91). Besides, the commercial laboratory Oncocyte has developed a panel of 43 gene expression biomarkers, PanC-Dx, to distinguish BC from non-cancerous conditions, showing good predictive values from urine samples (AUC = 0.91; sensitivity of 90% with a specificity of 82.5%) (Table 1) [48].

Besides instability and low abundance of circulating mRNAs, another problem associated to the use of mRNAs as biomarkers in liquid biopsy samples is the necessity of appropriate reference genes to compare the expression of target genes. Some studies have evaluated the expression of several potential housekeeping genes in urine samples, such as *PPIA, GAPDH, UBC, PGK1* and *ACTB* [132,136,137]. However, the potential of these and other genes as normalizers in biofluid samples should be studied more profoundly.

2.3.2. microRNAs

Over the last decade, microRNAs have represented a type of biomolecules widely studied as biomarkers in different pathologies, including several types of cancers [138,139]. Moreover, miRNAs expression is very homogeneous among individuals, showing specific expression profiles in different types of tissue [140]. Additionally, miRNAs are protected by a protein complex and they are usually included in exosomes, thereby preserving their integrity and avoiding RNase-mediated degradation [141,142]. Due to these properties, miRNAs are very stable in liquid biopsy samples, such as serum, plasma and urine [137,143], which makes them potential candidates as biomarkers in non-invasive diagnostic and prognostic methods. On the other hand, the new systems designed to perform RT-qPCR from miRNAs allow the study of a wide number of miRNAs from very small amounts of total RNA.

In BC, multiple studies have identified individual miRNAs or panels with predictive features. Some of the most relevant studies of miRNAs in urine samples are discussed next. Downregulation of miR-145 allows to distinguish BC patients from healthy controls (77.8% sensitivity and 61.1% specificity for NMIBC, AUC = 0.729; 84.1% and 61.1% for MIBC, respectively, AUC = 0.790) and shows correlation with tumour grade [144]. Furthermore, miR-106b and miR-146a-5p have shown to be upregulated in BC patients, correlating with tumour stage and with grade and invasion, respectively [145,146]. In addition, high expression of miR-452 and miR-222 (with respect to the miR-16 expression level as normalizer gene) has shown to have diagnostic value (AUC = 0.848 and AUC = 0.718, respectively) [147] and the miR-126: miR-152 ratio has also enabled the detection of BC (AUC = 0.768) [148]. Upregulation of miR-214 has been associated with NMIBC patients but not with tumour grade or stage. Curiously, BC patients with lower levels of miR-214 presented a higher risk of recurrence [149]. Zhang et al.

described that increased expression of miR-155 in urine is associated with tumour grade, stage, recurrence and invasion, allowing the discrimination of NMIBC patients, cystitis patients and healthy controls (80.2% sensitivity and 84.6% specificity) [150]. Besides, urine miR-200a has shown to have predictive properties, observing an association between low expression levels of this miRNA and high risk of recurrence in NMIBC patients [144]. Moreover, upregulation of miR-92a-3p and downregulation of miR-140-5p have been related to progression after recurrence [151].

On the other hand, there are some studies about miRNA expression in serum or plasma samples from BC patients, even though they are less frequent. High expression of miR-210 has been observed in serum of BC patients, correlating with tumour grade and stage and predicting progression (AUC = 0.898) [152]. In the case of plasma, expression of miR-19a is increased in tumour patients and associated with tumour grade [153], miR-200b is upregulated in MIBC, whilst miR-92 and miR-33 present inverse correlation with tumour stage [154].

Moreover, in the last years, several groups have developed multiple panels of miRNA expression, both in urine and in serum samples, to detect and monitor BC. Some of the main miRNA profiles are described in Table 2.

However, appropriate genes for normalization of miRNA expression in biofluids are unclear so far. In tissue samples, miRNA expression is usually normalized using the expression of small nuclear RNAs (snRNAs). Nevertheless, expression and stability of snRNAs is minimized in this type of sample [137], being inadequate as housekeeping genes. Although some authors have suggested some miRNAs, such as miR-16, miR-28-3p and miR-361-3p, as reference genes in urine samples [147,155], additional extensive studies are needed to determine specific housekeeping genes in the different types of liquid biopsies in this pathology. As observed for other tissues and disease conditions, specifically designed studies are required in order to find appropriate miRNAs, which do not show variation among the population to be separated (e.g., patients vs healthy controls, different disease state, metastatic vs non-metastatic disease), in serum and urine. In 2016, Martinez-Fernandez et al. described the use of two miRNAs, miR-193a and miR-448, as normalizers for urine studies [137]. However, these results still have to be validated in a well-designed clinical trial.

2.3.3. Long Non-Coding RNAs

Long non-coding RNAs (lncRNAs) are transcripts longer than 200 nucleotides that are not translated into protein and can modify gene expression at transcriptional, post-transcriptional and epigenetic levels [156]. Although lncRNAs have not been as widely studied as mRNAs or miRNAs, multiple studies have shown that expression of these molecules can be altered in cancer, promoting tumour development, progression and metastasis [157] and, therefore, their use as biomarkers in biofluids is of growing interest.

UCA1 (Urothelial cancer associated 1) is the most studied lncRNA in BC so far. Wang and collaborators determined that high expression of this lncRNA in urine sediments allows detection of high-grade superficial bladder tumours [158]. More recently, a meta-analysis of six studies, including 578 BC patients and 562 healthy controls, confirmed that upregulation of *UCA1* is able to predict BC (sensitivity of 81% and specificity of 86%, AUC = 0.88) [159]. Moreover, blood *UCA1* levels are upregulated in patients with metastatic BC after cisplatin treatment, increasing WNT6 protein expression and activating Wnt signalling, which results in cisplatin resistance [160]. Besides, overexpression of other lncRNAs, such as *HOTAIR, HOX-AS-2, MALAT1, HYMAI, LINC00477, LOC100506688* and *OTX2-AS1*, has been found in urine exosomes of high-grade MIBC patients [161]. On the other hand, other lncRNAs with biomarker potential are *ABHD11-AS1* and *H19* genes, whose increased expression has been associated with primary BC and early relapse, respectively, in tissue samples [162,163]. Future studies of these molecules in liquid biopsy samples of BC patients could be of great interest.

Table 2. Main miRNA panels for diagnosis, prognosis and recurrence surveillance of BC using liquid biopsy samples.

Studies [References]	Type of Sample	Clinical Application	miRNA Panels	Predictive Capacity
Sapre N. [164]	Urine	Recurrence surveillance	miR16, miR200c, miR205, miR21, miR221 and miR34a	Sensitivity = 88% Specificity = 48% AUC = **0.74**–0.85
Pardini B. [155]	Urine	Diagnostic and prognosis	<u>NMIBC G1 + G2 *</u>: miR-30a-5p, let-7c-5p, miR-486-5p, miR-205-5p and let-7i-5p <u>NMIBC G3 *</u>: miR-30a-5p, let-7c-5p, miR-486-5p, miR-21-5p, miR-106b-3p, miR-151a-3p, miR-200c-3p, miR-183-5p, miR-185-5p, miR-224-5p, miR-30c-2-5p and miR-10b-5p <u>MIBC *</u>: miR-30a-5p, let-7c-5p, miR-486-5p, miR-205-5p, miR-451a, miR-25-3p, miR-30a-5p and miR-7-1-5p	AUC = 0.73 AUC = 0.95 AUC = 0.99
Jiang X. [165]	Serum	Diagnostic	miR-152, miR-148b-3p, miR-3187-3p, miR-15b-5p, miR-27a-3p and miR-30a-5p	AUC = 0.899
Jiang X. [166]	Serum	Prognosis	<u>MIBC</u>: miR-422a-3p, miR-486-3p, miR-103a-3p and miR-27a-3p	AUC = **0.880**-0.894
Du L. [167]	Urine	Diagnostic	miR-7-5p, miR-22-3p, miR-29a-3p, miR-126-5p, miR-200a-3p, miR-375 and miR-423-5p	Sensitivity = 82-**85%** Specificity = 87-**96%** AUC = **0.916**-0.923
Urquidi V. [168]	Urine	Diagnostic	miR-652, miR-199a-3p, miR-140-5p, miR-93, miR-142-5p, miR-1305, miR-30a, miR-224, miR-96, miR-766, miR-223, miR-99b, miR-140-3p, let-7b, miR-141, miR-191, miR-146b-5p, miR-491-5p, miR-339-3p, miR-200c, miR-106b *, miR-143, miR-429, miR-222 and miR-200a	Sensitivity = 87% Specificity = 100% AUC = 0.982

* Including traditional BC risk factors (age and smoking status). Bold numbers indicate values from validation set.

In addition, expression of different types of cell-free RNAs can be combined to improve the accuracy of individual tests. Accordingly, Eissa and colleagues developed a panel from urine samples which combines the expression of one mRNA (*HYAL1*; Hyaluronoglucosaminidase 1), two miRNAs (miR-210 and miR-96) and one lncRNA (*UCA1*), thereby achieving a sensitivity of 100% and a specificity of 89.5% [169].

2.3.4. Other Non-Coding RNAs and Its Future Potential as Biomarkers

Additionally, other non-coding RNAs, such as piwi-interacting RNAs (piRNAs) and circular RNAs (circRNAs) have been linked to BC. Although these molecules and their roles in cancer have been only recently studied, they could be good candidates as new biomarkers.

piRNAs are short single strands (26–31 nucleotides) of non-coding RNAs which can repress the expression of target genes, mediated by their binding to PIWI proteins (members of Argonaute proteins subfamily) [170]. Recently, several studies have reported that piRNAs can be widely detected in human plasma. Besides, the expression of some piRNAs has been found to be deregulated in patients with colorectal, prostate and pancreatic cancer [171,172]. Downregulation of piRNA DQ594040 has been associated with BC, whereas its overexpression can inhibit cell proliferation and promote cell apoptosis by upregulation of the TNFSF4 protein [173]. However, specific piRNAs have not yet been found in liquid biopsies from patients with BC.

circRNAs are a type of RNA which are covalently closed in a loop at the 3′ and 5′ ends. For this reason, these RNAs are more resistant than linear RNAs to degradation mediated by exonucleases and, therefore, show a prolonged half-life [174]. Although intra- and extra-cellular roles of these molecules are still largely unknown, some of them have shown relevance in several cancer types [175,176]. Overexpression of some circRNAs, such as circTCF25, circRNA-MYLK, circRNA-CTDP1 and circRNA-PC, has been observed in BC tissue samples. These circRNAs competitively bind to tumour suppressor miRNAs, acting as RNAs sponge and inhibiting their function [177–179]. Stability and functional properties of circRNAs make them interesting molecules to use as biomarkers in liquid biopsy samples.

2.4. Proteins and Peptides

The presence of proteins in liquid biopsy in cancer patients was first published in 1847 by Dr. Henry Bence Jones (reviewed in Reference [180]). Proteins and peptides (protein mass < 15 kDa) might be great candidates as biomarkers, since they are directly related to the "real-time" dynamic molecular cell phenotype. Nevertheless, the relevance of proteins and peptides as potential biomarkers in liquid biopsies has only been extensively studied over the last decade, due to limited technological advances. In BC, proteomic blood analyses [181,182] are scarce compared to the multiple studies performed with urine [53,132,169,183–201]. Plasma comprises the highly complex human-derived proteome, including the presence of a wide variety of proteins, which results in challenges with regard to detection and analysis systems. On the other hand, the urine proteome has been broadly studied and well-characterized, providing reference standards for data comparison and validation in the discovery of BC diagnostic markers [202].

2.4.1. Peptide Biomarkers

In 2006, Theodorescu and colleagues have reported a diagnostic 22-peptide biomarker panel, using capillary electrophoresis coupled to mass spectrometry, which enables the differentiation between urinary BC patient samples and control samples (from prostate cancer, prostate hyperplasia, renal diseases and urinary tract infection), achieving 100% sensitivity and 73% specificity [195]. However, out of the 22 peptides, only fibrinopeptide A has been identified. Even though this peptide biomarker panel allows a good discrimination between advanced cancer and controls, less advanced tumours could not be correctly classified by this panel. Accordingly, the use of a predictive four polypeptide panel (fragments of membrane-associated progesterone receptor component 1, Collagen α-1 (I), Collagen α-1 (III) and Uromodulin) has been proposed as a relevant approach to distinguish between NMIBC and MIBC, reaching 92% sensitivity and 68% specificity [196]. Recently, the previously mentioned studies have been refined by Frantzi and collaborators, who discriminated two different panels using urine by performing a multi-centre study including 1357 patients. A 116-peptide biomarker panel (including identified Apolipoprotein A (APOA), β2-microglobulin, collagen fragments, fibrinogen A, Haemoglobin A, histidine-rich glycoprotein, insulin and small proline-rich protein 3) has been indicated for BC diagnosis, achieving 91% sensitivity and 68% specificity. The second panel has been proposed to encompass 106 peptide biomarkers (including identified ADAM22, ADAMTS1, Apolipoprotein A-1 (APOA-1), collagen fragments and HSPG2) allowing the detection of BC recurrences with 87% sensitivity and 51% specificity [197].

2.4.2. Protein Biomarkers

Multiple proteomic studies have identified proteins (mass >15 kDa) and modifications with diagnostic and prognostic value in BC. However, a large variability has been observed between individual biomarker studies, reflecting proteomic complexity and the excess of applied proteomic approaches. Additionally, suboptimal experimental design of the individual studies contributes to inter-study inconsistency. Nevertheless, reproducible findings have also been reported in several independent studies. Some of the most relevant analyses are discussed next.

Differential expression of urinary α-1-antitrypsin (A1AT) has been indicated between BC patients and hernia patients (AUC = 0.729) as well as between BC patients and healthy controls (74% sensitivity and 80% specificity, AUC = 0.820) [198,199]. The upregulation of A1AT in patients with BC has subsequently been emphasized in an analysis by Linden and colleagues (66% sensitivity and 85% specificity) [200]. Besides, several studies have shown an increased abundance of apolipoprotein E (APOE) (89% sensitivity and 31% specificity, AUC = 0.745–0.756) and fibrinogen β (AUC = 0.720–0.831) in BC urinary biopsies compared to control patients [200,201]. Additionally, multiple studies have validated the importance of different apoliprotein types, reporting an increased abundance of APOA-1 in urine of BC patients (89–94.6% sensitivity and 85–92% specificity) compared to control patients, as well as an upregulation of APOA-2 (AUC = 0.631–0.864) in BC patients compared to hernia patients [183,198,201]. Besides, the differential expression of urinary carbonic anhydrase I and S100A8 between BC patients and hernia patients (AUC = 0.837 and AUC = 0.836, respectively) has been reported [198]. Moreover, Ebbing and colleagues have performed a study, including 181 samples from BC, prostate and renal cancer patients as well as healthy controls, in order to study the heterodimer S100A8/S100A9, known as calprotectin [184]. They showed a significant increase of calprotectin in BC biopsies (AUC = 0.880, 81% sensitivity and 93% specificity) compared to samples of the above-mentioned other tumour types and healthy controls [184]. In addition, Miyake et al. reported an increased abundance of COL4A1, COL13A1 and the combination of both collagens (COL4A1 + COL13A1) in BC urinary biopsies compared to healthy controls (sensitivity 68.2%, 54.6% and 72.1%; specificity 68.9%, 77.1% and 65.6%, respectively) [203]. Besides, the diagnostic sensitivity of this protein combination has been found to improve with malignancy grade, observing a value of 57.4% for low-grade tumours versus 83.7% for high-grade tumours [203].

The identification of biomarkers related to BC aggressiveness has been described by a limited number of studies. Zoidakis et al. performed a study including 108 BC patient samples and 97 urinary biopsies from control patients with benign disease (for example urolithisasis, benign prostate hyperplasia, infection/inflammation or haematuria) and found a differential expression of myeloblastin, aminopeptidase N and profilin-1 [185]. In addition, Nuclear interacting factor 1/Zinc finger 335 (NIF-1) and histone H2B have been described to be differently abundant in urinary biopsies from MIBC patients, NMIBC patients and benign controls [186].

Additionally, multiple analyses have been performed using protein panels, which might enhance accuracy in BC detection. In 2012, Goodison and colleagues proposed the use of a diagnostic 8-protein biomarker panel (angiogenin (ANG), APOE, CA9, IL8, matrix metallopeptidase 9 (MMP9), MMP10, plasminogen activator inhibitor 1 (PAI-1) and vascular endothelial growth factor A (VEGFA)) to distinguish BC patients and healthy controls in a study encompassing 127 urine biopsies, achieving 92% sensitivity and 97% specificity (AUC = 0.980) [187]. Additionally, Rosser et al. showed that a similar protein biomarker panel, namely the previously described 8-protein biomarker panel without CA9, enables the differentiation between BC patients and patients with different urological disorders (74% sensitivity and 90% specificity) [188]. Besides, Urquidi and collaborators reported a 3-protein biomarker panel (PAI-1, CD44 antigen and C-C motif chemokine 18 (CCL18)) to discriminate BC patients from healthy controls [204]. In 2014, Rosser et al. described the combination of 10 proteins (ANG, APOE, CA9, IL8, MMP9, MMP10, SDC1, Serpin Family A Member 1 (SERPINA1), Serpin Family E Member 1 (SERPINE1) and VEGFA) as a potential biomarker panel to detect recurrent disease in urine (79% sensitivity and 88% specificity) [189]. Two years later, Shimizu and colleagues published a comparable study using a similar protein panel (including PAI-1 and A1AT instead of SERPINA1 and SERPINE1) which allowed the differentiation of BC patients from benign and healthy controls, achieving 85% sensitivity and 81% specificity [190]. Recently, Soukap and collaborators reported the value of a 2-protein biomarker panel (synuclein G and midkine) combined with cytology in BC detection (91.8% sensitivity and 97.5% specificity) and showed that the addition of CEACAM1 and ZAG2 proteins to this panel enables the prediction of BC recurrences, achieving 92.7% sensitivity and 90.2% specificity [191].

As previously mentioned, only a limited number of plasma proteomic studies have currently been reported. Bansal et al. have proposed two differently expressed proteins, S100A8 and S100A9, distinguishing BC patients from healthy controls (AUC = 0.850–0.856 and AUC = 0.902–0.957) [181,182]. Moreover, in pre-operative compared to post-operative BC sera samples, a significantly increased abundance of annexin V was observed as well as a reduction of CA1, S100A4, S100A8 and S100A9 [181]. An upregulation of CA1 has also been observed in BC patients compared to healthy controls (AUC = 0.891–0.908) [181,182].

Overall, the previously described studies emphasize the diagnostic value of protein biomarker panels and individual protein biomarkers. However, their clinical value is still compromised due to suboptimal experimental design including benign or healthy controls (instead of clinically relevant patients) in many of the reported analyses, resulting in over-representation of BC. Nevertheless, some FDA-approved and non-approved diagnostic protein biomarkers are currently commercially available for clinical practice in BC (Table 1) and will be discussed next.

One of the most extensively studied proteins in BC urinary biopsies is Nuclear Matrix Protein 22 (NMP22) and multiple studies have demonstrated the use of this protein as a diagnostic BC biomarker, achieving 75–100% sensitivity and 75.9–91.8% specificity [169,192–194]. Mowatt and colleagues reported a pooled data analysis, encompassing a total of 13885 patients from 41 studies, showing that the performance of biomarker NMP22 exceeds cytology in BC detection with regard to sensitivity of the approach (68% versus 44%), mainly due to an improved detection of low-grade tumours [50,205]. Two assays, NMP22 BC test kit and NMP22 BladderChek Test, are currently in clinical use to detect NMP22 in urine. The NMP22 BC test kit represents the original approach based on a quantitative sandwich enzyme-linked immunosorbent assay (ELISA) test using two antibodies and has been FDA-approved for BC surveillance achieving 40% sensitivity and 99% specificity [49] (Table 1). On the other hand, the NMP22 BladderChek Test relies on a qualitative approach designed as a point of care (POC) analysis. The NMP22 BladderChek Test has been approved by the FDA for both BC surveillance and BC diagnosis (68% sensitivity and 79% specificity) [50] (Table 1). Grossman and collaborators analysed the clinical accuracy of the NMP22 BladderChek Test in two multi-centre studies [206,207], showing an increased sensitivity compared to cytology (56% versus 16%, respectively) in patients with haematuria but it did not reach the level of specificity obtained by cytology (86% versus 99%, respectively) [207]. Additionally, a combination of NMP22 BladderChek Test and cystoscopy has been observed to significantly enhance the detection of BC recurrence (up to 99%) compared to cystoscopy alone (91%) [206].

Next to NMP22, the bladder tumour antigen (BTA) has been approved by the FDA as a diagnostic biomarker in BC [208,209]. A pooled data analysis of 23 studies encompassing a total of 2258 BC patients and 2994 non-cancer individuals has shown that BTA allows for the differentiation of BC patients, achieving a mean sensitivity of 64% and specificity of 76.6% [53]. Two assays, BTA stat and BTA TRAK, have been developed for the detection of BTA in urine. BTA TRAK is an ELISA based approach, which has been approved for BC diagnosis, achieving 66% sensitivity and 65% specificity [51,210] (Table 1). BTA stat represents a qualitative assay for POC analysis, accepted for BC diagnosis with 70% sensitivity and 75% specificity [51,210] (Table 1). Besides, it has to be taken into account that multiple studies excluded patients with benign genitourinary conditions and including these patients would drastically diminish the BTA test specificity [211]. Therefore, this biomarker has currently limited clinical value.

On the other hand, cytokeratin fragment 21.1 (CYFRA 21.1) represents an ELISA test detecting soluble cytokeratin 19 fragments [52]. Multiple studies have reported that CYFRA 21.1 allows differentiation between liquid biopsies of BC patients and patients with non-cancer conditions, achieving 70–90% sensitivity and 73–86% specificity (AUC = 0.87–0.90) [52,53,212]. The specificity of this test dramatically decreases with the inclusion of patients with history of BCG and radiotherapy, excluding current use of the CYFRA 21.1 assay as a BC surveillance test [213,214].

Additionally, bladder cancer rapid test represents an urinary BC (UBC) test based on the detection of soluble fragments of cytokeratin 8 and 18, either using a quantitative ELISA or qualitative POC assay [215]. Multiple reports have shown that the UBC test enables the discrimination of BC patients compared to non-cancer individuals with a mean sensitivity of 64.4% and specificity of 80.3% [53,215]. Subsequently, Babjuk et al. described an increase in sensitivity (79%) as well as a decrease in specificity (49%) for the UBC test, once patients with benign conditions or other urinary tract malignancies were included [216]. In these cases, the BTA tests exceed the UBC rapid test regarding their use in BC detection [216].

2.5. Metabolites

The application of metabolomics in cancer is increasing over the years as this approach has shown importance in the search for candidate biomarkers. Since tumour cells are known to have altered metabolic pathways, metabolites in body fluids could be promising for the assessment of pathology, progression and prognosis of cancer [217]. Moreover, metabolomics has recently proved to be useful in the area of biomarker discovery for cancers in which early diagnostic and prognostic is urgently needed, such as BC. Given that the bladder is in intimate contact with urine, this body fluid has been mined heavily for metabolite biomarkers [218].

The use of metabolomic analysis in BC has been primarily focused on the distinction between normal-appearing urothelium and BC. Zhou et al. found a urinary four-biomarker panel (5-hydroxyvaleric acid, cholesterol, 3-phosphoglyceric acid and glycolic acid) including important metabolic characteristics (e.g., organic acid metabolism, steroid hormone biosynthesis, glycolysis and glyoxylate metabolism) and defined this panel as a combinatorial biomarker for the differentiation between BC patients and healthy controls (AUC = 0.804 with 78.0% sensitivity and 70.3% specificity in the validation set) [219,220]. Besides, Huang and colleagues reported the elevation of component I and decrease of carnitine C9:1 in BC urine samples, compared to healthy controls, as a promising biomarker panel for the identification of BC patients (92.6% sensitivity and 96.9% specificity; AUC = 0.963) [221]. However, the structure and biological function of component I is still unclear and required to be studied as it has not been previously observed in nature. Nevertheless, carnitines are an example of disturbed fatty acid transportation, fatty acid-oxidation, or energy metabolism that is happening in tumour cells [221]. Supporting these findings, Ganti proposed that acylcarnitine appearance in BC patient urine samples varies widely in function of tumour grade, suggesting that consistently lower levels of acylcarnitines are present in the urinary biopsies of BC patients with low grade tumours as compared to both BC patients with high grade tumours as well as healthy controls [222]. These results have raised the possibility that fatty acid abnormalities might be involved in the pathogenesis of the tumour.

Moreover, Sahu and colleagues confirmed unique pathway alterations that differentiate MIBC and NMIBC [223]. MIBC appears to preferentially enhance cyclooxygenase (COX) and lipoxygenase (LOX) signalling (Eicosanoids, prostaglandins and tromboxanes (p-value < 0.004), increase heme catabolism (p = 0.0001) and alter nicotinamide adenine dinucleotide (NAD+) synthesis (kynurenine (p = 0.0212), anthranilate (p = 0.0111) and quinolate (p = 0.0015)) [223] with a possible influence in inflammatory cell regulation, cell proliferation and angiogenesis [224,225]. Supporting these results, Loras and colleagues were recently able to identify metabolites in urine enabling the discrimination of BC patients with a high sensitivity (87.9%) and specificity (100%) and a negative likelihood value of 0.1, as well high negative predictive values for low, low-intermediate and high-intermediate and high-risk patients [226]. Metabolomic analysis revealed altered phenylalanine, arginine, proline and tryptophan intermediate metabolism associated to NMIBC [226]. These studies suggest that different stages/grades of BC might generate distinct metabolic profiles, which might be due to the fact that cancer cells in advanced grades/stages require more energy for survival and continuous growing.

Next to the use of urinary analysis for the identification of metabolites as possible biomarkers, the evaluation of global serum profiles of BC, kidney cancer and non-cancer controls has revealed potential biomarkers for BC, including eicosatrienol (AUC = 0.98), azaprostanoic acid (AUC = 0.977), docosatrienol (AUC = 0.972), retinol (AUC = 0.801) and 14′-apo-beta-carotenal (AUC = 0.767) [227].

Overall, the BC metabolic signature is mainly characterized by alterations in metabolites related to energy metabolic pathways, amino acid and fatty acid metabolism, which are known to be crucial for cell proliferation as well as glutathione metabolism, a determinant in maintaining cellular redox balance [228]. However, the absence of a standard for sample acquisition, use of different platforms to profile metabolites, environmental stress and food intake strongly influence the composition of the metabolome and all these factors have led to a large diversity of metabolomic profiles obtained from different laboratories. These issues need to be considered, since they heavily affect the quality of the results by introducing bias and artefacts. Nevertheless, despite remaining challenges, metabolomics shows great clinical promise. The improved sensitivity, specificity of technics and the development of an in-depth reference metabolome may help to identify good metabolic biomarkers which can eventually be translated into the clinic.

2.6. Extracellular Vesicles

The concept of extracellular vesicles (EVs) has evolved from being considered garbage bags to the demonstration that extracellular vesicles could play very interesting roles and functions in cancer biology by promoting survival and growth of disseminated tumour cells; enhancing invasiveness; promoting angiogenesis, migration, tumour cell viability and inhibiting tumour cell apoptosis [229,230]. EVs include microvesicles, apoptotic bodies and exosomes, with the latter being mostly studied at present. Therefore, in this review, we will mainly focus on the potential of exosomes as cancer biomarkers in BC.

Exosomes are small (30–100 nm) membrane vesicles released into the extracellular environment due to fusion of multivesicular bodies with the plasma membrane. They were first described in 1983 in two different papers, published simultaneously [231,232] and currently tumour-released microvesicles, which are abundant in the body fluids of patients with cancer, are suggested to be involved in tumour progression [233]. Besides, it has been demonstrated that exosomes may help in immune response modulation, presentation of antigens to immune cells and intercellular communication through transfer of proteins, mRNAs and miRNAs, which could be a useful tool for diagnostic, predictive and prognostic purposes in different types of tumours. Regarding this, Valenti and colleagues showed that another kind of EVs, microvesicles, released by human melanoma and colorectal carcinoma cells, can promote the differentiation of monocytes to myeloid-derived suppressor cells, which support tumoral growth and immune escape [234].

Currently, there is an increasing interest in the application of exosomes as non-invasive cancer biomarkers and many studies have demonstrated that molecules, such as the lncRNAs *HOTAIR*, *HOX-AS-2*, among others and proteins, like EDIL3 and periostin, are significantly altered in patients with BC [161]. Therefore, EVs are proposed to be enriched in proteins that can be associated with signalling pathways related to tumorigenesis. In this way, Silvers reported that EVs collected from urine of six BC patients (pT1-pT3) showed, at least, a fifteen fold enrichment in the protein levels of β-Hexosaminidase (HEXB), S100A4 and Staphylococcal nuclease and tumour domain containing 1 (SND1) compared to the urinary protein levels of six healthy volunteers ($p < 0.05$) [235]. However, despite these promising preliminary results, the size of this study population is confined and additional extensive research is required for the validation of these data.

Furthermore, based on their stability in body fluids, especially exosomal miRNAs are discussed to be useful diagnostic and prognostic biomarkers in liquid biopsies. Baumgart and colleagues showed that exosomes from invasive BC cell lines, compared to non-invasive BC cell lines, are characterized by a specific miRNA signature which could play a role in the modification of the tumour microenvironment ($p < 0.05$; FC > 1.5) [236]. These results confirmed the hypothesis that the molecular content of exosomes is, at least in part, similar to that of host cells and reflects their cellular properties. However, Baumgart also analysed urinary exosomes from BC patients and they exhibited only in part the miRNA alterations detected in cell line exosomes [236]. Therefore, further analyses will have to clarify the functional relevance of exosomal miRNAs and their role as molecular markers in liquid biopsies.

Even though EVs are a promising source of cancer biomarkers, few studies have been done and no exosomal biomarkers have been implemented in BC clinical practice so far. In general, the interest in EVs is growing but the introduction as established predictive biomarkers has been hampered by challenges in exosome isolation and characterization, indicating the need for new sensitive platforms which allow more accurate isolation and detection methods. Furthermore, the use of an efficient, rapid and reproducible isolation method is fundamental for analytical reproducibility.

3. Summary and Discussion

Among body fluids, urine and saliva are the most attractive fluids for liquid biopsy due to their accessibility and low invasiveness of collection. As somatic alterations detected in ctDNA are reflective for those present in tumour tissue, the ctDNA profile could be a practical method for obtaining the tumour genome independently of direct tissue sequencing. Additionally, mutations in ctDNA of cancer patients could be detected over one year prior to clinical diagnosis, which emphasizes the great potential of liquid biopsy for the detection of cancer at early stages [98,237,238]. At present, there are several diagnostic kits based on the detection of mutations in liquid biopsy samples using ctDNA or CTCs from the bloodstream. Most of them have been designed for blood/plasma/serum samples using qPCR and NGS techniques. Only the diagnostic kit Trovera (initially designed for the identification of mutations in *BRAF, KRAS, EGFR* in plasma samples; Trovagene) is marketed for both plasma and urine samples. A diagnostic alternative is based on the detection of both circulating RNA and extracellular vesicles (such as exosomes), for which multiple diagnostic kits are brought on the market in order to detect and monitor prostate (like ExoDx Prostate; IntelliScore) or bladder (like CxBladder; Pacific Edge, among others) cancer in urine samples.

Although it is true that urine can reflect genetic alterations of a large number of solid tumours [239], it will probably be more relevant for the diagnosis and monitoring of tumours of the genitourinary tract. In these cases, the content of nucleic acids from the tumour cells is released directly into the urine, which minimalizes the DNA/RNA contamination background of blood cells as observed in plasma (Figure 3) [240].

As previously mentioned, the high recurrence rate and the need for expensive diagnostic and monitoring methods, such as cystoscopy, make BC the most expensive human cancer from diagnosis to death. For this reason, efforts to develop diagnostic, prognostic and follow-up systems for BC have been enormous in recent years, with various systems published for liquid biopsy samples. Accordingly, several diagnostic laboratories have launched different diagnostic and monitoring systems for BC patients, which are based on the determination of gene expression or protein biomarkers in urine samples (Table 1). Moreover, the identification of metabolites as potential biomarker in BC liquid biopsy has also been explored. Several authors have found specific metabolites that are able to identify patients with BC, even before appearance of the first clinical symptoms of this disease [241]. However, the main concern regarding metabolomics in urine as a diagnostic system is the variability of glomerular filtration, both with medication and dietary habits as the main confounding factors [242,243]. Therefore, large cohort studies and standardization of sample taking and processing procedures will be necessary to finally establish metabolomics as a diagnostic approach.

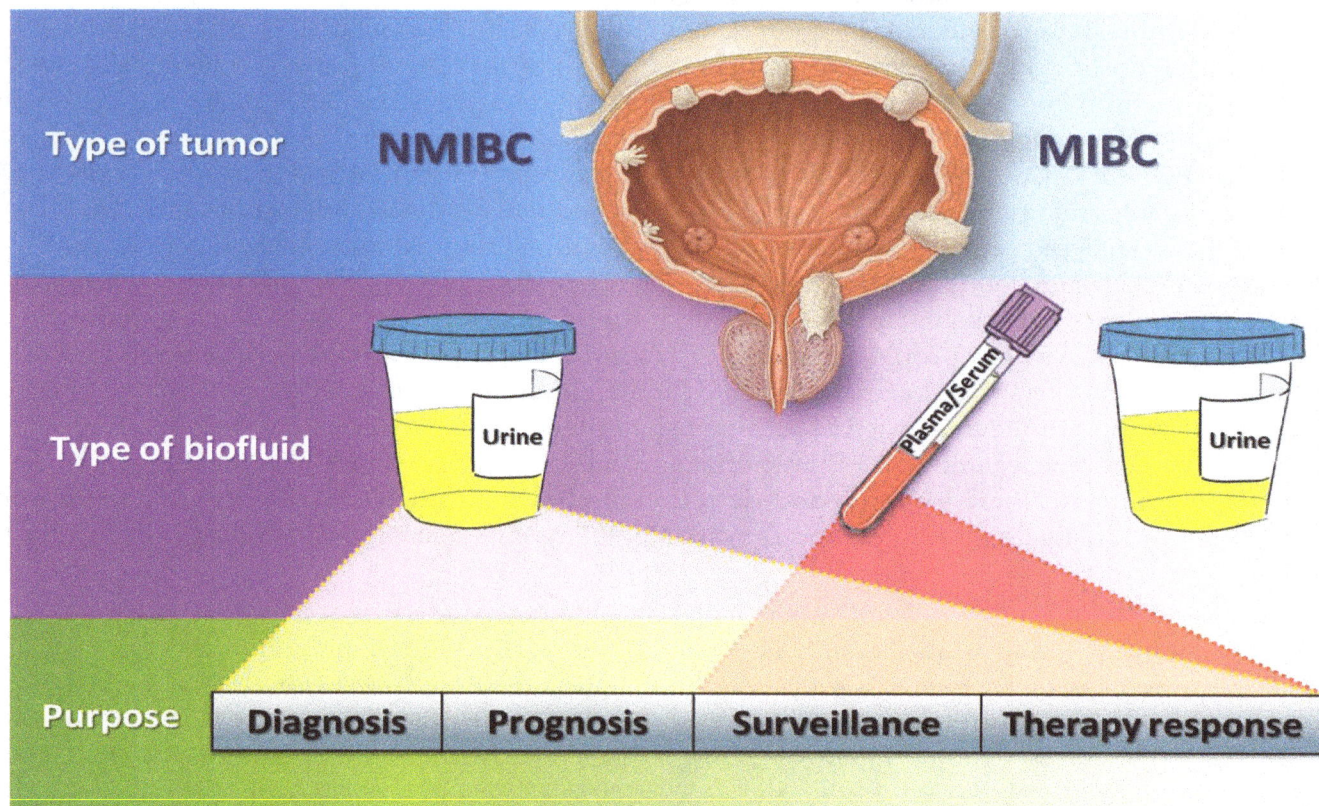

Figure 3. Hypothetical flowchart of liquid biopsies management in BC. In NMIBC patients, urine could be the best type of biofluid for diagnosis, prognosis, surveillance and therapy response due to its intimate contact with the tumour, whilst in MIBC patients, though urine could also be used, plasma and serum acquire more importance to monitor patients.

Regarding MIBC patient follow-up, it should be taken into account that, even though cystectomy is performed in most cases, progression of bladder tumours is produced by metastasis in other tissues and organs. In case of metastatic tumours, blood becomes perhaps the most appropriate fluid for follow-up and to explore possible therapies once progression of the disease is established (Figure 3). Therefore, the determination of mutations or alterations of gene expression patterns has been explored from both ctDNA in plasma/serum and from the isolation of CTCs in the bloodstream (reviewed in [244–246]). However, care must be taken with predictions regarding the future of these new technologies and the studies that support them. Some of the current FDA-approved systems for the diagnosis and monitoring of BC do not meet sensitivity and specificity requirements (e.g., the NMP22 determination), whereas other tests have such high costs that their use in daily health practice is limited (e.g., the UroVysion test). Consequently, there is an urgent need for suitable studies in order to validate biomarkers for early detection. Nevertheless, conventional case-control studies have proven not to be adequate, emphasizing the importance of prospective cohort studies, consisting of serial samples at different time points from a person at-risk, as well as large randomized trials, validating biomarker clinical benefit compared to actual gold standard methods. Additionally, a coherent and comprehensive set of guidelines must be delineated to ensure success once an approach is approved for clinical set-up. For example, Pepe et al. described a prospective randomized open blinded end-point (PROBE) study design which takes into account components related to the clinical context and outcomes, criteria for measuring biomarker performance, the biomarker test itself and the size of the study as a guidance for the design of a biomarker accuracy study [247]. Besides, sample repositories (crucial for the discovery and evaluation of biomarkers with potential use in clinical medicine) should follow this design strategy in order to maximize biomarker values.

4. Concluding Remarks

In general, physicians and researchers agree that liquid biopsy is the most promising strategy for diagnostics, selection of treatments and follow-up in various tumour types. However, it is important that the development of these new diagnostic and follow-up systems come together with the appropriate proposals for changes in the therapeutic procedure, either with a better characterization of the patients or with an adequate proposal of an effective treatment line. On the other hand, the lack of validation of these systems, which are capable of detecting a tumour burden much smaller than the imaging technologies, currently prevents them from clinical practice, since they can generate great anxiety among patients and possibly lead to overtreatment of the patient. Therefore, more studies with long follow-up periods and large cohorts are required to demonstrate that the positive result in a liquid biopsy test is valid as a starting point to initiate or change an oncologic treatment. However, despite the difficulties and current limitations in liquid biopsy technologies and the current lack of robust and confident methodologies that unequivocally allow diagnosis, prognosis or detection of therapy response, with the current accumulation of clinical evidence, we are convinced that it will only be a matter of time until liquid biopsy replaces tissue biopsy in all solid tumours.

Author Contributions: All authors contributed equally to review the current literature and write specific sections. The whole work was coordinated by J.M.P. and C.S.-C. All the authors agreed with the final version.

References

1. Ferlay, J.; Soerjomataram, I.; Dikshit, R.; Eser, S.; Mathers, C.; Rebelo, M.; Parkin, D.M.; Forman, D.; Bray, F. Cancer incidence and mortality worldwide: Sources, methods and major patterns in GLOBOCAN 2012. *Int. J. Cancer* **2015**, *136*, E359–E386. [CrossRef] [PubMed]
2. Witjes, J.A.; Lebret, T.; Compérat, E.M.; Cowan, N.C.; de Santis, M.; Bruins, H.M.; Hernández, V.; Espinós, E.L.; Dunn, J.; Rouanne, M.; et al. Updated 2016 EAU guidelines on guscle-invasive and metastatic bladder cancer. *Eur. Urol.* **2017**, *71*, 462–475. [CrossRef] [PubMed]
3. Babjuk, M.; Böhle, A.; Burger, M.; Capoun, O.; Cohen, D.; Compérat, E.M.; Hernández, V.; Kaasinen, E.; Palou, J.; Rouprêt, M.; et al. EAU guidelines on non-muscle-invasive urothelial carcinoma of the bladder: Update 2016. *Eur. Urol.* **2017**, *71*, 447–461. [CrossRef] [PubMed]
4. Babjuk, M. Trends in bladder cancer incidence and mortality: Success or disappointment? *Eur. Urol.* **2017**, *71*, 109–110. [CrossRef] [PubMed]
5. Robertson, A.G. Comprehensive molecular characterization of muscle-invasive bladder cancer. *Cell* **2017**, *171*, 540–556. [CrossRef] [PubMed]
6. Berdik, C. Unlocking bladder cancer. *Nature* **2017**, *551*, S34–S35. [CrossRef] [PubMed]
7. Humphrey, P.A.; Moch, H.; Cubilla, A.L.; Ulbright, T.M.; Reuter, V.E. The 2016 WHO Classification of tumours of the urinary system and male genital organs—Part B: Prostate and bladder tumours. *Eur. Urol.* **2016**, *70*, 106–119. [CrossRef] [PubMed]

8.   Noone, A.; Howlader, N.; Krapcho, M.; Miller, D.; Brest, A.; Yu, M.; Ruhl, J.; Tatalovich, Z.; Mariotto, A.; Lewis, D.; et al. SEER Cancer Statistics Review, 1975–2015. National Cancer Institute: Bethesda, MD. Available online: https://seer.cancer.gov/csr/1975_2015/ (accessed on 12 August 2018).

9.   Knowles, M.A.; Hurst, C.D. Molecular biology of bladder cancer: New insights into pathogenesis and clinical diversity. *Nat. Rev. Cancer* **2015**, *15*, 25. [CrossRef] [PubMed]

10. Pietzak, E.J.; Bagrodia, A.; Cha, E.K.; Drill, E.N.; Iyer, G.; Isharwal, S.; Ostrovnaya, I.; Baez, P.; Li, Q.; Berger, M.F.; et al. Next-generation sequencing of nonmuscle invasive bladder cancer reveals potential biomarkers and rational therapeutic targets. *Eur. Urol.* **2017**, *6*, 952–959. [CrossRef] [PubMed]

11. Van Rhijn, B.W.G.; Burger, M.; Lotan, Y.; Solsona, E.; Stief, C.G.; Sylvester, R.J.; Witjes, J.A.; Zlotta, A.R. Recurrence and progression of disease in non-muscle-invasive bladder cancer: From epidemiology to treatment strategy. *Eur. Urol.* **2009**, *56*, 430–442. [CrossRef] [PubMed]

12. Sylvester, R.J.; Oosterlinck, W.; Witjes, J.A. The schedule and duration of intravesical chemotherapy in patients with non-muscle-invasive bladder cancer: A systematic review of the published results of randomized clinical trials. *Eur. Urol.* **2008**, *53*, 709–719. [CrossRef] [PubMed]

13. Shariat, S.F.; Zippe, C.; Lübecke, G.; Boman, H.; Sanchez-Carbayo, M.; Casella, R.; Mian, C.; Friedrich, M.G.; Eissa, S.; Akaza, H.; et al. Nomograms including nuclear matrix protein 22 for prediction of disease recurrence and progression in patients with Ta, T1 or CIS transitional cell carcinoma of the bladder. *J. Urol.* **2005**, *173*, 1518–1525. [CrossRef] [PubMed]

14. Lee, D.J.; Chang, S.S. Cost Considerations in the Management of Bladder Cancer. *Urol. Times.* Available online: http://www.urologytimes.com/modern-medicine-feature-articles/cost-considerations-management-bladder-cancer (accessed on 16 October 2017).

15. Mariotto, A.B.; Yabroff, K.R.; Shao, Y.; Feuer, E.J.; Brown, M.L. Projections of the cost of cancer care in the United States: 2010–2020. *J. Natl. Cancer Inst.* **2011**, *103*, 117–128. [CrossRef] [PubMed]

16. Leal, J.; Luengo-Fernandez, R.; Sullivan, R.; Witjes, J.A. Economic Burden of Bladder Cancer across the European Union. *Eur. Urol.* **2016**, *69*, 438–447. [CrossRef] [PubMed]

17. Wolff, E.M.; Liang, G.; Jones, P.A. Mechanisms of disease: Genetic and epigenetic alterations that drive bladder cancer. *Nat. Clin. Pract. Urol.* **2005**, *2*, 502. [CrossRef] [PubMed]

18. Burger, M.; Catto, J.W.F.; Dalbagni, G.; Grossman, H.B.; Herr, H.; Karakiewicz, P.; Kassouf, W.; Kiemeney, L.A.; La Vecchia, C.; Shariat, S.; et al. Epidemiology and risk factors of urothelial bladder cancer. *Eur. Urol.* **2013**, *63*, 234–241. [CrossRef] [PubMed]

19. Griffiths, G.; Hall, R.; Sylvester, R.; Raghavan, D.; Parmar, M. International phase III trial assessing neoadjuvant cisplatin, methotrexate, and vinblastine chemotherapy for muscle-invasive bladder cancer: Long-term results of the BA06 30894 trial. *J. Clin. Oncol.* **2011**, *29*, 2171–2177. [CrossRef] [PubMed]

20. Advanced Bladder Cancer (ABC) Meta-Analysis Collaboration. Neoadjuvant chemotherapy in invasive bladder cancer: Update of a systematic review and meta-analysis of individual patient data advanced bladder cancer (ABC) meta-analysis collaboration. *Eur. Urol.* **2005**, *48*, 202–205. [CrossRef] [PubMed]

21. Yuh, B.E.; Ruel, N.; Wilson, T.G.; Vogelzang, N.; Pal, S.K. Pooled analysis of clinical outcomes with neoadjuvant cisplatin and gemcitabine chemotherapy for muscle invasive bladder cancer. *J. Urol.* **2013**, *189*, 1682–1686. [CrossRef] [PubMed]

22. Stenzl, A.; Cowan, N.C.; de Santis, M.; Kuczyk, M.A.; Merseburger, A.S.; Ribal, M.J.; Sherif, A.; Witjes, J.A. Treatment of muscle-invasive and metastatic bladder cancer: Update of the EAU guidelines. *Actas Urol. Españolas* **2012**, *36*, 449–460. [CrossRef]

23. Pal, S.K.; Milowsky, M.I.; Plimack, E.R. Optimizing systemic therapy for bladder cancer. *J. Natl. Compr. Cancer Netw.* **2013**, *11*, 793–804. [CrossRef]

24. Bellmunt, J.; de Wit, R.; Vaughn, D.J.; Fradet, Y.; Lee, J.-L.; Fong, L.; Vogelzang, N.J.; Climent, M.A.; Petrylak, D.P.; Choueiri, T.K.; et al. Pembrolizumab as Second-Line Therapy for Advanced Urothelial Carcinoma. *N. Engl. J. Med.* **2017**, *376*, 1015–1026. [CrossRef] [PubMed]

25. Powles, T.; Eder, J.P.; Fine, G.D.; Braiteh, F.S.; Loriot, Y.; Cruz, C.; Bellmunt, J.; Burris, H.A.; Petrylak, D.P.; Teng, S.L.; et al. MPDL3280A (anti-PD-L1) treatment leads to clinical activity in metastatic bladder cancer. *Nature* **2014**, *515*, 558–562. [CrossRef] [PubMed]

26. Blick, C.G.T.; Nazir, S.A.; Mallett, S.; Turney, B.W.; Onwu, N.N.; Roberts, I.S.D.; Crew, J.P.; Cowan, N.C. Evaluation of diagnostic strategies for bladder cancer using computed tomography (CT) urography, flexible cystoscopy and voided urine cytology: Results for 778 patients from a hospital haematuria clinic. *BJU Int.* **2012**, *110*, 84–94. [CrossRef] [PubMed]

27. Van Rhijn, B.W.G.; van der Poel, H.G.; van der Kwast, T.H. Cytology and Urinary Markers for the Diagnosis of Bladder Cancer. *Eur. Urol. Suppl.* **2009**, *8*, 536–541. [CrossRef]

28. Fradet, Y.; Lockhard, C. Performance characteristics of a new monoclonal antibody test for bladder cancer: ImmunoCyt trade mark. *Can. J. Urol.* **1997**, *4*, 400–405. [PubMed]

29. He, H.; Han, C.; Hao, L.; Zang, G. ImmunoCyt test compared to cytology in the diagnosis of bladder cancer: A meta-analysis. *Oncol. Lett.* **2016**, *12*, 83–88. [CrossRef] [PubMed]

30. Glatz, K.; Willi, N.; Glatz, D.; Barascud, A.; Grilli, B.; Herzog, M.; Dalquen, P.; Feichter, G.; Gasser, T.C.; Sulser, T.; et al. An international telecytologic quiz on urinary cytology reveals educational deficits and absence of a commonly used classification system. *Am. J. Clin. Pathol.* **2006**, *126*, 294–301. [CrossRef] [PubMed]

31. Kehinde, E.O.; Al-Mulla, F.; Kapila, K.; Anim, J.T. Comparison of the sensitivity and specificity of urine cytology, urinary nuclear matrix protein-22 and multitarget fluorescence in situ hybridization assay in the detection of bladder cancer. *Scand. J. Urol. Nephrol.* **2011**, *45*, 113–121. [CrossRef] [PubMed]

32. O'Sullivan, P.; Sharples, K.; Dalphin, M.; Davidson, P.; Gilling, P.; Cambridge, L.; Harvey, J.; Toro, T.; Giles, N.; Luxmanan, C.; et al. A Multigene Urine Test for the Detection and Stratification of Bladder Cancer in Patients Presenting with Hematuria. *J. Urol.* **2012**, *188*, 741–747. [CrossRef] [PubMed]

33. Loidl, W.; Schmidbauer, J.; Susani, M.; Marberger, M. Flexible cystoscopy assisted by hexaminolevulinate induced fluorescence: A new approach for bladder cancer detection and surveillance? *Eur. Urol.* **2005**, *47*, 323–326. [CrossRef] [PubMed]

34. Crowley, E.; Di Nicolantonio, F.; Loupakis, F.; Bardelli, A. Liquid biopsy: Monitoring cancer-genetics in the blood. *Nat. Rev. Clin. Oncol.* **2013**, *10*, 472–484. [CrossRef] [PubMed]

35. Bardelli, A.; Pantel, K. Liquid Biopsies, What We Do Not Know (Yet). *Cancer Cell* **2017**, *31*, 172–179. [CrossRef] [PubMed]

36. Di Meo, A.; Bartlett, J.; Cheng, Y.; Pasic, M.D.; Yousef, G.M. Liquid biopsy: A step forward towards precision medicine in urologic malignancies. *Mol. Cancer* **2017**, *16*, 80. [CrossRef] [PubMed]

37. Heitzer, E.; Perakis, S.; Geigl, J.B.; Speicher, M.R. The potential of liquid biopsies for the early detection of cancer. *NPJ Precis. Oncol.* **2017**, *1*, 36. [CrossRef] [PubMed]

38. Khetrapal, P.; Lee, M.W.L.; Tan, W.S.; Dong, L.; de Winter, P.; Feber, A.; Kelly, J.D. The role of circulating tumour cells and nucleic acids in blood for the detection of bladder cancer: A systematic review. *Cancer Treat. Rev.* **2018**, *66*, 56–63. [CrossRef] [PubMed]

39. Siravegna, G.; Marsoni, S.; Siena, S.; Bardelli, A. Integrating liquid biopsies into the management of cancer. *Nat. Rev. Clin. Oncol.* **2017**, *14*, 531–548. [CrossRef] [PubMed]

40. Wan, J.C.M.; Massie, C.; Garcia-Corbacho, J.; Mouliere, F.; Brenton, J.D.; Caldas, C.; Pacey, S.; Baird, R.; Rosenfeld, N. Liquid biopsies come of age: Towards implementation of circulating tumour DNA. *Nat. Rev. Cancer* **2017**, *17*, 223–238. [CrossRef] [PubMed]

41. Mandel, P.; Metais, P. Les acides nucléiques du plasma sanguin chez l'homme. *C. R. Seances Soc. Biol. Fil.* **1948**, *142*, 241–243. [PubMed]

42. Hajdinjak, T. UroVysion FISH test for detecting urothelial cancers: Meta-analysis of diagnostic accuracy and comparison with urinary cytology testing. *Urol. Oncol. Semin. Orig. Investig.* **2008**, *26*, 646–651. [CrossRef] [PubMed]

43. Feber, A.; Dhami, P.; Dong, L.; de Winter, P.; Tan, W.S.; Martínez-Fernández, M.; Paul, D.S.; Hynes-Allen, A.; Rezaee, S.; Gurung, P.; et al. UroMark-a urinary biomarker assay for the detection of bladder cancer. *Clin. Epigenet.* **2017**, *9*, 8. [CrossRef] [PubMed]

44. Zhang, Z.; Fan, W.; Deng, Q.; Tang, S.; Wang, P.; Xu, P.; Wang, J.; Yu, M. The prognostic and diagnostic value of circulating tumor cells in bladder cancer and upper tract urothelial carcinoma: A meta-analysis of 30 published studies. *Oncotarget* **2017**, *8*, 59527. [CrossRef] [PubMed]

45. Lotan, Y.; O'Sullivan, P.; Raman, J.D.; Shariat, S.F.; Kavalieris, L.; Frampton, C.; Guilford, P.; Luxmanan, C.; Suttie, J.; Crist, H.; et al. Clinical comparison of noninvasive urine tests for ruling out recurrent urothelial carcinoma. *Urol. Oncol. Semin. Orig. Investig.* **2017**, *35*, 531. [CrossRef] [PubMed]

46.   Valenberg FJP, V. Validation of a mRNA-based urine test for bladder cancer detection in patients with hematuria. *Eur. Urol.* **2017**, *16*, e190–e191. [CrossRef]

47.   Pichler, R.; Fritz, J.; Tulchiner, G.; Klinglmair, G.; Soleiman, A.; Horninger, W.; Klocker, H.; Heidegger, I. Increased accuracy of a novel mRNA-based urine test for bladder cancer surveillance. *BJU Int.* **2018**, *121*, 29–37. [CrossRef] [PubMed]

48.   Chapman, K. Positive Clinical Results of OncoCyte's PanC-Dx^TM Diagnostic Test Demonstrate High Level of Sensitivity and Specificity in Non-Invasive Detection of Bladder Cancer—OncoCyte Corporation. In Proceedings of the American Association for Cancer Research 2015 Annual Meeting, Philadelphia, PA, USA, 19 April 2015.

49.   Hatzichristodoulou, G.; Kubler, H.; Schwaibold, H.; Wagenpfeil, S.; Eibauer, C.; Hofer, C.; Gschwend, J.; Treiber, U. Nuclear matrix protein 22 for bladder cancer detection: Comparative analysis of the BladderChek® and ELISA. *Anticancer Res.* **2012**, *32*, 5093–5097. [PubMed]

50.   Mowatt, G.; Zhu, S.; Kilonzo, M.; Boachie, C.; Fraser, C.; Griffiths, T.R.L.; N'Dow, J.; Nabi, G.; Cook, J.; Vale, L. Systematic review of the clinical effectiveness and cost-effectiveness of photodynamic diagnosis and urine biomarkers (FISH, ImmunoCyt, NMP22) and cytology for the detection and follow-up of bladder cancer. *Health Technol. Assess.* **2010**, *14*, 1–331. [CrossRef] [PubMed]

51.   Glas, A.S.; Roos, D.; Deutekom, M.; Zwinderman, A.H.; Bossuyt, P.M.M.; Kurth, K.H. Tumor Markers in the Diagnosis of Primary Bladder Cancer. A Systematic Review. *J. Urol.* **2003**, *169*, 1975–1982. [CrossRef] [PubMed]

52.   Huang, Y.-L.; Chen, J.; Yan, W.; Zang, D.; Qin, Q.; Deng, A.-M. Diagnostic accuracy of cytokeratin-19 fragment (CYFRA 21–21) for bladder cancer: A systematic review and meta-analysis. *Tumor Biol.* **2015**, *36*, 3137–3145. [CrossRef] [PubMed]

53.   D'Costa, J.J.; Goldsmith, J.C.; Wilson, J.S.; Bryan, R.T.; Ward, D.G. A Systematic Review of the Diagnostic and Prognostic Value of Urinary Protein Biomarkers in Urothelial Bladder Cancer. *Bladder Cancer* **2016**, *2*, 301–317. [CrossRef] [PubMed]

54.   Ashworth, T.R. A case of cancer in which cells similar to those in the tumours were seen in the blood after death. *Aust. Med. J.* **1869**, *14*, 146–147.

55.   Stoecklein, N.H.; Fischer, J.C.; Niederacher, D.; Terstappen, L.W. Challenges for CTC-based liquid biopsies: Low CTC frequency and diagnostic leukapheresis as a potential solution. *Expert Rev. Mol. Diagn.* **2016**, *16*, 147–164. [CrossRef] [PubMed]

56.   Harouaka, R.; Kang, Z.; Zheng, S.-Y.; Cao, L. Circulating tumor cells: Advances in isolation and analysis, and challenges for clinical applications. *Pharmacol. Ther.* **2014**, *141*, 209–221. [CrossRef] [PubMed]

57.   Lv, Q.; Gong, L.; Zhang, T.; Ye, J.; Chai, L.; Ni, C.; Mao, Y. Prognostic value of circulating tumor cells in metastatic breast cancer: A systemic review and meta-analysis. *Clin. Transl. Oncol.* **2016**, *18*, 322–330. [CrossRef] [PubMed]

58.   Huang, X.; Gao, P.; Sun, J.; Chen, X.; Song, Y.; Zhao, J.; Xu, H.; Wang, Z. Clinicopathological and prognostic significance of circulating tumor cells in patients with gastric cancer: A meta-analysis. *Int. J. Cancer* **2015**, *136*, 21–33. [CrossRef] [PubMed]

59.   Rahbari, N.N.; Aigner, M.; Thorlund, K.; Mollberg, N.; Motschall, E.; Jensen, K.; Diener, M.K.; Büchler, M.W.; Koch, M.; Weitz, J. Meta-analysis Shows That Detection of Circulating Tumor Cells Indicates Poor Prognosis in Patients With Colorectal Cancer. *Gastroenterology* **2010**, *138*, 1714.e13–1726.e13. [CrossRef] [PubMed]

60.   Wang, S.; Zheng, G.; Cheng, B.; Chen, F.; Wang, Z.; Chen, Y.; Wang, Y.; Xiong, B. Circulating Tumor Cells (CTCs) Detected by RT-PCR and Its Prognostic Role in Gastric Cancer: A Meta-Analysis of Published Literature. *PLoS ONE* **2014**, *9*, e99259. [CrossRef] [PubMed]

61.   Naoe, M.; Ogawa, Y.; Morita, J.; Omori, K.; Takeshita, K.; Shichijyo, T.; Okumura, T.; Igarashi, A.; Yanaihara, A.; Iwamoto, S.; et al. Detection of circulating urothelial cancer cells in the blood using the CellSearch System. *Cancer* **2007**, *109*, 1439–1445. [CrossRef] [PubMed]

62.   Neumann, M.H.D.; Bender, S.; Krahn, T.; Schlange, T. ctDNA and CTCs in Liquid Biopsy—Current Status and Where We Need to Progress. *Comput. Struct. Biotechnol. J.* **2018**, *16*, 190–195. [CrossRef] [PubMed]

63.   Yoo, C.E.; Park, J.-M.; Moon, H.-S.; Joung, J.-G.; Son, D.-S.; Jeon, H.-J.; Kim, Y.J.; Han, K.-Y.; Sun, J.-M.; Park, K.; et al. Vertical Magnetic Separation of Circulating Tumor Cells for Somatic Genomic-Alteration Analysis in Lung Cancer Patients OPEN. *Nat. Publ. Gr.* **2016**, *6*, 37392. [CrossRef]

64. Yap, T.A.; Lorente, D.; Omlin, A.; Olmos, D.; de Bono, J.S. Circulating tumor cells: A multifunctional biomarker. *Clin. Cancer Res.* **2014**, *20*, 2553–2568. [CrossRef] [PubMed]

65. Wang, L.; Balasubramanian, P.; Chen, A.P.; Kummar, S.; Evrard, Y.A.; Kinders, R.J. Promise and limits of the CellSearch platform for evaluating pharmacodynamics in circulating tumor cells. *Semin. Oncol.* **2016**, *43*, 464–475. [CrossRef] [PubMed]

66. Hillig, T.; Nygaard, A.B.; Nekiunaite, L.; Klingelhöfer, J.; Sölétormos, G. In vitro validation of an ultra-sensitive scanning fluorescence microscope for analysis of circulating tumor cells. *APMIS* **2014**, *122*, 545–551. [CrossRef] [PubMed]

67. Hillig, T.; Horn, P.; Nygaard, A.B.; Haugaard, A.S.; Nejlund, S.; Brandslund, I.; Sölétormos, G. In vitro detection of circulating tumor cells compared by the CytoTrack and CellSearch methods. *Tumor Biol.* **2015**, *36*, 4597–4601. [CrossRef] [PubMed]

68. Frandsen, A.S.; Fabisiewicz, A.; Jagiello-Gruszfeld, A.; Haugaard, A.S.; Petersen, L.M.; Brandt Albrektsen, K.; Nejlund, S.; Smith, J.; Stender, H.; Hillig, T.; Sölétormos, G. Retracing Circulating Tumour Cells for Biomarker Characterization after Enumeration. *J. Circ. Biomark.* **2015**, *4*, 5. [CrossRef] [PubMed]

69. Riethdorf, S.; Soave, A.; Rink, M. The current status and clinical value of circulating tumor cells and circulating cell-free tumor DNA in bladder cancer. *Transl. Androl. Urol.* **2017**, *6*, 1090. [CrossRef] [PubMed]

70. Werner, S.L.; Graf, R.P.; Landers, M.; Valenta, D.T.; Schroeder, M.; Greene, S.B.; Bales, N.; Dittamore, R.; Marrinucci, D. Analytical Validation and Capabilities of the Epic CTC Platform: Enrichment-Free Circulating Tumour Cell Detection and Characterization. *J. Circ. Biomark.* **2015**, *4*, 4. [CrossRef] [PubMed]

71. Marrinucci, D.; Bethel, K.; Kolatkar, A.; Luttgen, M.S.; Malchiodi, M.; Baehring, F.; Voigt, K.; Lazar, D.; Nieva, J.; Bazhenova, L.; et al. Fluid biopsy in patients with metastatic prostate, pancreatic and breast cancers. *Phys. Biol.* **2012**, *9*, 016003. [CrossRef] [PubMed]

72. Greene, B.T.; Hughes, A.D.; King, M.R. Circulating tumor cells: The substrate of personalized medicine? *Front. Oncol.* **2012**, *2*, 69. [CrossRef] [PubMed]

73. Stratmann, A.; Fischer, J.C.; Niederacher, D.; Raba, K.; Schmitz, A.; Kim, P.S.; Singh, S.; Stoecklein, N.H.; Krahn, T. A comprehensive comparison of circulating tumor cell capturing technologies by apheresis of cancer patients. *J. Clin. Oncol.* **2012**, *30*, e21017. [CrossRef]

74. Stoecklein, N.H.; Niederacher, D.; Topp, S.A.; Zacarias Föhrding, L.; Vay, C. Effect of leukapheresis on efficient CTC enrichment for comprehensive molecular characterization and clinical diagnostics. *J. Clin. Oncol.* **2012**, *30*, e21020. [CrossRef]

75. Lu, J.J.; Kakehi, Y.; Takahashi, T.; Wu, X.X.; Yuasa, T.; Yoshiki, T.; Okada, Y.; Terachi, T.; Ogawa, O. Detection of circulating cancer cells by reverse transcription-polymerase chain reaction for uroplakin II in peripheral blood of patients with urothelial cancer. *Clin. Cancer Res.* **2000**, *6*, 3166–3171. [PubMed]

76. Flaig, T.W.; Wilson, S.; van Bokhoven, A.; Varella-Garcia, M.; Wolfe, P.; Maroni, P.; Genova, E.E.; Morales, D.; Lucia, M.S. Detection of circulating tumor cells in metastatic and clinically localized urothelial carcinoma. *Urology* **2011**, *78*, 863–867. [CrossRef] [PubMed]

77. Busetto, G.M.; Ferro, M.; Del Giudice, F.; Antonini, G.; Chung, B.I.; Sperduti, I.; Giannarelli, D.; Lucarelli, G.; Borghesi, M.; Musi, G.; et al. The Prognostic Role of Circulating Tumor Cells (CTC) in High-risk Non–muscle-invasive Bladder Cancer. *Clin. Genitourin. Cancer* **2017**, *15*, e661–e666. [CrossRef] [PubMed]

78. Leon, S.A.; Shapiro, B.; Sklaroff, D.M.; Yaros, M.J. Free DNA in the serum of cancer patients and the effect of therapy. *Cancer Res.* **1977**, *37*, 646–650. [PubMed]

79. Thierry, A.R.; Messaoudi, S.E.; Gahan, P.B.; Anker, P.; Stroun, M. Origins, structures, and functions of circulating DNA in oncology. *Cancer Metastasis Rev.* **2016**, *35*, 347–376. [CrossRef] [PubMed]

80. Sun, K.; Jiang, P.; Chan, K.C.A.; Wong, J.; Cheng, Y.K.Y.; Liang, R.H.S.; Chan, W.; Ma, E.S.K.; Chan, S.L.; Cheng, S.H.; et al. Plasma DNA tissue mapping by genome-wide methylation sequencing for noninvasive prenatal, cancer, and transplantation assessments. *Proc. Natl. Acad. Sci. USA* **2015**, *112*, E5503–E5512. [CrossRef] [PubMed]

81. Stroun, M.; Anker, P.; Maurice, P.; Lyautey, J.; Lederrey, C.; Beljanski, M. Neoplastic Characteristics of the DNA Found in the Plasma of Cancer Patients. *Oncology* **1989**, *46*, 318–322. [CrossRef] [PubMed]

82. Sidransky, D.; Von Eschenbach, A.; Tsai, Y.C.; Jones, P.; Summerhayes, I.; Marshall, F.; Paul, M.; Green, P.; Hamilton, S.R.; Frost, P. Identification of p53 gene mutations in bladder cancers and urine samples. *Science* **1991**, *252*, 706–709. [CrossRef]

83. Sorenson, G.D.; Pribish, D.M.; Valone, F.H.; Memoli, V.A.; Bzik, D.J.; Yao, S.L. Soluble Normal and Mutated Dna-Sequences from Single-Copy Genes in Human Blood. *Cancer Epidemiol. Biomark. Prev.* **1994**, *3*, 67–71.

84. Parkinson, C.A.; Gale, D.; Piskorz, A.M.; Biggs, H.; Hodgkin, C.; Addley, H.; Freeman, S.; Moyle, P.; Sala, E.; Sayal, K.; et al. Exploratory Analysis of TP53 Mutations in Circulating Tumour DNA as Biomarkers of Treatment Response for Patients with Relapsed High-Grade Serous Ovarian Carcinoma: A Retrospective Study. *PLoS Med.* **2016**, *13*, e1002198. [CrossRef] [PubMed]

85. Vandekerkhove, G.; Todenhöfer, T.; Annala, M.; Struss, W.J.; Wong, A.; Beja, K.; Ritch, E.; Brahmbhatt, S.; Volik, S.V.; Hennenlotter, J.; et al. Circulating tumor DNA reveals clinically actionable somatic genome of metastatic bladder cancer. *Clin. Cancer Res.* **2017**, *23*, 6487–6497. [CrossRef] [PubMed]

86. Todenhöfer, T.; Struss, W.J.; Seiler, R.; Wyatt, A.W.; Black, P.C. Liquid Biopsy-Analysis of Circulating Tumor DNA (ctDNA) in Bladder Cancer. *Bladder Cancer* **2018**, *4*, 19–29. [CrossRef] [PubMed]

87. Hegemann, M.; Stenzl, A.; Bedke, J.; Chi, K.N.; Black, P.C.; Todenhöfer, T. Liquid biopsy: Ready to guide therapy in advanced prostate cancer? *BJU Int.* **2016**, *118*, 855–863. [CrossRef] [PubMed]

88. Alix-Panabieres, C.; Pantel, K. Clinical Applications of Circulating Tumor Cells and Circulating Tumor DNA as Liquid Biopsy. *Cancer Discov.* **2016**, *6*, 479–491. [CrossRef] [PubMed]

89. Swisher, E.M.; Wollan, M.; Mahtani, S.M.; Willner, J.B.; Garcia, R.; Goff, B.A.; King, M.-C. Tumor-specific p53 sequences in blood and peritoneal fluid of women with epithelial ovarian cancer. *Am. J. Obstet. Gynecol.* **2005**, *193*, 662–667. [CrossRef] [PubMed]

90. Kimura, H.; Kasahara, K.; Kawaishi, M.; Kunitoh, H.; Tamura, T.; Holloway, B.; Nishio, K. Detection of epidermal growth factor receptor mutations in serum as a predictor of the response to gefitinib in patients with non-small-cell lung cancer. *Clin. Cancer Res.* **2006**, *12*, 3915–3921. [CrossRef] [PubMed]

91. Sozzi, G.; Musso, K.; Ratliffe, C. Detection of microsatellite alterations in plasma DNA of non-small cell lung cancer patients: A prospect for early diagnosis. *Clin. Cancer Res.* **1999**, 2689–2692.

92. Diaz, L.A.; Bardelli, A.; Bardelli, A. Liquid biopsies: Genotyping circulating tumor DNA. *J. Clin. Oncol.* **2014**, *32*, 579–586. [CrossRef] [PubMed]

93. Forshew, T.; Murtaza, M.; Parkinson, C.; Gale, D.; Tsui, D.W.Y.; Kaper, F.; Dawson, S.-J.; Piskorz, A.M.; Jimenez-Linan, M.; Bentley, D.; et al. Noninvasive Identification and Monitoring of Cancer Mutations by Targeted Deep Sequencing of Plasma DNA. *Sci. Transl. Med.* **2012**, *4*, 136ra68. [CrossRef] [PubMed]

94. Leary, R.J.; Sausen, M.; Kinde, I.; Papadopoulos, N.; Carpten, J.D.; Craig, D.; O'shaughnessy, J.; Kinzler, K.W.; Parmigiani, G.; Vogelstein, B.; et al. Detection of Chromosomal Alterations in the Circulation of Cancer Patients with Whole-Genome Sequencing. *Sci. Transl. Med.* **2012**, *28*, 162ra154. [CrossRef] [PubMed]

95. Chan, K.C.A.; Jiang, P.; Zheng, Y.W.L.; Liao, G.J.W.; Sun, H.; Wong, J.; Siu, S.S.N.; Chan, W.C.; Chan, S.L.; Chan, A.T.C.; et al. Cancer genome scanning in plasma: Detection of tumor-associated copy number aberrations, single-nucleotide variants, and tumoral heterogeneity by massively parallel sequencing. *Clin. Chem.* **2013**, *59*, 211–224. [CrossRef] [PubMed]

96. Murtaza, M.; Dawson, S.-J.; Tsui, D.W.Y.; Gale, D.; Forshew, T.; Piskorz, A.M.; Parkinson, C.; Chin, S.-F.; Kingsbury, Z.; Wong, A.S.C.; et al. Non-invasive analysis of acquired resistance to cancer therapy by sequencing of plasma DNA. *Nature* **2013**, *497*, 108–112. [CrossRef] [PubMed]

97. Lebofsky, R.; Decraene, C.; Bernard, V.; Kamal, M.; Blin, A.; Leroy, Q.; Rio Frio, T.; Pierron, G.; Callens, C.; Bieche, I.; et al. Circulating tumor DNA as a non-invasive substitute to metastasis biopsy for tumor genotyping and personalized medicine in a prospective trial across all tumor types. *Mol. Oncol.* **2015**, *9*, 783–790. [CrossRef] [PubMed]

98. Olsson, E.; Winter, C.; George, A.; Chen, Y.; Howlin, J.; Eric Tang, M.-H.; Dahlgren, M.; Schulz, R.; Grabau, D.; van Westen, D.; et al. Serial monitoring of circulating tumor DNA in patients with primary breast cancer for detection of occult metastatic disease. *EMBO Mol. Med.* **2015**, *7*, 1034–1047. [CrossRef] [PubMed]

99. Diehl, F.; Li, M.; Dressman, D.; He, Y.; Shen, D.; Szabo, S.; Diaz, L.A.; Goodman, S.N.; David, K.A.; Juhl, H.; et al. Detection and quantification of mutations in the plasma of patients with colorectal tumors. *Proc. Natl. Acad. Sci. USA* **2005**, *102*, 16368–16373. [CrossRef] [PubMed]

100. Li, M.; Diehl, F.; Dressman, D.; Vogelstein, B.; Kinzler, K.W. BEAMing up for detection and quantification of rare sequence variants. *Nat. Methods* **2006**, *3*, 95–97. [CrossRef] [PubMed]

101. Newman, A.M.; Bratman, S.V.; To, J.; Wynne, J.F.; Eclov, N.C.W.; Modlin, L.A.; Liu, C.L.; Neal, J.W.; Wakelee, H.A.; Merritt, R.E.; et al. An ultrasensitive method for quantitating circulating tumor DNA with broad patient coverage. *Nat. Med.* **2014**, *20*, 548–554. [CrossRef] [PubMed]

102. Patel, K.M.; Van Der Vos, K.E.; Smith, C.G.; Mouliere, F.; Tsui, D.; Morris, J.; Chandrananda, D.; Marass, F.; Van Den Broek, D.; Neal, D.E.; et al. Association of plasma and urinary mutant DNA with clinical outcomes in muscle invasive bladder cancer. *Sci. Rep.* **2017**, *7*. [CrossRef] [PubMed]

103. Christensen, E.; Birkenkamp-Demtröder, K.; Nordentoft, I.; Høyer, S.; van der Keur, K.; van Kessel, K.; Zwarthoff, E.; Agerbæk, M.; Ørntoft, T.F.; Jensen, J.B.; et al. Liquid Biopsy Analysis of FGFR3 and PIK3CA Hotspot Mutations for Disease Surveillance in Bladder Cancer. *Eur. Urol.* **2017**, *71*, 961–969. [CrossRef] [PubMed]

104. Gormally, E.; Vineis, P.; Matullo, G.; Veglia, F.; Caboux, E.; Le Roux, E.; Peluso, M.; Garte, S.; Guarrera, S.; Munnia, A.; et al. *TP53* and *KRAS2* Mutations in Plasma DNA of Healthy Subjects and Subsequent Cancer Occurrence: A Prospective Study. *Cancer Res.* **2006**, *66*, 6871–6876. [CrossRef] [PubMed]

105. Utting, M.; Werner, W.; Dahse, R.; Schubert, J.; Junker, K. Microsatellite analysis of free tumor DNA in urine, serum, and plasma of patients: A minimally invasive method for the detection of bladder cancer. *Clin. Cancer Res.* **2002**, *8*, 35–40. [PubMed]

106. Christensen, M.; Wolf, H.; Orntoft, T.F. Microsatellite alterations in urinary sediments from patients with cystitis and bladder cancer. *Int. J. Cancer* **2000**, *85*, 614–617. [CrossRef]

107. Domínguez, G.; Carballido, J.; Silva, J.; Silva, J.M.; Garcı, J.M.; Mene, J. p14ARF Promoter Hypermethylation in Plasma DNA as an Indicator of Disease Recurrence in Bladder Cancer Patients Advances in Brief p14ARF Promoter Hypermethylation in Plasma DNA as an Indicator of Disease Recurrence in Bladder. *Clin. Cancer Res.* **2002**, *8*, 980–985. [PubMed]

108. Dahse, R.; Utting, M.; Werner, W.; Schimmel, B.; Claussen, U.; Junker, K. TP53 alterations as a potential diagnostic marker in superficial bladder carcinoma and in patients serum, plasma and urine samples. *Int. J. Oncol.* **2002**, *20*, 107–115. [CrossRef] [PubMed]

109. Wang, Y.; Yu, Y.; Ye, R.; Zhang, D.; Li, Q.; An, D.; Fang, L.; Lin, Y.; Hou, Y.; Xu, A.; et al. An epigenetic biomarker combination of PCDH17 and POU4F2 detects bladder cancer accurately by methylation analyses of urine sediment DNA in Han Chinese. *Oncotarget* **2016**, *7*, 2754–2764. [CrossRef] [PubMed]

110. Renard, I.; Joniau, S.; van Cleynenbreugel, B.; Collette, C.; Naômé, C.; Vlassenbroeck, I.; Nicolas, H.; de Leval, J.; Straub, J.; Van Criekinge, W.; et al. Identification and Validation of the Methylated TWIST1 and NID2 Genes through Real-Time Methylation-Specific Polymerase Chain Reaction Assays for the Noninvasive Detection of Primary Bladder Cancer in Urine Samples. *Eur. Urol.* **2010**, *58*, 96–104. [CrossRef] [PubMed]

111. Dulaimi, E.; Uzzo, R.G.; Greenberg, R.E.; Al-Saleem, T.; Cairns, P. Detection of bladder cancer in urine by a tumor suppressor gene hypermethylation panel. *Clin. Cancer Res.* **2004**, *10*, 1887–1893. [CrossRef] [PubMed]

112. Hoque, M.O.; Begum, S.; Topaloglu, O.; Chatterjee, A.; Rosenbaum, E.; Van Criekinge, W.; Westra, W.H.; Schoenberg, M.; Zahurak, M.; Goodman, S.N.; et al. Quantitation of Promoter Methylation of Multiple Genes in Urine DNA and Bladder Cancer Detection. *JNCI J. Natl. Cancer Inst.* **2006**, *98*, 996–1004. [CrossRef] [PubMed]

113. Ellinger, J.; El Kassem, N.; Heukamp, L.C.; Matthews, S.; Cubukluoz, F.; Kahl, P.; Perabo, F.G.; Müller, S.C.; von Ruecker, A.; Bastian, P.J. Hypermethylation of Cell-Free Serum DNA Indicates Worse Outcome in Patients With Bladder Cancer. *J. Urol.* **2008**, *179*, 346–352. [CrossRef] [PubMed]

114. Kim, Y.K.; Kim, W.J. Epigenetic markers as promising prognosticators for bladder cancer. *Int. J. Urol.* **2009**, *16*, 17–22. [CrossRef] [PubMed]

115. Kitchen, M.O.; Bryan, R.T.; Emes, R.D.; Luscombe, C.J.; Cheng, K.; Zeegers, M.P.; James, N.D.; Gommersall, L.M.; Fryer, A.A. HumanMethylation450K Array–Identified Biomarkers Predict Tumour Recurrence/Progression at Initial Diagnosis of High-risk Non-muscle Invasive Bladder Cancer. *Biomark. Cancer* **2018**, *10*. [CrossRef] [PubMed]

116. Phé, V.; Cussenot, O.; Rouprêt, M. Interest of methylated genes as biomarkers in urothelial cell carcinomas of the urinary tract. *BJU Int.* **2009**, *104*, 896–901. [CrossRef] [PubMed]

117. Lotan, Y.; Bensalah, K.; Ruddell, T.; Shariat, S.F.; Sagalowsky, A.I.; Ashfaq, R. Prospective Evaluation of the Clinical Usefulness of Reflex Fluorescence In Situ Hybridization Assay in Patients With Atypical Cytology for the Detection of Urothelial Carcinoma of the Bladder. *J. Urol.* **2008**, *179*, 2164–2169. [CrossRef] [PubMed]

118. Funaki, N.O.; Tanaka, J.; Kasamatsu, T.; Ohshio, G.; Hosotani, R.; Okino, T.; Imamura, M. Identification of carcinoembryonic antigen mRNA in circulating peripheral blood of pancreatic carcinoma and gastric carcinoma patients. *Life Sci.* **1996**, *59*, 2187–2199. [CrossRef]

119. Lo, K.W.; Lo, Y.M.; Leung, S.F.; Tsang, Y.S.; Chan, L.Y.; Johnson, P.J.; Hjelm, N.M.; Lee, J.C.; Huang, D.P. Analysis of cell-free Epstein-Barr virus associated RNA in the plasma of patients with nasopharyngeal carcinoma. *Clin. Chem.* **1999**, *45*, 1292–1294. [PubMed]

120. Kopreski, M.S.; Benko, F.A.; Kwak, L.W.; Gocke, C.D. Detection of tumor messenger RNA in the serum of patients with malignant melanoma. *Clin. Cancer Res.* **1999**, *5*, 1961–1965. [PubMed]

121. Silva, J.; García, V.; García, J.M.; Peña, C.; Domínguez, G.; Díaz, R.; Lorenzo, Y.; Hurtado, A.; Sánchez, A.; Bonilla, F. Circulating *Bmi-1* mRNA as a possible prognostic factor for advanced breast cancer patients. *Breast Cancer Res.* **2007**, *9*, R55. [CrossRef] [PubMed]

122. García, V.; García, J.M.; Peña, C.; Silva, J.; Domínguez, G.; Lorenzo, Y.; Diaz, R.; Espinosa, P.; de Sola, J.G.; Cantos, B.; Bonilla, F. Free circulating mRNA in plasma from breast cancer patients and clinical outcome. *Cancer Lett.* **2008**, *263*, 312–320. [CrossRef] [PubMed]

123. Garcia, V.; Garcia, J.M.; Silva, J.; Martin, P.; Peña, C.; Dominguez, G.; Diaz, R.; Herrera, M.; Maximiano, C.; Sabin, P.; et al. Extracellular Tumor-Related mRNA in Plasma of Lymphoma Patients and Survival Implications. *PLoS ONE* **2009**, *4*, e8173. [CrossRef] [PubMed]

124. March-Villalba, J.A.; Martínez-Jabaloyas, J.M.; Herrero, M.J.; Santamaria, J.; Aliño, S.F.; Dasí, F. Cell-Free Circulating Plasma hTERT mRNA Is a Useful Marker for Prostate Cancer Diagnosis and Is Associated with Poor Prognosis Tumor Characteristics. *PLoS ONE* **2012**, *7*, e43470. [CrossRef] [PubMed]

125. Deligezer, U.; Erten, N.; Akisik, E.E.; Dalay, N. Circulating fragmented nucleosomal DNA and caspase-3 mRNA in patients with lymphoma and myeloma. *Exp. Mol. Pathol.* **2006**, *80*, 72–76. [CrossRef] [PubMed]

126. Reddi, K.K.; Holland, J.F. Elevated serum ribonuclease in patients with pancreatic cancer. *Proc. Natl. Acad. Sci. USA* **1976**, *73*, 2308–2310. [CrossRef] [PubMed]

127. Chomczynski, P.; Wilfinger, W.W.; Eghbalnia, H.R.; Kennedy, A.; Rymaszewski, M.; Mackey, K. Inter-Individual Differences in RNA Levels in Human Peripheral Blood. *PLoS ONE* **2016**, *11*, e0148260. [CrossRef] [PubMed]

128. Malentacchi, F.; Vinci, S.; Della Melina, A.; Kuncova, J.; Villari, D.; Nesi, G.; Selli, C.; Orlando, C.; Pazzagli, M.; Pinzani, P. Urinary carbonic anhydrase IX splicing messenger RNA variants in urogenital cancers. *Urol. Oncol. Semin. Orig. Investig.* **2016**, *34*, 292.e9–292.e16. [CrossRef] [PubMed]

129. Kim, W.T.; Jeong, P.; Yan, C.; Kim, Y.H.; Lee, I.-S.; Kang, H.-W.; Kim, Y.-J.; Lee, S.-C.; Kim, S.J.; Kim, Y.T.; et al. UBE2C cell-free RNA in urine can discriminate between bladder cancer and hematuria. *Oncotarget* **2016**, *7*, 58193–58202. [CrossRef] [PubMed]

130. Guo, B.; Luo, C.; Xun, C.; Xie, J.; Wu, X.; Pu, J. Quantitative detection of cytokeratin 20 mRNA in urine samples as diagnostic tools for bladder cancer by real-time PCR. *Exp. Oncol.* **2009**, *31*, 43–47. [PubMed]

131. Bacchetti, T.; Sartini, D.; Pozzi, V.; Cacciamani, T.; Ferretti, G.; Emanuelli, M. Exploring the role of Paraoxonase-2 in bladder cancer: Analyses performed on tissue samples, urines and cell culturess. *Oncotarget* **2017**, *8*, 28785–28795. [CrossRef] [PubMed]

132. Urquidi, V.; Goodison, S.; Cai, Y.; Sun, Y.; Rosser, C.J. A Candidate Molecular Biomarker Panel for the Detection of Bladder Cancer. *Cancer Epidemiol. Biomark. Prev.* **2012**, *21*, 2149–2158. [CrossRef] [PubMed]

133. Mengual, L.; Burset, M.; Ribal, M.J.; Ars, E.; Marin-Aguilera, M.; Fernandez, M.; Ingelmo-Torres, M.; Villavicencio, H.; Alcaraz, A. Gene Expression Signature in Urine for Diagnosing and Assessing Aggressiveness of Bladder Urothelial Carcinoma. *Clin. Cancer Res.* **2010**, *16*, 2624–2633. [CrossRef] [PubMed]

134. Urquidi, V.; Netherton, M.; Gomes-Giacoia, E.; Serie, D.; Eckel-Passow, J.; Rosser, C.J.; Goodison, S. Urinary mRNA biomarker panel for the detection of urothelial carcinoma. *Oncotarget* **2016**, *7*, 38731–38740. [CrossRef] [PubMed]

135. Kavalieris, L.; O'Sullivan, P.; Frampton, C.; Guilford, P.; Darling, D.; Jacobson, E.; Suttie, J.; Raman, J.D.; Shariat, S.F.; Lotan, Y. Performance Characteristics of a Multigene Urine Biomarker Test for Monitoring for Recurrent Urothelial Carcinoma in a Multicenter Study. *J. Urol.* **2017**, *197*, 1419–1426. [CrossRef] [PubMed]

136. Goodison, S.; Rosser, C.J. Bladder Cancer Detection Composition Kit, and Associated Methods. Google Patents WO2014042763A1, 18 July 2013.

137. Martínez-Fernández, M.; Paramio, J.M.; Dueñas, M. RNA Detection in Urine: From RNA Extraction to Good Normalizer Molecules. *J. Mol. Diagn.* **2016**, *18*, 15–22. [CrossRef] [PubMed]

138. Romero-Cordoba, S.L.; Salido-Guadarrama, I.; Rodriguez-Dorantes, M.; Hidalgo-Miranda, A. miRNA biogenesis: Biological impact in the development of cancer. *Cancer Biol. Ther.* **2014**, *15*, 1444–1455. [CrossRef] [PubMed]

139. Chan, B.; Manley, J.; Lee, J.; Singh, S.R. The emerging roles of microRNAs in cancer metabolism. *Cancer Lett.* **2015**, *356*, 301–308. [CrossRef] [PubMed]

140. Liang, Y.; Ridzon, D.; Wong, L.; Chen, C. Characterization of microRNA expression profiles in normal human tissues. *BMC Genom.* **2007**, *8*, 166. [CrossRef] [PubMed]

141. Ge, Q.; Zhou, Y.; Lu, J.; Bai, Y.; Xie, X.; Lu, Z. miRNA in Plasma Exosome is Stable under Different Storage Conditions. *Molecules* **2014**, *19*, 1568–1575. [CrossRef] [PubMed]

142. Mitchell, P.S.; Parkin, R.K.; Kroh, E.M.; Fritz, B.R.; Wyman, S.K.; Pogosova-Agadjanyan, E.L.; Peterson, A.; Noteboom, J.; O'Briant, K.C.; Allen, A.; et al. Circulating microRNAs as stable blood-based markers for cancer detection. *Proc. Natl. Acad. Sci. USA* **2008**, *105*, 10513–10518. [CrossRef] [PubMed]

143. Weber, J.A.; Baxter, D.H.; Zhang, S.; Huang, D.Y.; How Huang, K.; Jen Lee, M.; Galas, D.J.; Wang, K. The MicroRNA Spectrum in 12 Body Fluids. *Clin. Chem.* **2010**, *56*, 1733–1741. [CrossRef] [PubMed]

144. Yun, S.J.; Jeong, P.; Kim, W.-T.; Kim, T.H.; Lee, Y.-S.; Song, P.H.; Choi, Y.-H.; Kim, I.Y.; Moon, S.-K.; Kim, W.-J.; et al. Cell-free microRNAs in urine as diagnostic and prognostic biomarkers of bladder cancer. *Int. J. Oncol.* **2012**, *41*, 1871–1878. [CrossRef] [PubMed]

145. Zhou, X.; Zhang, X.; Yang, Y.; Li, Z.; Du, L.; Dong, Z.; Qu, A.; Jiang, X.; Li, P.; Wang, C. Urinary cell-free microRNA-106b as a novel biomarker for detection of bladder cancer. *Med. Oncol.* **2014**, *31*, 197. [CrossRef] [PubMed]

146. Sasaki, H.; Yoshiike, M.; Nozawa, S.; Usuba, W.; Katsuoka, Y.; Aida, K.; Kitajima, K.; Kudo, H.; Hoshikawa, M.; Yoshioka, Y.; et al. Expression Level of Urinary MicroRNA-146a-5p Is Increased in Patients With Bladder Cancer and Decreased in Those After Transurethral Resection. *Clin. Genitourin. Cancer* **2016**, *14*, e493–e499. [CrossRef] [PubMed]

147. Puerta-Gil, P.; García-Baquero, R.; Jia, A.Y.; Ocaña, S.; Alvarez-Múgica, M.; Alvarez-Ossorio, J.L.; Cordon-Cardo, C.; Cava, F.; Sánchez-Carbayo, M. miR-143, miR-222, and miR-452 Are Useful as Tumor Stratification and Noninvasive Diagnostic Biomarkers for Bladder Cancer. *Am. J. Pathol.* **2012**, *180*, 1808–1815. [CrossRef] [PubMed]

148. Hanke, M.; Hoefig, K.; Merz, H.; Feller, A.C.; Kausch, I.; Jocham, D.; Warnecke, J.M.; Sczakiel, G. A robust methodology to study urine microRNA as tumor marker: MicroRNA-126 and microRNA-182 are related to urinary bladder cancer. *Urol. Oncol. Semin. Orig. Investig.* **2010**, *28*, 655–661. [CrossRef] [PubMed]

149. Kim, S.M.; Kang, H.W.; Kim, W.T.; Kim, Y.-J.; Yun, S.J.; Lee, S.-C.; Kim, W.-J. Cell-Free microRNA-214 From Urine as a Biomarker for Non-Muscle-Invasive Bladder Cancer. *Korean J. Urol.* **2013**, *54*, 791. [CrossRef] [PubMed]

150. Zhang, X.; Zhang, Y.; Liu, X.; Fang, A.; Wang, J.; Yang, Y.; Wang, L.; Du, L.; Wang, C.; Zhang, X.; et al. Direct quantitative detection for cell-free miR-155 in urine: A potential role in diagnosis and prognosis for non-muscle invasive bladder cancer. *Oncotarget* **2016**, *7*, 3255–3266. [CrossRef] [PubMed]

151. Ingelmo-Torres, M.; Lozano, J.J.; Izquierdo, L.; Carrion, A.; Costa, M.; Gomez, L.; Ribal, M.J.; Alcaraz, A.; Mengual, L. Urinary cell microRNA-based prognostic classifier for non-muscle invasive bladder cancer. *Oncotarget* **2017**, *8*, 18238–18247. [CrossRef] [PubMed]

152. Yang, Y.; Qu, A.; Liu, J.; Wang, R.; Liu, Y.; Li, G.; Duan, W.; Fang, Q.; Jiang, X.; Wang, L.; et al. Serum miR-210 Contributes to Tumor Detection, Stage Prediction and Dynamic Surveillance in Patients with Bladder Cancer. *PLoS ONE* **2015**, *10*, e0135168. [CrossRef] [PubMed]

153. Feng, Y.; Liu, J.; Kang, Y.; He, Y.; Liang, B.; Yang, P.; Yu, Z. miR-19a acts as an oncogenic microRNA and is up-regulated in bladder cancer. *J. Exp. Clin. Cancer Res.* **2014**, *33*, 67. [CrossRef] [PubMed]

154. Adam, L.; Wszolek, M.F.; Liu, C.-G.; Jing, W.; Diao, L.; Zien, A.; Zhang, J.D.; Jackson, D.; Dinney, C.P.N. Plasma microRNA profiles for bladder cancer detection. *Urol. Oncol. Semin. Orig. Investig.* **2013**, *31*, 1701–1708. [CrossRef] [PubMed]

155. Pardini, B.; Cordero, F.; Naccarati, A.; Viberti, C.; Birolo, G.; Oderda, M.; Di Gaetano, C.; Arigoni, M.; Martina, F.; Calogero, R.A.; et al. microRNA profiles in urine by next-generation sequencing can stratify bladder cancer subtypes. *Oncotarget* **2018**, *9*, 20658–20669. [CrossRef] [PubMed]

156. Wang, K.C.; Chang, H.Y. Molecular mechanisms of long noncoding RNAs. *Mol. Cell* **2011**, *43*, 904–914. [CrossRef] [PubMed]

157. Schmitt, A.M.; Chang, H.Y. Long Noncoding RNAs in Cancer Pathways. *Cancer Cell* **2016**, *29*, 452–463. [CrossRef] [PubMed]

158. Wang, X.-S.; Zhang, Z.; Wang, H.-C.; Cai, J.-L.; Xu, Q.-W.; Li, M.-Q.; Chen, Y.-C.; Qian, X.-P.; Lu, T.-J.; Yu, L.-Z.; et al. Rapid Identification of UCA1 as a Very Sensitive and Specific Unique Marker for Human Bladder Carcinoma. *Clin. Cancer Res.* **2006**, *12*, 4851–4858. [CrossRef] [PubMed]

159. Cui, X.; Jing, X.; Long, C.; Yi, Q.; Tian, J.; Zhu, J. Accuracy of the urine UCA1 for diagnosis of bladder cancer: A meta-analysis. *Oncotarget* **2017**, *8*, 35222–35233. [CrossRef] [PubMed]

160. Fan, Y.; Shen, B.; Tan, M.; Mu, X.; Qin, Y.; Zhang, F.; Liu, Y. Long non-coding RNA UCA1 increases chemoresistance of bladder cancer cells by regulating Wnt signaling. *FEBS J.* **2014**, *281*, 1750–1758. [CrossRef] [PubMed]

161. Berrondo, C.; Flax, J.; Kucherov, V.; Siebert, A.; Osinski, T.; Rosenberg, A.; Fucile, C.; Richheimer, S.; Beckham, C.J. Expression of the Long Non-Coding RNA HOTAIR Correlates with Disease Progression in Bladder Cancer and Is Contained in Bladder Cancer Patient Urinary Exosomes. *PLoS ONE* **2016**, *11*, e0147236. [CrossRef] [PubMed]

162. Chen, M.; Li, J.; Zhuang, C.; Cai, Z. Increased lncRNA ABHD11-AS1 represses the malignant phenotypes of bladder cancer. *Oncotarget* **2017**, *8*, 28176–28186. [CrossRef] [PubMed]

163. Ariel, I.; Sughayer, M.; Fellig, Y.; Pizov, G.; Ayesh, S.; Podeh, D.; Libdeh, B.A.; Levy, C.; Birman, T.; Tykocinski, M.L.; et al. The imprinted *H19* gene is a marker of early recurrence in human bladder carcinoma. *Mol. Pathol.* **2000**, *53*, 320–323. [CrossRef] [PubMed]

164. Sapre, N.; Macintyre, G.; Clarkson, M.; Naeem, H.; Cmero, M.; Kowalczyk, A.; Anderson, P.D.; Costello, A.J.; Corcoran, N.M.; Hovens, C.M. A urinary microRNA signature can predict the presence of bladder urothelial carcinoma in patients undergoing surveillance. *Br. J. Cancer* **2016**, *114*, 454–462. [CrossRef] [PubMed]

165. Jiang, X.; Du, L.; Wang, L.; Li, J.; Liu, Y.; Zheng, G.; Qu, A.; Zhang, X.; Pan, H.; Yang, Y.; et al. Serum microRNA expression signatures identified from genome-wide microRNA profiling serve as novel noninvasive biomarkers for diagnosis and recurrence of bladder cancer. *Int. J. Cancer* **2015**, *136*, 854–862. [CrossRef] [PubMed]

166. Jiang, X.; Du, L.; Duan, W.; Wang, R.; Yan, K.; Wang, L.; Li, J.; Zheng, G.; Zhang, X.; Yang, Y.; et al. Serum microRNA expression signatures as novel noninvasive biomarkers for prediction and prognosis of muscle-invasive bladder cancer. *Oncotarget* **2016**, *7*, 36733–36742. [CrossRef] [PubMed]

167. Du, L.; Jiang, X.; Duan, W.; Wang, R.; Wang, L.; Zheng, G.; Yan, K.; Wang, L.; Li, J.; Zhang, X.; et al. Cell-free microRNA expression signatures in urine serve as novel noninvasive biomarkers for diagnosis and recurrence prediction of bladder cancer. *Oncotarget* **2017**, *8*, 40832–40842. [CrossRef] [PubMed]

168. Urquidi, V.; Netherton, M.; Gomes-Giacoia, E.; Serie, D.J.; Eckel-Passow, J.; Rosser, C.J.; Goodison, S. A microRNA biomarker panel for the non-invasive detection of bladder cancer. *Oncotarget* **2016**, *7*, 86290–86299. [CrossRef] [PubMed]

169. Eissa, S.; Matboli, M.; Essawy, N.O.E.; Kotb, Y.M. Integrative functional genetic-epigenetic approach for selecting genes as urine biomarkers for bladder cancer diagnosis. *Tumor Biol.* **2015**, *36*, 9545–9552. [CrossRef] [PubMed]

170. Siomi, M.C.; Sato, K.; Pezic, D.; Aravin, A.A. PIWI-interacting small RNAs: The vanguard of genome defence. *Nat. Rev. Mol. Cell Biol.* **2011**, *12*, 246–258. [CrossRef] [PubMed]

171. Yuan, T.; Huang, X.; Woodcock, M.; Du, M.; Dittmar, R.; Wang, Y.; Tsai, S.; Kohli, M.; Boardman, L.; Patel, T.; et al. Plasma extracellular RNA profiles in healthy and cancer patients. *Sci. Rep.* **2016**, *6*, 19413. [CrossRef] [PubMed]

172. Freedman, J.E.; Gerstein, M.; Mick, E.; Rozowsky, J.; Levy, D.; Kitchen, R.; Das, S.; Shah, R.; Danielson, K.; Beaulieu, L.; et al. Diverse human extracellular RNAs are widely detected in human plasma. *Nat. Commun.* **2016**, *7*, 11106. [CrossRef] [PubMed]

173. Chu, H.; Hui, G.; Yuan, L.; Shi, D.; Wang, Y.; Du, M.; Zhong, D.; Ma, L.; Tong, N.; Qin, C.; et al. Identification of novel piRNAs in bladder cancer. *Cancer Lett.* **2015**, *356*, 561–567. [CrossRef] [PubMed]

174. Jeck, W.R.; Sharpless, N.E. Detecting and characterizing circular RNAs. *Nat. Biotechnol.* **2014**, *32*, 453–461. [CrossRef] [PubMed]

175. Kristensen, L.S.; Hansen, T.B.; Venø, M.T.; Kjems, J. Circular RNAs in cancer: Opportunities and challenges in the field. *Oncogene* **2018**, *37*, 555–565. [CrossRef] [PubMed]

176. Zhang, Y.; Liang, W.; Zhang, P.; Chen, J.; Qian, H.; Zhang, X.; Xu, W. Circular RNAs: Emerging cancer biomarkers and targets. *J. Exp. Clin. Cancer Res.* **2017**, *36*, 152. [CrossRef] [PubMed]

177. Zhong, Z.; Lv, M.; Chen, J. Screening differential circular RNA expression profiles reveals the regulatory role of circTCF25-miR-103a-3p/miR-107-CDK6 pathway in bladder carcinoma. *Sci. Rep.* **2016**, *6*, 30919. [CrossRef] [PubMed]

178. Zhong, Z.; Huang, M.; Lv, M.; He, Y.; Duan, C.; Zhang, L.; Chen, J. Circular RNA MYLK as a competing endogenous RNA promotes bladder cancer progression through modulating VEGFA/VEGFR2 signaling pathway. *Cancer Lett.* **2017**, *403*, 305–317. [CrossRef] [PubMed]

179. Huang, M.; Zhong, Z.; Lv, M.; Shu, J.; Tian, Q.; Chen, J. Comprehensive analysis of differentially expressed profiles of lncRNAs and circRNAs with associated co-expression and ceRNA networks in bladder carcinoma. *Oncotarget* **2016**, *7*, 47186–47200. [CrossRef] [PubMed]

180. Chander, Y.; Subramanya, H. Serological tumor markers—Their role. *Med. J. Armed Forces India* **2000**, *56*, 279–281. [CrossRef]

181. Bansal, N.; Gupta, A.K.; Gupta, A.; Sankhwar, S.N.; Mahdi, A.A. Serum-based protein biomarkers of bladder cancer: A pre- and post-operative evaluation. *J. Pharm. Biomed. Anal.* **2016**, *124*, 22–25. [CrossRef] [PubMed]

182. Bansal, N.; Gupta, A.; Sankhwar, S.N.; Mahdi, A.A. Low- and high-grade bladder cancer appraisal via serum-based proteomics approach. *Clin. Chim. Acta* **2014**, *436*, 97–103. [CrossRef] [PubMed]

183. Chen, Y.T.; Chen, C.L.; Chen, H.W.; Chung, T.; Wu, C.C.; Chen, C.D.; Hsu, C.W.; Chen, M.C.; Tsui, K.H.; Chang, P.L.; Chang, Y.S.; Yu, J.S. Discovery of novel bladder cancer biomarkers by comparative urine proteomics using iTRAQ technology. *J. Proteome Res.* **2010**, *11*, 5803–5815. [CrossRef] [PubMed]

184. Ebbing, J.; Mathia, S.; Seibert, F.S.; Pagonas, N.; Bauer, F.; Erber, B.; Günzel, K.; Kilic, E.; Kempkensteffen, C.; Miller, K.; et al. Urinary calprotectin: A new diagnostic marker in urothelial carcinoma of the bladder. *World J. Urol.* **2014**, *32*, 1485–1492. [CrossRef] [PubMed]

185. Zoidakis, J.; Makridakis, M.; Zerefos, P.G.; Bitsika, V.; Esteban, S.; Frantzi, M.; Stravodimos, K.; Anagnou, N.P.; Roubelakis, M.G.; Sanchez-Carbayo, M.; et al. Profilin 1 is a Potential Biomarker for Bladder Cancer Aggressiveness. *Mol. Cell. Proteom.* **2012**, *11*, M111.009449. [CrossRef] [PubMed]

186. Frantzi, M.; Zoidakis, J.; Papadopoulos, T.; Zürbig, P.; Katafigiotis, I.; Stravodimos, K.; Lazaris, A.; Giannopoulou, I.; Ploumidis, A.; Mischak, H.; et al. IMAC fractionation in combination with LC-MS reveals H2B and NIF-1 peptides as potential bladder cancer biomarkers. *J. Proteome Res.* **2013**, *12*, 3969–3979. [CrossRef] [PubMed]

187. Goodison, S.; Chang, M.; Dai, Y.; Urquidi, V.; Rosser, C.J. A Multi-Analyte Assay for the Non-Invasive Detection of Bladder Cancer. *PLoS ONE* **2012**, *7*, e47469. [CrossRef] [PubMed]

188. Rosser, C.J.; Ross, S.; Chang, M.; Dai, Y.; Mengual, L.; Zhang, G.; Kim, J.; Urquidi, V.; Alcaraz, A.; Goodison, S. Multiplex protein signature for the detection of bladder cancer in voided urine samples. *J. Urol.* **2013**, *190*, 2257–2262. [CrossRef] [PubMed]

189. Rosser, C.J.; Chang, M.; Dai, Y.; Ross, S.; Mengual, L.; Alcaraz, A.; Goodison, S. Urinary Protein Biomarker Panel for the Detection of Recurrent Bladder Cancer. *Cancer Epidemiol. Biomark. Prev.* **2014**, *23*, 247–253. [CrossRef] [PubMed]

190. Shimizu, Y.; Furuya, H.; Bryant Greenwood, P.; Chan, O.; Dai, Y.; Thornquist, M.D.; Goodison, S.; Rosser, C.J. A multiplex immunoassay for the non-invasive detection of bladder cancer. *J. Transl. Med.* **2016**, *14*, 31. [CrossRef] [PubMed]

191. Soukup, V.; Kalousová, M.; Capoun, O.; Sobotka, R.; Breyl, Z.; Pešl, M.; Zima, T.; Hanuš, T. Panel of Urinary Diagnostic Markers for Non-Invasive Detection of Primary and Recurrent Urothelial Urinary Bladder Carcinoma. *Urol. Int.* **2015**, *95*, 56–64. [CrossRef] [PubMed]

192. Jamshidian, H.; Kor, K.; Djalali, M. Urine concentration of nuclear matrix protein 22 for diagnosis of transitional cell carcinoma of bladder. *Urol. J.* **2008**, *5*, 243–247. [PubMed]

193. Soloway, M.S.; Briggman, V.; Carpinito, G.A.; Chodak, G.W.; Church, P.A.; Lamm, D.L.; Lange, P.; Messing, E.; Pasciak, R.M.; Reservitz, G.B.; et al. Use of a new tumor marker, urinary NMP22, in the detection of occult or rapidly recurring transitional cell carcinoma of the urinary tract following surgical treatment. *J. Urol.* **1996**, *156*, 363–367. [CrossRef]

194. Zippe, C.; Pandrangi, L.; Agarwal, A. NMP22 Is a Sensitive, Cost-Effective Test in Patients At Risk for Bladder Cancer. *J. Urol.* **1999**, *161*, 62–65. [CrossRef]

195. Theodorescu, D.; Wittke, S.; Ross, M.M.; Walden, M.; Conaway, M.; Just, I.; Mischak, H.; Frierson, H.F. Discovery and validation of new protein biomarkers for urothelial cancer: A prospective analysis. *Lancet Oncol.* **2006**, *7*, 230–240. [CrossRef]

196. Schiffer, E.; Vlahou, A.; Petrolekas, A.; Stravodimos, K.; Tauber, R.; Geschwend, J.E.; Neuhaus, J.; Stolzenburg, J.U.; Conaway, M.R.; Mischak, H.; et al. Prediction of muscle-invasive bladder cancer using urinary proteomics. *Clin. Cancer Res.* **2009**, *15*, 4935–4943. [CrossRef] [PubMed]

197. Frantzi, M.; Van Kessel, K.E.; Zwarthoff, E.C.; Marquez, M.; Rava, M.; Malats, N.; Merseburger, A.S.; Katafigiotis, I.; Stravodimos, K.; Mullen, W.; et al. Development and validation of urine-based peptide biomarker panels for detecting bladder cancer in a multi-center study. *Clin. Cancer Res.* **2016**, *22*, 4077–4086. [CrossRef] [PubMed]

198. Chen, C.L.; Lai, Y.F.; Tang, P.; Chien, K.Y.; Yu, J.S.; Tsai, C.H.; Chen, H.W.; Wu, C.C.; Chung, T.; Hsu, C.W.; et al. Comparative and targeted proteomic analyses of urinary microparticles from bladder cancer and hernia patients. *J. Proteome Res.* **2012**, *11*, 5611–5629. [CrossRef] [PubMed]

199. Yang, N.; Feng, S.; Shedden, K.; Xie, X.; Liu, Y.; Rosser, C.J.; Lubman, D.M.; Goodison, S. Urinary Glycoprotein Biomarker Discovery for Bladder Cancer Detection using LC-MS/MS and Label-free Quantification. *Clin. Cancer Res.* **2011**, *17*, 247–253. [CrossRef] [PubMed]

200. Lindén, M.; Lind, S.B.; Mayrhofer, C.; Segersten, U.; Wester, K.; Lyutvinskiy, Y.; Zubarev, R.; Malmström, P.U.; Pettersson, U. Proteomic analysis of urinary biomarker candidates for nonmuscle invasive bladder cancer. *Proteomics* **2012**, *12*, 135–144. [CrossRef] [PubMed]

201. Chen, C.L.; Lin, T.S.; Tsai, C.H.; Wu, C.C.; Chung, T.; Chien, K.Y.; Wu, M.; Chang, Y.S.; Yu, J.S.; Chen, Y.T. Identification of potential bladder cancer markers in urine by abundant-protein depletion coupled with quantitative proteomics. *J. Proteom.* **2013**, *85*, 28–43. [CrossRef] [PubMed]

202. Mischak, H.; Kolch, W.; Aivaliotis, M.; Bouyssié, D.; Dihazi, H.; Dihazi, G.H.; Franke, J.; Garin, J.; Gonzalez, A.; Peredo, D.; et al. Comprehensive human urine standards for comparability and standardization in clinical proteome analysis. *Proteom. Clin. Appl.* **2010**, *4*, 464–478. [CrossRef] [PubMed]

203. Miyake, M.; Morizawa, Y.; Hori, S.; Tatsumi, Y.; Onishi, S.; Owari, T.; Iida, K.; Onishi, K.; Gotoh, D.; Nakai, Y.; et al. Diagnostic and prognostic role of urinary collagens in primary human bladder cancer. *Cancer Sci.* **2017**, *108*, 2221–2228. [CrossRef] [PubMed]

204. Urquidi, V.; Kim, J.; Chang, M.; Dai, Y.; Rosser, C.J.; Goodison, S. CCL18 in a multiplex urine-based assay for the detection of bladder cancer. *PLoS ONE* **2012**, *7*, e37797. [CrossRef] [PubMed]

205. Hwang, E.C.; Choi, H.S.; Jung, S., II; Kwon, D.D.; Park, K.; Ryu, S.B. Use of the NMP22 BladderChek test in the diagnosis and follow-up of urothelial cancer: A cross-sectional study. *Urology* **2011**, *77*, 154–159. [CrossRef] [PubMed]

206. Barton Grossman, H.; Soloway, M.; Messing, E.; Katz, G.; Stein, B.; Kassabian, V.; Shen, Y. Surveillance for recurrent bladder cancer using a point-of-care proteomic assay. *J. Am. Med. Assoc.* **2006**, *295*, 299–305. [CrossRef] [PubMed]

207. Grossman, H. Detection of bladder cancer using a proteomic assay. *JAMA* **2005**, *293*, 2467. [CrossRef] [PubMed]

208. Kinders, R.; Jones, T.; Root, R.; Bruce, C.; Murchison, H.; Corey, M.; Williams, L.; Enfield, D.; Hass, G.M. Complement factor H or a related protein is a marker for transitional cell cancer of the bladder. *Clin. Cancer Res.* **1998**, *4*, 2511–2520. [PubMed]

209. Malkowicz, S.B. The application of human complement factor H-related protein (BTA TRAK) in monitoring patients with bladder cancer. *Urol. Clin. N. Am.* **2000**, *27*, 63–73. [CrossRef]

210. Guo, A.; Wang, X.; Gao, L.; Shi, J.; Sun, C.; Wan, Z. Bladder tumour antigen (BTA stat) test compared to the urine cytology in the diagnosis of bladder cancer: A meta-analysis. *J. Can. Urol. Assoc.* **2014**, *8*, E347. [CrossRef] [PubMed]

211. Raitanen, M. The role of BTA stat test in follow-up of patients with bladder cancer: Results from Finn Bladder studies. *World J. Urol.* **2008**, *26*, 45–50. [CrossRef] [PubMed]

212. Jeong, S.; Park, Y.; Cho, Y.; Kim, Y.R.; Kim, H.S. Diagnostic values of urine CYFRA21-1, NMP22, UBC, and FDP for the detection of bladder cancer. *Clin. Chim. Acta* **1970**, *414*, 93–100. [CrossRef] [PubMed]

213. Nisman, B.; Yutkin, V.; Peretz, T.; Shapiro, A.; Barak, V.; Pode, D. The follow-up of patients with non-muscle-invasive bladder cancer by urine cytology, abdominal ultrasound and urine CYFRA 21-1: A pilot study. *Anticancer Res.* **2009**, *29*, 4281–4285. [PubMed]

214. Fernandez-Gomez, J.; Rodríguez-Martínez, J.J.; Barmadah, S.E.; García Rodríguez, J.; Allende, D.M.; Jalon, A.; Gonzalez, R.; Álvarez-Múgica, M. Urinary CYFRA 21.1 Is Not a Useful Marker for the Detection of Recurrences in the Follow-Up of Superficial Bladder Cancer. *Eur. Urol.* **2007**, *51*, 1267–1274. [CrossRef] [PubMed]

215. Hakenberg, O.W.; Fuessel, S.; Richter, K.; Froehner, M.; Oehlschlaeger, S.; Rathert, P.; Meye, A.; Wirth, M.P. Qualitative and quantitative assessment of urinary cytokeratin 8 and 18 fragments compared with voided urine cytology in diagnosis of bladder carcinoma. *Urology* **2004**, *64*, 1121–1126. [CrossRef] [PubMed]

216. Babjuk, M.; Koštířová, M.; Mudra, K.; Pecher, S.; Smolová, H.; Pecen, L.; Ibrahim, Z.; Dvořáček, J.; Jarolím, L.; Novák, J.; Zima, T. Qualitative and quantitative detection of urinary human complement factor H-related protein (BTA stat and BTA TRAK) and fragments of cytokeratins 8, 18 (UBC rapid and UBC IRMA) as markers for transitional cell carcinoma of the bladder. *Eur. Urol.* **2002**, *41*, 34–39. [CrossRef]

217. Cheng, Y.; Yang, X.; Deng, X.; Zhang, X.; Li, P.; Tao, J.; Qin, C.; Wei, J.; Lu, Q. Metabolomics in bladder cancer: A systematic review. *Int. J. Clin. Exp. Med.* **2015**, *8*, 11052–11063. [PubMed]

218. Bauça, J.M.; Martínez-Morillo, E.; Diamandis, E.P. Peptidomics of urine and other biofluids for cancer diagnostics. *Clin. Chem.* **2014**, *60*, 1052–1061. [CrossRef] [PubMed]

219. Jin, X.; Yun, S.J.; Jeong, P.; Kim, I.Y.; Kim, W.-J.; Park, S. Diagnosis of bladder cancer and prediction of survival by urinary metabolomics. *Oncotarget* **2014**, *5*, 1635–1645. [CrossRef] [PubMed]

220. Zhou, Y.; Song, R.; Ma, C.; Zhou, L.; Liu, X.; Yin, P.; Zhang, Z.; Sun, Y.; Xu, C.; Lu, X.; et al. Discovery and validation of potential urinary biomarkers for bladder cancer diagnosis using a pseudotargeted GC-MS metabolomics method. *Oncotarget* **2017**, *8*, 20719–20728. [CrossRef] [PubMed]

221. Huang, Z.; Lin, L.; Gao, Y.; Chen, Y.; Yan, X.; Xing, J.; Hang, W. Bladder Cancer Determination Via Two Urinary Metabolites: A Biomarker Pattern Approach. *Mol. Cell. Proteom.* **2011**, *10*, mcp.M111.007922. [CrossRef] [PubMed]

222. Ganti, S.; Taylor, S.L.; Kim, K.; Hoppel, C.L.; Guo, L.; Yang, J.; Evans, C.; Weiss, R.H. Urinary acylcarnitines are altered in human kidney cancer. *Int. J. Cancer* **2012**, *130*, 2791–2800. [CrossRef] [PubMed]

223. Sahu, D.; Lotan, Y.; Wittmann, B.; Neri, B.; Hansel, D.E. Metabolomics analysis reveals distinct profiles of nonmuscle-invasive and muscle-invasive bladder cancer. *Cancer Med.* **2017**, *6*, 2106–2120. [CrossRef] [PubMed]

224. Madka, V.; Mohammed, A.; Li, Q.; Zhang, Y.; Patlolla, J.M.R.; Biddick, L.; Lightfoot, S.; Wu, X.R.; Steele, V.; Kopelovich, L.; et al. Chemoprevention of urothelial cell carcinoma growth and invasion by the dual COX-LOX inhibitor licofelone in UPII-SV40T transgenic mice. *Cancer Prev. Res.* **2014**, *7*, 708–716. [CrossRef] [PubMed]

225. Miyata, Y.; Kanda, S.; Mitsunari, K.; Asai, A.; Sakai, H. Heme oxygenase-1 expression is associated with tumor aggressiveness and outcomes in patients with bladder cancer: A correlation with smoking intensity. *Transl. Res.* **2014**, *164*, 468–476. [CrossRef] [PubMed]

226. Loras, A.; Trassierra, M.; Castell, J.V. Bladder cancer recurrence surveillance by urine metabolomics analysis. *Sci. Rep.* **2018**, *8*, 9172. [CrossRef] [PubMed]

227. Lin, L.; Huang, Z.; Gao, Y.; Chen, Y.; Hang, W.; Xing, J.; Yan, X. LC-MS-based serum metabolic profiling for genitourinary cancer classification and cancer type-specific biomarker discovery. *Proteomics* **2012**, *12*, 2238–2246. [CrossRef] [PubMed]

228. Rodrigues, D.; Jerónimo, C.; Henrique, R.; Belo, L.; de Lourdes Bastos, M.; de Pinho, P.G.; Carvalho, M. Biomarkers in bladder cancer: A metabolomic approach using in vitro and ex vivo model systems. *Int. J. Cancer* **2016**, *139*, 256–268. [CrossRef] [PubMed]

229. Franzen, C.A.; Blackwell, R.H.; Todorovic, V.; Greco, K.A.; Foreman, K.E.; Flanigan, R.C.; Kuo, P.C.; Gupta, G.N. Urothelial cells undergo epithelial-to-mesenchymal transition after exposure to muscle invasive bladder cancer exosomes. *Oncogenesis* **2015**, *4*, e163-10. [CrossRef] [PubMed]

230. Reclusa, P.; Taverna, S.; Pucci, M.; Durendez, E.; Calabuig, S.; Manca, P.; Serrano, M.J.; Sober, L.; Pauwels, P.; Russo, A.; et al. Exosomes as diagnostic and predictive biomarkers in lung cancer. *J. Thorac. Dis.* **2017**, *9*, S1373–S1382. [CrossRef] [PubMed]

231. Johnstone, R.M.; Adam, M.; Pan, B.T. The fate of the transferrin receptor during maturation of sheep reticulocytes in vitro. *Can. J. Biochem. Cell Biol.* **1984**, *62*, 1246–1254. [CrossRef] [PubMed]

232. Harding, C.; Heuser, J.; Stahl, P. Receptor-mediated endocytosis of transferrin and recycling of the transferrin receptor in rat reticulocytes. *J. Cell Biol.* **1983**, *97*, 329–339. [CrossRef] [PubMed]

233. Iero, M.; Valenti, R.; Huber, V.; Filipazzi, P.; Parmiani, G.; Fais, S.; Rivoltini, L. Tumour-released exosomes and their implications in cancer immunity. *Cell Death Differ.* **2008**, *15*, 80–88. [CrossRef] [PubMed]

234. Valenti, R.; Huber, V.; Iero, M.; Filipazzi, P.; Parmiani, G.; Rivoltini, L. Tumor-released microvesicles as vehicles of immunosuppression. *Cancer Res.* **2007**, *67*, 2912–2915. [CrossRef] [PubMed]

235. Silvers, C.R.; Miyamoto, H.; Messing, E.M.; Netto, G.J.; Lee, Y.-F. Characterization of urinary extracellular vesicle proteins in muscle-invasive bladder cancer. *Oncotarget* **2017**, *8*, 91199–91208. [CrossRef] [PubMed]

236. Baumgart, S.; Hölters, S.; Ohlmann, C.-H.; Bohle, R.; Stöckle, M.; Ostenfeld, M.S.; Dyrskjøt, L.; Junker, K.; Heinzelmann, J. Exosomes of invasive urothelial carcinoma cells are characterized by a specific miRNA expression signature. *Oncotarget* **2017**, *8*, 58278–58291. [CrossRef] [PubMed]

237. Mao, L.; Hruban, R.H.; Boyle, J.O.; Tockman, M.; Sidransky, D. Detection of Oncogene Mutations in Sputum Precedes Diagnosis of Lung Cancer Advances in Brief Detection of Oncogene Mutations in Sputum Precedes Diagnosis of Lung Cancer1. *Cancer* **1994**, *54*, 1634–1637.

238. Wyatt, A.W.; Annala, M.; Aggarwal, R.; Beja, K.; Feng, F.; Youngren, J.; Foye, A.; Lloyd, P.; Nykter, M.; Beer, T.M.; et al. Concordance of Circulating Tumor DNA and Matched Metastatic Tissue Biopsy in Prostate Cancer. *J. Natl. Cancer Inst.* **2017**, *109*, 78–86. [CrossRef] [PubMed]

239. Su, Y.-H.; Wang, M.; Brenner, D.E.; Ng, A.; Melkonyan, H.; Umansky, S.; Syngal, S.; Block, T.M. Human urine contains small, 150 to 250 nucleotide-sized, soluble DNA derived from the circulation and may be useful in the detection of colorectal cancer. *J. Mol. Diagn.* **2004**, *6*, 101–107. [CrossRef]

240. Peng, M.; Chen, C.; Hulbert, A.; Brock, M.V.; Yu, F. Non-blood circulating tumor DNA detection in cancer. *Oncotarget* **2017**, *8*, 69162–69173. [CrossRef] [PubMed]

241. Shao, C.-H.; Chen, C.-L.; Lin, J.-Y.; Chen, C.-J.; Fu, S.-H.; Chen, Y.-T.; Chang, Y.-S.; Yu, J.-S.; Tsui, K.-H.; Juo, C.-G.; et al. Metabolite marker discovery for the detection of bladder cancer by comparative metabolomics. *Oncotarget* **2017**, *8*, 38802–38810. [CrossRef] [PubMed]

242. Maher, A.D.; Zirah, S.F.M.; Holmes, E.; Nicholson, J.K. Experimental and Analytical Variation in Human Urine in ^{1}H NMR Spectroscopy-Based Metabolic Phenotyping Studies. *Anal. Chem.* **2007**, *79*, 5204–5211. [CrossRef] [PubMed]

243. Walsh, M.C.; Brennan, L.; Pujos-Guillot, E.; Sébédio, J.-L.; Scalbert, A.; Fagan, A.; Higgins, D.G.; Gibney, M.J. Influence of acute phytochemical intake on human urinary metabolomic profiles. *Am. J. Clin. Nutr.* **2007**, *86*, 1687–1693. [CrossRef] [PubMed]

244. Thoma, C. Bladder cancer: The promise of liquid biopsy ctDNA analysis. *Nat. Rev. Urol.* **2017**, *14*, 580–581. [CrossRef] [PubMed]

245. Yang, Y.; Miller, C.R.; Lopez-Beltran, A.; Montironi, R.; Cheng, M.; Zhang, S.; Koch, M.O.; Kaimakliotis, H.Z.; Cheng, L. Liquid Biopsies in the Management of Bladder Cancer: Next-Generation Biomarkers for Diagnosis, Surveillance, and Treatment-Response Prediction. *Crit. Rev. Oncog.* **2017**, *22*, 389–401. [CrossRef] [PubMed]

246. Chalfin, H.J.; Kates, M.; van der Toom, E.E.; Glavaris, S.; Verdone, J.E.; Hahn, N.M.; Pienta, K.J.; Bivalacqua, T.J.; Gorin, M.A. Characterization of Urothelial Cancer Circulating Tumor Cells with a Novel Selection-Free Method. *Urology* **2018**, *115*, 82–86. [CrossRef] [PubMed]

247. Pepe, M.S.; Etzioni, R.; Feng, Z.; Potter, J.D.; Thompson, M.L.; Thornquist, M.; Winget, M.; Yasui, Y. Phases of biomarker development for early detection of cancer. *J. Natl. Cancer Inst.* **2001**, *93*, 1054–1061. [CrossRef] [PubMed]

4

Histone Demethylase KDM7A Regulates Androgen Receptor Activity and its Chemical Inhibitor TC-E 5002 Overcomes Cisplatin-Resistance in Bladder Cancer Cells

Kyoung-Hwa Lee [1,†], Byung-Chan Kim [1,†], Seung-Hwan Jeong [2], Chang Wook Jeong [1], Ja Hyeon Ku [1], Hyeon Hoe Kim [1] and Cheol Kwak [1,3,*]

[1] Department of Urology, Seoul National University Hospital, Seoul 03080, Korea; lee12042@snu.ac.kr (K.-H.L.); dalkyal12@gmail.com (B.-C.K.); drboss@gmail.com (C.W.J.); randyku@hanmail.net (J.H.K.); hhkim@snu.ac.kr (H.H.K.)
[2] Graduate School of Medical Science and Engineering, Korea Advanced Institute of Science and Technology (KAIST), Daejeon 34052, Korea; 11shjeong@gmail.com
[3] Department of Urology, Seoul National University College of Medicine, Seoul 03080, Korea
* Correspondence: mdrafael@snu.ac.kr
† These authors contributed equally to this work.

Abstract: Histone demethylase KDM7A regulates many biological processes, including differentiation, development, and the growth of several cancer cells. Here, we have focused on the role of KDM7A in bladder cancer cells, especially under drug-resistant conditions. When the *KDM7A* gene was knocked down, bladder cancer cell lines showed impaired cell growth, increased cell death, and reduced rates of cell migration. Biochemical studies revealed that KDM7A knockdown in the bladder cancer cells repressed the activity of androgen receptor (AR) through epigenetic regulation. When we developed a cisplatin-resistant bladder cancer cell line, we found that AR expression was highly elevated. Upon treatment with TC-E 5002, a chemical inhibitor of KDM7A, the cisplatin-resistant bladder cancer cells, showed decreased cell proliferation. In the mouse xenograft model, KDM7A knockdown or treatment with its inhibitor reduced the growth of the bladder tumor. We also observed the upregulation of KDM7A expression in patients with bladder cancer. The findings suggest that histone demethylase KDM7A mediates the growth of bladder cancer. Moreover, our findings highlight the therapeutic potential of the KMD7A inhibitor, TC-E 5002, in patients with cisplatin-resistant bladder cancer.

Keywords: bladder cancer; KDM7A; histone demethylase; TC-E 5002; androgen receptor; drug resistance

1. Introduction

Bladder cancer (BCa) is one of the most common cancers in men, resulting in a reported 8470 new cases and over 17,670 deaths in the United States in 2019 [1]. BCa has a high prevalence of recurrence and metastatic spread, and the 5-year survival rate has remained relatively low, despite the advances in various surgical and chemotherapeutic treatment options [2]. The incidence of BCa is three times higher in men than women, and is the 4th and 11th most common cancer in men and women, respectively [3]. The variation in prevalence depending on gender has prompted a number of studies into the role of sex hormone receptors in BCa. Notably, emerging evidence has supported a role for the androgen receptor (AR) in BCa [4]. AR is a well-known transcription factor that responds to male sex hormones, and controls prostate cancer development and metastasis [5,6]. Recently, many studies have highlighted its role in other cancer types, including colon [7], breast [8], stomach [9], and bladder cancer [10–13]. A reduced incidence of N-butyl-N-(4-hydroxybutyl)-nitrosamine (BBN)-induced BCa has been reported in both full-body [14] as well as urothelial-specific [15] AR knock-out mice models. Recent preclinical studies have suggested that the androgen-mediated AR signaling promotes bladder cancer progression, and blocking this signaling with enzalutamide can strongly impair bladder cancer cell growth [16–18]. Another recent study has shed light on the role of the AR in cisplatin-resistant bladder cancer [19]. It is also reported that the anti-androgenic drug hydroxyflutamide increased cisplatin sensitivity in cisplatin-resistant bladder cancer cell line T24.

Since AR is a transcription factor, controlling its transcriptional activity can be a major target for anti-cancer drug development. Among the mechanisms known to regulate transcriptional activity, epigenetic regulation, including DNA methylation and histone modification, plays a key role in cancer development [20,21]. Specifically, histone methylation on lysine residues of histone H3 or H4 are known to modify transcriptional activity, depending on the residues modified. Methylation on lysine 4 (H3K4) or 36 (H3K36) is usually associated with transcriptional activation, while H3K9 and H3K27 methylation are frequently linked with gene silencing, and are hallmarks of chromatin condensation [22,23]. Each methylase and demethylase has specific target promoters; therefore, inhibitors can be used for targeting the regulation of a specific gene. Since the epigenetic modifications play important roles in cancer formation, malignancy, and metastasis, targeting the epigenetic enzymes would be a promising approach in cancer therapy. Indeed, epigenetic processes which control AR activity have been reported to play a role in prostate cancer development [24,25]. For the regulation of histone methylation on its target promoters, AR is known to interact with several enzymes, including LSD1, KDM4B, KDM5B, EZH2, SMYD3, PRMT5, and KDM7A [26–32].

Among the histone modifying enzymes, the enzyme KDM7A belongs to a family of plant homeodomain finger proteins, that contain a plant homeodomain (PHD) and a JmjC domain. The methyl groups of the lysine at positions 9 and 27 in histone 3 can be removed by the JmjC domain-containing family of proteins [33]. Since the methylation of H3K9 and H3K27 represent the repression of gene expression, their demethylation activates target gene transcription. Previous studies have shown that KDM7A regulates bone development, adipogenesis, inflammation, as well as the development of various types of cancers [34–36]. A recently published paper from our research group described the H3K27 demethylase activity of KDM7A on the response elements of AR target genes in prostate cancer [32]. The study presents a detailed account of the physical interaction of KDM7A with AR, using the immune-precipitation method. Furthermore, we found that KDM7A directly binds to the androgen response element (ARE) sequences of AR target genes, including KLK3, KLK2, and TMPRSS2. An increase in the histone H3K27 di-methylation of those ARE sequences and a decrease in the AR activity was also observed in KDM7A knockdown prostate cells. The existence of a KDM7A chemical inhibitor further highlighted the value of this data, owing to its clinical application as an anti-cancer drug.

In the present study, we have further investigated the role of KDM7A in the epigenetic regulation of AR in BCa, with a focus on the regulation of AR activity in the cisplatin-resistant bladder cancer cells.

2. Results

2.1. KDM7A Regulates AR Transcription Activity in Bladder Cancer Cells

In order to investigate the possible role of KDM7A demethylase in the functioning of AR in bladder cancer cells, we first compared the AR expression levels in various bladder cancer cell lines, including

253J, RT4, T24, and J82. As expected, the levels of AR mRNA and protein in bladder cancer cells were quite low compared to that in LNCaP prostate cancer cells (Supplemental Figure S1A,B). Nonetheless, we were able to detect AR mRNA and protein in the bladder cancer cells that we tested, with the levels found to be comparable among them. Since a previous study has reported the development of cisplatin-resistant T24 cells [19], we selected this cell line for our experiments. We also included another bladder cancer cell line, J82, in order to demonstrate data reproducibility. To analyze the function of KDM7A histone demethylase in bladder cancer cells, we produced KDM7A knock-down bladder cell lines (T24 and J82), using a lenti-viral shRNA expression system. After antibiotics selection, efficient knock-down of the gene expression was confirmed by Western blotting and reverse transcriptase quantitative PCR (RT-qPCR) (Figure 1A). Since KDM7A is known to regulate AR activity in prostate cancer cells [32], we speculated that it may control AR activity as an epigenetic regulator in bladder cancer cells. Our studies showed that the levels of both AR mRNA and protein were regulated by KDM7A, before and after dihydrotestosterone (DHT) induction (Figure 1B, Supplemental Figure S2), even though we had expected changes only in the protein activity. A possible explanation could be the autoregulatory effect of AR on its own promoter [37]. In order to measure AR activity in KDM7A knock-down cells, the expression of previously reported downstream target genes of AR was screened using RT-qPCR [38–43]. The relative mRNA levels of these genes, compared with those of LNCaP, are listed in Supplemental Figure S1C. The PCR signals of six genes (*KLK3, TMPRSS2, KLK4, IGF1R, VEGF,* and *MYC*) were successfully amplified in bladder cancer cell lines. The mRNA levels of these AR target genes were elevated after DHT treatment, and this induction was reduced in KDM7A knock-down stable cells (Figure 1C).

2.2. KDM7A Regulates AR Transcription Activity via Epigenetic Regulation of AR Target Gene Promoters

Next, we analyzed the histone methylation status in KDM7A knock-down cells. The cell extracts from each of the cell lines were analyzed with specific antibodies for diverse histone methylation sites (Figure 2A). Among the sites tested, only H3K27 di-methylated lysine was elevated in KDM7A knock-down cells. The AR activity can be measured as the extent of binding of AR onto target promoters. We, therefore, analyzed the binding efficiency of AR to its target promoters, using the chromatin immunoprecipitation (ChIP) experiment. The T24 bladder cancer cells expressing control or KDM7A shRNA were treated with DHT, sonicated, and the chromatin was precipitated with AR antibody. The promoter binding by AR on the indicated genes was detected with IP PCR. The precise location of the PCR primers for each of the gene promoters is described in Supplemental Figure S3. Induction with DHT was shown to increase the binding of AR to these promoters, while this induction was abolished in the KDM7A knock-down cells (Figure 2B). We next attempted to investigate methylation statuses on AR responsive promoters in the KDM7A knock-down cells. Based on the changes in methylation (Figure 2A), we used H3K27 di-methyl-specific histone antibodies for immunoprecipitations, and H3K27 methylation was found to be increased in KDM7A knock-down bladder cells, before and after DHT induction (Figure 2C). Our data confirmed the molecular function of KDM7A on AR transcription factor activity in bladder cancer cells.

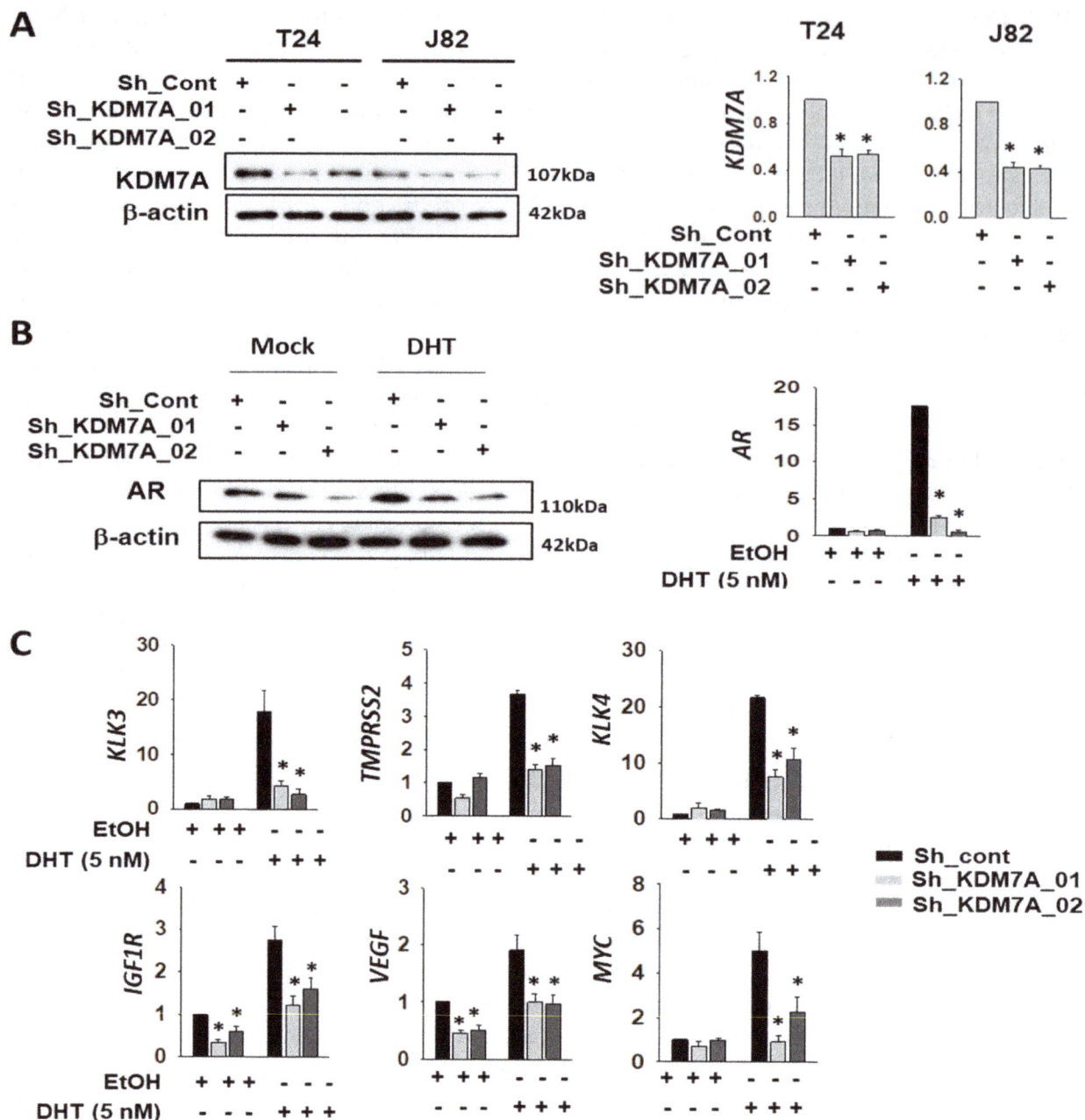

Figure 1. Histone demethylase KDM7A is required for AR activity in bladder cancer cells. (**A**) The efficiency of KDM7A knock-down was measured by comparing protein levels of KDM7A in the indicated cell lines, expressing control or two different shRNAs. Whole-cell lysates were analyzed with the indicated antibodies (left). The mRNA levels of KDM7A were measured by RT-qPCR method in the KDM7A knock-down cell lines (right graphs). Bars represent the means ± SD of three independent experiments, and * denotes $p < 0.05$ (student t-test) versus the control shRNA (sh-cont) group. (**B**) The AR protein levels in KDM7A knock-down T24 cells treated with dihydrotestosterone (DHT) were analyzed with indicated antibodies (left). The mRNA levels of AR in T24 cells after DHT induction were measured by RT-qPCR (right graph). Bars represent the means ± SD of three independent experiments, and * denotes $p < 0.05$ (student t-test) versus the control shRNA (sh-cont) group. (**C**) The mRNA levels of AR downstream genes were measured by RT-qPCR method in KDM7A knock-down T24 cell lines. Bars represent mean ± SD of three independent experiments. * $p < 0.05$ (Student's t-test), versus the control shRNA (sh-cont) group.

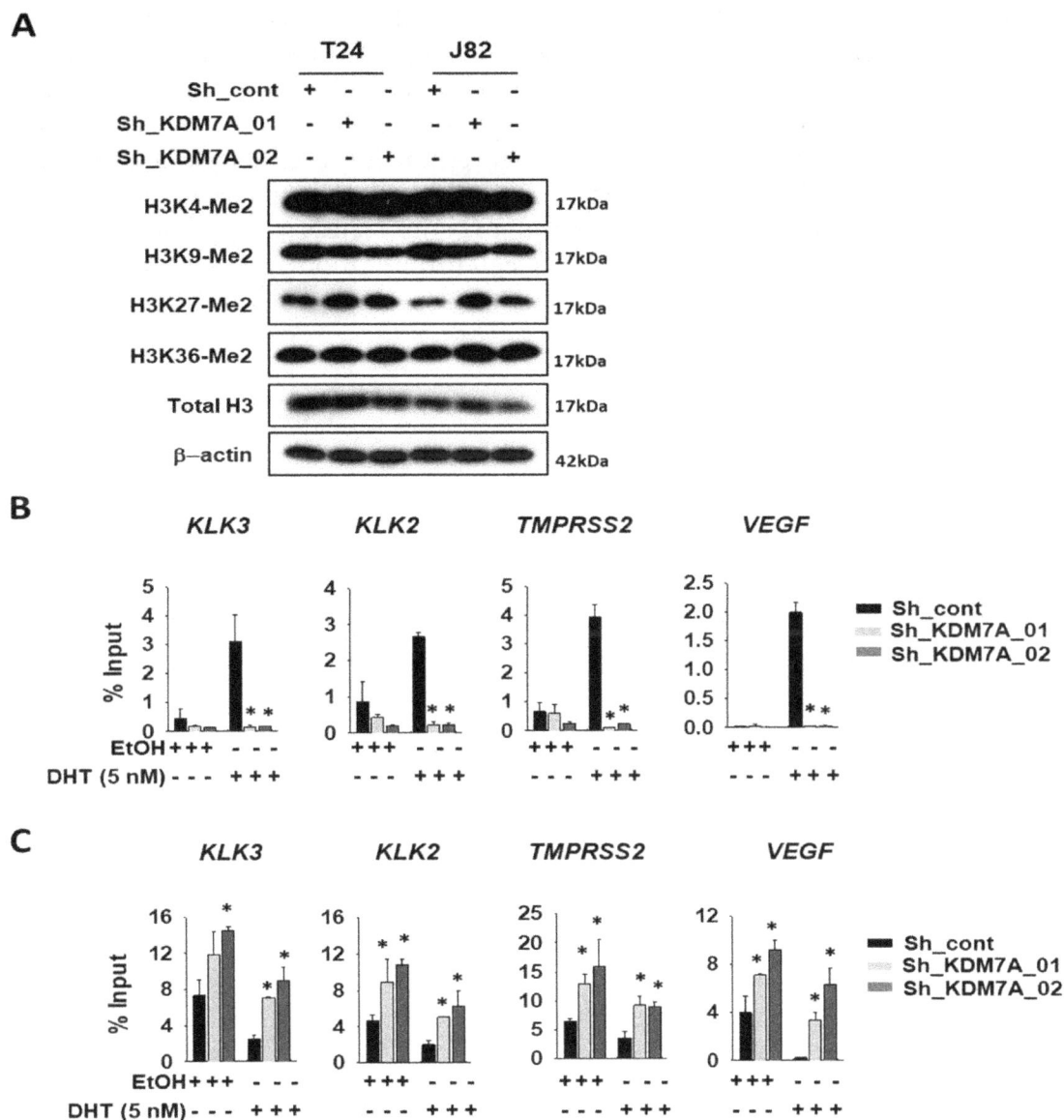

Figure 2. KDM7A directly binds on androgen receptor (AR) downstream gene promoters, and regulates H3K27 methylation. (**A**) Histone methylation status in KDM7A knock-down cells was analyzed with the indicated antibodies. T24 cells expressing control or KMD7A shRNA were treated with 5 nM DHT for 1 day, and the sonicated chromatins were immune-precipitated with anti-AR (**B**) or anti-H3K27 di-methyl (**C**) antibody. Immunoprecipitated DNAs were subjected to qPCR with the indicated gene promoter sequence primers. Bars represent means ± SD of three independent experiments. * $p < 0.05$ (Student's t-test), versus the control shRNA (sh-cont) group.

2.3. KDM7A is Required for Bladder Cancer Cell Growth and Apoptosis Inhibition

Since AR is known to be essential for cell growth in many cancers, we treated AR siRNA or enzalutamide, to confirm the growth inhibition effect on bladder cancer cell growth (Supplemental Figure S4). Next, we measured cell proliferation in both control and KDM7A knock-down cells. Although the morphology of KDM7A knock-down cells was not different from control cells (Supplemental Figure S5), the rate of cell proliferation in KDM7A knock-down bladder cancer cells was reduced compared to that of control shRNA-expressing cells (Figure 3A). When we seeded the same number of cells in cell culture dishes, knock-down cells showed a reduction in colony numbers and size compared to control cells (Figure 3B). We next observed the expression levels of cell cycle proteins in KDM7A knock-down cells (Figure 3C). Previous studies have reported that AR regulates cell cycle by controlling cyclin D1 [44], and cyclin B1 is a direct target of AR [45]. We observed a decrease in the cyclin B1 protein levels in KDM7A knock-down bladder cancer cells, which is consistent with the cell proliferation rate difference data in Figure 3A,B. It was observed that the decrease in cyclin D1 is not as obvious as that in cyclin B1 in our experimental conditions. Since AR is known to inhibit apoptosis induced by cytotoxic stimuli [46], we measured the levels of apoptotic proteins in KDM7A knock-down cells treated with the anti-cancer drug cisplatin (Figure 3D). We observed an increase in the PARP and caspase 3 cleavage products compared to control shRNA-expressing cells. These results strongly suggest that KDM7A regulates the rate of cell proliferation and drug-induced apoptosis in bladder cancer cells.

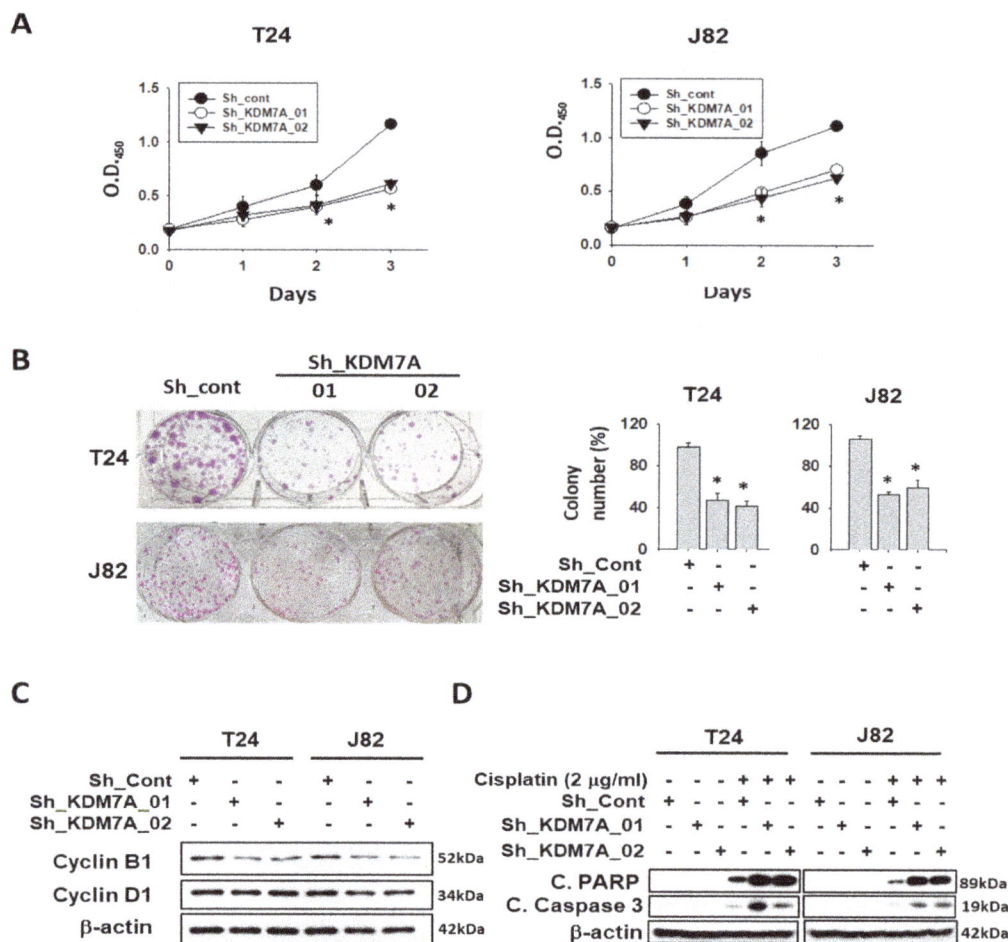

Figure 3. Histone demethylase KDM7A is required for the cell proliferation and apoptosis inhibition in bladder cancer cell lines. (**A**) The time dependent viability changes of control shRNA and KDM7A shRNA expressing bladder cancer cell lines were measured using EZ-Cytox solution. Bars represent means ± SD of three independent experiments. * $p < 0.05$ (Student's t-test) versus the control shRNA (sh-cont) group. (**B**) Crystal violet staining for colonies from the same number of indicated shRNA-expressing stable cells. The average number of colonies is shown in the right panel. Bars represent means ± SD of three independent experiments. * $p < 0.05$ (Student's t-test) versus the sh-cont group. (**C**) The levels of cell cycle-related proteins were measured from the whole cell extracts of control and KDM7A knock-down cells. (**D**) The apoptotic proteins were detected in the cisplatin-treated KDM7A knock-down bladder cells. Whole-cell lysates were analyzed with the indicated antibodies.

2.4. KDM7A Facilitates Migration and Invasion of Bladder Cancer Cells

One of the major functions of AR in cancer progression is to facilitate cell migration and metastasis. It was observed that AR inhibition by enzalutamide affected the migration of bladder cancer cells

(Supplemental Figure S6). To verify the effect of KDM7A in bladder cancer cell migration and metastasis, we measured migration and invasion in KDM7A knock-down T24 and J82 bladder cancer cells. One day after scratch, KDM7A knock-down cells showed decreased mobility when compared to control cells (Figure 4A). We demarcated the wound margin with a yellow line for better visualization, and added the original pictures and quantification of remaining scratched areas after the indicated times in Supplemental Figure S7. The cell invasion assay using Matrigel Transwell showed the decreased invasion of KDM7A knock-down cells compared to control cells (Figure 4B). To elucidate the molecular mechanism of this decrease in cell migration, we measured the expression of several epithelial-mesenchymal transition (EMT) markers in KDM7A knock-down cells. Although a decrease in the protein levels of N-cadherin and vimentin, the epithelial markers, was observed only in J82 cells (Figure 4C, Supplemental Figure S8), the mRNA expression levels of them were reduced in both T24 and J82 cells (Figure 4D). The protein and mRNA levels of mesenchymal marker E-cadherin were elevated in KDM7A knock-down cells in both T24 and J82 cells (Figure 4C,D, Supplemental Figure S8). The findings suggest that KDM7A is required for cell migration and EMT transition in bladder cancer cells.

2.5. Enzalutamide and a KDM7A Inhibitor Decrease the Proliferation of Cisplatin-resistant Bladder Cancer Cells

The effect of AR induction on the cisplatin resistance process of bladder cancer has been previously reported [19]. Therefore, we wanted to explore the possibility of AR regulation as a target for overcoming the drug resistance of bladder cancer. Initially, we established a cisplatin-resistant T24 (CR-T24) bladder cancer cell line. After 2 months of exposure to increasing concentrations of cisplatin, we obtained T24 cells that survived in 2 μM cisplatin (Figure 5A). To compare the AR protein levels between original and CR-T24 cells, we compared their nuclear extracts, since the active form of AR protein occurs only in the nuclear fraction. We used the Lamin B1 antibody as the loading control of the nuclear extract, and for establishing the purity of the fraction, while GAPDH acted as the loading control of the cytosolic fraction. In addition to an increase in the total AR protein level, our study found that the level of active AR protein was higher in the nuclear fraction of CR-T24 when compared to the parental cells (Figure 5B). The protein level of KDM7A in CR-T24 cells decreased in the cytosolic fraction, but remained the same in nuclear fraction. The AR protein level in CR-T24 cells was found to be elevated before and after DHT treatment (Figure 5C), as reported previously [19]. The mRNA levels of several AR target genes also showed an increase, when compared to the parental T24 cells before and after DHT treatment (Figure 5D), suggesting that the elevated AR has functional activity. After confirming an increase in AR activity in CR-T24 cells, we utilized the KDM7A inhibitor TC-E 5002, in conjunction with AR antagonist enzalutamide, to evaluate the role of KDM7A on bladder cancer growth and drug resistance in terms of the AR pathway. Cell viability was tested in parental and CR-T24 cells in the presence of enzalutamide and/or TC-E 5002 (Figure 5E). In order to obtain a clearer picture of the changes in cell viability, we used a non-toxic dose and time of enzalutamide or TC-E 5002 when treated to parental T24 cells. CR-T24 cells were found to be more sensitive to a single treatment with enzalutamide or TC-E 5002 than parental cells. Moreover, when CR-T24 cells were treated with both enzalutamide and TC-E 5002, fewer cells survived compared to the single drug treatments. The anti-cancer effect of this co-treatment was significantly greater in CR-T24 compared to the parental T24 cells. Finally, we investigated the involvement of cellular signaling pathways involved in the anti-cancer effect of AR and/or KDM7A inhibitors on CR-T24 cells. Of the several pathways tested, Akt signaling pathway molecules were significantly decreased upon treatment with AR and/or KDM7A inhibitor. In our experiments, the total and phosphorylated protein levels of Akt and mTOR in T24 cells were decreased after enzalutamide and/or TC-E 5002 treatment. The changes were more significant in CR-T24 compared to the parental cells, and the effect was synergistically increased in co-treatment (Figure 5F; Supplemental Figure S9A). Upon cisplatin treatment, we observed the synergistic effect of two drugs on apoptosis signaling induction in the parental T24 cells, although the resistant cells did not show the apoptosis induction (Supplemental Figure S9B). For studying the changes in cell migration ability in CR-T24 cells, we performed a wound healing assay using both the cell lines treated with AR and/or KDM7A inhibitors (Supplemental Figure S10). The findings showed a decrease in the migration of cells upon treatment with AR and/or KDM7A inhibitors, in both original as well as CR-T24 cells.

2.6. KDM7A Knock-Down Attenuated Tumor Growth in Orthotopic Bladder Cancer Xenograft Model

To investigate the role of KDM7A in bladder tumor growth in vivo, we stably incorporated a luciferase-expressing vector into KDM7A shRNA-expressing bladder cancer cell lines and control cell line. After their inoculation into the bladders of NOD scid gamma (NSG) immune-deficient mice, the growth of the cancer cells was monitored using luciferase signal. The growth of bladder tumors was consistently higher in control cells compared to KMD7A knock-down cells (Figure 6A, Supplemental Figure S11). On the day of sacrifice, the tumors were extracted and the luminescence in control tumors was seen to be significantly higher than in KDM7A knock-down tumors (Figure 6B). Immunostaining of proliferation marker Ki-67 was used to evaluate the aggressiveness of the tumor (Figure 6C). The control tumor was positive for Ki-67, while the KDM7A knock-down tumor was found to be negative. The expression of vascular endothelial growth factor (VEGF) was detected in control tumor, but not in KDM7A knock-down tumors. These results implied that the growth and migration capability of bladder tumor is highly affected by the expression of KDM7A in vivo.

2.7. TC-E 5002 Treatment of Xenografted Bladder Tumors Reduced the Tumor Size

In the prostate study, we found that the KDM7A inhibitor TC-E 5002 effectively reduced tumor cell growth and migration in vitro [32]. In order to assess the in vivo effect of TC-E 5002 on bladder cancer development, we subcutaneously injected the T24 cells in the flanks of the NSG mice. After the tumor volume had reached 200 mm^3, the mice were divided into 2 groups and injected with the vehicle or TC-E 5002 intraperitoneally daily for 8 days. After day 8, we observed a difference in the tumor sizes between the two groups (Figure 7A). The tumors excised from mice treated with TC-E 5002 weighed lesser than those excised from control mice (Figure 7B). Suppression of the AR activity by TC-E 5002 treatment was evident from the protein and mRNA expression levels of AR-dependent genes in the individual tumors (Figure 7 C,D). In tumors treated with TC-E 5002, the expression of the cell-cycle marker Ki-67 and VEGF protein were decreased, while the expression of the apoptotic DNA-fragmentation marker TUNEL was increased (Figure 7E). Our data exemplified the potential applications of TC-E 5002 in bladder cancer treatment in vivo.

2.8. KDM7A Protein and mRNA Level Were Elevated in Bladder Cancer Patients

In order to analyze KDM7A expression in bladder cancer patients, we performed immunohistochemistry (IHC) of KDM7A using tissue microarray. The results showed a higher level of KMD7A in tumor tissues compared to normal bladder tissue (Figure 8A). In the next step, patient tissue samples were collected, and the KDM7A protein and mRNA levels were analyzed. The protein (Figure 8B, Table 1) and mRNA (Figure 8C, Table 1) levels were significantly higher in tumor samples compared to normal bladder tissue from the same patients. Upon quantification of the signal from Western blot for KDM7A and its comparison with the tumor stages, the results were not statistically significant, which might be due to the small sample size (Supplemental Figure S12). Next, we evaluated the correlation between mRNA expression level of KDM7A and clinical outcome using a Kaplan–Meier plotter in public database (www.kmplot.com). We examined the prognostic value of KDM7A expression at each tumor stage, and in both men and women, in the bladder cancer database using KDM7A as the 'key gene' for data mining. High *KDM7A* mRNA expression was associated with significantly worse overall survival (OS) in men with stage 2 bladder cancer (Figure 8D). However, we were not able to identify a correlation in other stages of male cancer patients (Supplemental Figures S13 and S14), or in any stages of female patients.

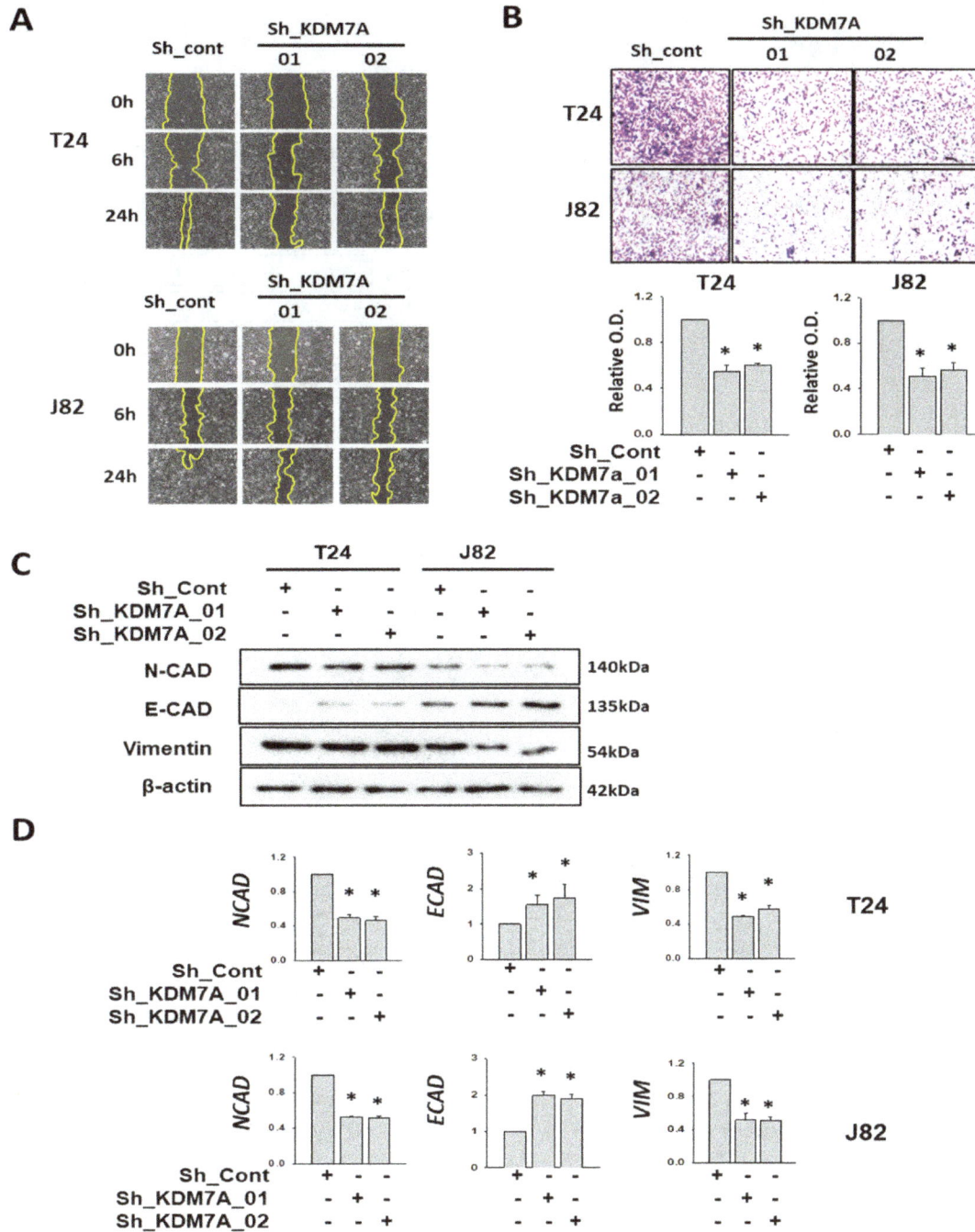

Figure 4. KDM7A knock-down reduced cell mobility and EMT-related gene expressions in bladder cancer cells. (**A**) Scratch-wounding cell migration assay of the control and KDM7A shRNA-expressing cells was performed for the indicated time. The wound margin is marked with a yellow line. (**B**) The Transwell assay of the same number of control and KDM7A shRNA-expressing cells. At 48 h after plating, cells that had migrated to the underside of the filters were fixed and stained with crystal violet. Photographs were taken and the relative cell migration was determined by measuring OD_{495} after extraction. Bars represent means ± SD of three independent experiments. * $p < 0.05$ (Student's t-test) versus the control shRNA (sh-cont) group. (**C**) The protein levels of indicated EMT markers were measured from the whole cell extracts of control or KDM7A knock-down cells. (**D**) The mRNA levels of the indicated EMT marker genes were measured from cell lines with control or KDM7A shRNA expression. Bars represent means ± SD of three independent experiments * $p < 0.05$ (Student's t-test) versus the sh-cont group.

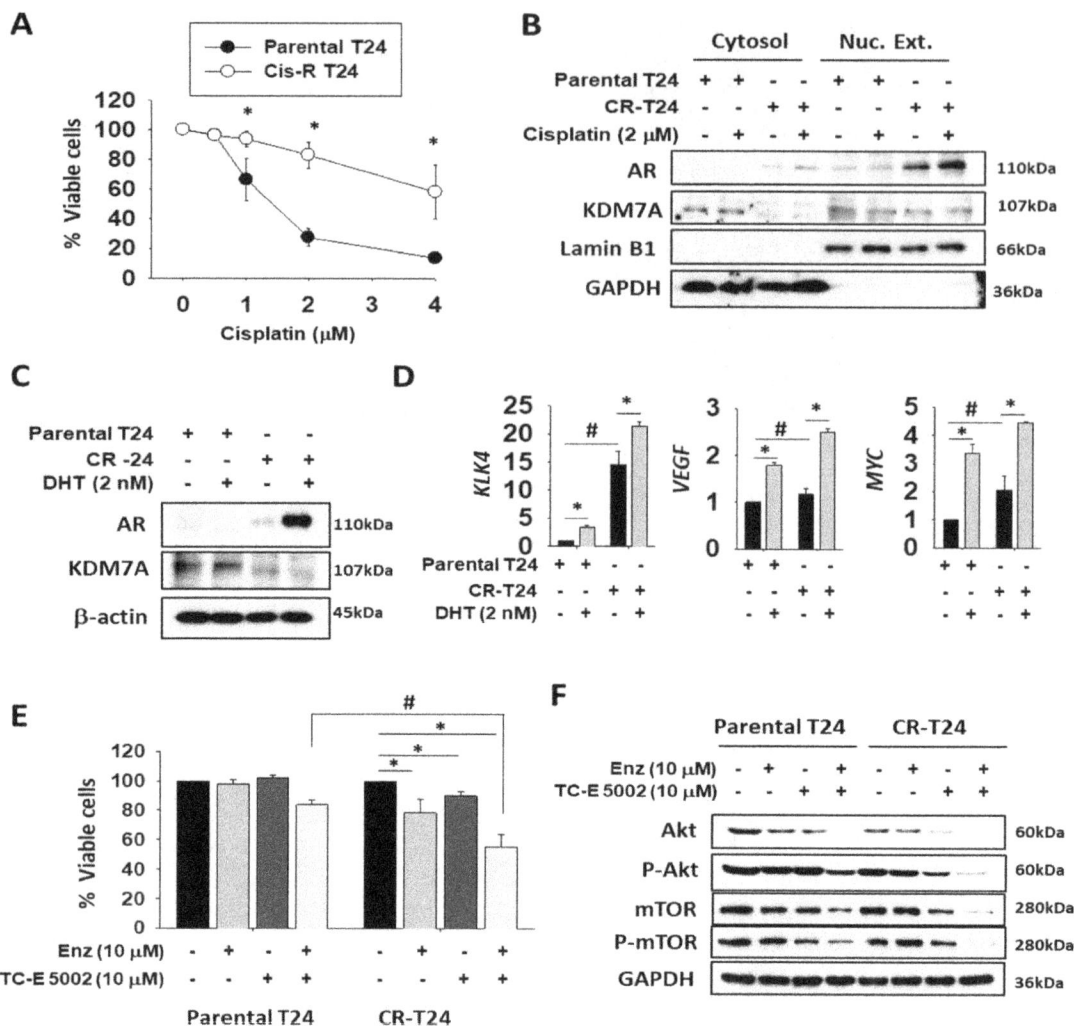

Figure 5. Nuclear localization and activity of AR were elevated in cisplatin-resistant T24 (CR-T24) cells, and treatment with enzalutamide and KDM7A inhibitor reduced the growth of CR-T24 bladder cancer cells. (**A**) Viability of parental and CR-T24 cells after treatment with the indicated concentrations of cisplatin for 3 days. Bars represent means ± SD of three independent experiments. * $p < 0.05$ (Student's *t*-test) versus parental cells. (**B**) Western blots of the indicated proteins from parental and CR-T24 cells. The cytosolic and nuclear fractions from each cell line were extracted and blotted with the indicated antibodies. Lamin B1 immunostaining served as the nuclear protein loading control and GAPDH immunostaining as cytoplasmic control. (**C**) Western blots of AR and KDM7A proteins from parental and CR-24 cells, before and after 5α-dihydrotestosterone (DHT) treatment. (**D**) mRNA levels of the indicated genes were measured from parental and CR-T24 cells. Bars represent means ± SD of three independent experiments. * $p < 0.05$ (Student's *t*-test), versus the mock-treated group. # $p < 0.05$ (Student's t-test) versus parental T24 cells. (**E**) Cell viability changes after 3 days of treatment with the indicated drugs on parental or CR-T24 cells. Bars represent means ± SD of three independent experiments. * $p < 0.05$ (Student's *t*-test) versus the mock-treated group. # $p < 0.05$ (Student's *t*-test) versus parental T24 cells. (**F**) Levels of the indicated proteins were measured from whole cell extracts of parental and CR-T24 cells, treated with either enzalutamide and/or TC-E 5002 for 2 days.

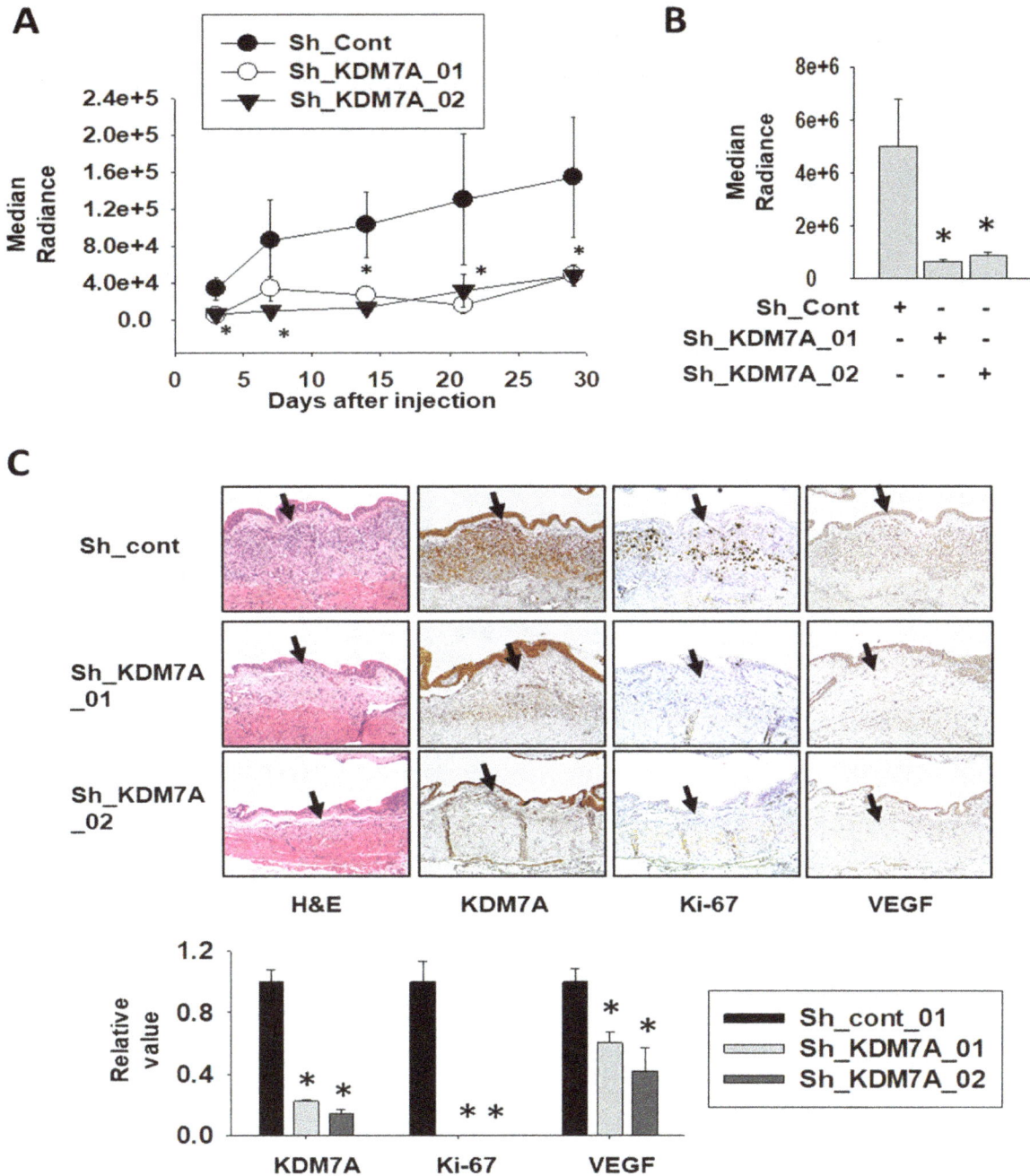

Figure 6. Attenuation of KDM7A expression reduces bladder tumor growth in orthotopic xenograft model. (**A**) Bioluminescent flux plot quantifying tumors in response to control or KDM7A shRNA-expressing T24 cells xenografted into mouse bladder. Error bars represent means ± SEM of each group ($n = 5$). * $p < 0.05$ (Student's t-test) versus the control shRNA (sh-cont) group. (**B**) Bioluminescent flux plot from the extracted bladder from each group. Error bars represent means ± SEM of each group ($n = 5$). * $p < 0.05$ (Student's t-test) versus the sh-cont group. (**C**) Representative hematoxylin-eosin staining and immunohistochemistry images of the orthotopically implanted bladder tumors. Arrow indicates tumor area of the mouse bladder. Positive signal was calculated from at least 3 independent areas, and relative values were plotted. Error bars represent means ± SEM of each group ($n = 5$). * $p < 0.05$ (Student's t-test) versus the sh-cont group.

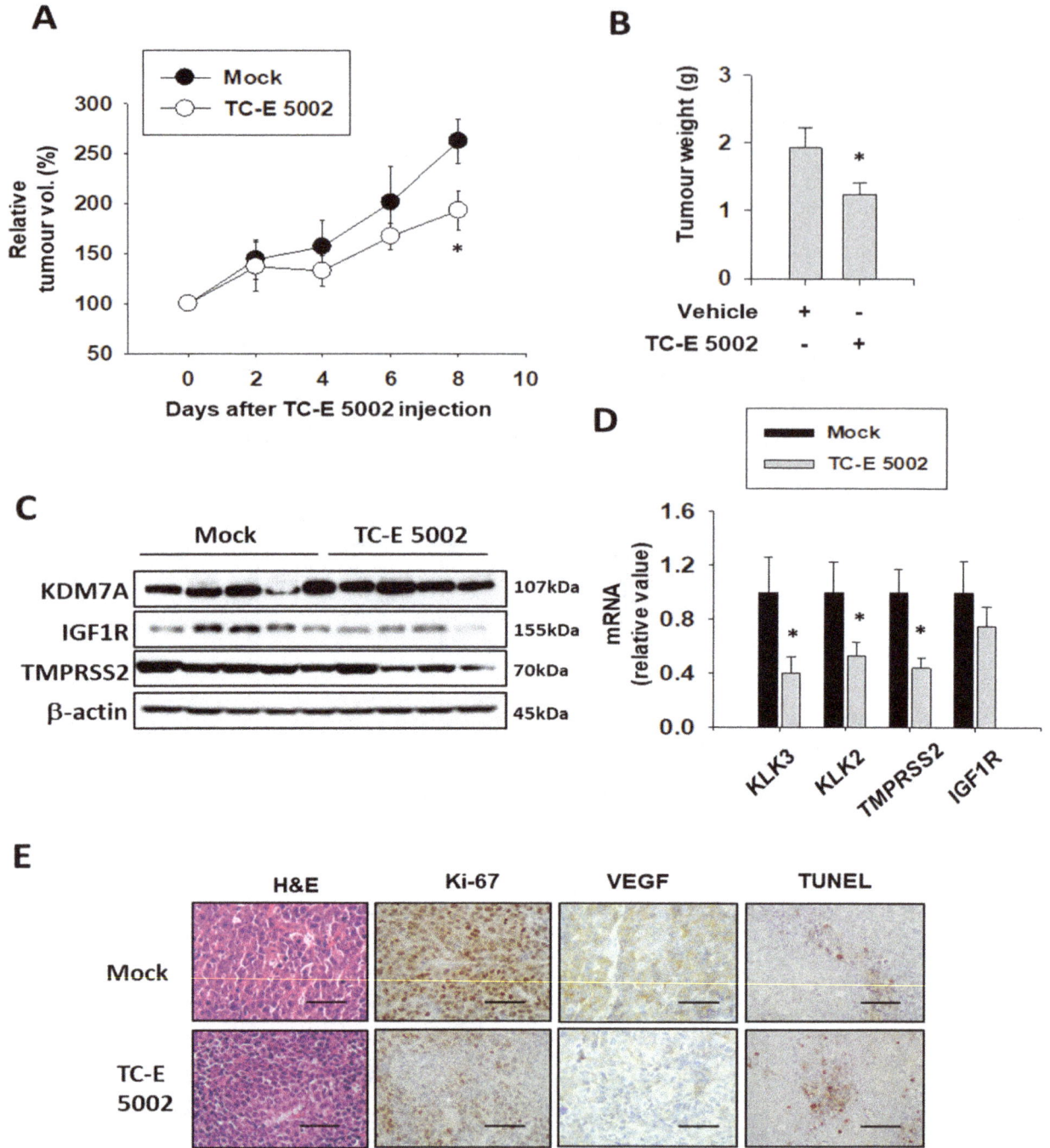

Figure 7. Effect of TC-E 5002 treatment on bladder tumor growth in the xenograft model in NSG mice. (**A**) Relative tumor volume in animals treated with vehicle or TC-E 5002 (10 mg/kg per day). Intraperitoneal drug treatment was started when the average tumor volume reached 200 mm^3 and continued every day for 8 days. Error bars represent means ± SEM for each group ($n = 5$). * $p < 0.05$ (Student's t-test) versus the vehicle-treated group. (**B**) Weight of tumors excised from animals treated with the vehicle or TC-E 5002. Error bars represent means ± SEM for each group ($n = 5$). * $p < 0.05$ (Student's t-test) versus the vehicle-treated group. (**C**) Total protein was extracted from each xenografted tumor, and Western blotting was performed using the indicated antibodies. (**D**) Total RNA was extracted from each xenografted tumor, and the indicated mRNA levels were measured. Bars represent means ± SEM for each group ($n = 5$). * $p < 0.05$ (Student's t-test) versus the vehicle-treated group. (**E**) Representative hematoxylin-eosin staining and immunohistochemistry images of the excised tumors. Scale bar is 20 µm.

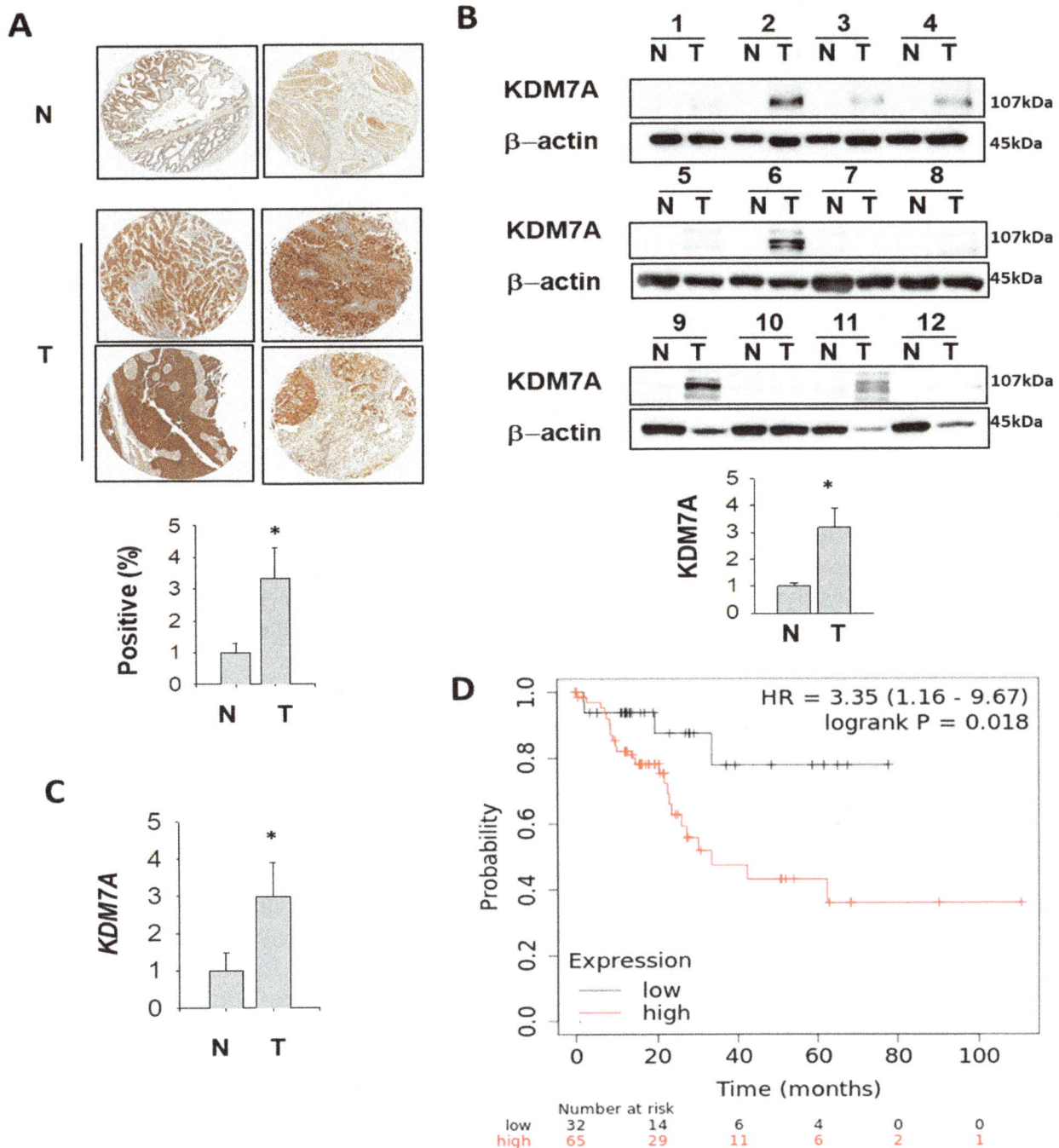

Figure 8. KDM7A is up-regulated in bladder cancer patients (**A**) Representative images of KDM7A expression in bladder tumor and normal tissue arrays (upper figures). N, normal bladder tissue; T, bladder tumor tissue. The expression level of KDM7A from 25 different bladder tumors and 6 normal tissues were calculated and plotted (below graph). * $p < 0.05$ (Student's t-test) between two groups. (**B**) Bladder tumor (T) and adjacent normal (N) tissues were subjected to Western blotting using the KDM7A and beta actin antibodies. Protein bands were analyzed densitometrically and protein levels normalized to beta actin levels were plotted in the lower graph. * $p < 0.05$ (Student's t-test) between two groups. (**C**) Comparison of KDM7A mRNA expression levels between normal and tumor bladder tissues. * $p < 0.05$ (Student's t-test) between two groups. (**D**) A survival curve was plotted for male bladder cancer patients with cancer stage 2 ($n = 97$). Data were analyzed using the Kaplan–Meier Plotter (www.kmplot.com). Patients with expression above the median are indicated in red line, and patients with expressions below the median in black line. HR means hazard ratio.

Table 1. Demographics of patients used for tissue extract.

No.	Age	Sex	T Stage
1	66	M	T2bN0(0/21) LVI necrosis
2	73	F	T2aN0(0/16)
3	58	M	TaN0(0/25) CIS
4	56	F	T1N0(0/37)
5	84	M	T4aN0(0/1) LVI, Perineural invasion
6	67	M	TaN0(0/26)
7	64	M	T3aN2(2/7) LVI, Perineural invasion
8	75	M	T3bN1(1/17), Perineural invasion
9	72	M	T2aN0(0/14)
10	70	M	T3aN0(0/15) Lymphatic invasion
11	61	M	T4aN2(3/17), LVI Perineural invasion, necrosis
12	63	M	T3aN0(0/13)

3. Discussion

Although the epigenetic regulation of AR has been extensively studied in prostate cancer, a growing body of evidence has suggested a role for AR in other cancers, including colon, breast, and bladder cancer. Because anti-cancer drugs targeting AR have been well-characterized in prostate cancer, existing drugs can be explored as potential treatment options for other AR-positive cancers as well. In this paper, we focused on the AR function in bladder cancer, because of its high malignant character, which is known to be related to AR malfunction.

KDM7A histone demethylase is known to act on H3K27 residues, which function as repressive marks of transcription. Consequently, lowering KDM7A activity results in H3K27 methylation on chromatin and reduced gene transcription. We had previously showed that AR binding to KLK3, KLK2, and TMPRSS2 gene promoters was decreased in KDM7A knock-down prostate cells, and the expression levels of these genes were also reduced. More importantly, the effect of the KDM7A inhibitor TC-E 5002 on prostate cancer cell proliferation was analyzed, and we observed that prostate cancer cell growth was reduced on treatment with TC-E 5002 treatment. In the present study, we found that the bladder cancer cells expressing KDM7A shRNA also showed decreased cell proliferation. As expected, the AR expression in bladder cancer cells was lower than that of prostate cells (Supplemental Figure S1). Therefore, the effect of KDM7A knockdown was not as dramatic as in prostate cells. However, the reduction of bladder cancer cell growth, migration and metastatic abilities was found to be statistically significant. On the other hand, when we used TC-E 5002, a chemical inhibitor of KDM7A, we detected a relatively small effect on T24 bladder cancer cell growth (Figure 5E) compared to the inhibition effect of KDM7A knock-down (Figure 3A). This could be because the selected TC-E 5002 treatment time and concentration were not high enough to kill the original T24 cells, since we wanted to see the effect of TC-E 5002 and/or enzalutamide on CR-T24 cells. When we continued TC-E 5002 treatment for longer durations and using higher doses, more cell death was achieved. Since many in vitro studies have shown the anti-cancer effect of enzalutamide in bladder cancer, including drug-resistant conditions [16–19], co-treatment of TC-E 5002 together with enzalutamide was performed to study the effect on cisplatin-resistant bladder cancer cells. As we can see in the right part of graph in Figure 5E, CR-T24 cells, which had elevated AR expression, died more efficiently upon TC-E 5002 treatment. In addition to cisplatin-resistant T24 [19], gemcitabine-resistant T24 has also been reported to show increased AR expression [17]. Therefore, it would be interesting to investigate whether treatment of gemcitabine-resistant cells with TC-E 5002 has the same effect. In particular, the effect of co-treatment with enzalutamide and TC-E 5002 on CR-T24 bladder cancer cell line could be useful for understanding the value of this treatment in drug-resistant bladder cancer. In addition to testing TC-E 5002 in vitro in cell culture, our in vivo data using the xenograft bladder tumors illustrated the future possibility of applying the drug clinically.

Although we focused only on demonstrating the role of KDM7A in regulating AR activity, we cannot rule out the possibility that KDM7A acts on other factors, regulating the cell cycle, or that our results are owing to the non-specific knockdown effect of KDM7A. This is because the AR expression level of the cell lines that we used was notably lower than that of prostate cancer, and the repressive effect on neoplasia was relatively strong. Factors other than AR may include KLF4 and c-MYC, which were found to be involved in breast cancer stem cell maintenance [34]. The use of only two bladder cell lines with undifferentiated character may also limit the universality of our data. Therefore, it would be interesting to study the function of KDM7A in other differentiated cancer cells.

Our finding that the protein and mRNA levels of KDM7A are increased in bladder cancer tissues (Figure 8) may point to elevated AR activity in the cancer. Based on our results, it is possible that KDM7A controls AR activity as an epigenetic co-activator during cancer progression. Most importantly, the KDM7A protein level increased in tumor tissues compared to matching normal tissues (Figure 8B). However, the correlation of KDM7A expression level with each cancer stage was not statistically significant, perhaps due to the small number of cases for each stage (Supplemental Figure S12). Nonetheless, the fact that we identified a correlation between high KDM7A mRNA levels and cancer-dependent deaths only in men (Figure 8D), but not in women, may explain the AR dependency of this effect. Interestingly, this correlation was lost in men with higher grades of cancer (grade 3 and 4; Supplement Supplement Figures S13 and S14), which may be due to the AR loss-of-function during the progression of bladder cancer. Given that this phenomenon is widely reported in prostate cancer, a similar mechanism may exist in bladder cancer. For the early stage male bladder cancer patients, it would be interesting to explore whether an AR antagonist can be used as an anti-cancer drug upon screening KMD7A expression levels. In addition, the regulation of other transcription factors besides AR, which are under the control of KDM7A, should be considered.

An increasing number of histone-modifying enzymes have been shown to be important for bladder cancer development. Among them, the knock-down of LSD1 was found to effectively repress bladder cancer growth, and this effect was confirmed to be associated with AR activity regulation [47]. Additionally, it has been shown that the up-regulation of histone methyl transferase SMYD3 promotes bladder cancer progression. It is worth noting that, although the authors demonstrated that SMYD3 physically interacted with the BCLAF1 promoter [48], it is possible that SMYD3 may regulate bladder cancer growth *via* AR, because of its previously reported interaction with the receptor [30]. Our data point to the possibility that KDM7A may regulate AR in bladder cancer together with the above-mentioned co-regulators. Investigating potential interactions of the above-mentioned co-factors with KDM7A on the AR-regulated gene promoters would lead to a better understanding of the mechanism.

The anti-cancer effect of many histone methylase or demethylase inhibitors have been reported in bladder cancer, and many of them are presently being developed for cancer treatment [49]. Based on our data, we suggest that KDM7A inhibitor TC-E 5002 could be added to this list. Although further in-depth research is needed to validate the results of our study, our findings suggest that KDM7A could be a new target for treating bladder cancer and overcoming drug resistance, in conjunction with an AR inhibitor.

4. Materials and Methods

4.1. Materials

RPMI-1640, DMEM, trypsin, anti-biotics, Trizol and Lipofectamine 2000 were purchased from Invitrogen (Carlsbad, CA, USA). Fetal bovine serum and culture media were obtained from HyClone Laboratories Inc. (South Logan, UT, USA). The detailed information of all primary antibodies is listed in Supplemental Table S1.

4.2. Cell Lines, Plasmids, Virus Production and Infection

The T24, J82, and 293T cell lines were purchased from the American Type Culture Collection (Rockville, MD). T24 and J82 cells were cultured in RPMI-1640, and 293T cells for lentiviral package were cultured in DMEM medium at 37 °C in 5% CO_2, which was supplemented with 10% fetal bovine serum. For gene silencing, the control or KDM7A shRNA expressing lenti-virus packaging and stable cell line establishment were performed as described [32]. The oligo sequence used for KDM7A shRNA 01 cloning is 5′-CCGGTGGATTTGATGTCCCTATTATCTCGAGATAATAGGGACATCAAATCCAT TTTT-3′, and for shRNA 02 sequence is 5′-CCGGTTAGACCTGGACACCTTATTACTCGAGTAATAA GGTGTCCAGGTCTAATTTTT-3′. The oligo sequence for control shRNA cloning is 5′-CCGGCGTGA TCTTCACCGACAAGATCTCGAGATCTTGTCGGTGAAGATCACGTTTTT-3′. FUGW-luc vector (from the Molecular Imaging and Neurovascular Research Laboratory, Dongguk University Ilsan Hospital, Goyang, Korea) expressing cells were produced as described below. FUGW-luc vector was cut with XhoI enzyme and transfected into the T24 cell line, expressing either control vector or KMD7A shRNA vector. The cells with FUGW-luc incorporation were sorted with GFP channel using BD FACSAria II (BD Biosciences, Franklin Lakes, NJ, USA).

4.3. Colony Formation Assay and Cell Viability Assay

For the colony formation assay, 1000 cells were plated in 6-well plates. The cells were cultured for 14 days and stained with 0.1% crystal violet. The cell colonies were photographed, and the number of colonies comprising more than 50 individual cells was counted using SZX7 stereo microscope (Olympus, Tokyo, Japan). For the cell viability assay, cells (2000 to 3000 cells/well) were dispensed in 100 µL culture medium in a 96-well plate, and incubated for the indicated time. EZ-Cytox cell viability kit (Daeil-Lab, Seoul, Korea) solution (10 µL) was mixed with the culture medium in each well of the plate. Samples were incubated for 1 h at 37 °C, and the absorbance of each sample at 450 nm was measured using a microplate reader (PerkinElmer, Waltham, MA, USA).

4.4. RNA Isolation and the Real-Time Quantitative Polymerase Chain Reaction (RT-qPCR)

The total cellular RNA was extracted using the Trizol reagent (Ambion, Austin, TX, USA), according to the manufacturer's instructions. For the induction of AR activity, 5 nM 5α-dihydrotestosterone (DHT) was added after one day of serum deprivation. For each reverse-transcription reaction, 1 µg of total RNA was used for cDNA synthesis, using the MultiScribe Reverse Transcription Kit from Life Technologies (Carlsbad, CA, USA). RT-qPCR was performed using the EvaGreen qPCR Master Mix Kit from Applied Biological Materials Inc. (Richmond, BC, Canada) and a StepOne™ Real-Time PCR System (Applied Biosystems, Foster City, CA, USA). The quantity of 18S ribosomal RNA was measured as an internal control. The sequences of the primers used for RT-qPCR are listed in Supplemental Table S2.

4.5. Wound Healing and Cell Invasion Assays

The wound healing assay was performed on 100% confluent cells, plated into 6-well culture plates. Straight scratches were made by using a pipette tip. The cells were washed twice to remove debris, followed by the addition of fresh medium. The cells were incubated in a 5% CO_2 environment at 37 °C, and observed using a SZX7 stereo microscope at the indicated time. The scratched areas were measured using ImageJ program (ver. 1.43u; www.rsb.info.nih.gov/ij). For the invasion assay, cells (5×10^4/well) were plated in the upper chambers of Transwells without serum, using Matrigel-coated polycarbonate membranes (Corning, Big Flats, NY, USA). The basal medium containing 10% fetal bovine serum was added into the lower chambers, as a chemoattractant for cell migration. After 48-h, non-migrated cells were removed from the upper chambers, while cells that migrated through chambers were fixed using 10% ethanol (Sigma-Aldrich). After cells were stained with the 0.01% crystal violet solution (Sigma-Aldrich), migrated cells were randomly counted in five different microscopic fields at 20× magnification.

4.6. Human Ethics Approval and Collection of Human Tissues

The frozen tissues from bladder cancer patients were collected from Seoul Nation University Hospital Tissue Bank, with the approval of Institutional Review Board No. H-1004-037-315 (Date of approval: 06/11/2010). The demographic data of each patient are shown in Table 1. Tumor tissues and matching normal tissues from the same patient were identified from the pathology results. For Western blotting, 50–200 mg of tissues was ground in liquid nitrogen and lysed with RIPA buffer.

4.7. Animal Studies and In Vivo Bioluminescent Imaging

All animal experiments were performed in accordance with the Seoul National University Hospital institutional guidelines, under IACUC protocol No.16-0167-C2A0 (Date of approval: 07/20/2018). NOD scid gamma (NSG) mice were bred and maintained under specific pathogen-free (SPF) conditions. For generating orthotopic tumors, 1×10^5 T24 human bladder cells expressing the indicated shRNA and Luciferase expression vector were injected into the bladder of six-week-old male NSG mice ($n = 5$ for each group). For injection, the cells were suspended with 100 µL of 50 % Matrigel (BD Biosciences) in complete media. The mice from each group were injected intraperitoneally with 150 mg/kg D-luciferin (Promega, Madison, WI, USA), 15 min before acquiring the image. After anesthetizing the mice using 1–3% isoflurane, the photons emitted from the tumor were detected with Xenogen IVIS imaging system 200 (Alameda, CA, USA) as described. The image acquisition period was 1 s. Living Image (Version 2.20, Xenogen) was used to quantify signals emitted from the regions of interest. The mice were sacrificed after 30 days of tumor implantation, and bladder tumor was fixed in 4% paraformaldehyde at 4 °C and embedded in paraffin. The specimens were subjected to IHC with the indicated antibodies. For subcutaneous xenografting, six-week-old male NSG mice were injected, in their lower flanks, with 1×10^7 T24 cells in 100 µL of 50% (v/v) Matrigel ($n = 5$ for each group). When the average tumor volume reached 200 mm^3, mice were randomly assigned into two groups and injected intraperitoneally everyday with vehicle (0.05 mL; 90% corn-oil and 10% DMSO (v/v)) or 10 mg/kg TC-E 5002 in the same vehicle, respectively. The tumors were measured every other day, and at the end of 8 days of treatment, the mice were sacrificed, and the tumors were excised, weighed, and either frozen or fixed in formalin for further analyses.

4.8. Western Blotting

The cells (5×10^6) and ground tissue (50–200 mg) were lysed in 1ml RIPA buffer (150 mM NaCl, 50 mM Tris-HCl [pH 7.2], 0.5% NP-40, 1% Triton X-100, and 1% sodium deoxycholate), containing a protease/phosphatase inhibitor cocktail (Sigma-Aldrich, St. Louis, MO, USA). For the induction of AR activity, 5 nM 5α-dihydrotestosterone (DHT) was added after one day of serum deprivation. The cell lysates were separated on sodium dodecyl sulfate-polyacrylamide gels and transferred to an Immobilon-P membrane (Millipore, Darmstadt, Germany). The membranes were blocked with 5% skim milk in 0.1% Tween-20 for 1 h, followed by overnight incubation at 4 °C with the indicated primary antibodies. The membranes were incubated with a horseradish peroxidase-conjugated secondary antibody (1:5000) for 1 h and developed using the ECL-Plus Kit (Thermo Scientific, Rockford, IL, USA).

4.9. Immunohistochemical Staining and Analysis

Bladder cancer tissue microarrays purchased from SuperBioChips Laboratories (Seoul, Korea) were stained with an anti-KDM7A antibody. The slides were incubated with an anti-Rabbit IgG secondary antibody and hematoxylin and eosin (nuclear staining dye). The expression level of KDM7A from 25 different bladder tumors and 6 normal tissues was calculated and plotted. The expression of KDM7A positive cells was evaluated using the Cytoplasmic V2.0 algorithm in Aperio ImageScope software (Leica, Nussloch, Germany), and logistic regression analysis was used to compare the expression patterns between groups. Mouse tumor tissues were fixed in paraffin after formaldehyde fixation. Mouse tissue slides were deparaffinized and stained with indicated antibodies, and the slides were photographed under a Leica microscope (Wetzlar, Germany). Positive signals were counted from at least 3 different fields of the same area, and relative values were calculated.

4.10. The Kaplan–Meier Plotter

The prognostic significance of the mRNA expression of KDM7A was evaluated using the Kaplan–Meier plotter (www.kmplot.com), an online database comprising gene expression data and clinical data. In order to assess the prognostic value of the KDM7A gene, the patient samples were divided into two cohorts according to the median expression level of the gene (high vs. low expression). We analyzed overall survival (OS) of bladder cancer patients by the Kaplan–Meier survival plot. KDM7A gene was uploaded into the database to obtain the Kaplan–Meier survival plot, in which the number-at-risk was shown below the main plot. Log rank p-value and hazard ratio (HR) with 95% confidence intervals were calculated and displayed on the webpage. We exported the plot data as a PowerPoint file.

4.11. Statistical Analyses

All data were analyzed using Microsoft Excel 2010 software, unless otherwise stated. Continuous variables were analyzed using Student's t-test if the data were normally distributed. All statistical tests were two-sided. Differences were considered significant in cases where p values were <0.05.

Supplementary Materials:
Figure S1. AR expression in bladder cell lines. Figure S2. AR expression levels in KDM7A knockdown J82 cells. Figure S3. The primer positions for ChIP-qPCR in the indicated gene promoters are illustrated. Figure S4. AR inhibition reduced cell viability of bladder cancer cells. Figure S5. T24 and J82 bladder cancer cells expressing KDM7A shRNAs or treated with TC-E 5002 photographed under phase contrast microscope. Figure S6. Enzalutamide treatment reduced cell mobility in bladder cancer cells. Figure S7. KDM7A knock-down reduced cell mobility in bladder cancer cells. Figure S8. Protein bands from Figure 4C were analyzed densitometrically and protein levels were normalized to beta-actin levels. Figure S9. The enzalutamide and TC-E 5002 treatment reduces cell growth and increased apoptosis in cisplatin resistant T24 cells. Figure S10. Enzalutamide and TC-E 5002 treatment reduced cell mobility in bladder cancer cells. Figure S11. IVIS images demonstrating tumor formation on the day of sacrifice. Figure S12. KDM7A protein expression in human bladder tumor tissues and normal tissues from the same patient. Figure S13. Survival curve was plotted for male bladder cancer patients with cancer stage 3. Figure S14. A survival curve was plotted for male bladder cancer patients with cancer stage 4. Table S1. The company and catalog numbers of antibodies. Table S2. Oligonucleotide sequences for RT-PCR and ChIP-PCR.

Author Contributions: Conceptualization, K.-H.L. and C.K.; Data curation, K.-H.L. and B.-C.K.; Funding acquisition, K.-H.L. and C.K.; Writing—original draft, K.-H.L.; Writing—review and editing, S.-H.J., C.W.J., J.H.K., H.H.K. and C.K. All authors have read and agreed to the published version of the manuscript.

Abbreviations

AR	androgen receptor
BCa	bladder cancer
CBP	CREB-binding protein
ChIP	chromatin immunoprecipitation
DHT	dihydrotestosterone
ECAD	E-cadherin
EMT	epithelial-mesenchymal transition
EZH2	enhancer of zeste homolog 2

HAT   histone acetyltransferase
IGF1R   insulin-like growth factor 1 receptor
KDM   lysine demethylase
KLK   kallikrein related peptidase
LSD1   lysine-specific histone demethylase 1
NCAD   N-cadherin
PCAF   P300/CBP-associated factor
PSA   prostate specific antigen
PHD   plant homeodomain
SET   su(var)3-9, enhancer-of-zeste and trithorax
SRC   steroid receptor coactivator proteins
VEGF   vascular endothelial growth factor

References

1.   Siegel, R.L.; Miller, K.D.; Jemal, A. Cancer statistics, 2019. *CA Cancer J. Clin.* **2019**, *69*, 7–34. [CrossRef] [PubMed]

2.   Sievert, K.D.; Amend, B.; Nagele, U.; Schilling, D.; Bedke, J.; Horstmann, M.; Hennenlotter, J.; Kruck, S.; Stenzl, A. Economic aspects of bladder cancer: What are the benefits and costs? *World J. Urol.* **2009**, *27*, 295–300. [CrossRef] [PubMed]

3.   Dobruch, J.; Daneshmand, S.; Fisch, M.; Lotan, Y.; Noon, A.P.; Resnick, M.J.; Shariat, S.F.; Zlotta, A.R.; Boorjian, S.A. Gender and Bladder Cancer: A Collaborative Review of Etiology, Biology, and Outcomes. *Eur. Urol.* **2016**, *69*, 300–310. [CrossRef] [PubMed]

4.   Chen, J.; Cui, Y.; Li, P.; Liu, L.; Li, C.; Zu, X. Expression and clinical significance of androgen receptor in bladder cancer: A meta-analysis. *Mol. Clin. Oncol.* **2017**, *7*, 919–927. [CrossRef]

5.   Claps, M.; Petrelli, F.; Caffo, O.; Amoroso, V.; Roca, E.; Mosca, A.; Maines, F.; Barni, S.; Berruti, A. Testosterone Levels and Prostate Cancer Prognosis: Systematic Review and Meta-analysis. *Clin. Genitourin. Cancer* **2018**, *16*, 165–175. [CrossRef]

6.   Sumanasuriya, S.; De Bono, J. Treatment of Advanced Prostate Cancer-A Review of Current Therapies and Future Promise. *Cold Spring Harb. Perspect. Med.* **2018**, *8*, a030635. [CrossRef]

7.   Roshan, M.H.; Tambo, A.; Pace, N.P. The role of testosterone in colorectal carcinoma: Pathomechanisms and open questions. *EPMA J.* **2016**, *7*, 22. [CrossRef]

8.   Ricciardelli, C.; Bianco-Miotto, T.; Jindal, S.; Butler, L.M. The Magnitude of Androgen Receptor Positivity in Breast Cancer is Critical for Reliable Prediction of Disease Outcome. *Clin. Cancer Res.* **2018**, *24*, 2328–2341. [CrossRef]

9.   Zhang, B.G.; Du, T.; Zang, M.D.; Chang, Q.; Fan, Z.Y.; Li, J.F.; Yu, B.Q.; Su, L.P.; Li, C.; Yan, C.; et al. Androgen receptor promotes gastric cancer cell migration and invasion via AKT-phosphorylation dependent upregulation of matrix metalloproteinase 9. *Oncotarget* **2014**, *5*, 10584–10595. [CrossRef]

10. Li, Y.; Izumi, K.; Miyamoto, H. The role of the androgen receptor in the development and progression of bladder cancer. *Jpn. J. Clin. Oncol.* **2012**, *42*, 569–577. [CrossRef]

11. Zhuang, Y.H.; Blauer, M.; Tammela, T.; Tuohimaa, P. Immunodetection of androgen receptor in human urinary bladder cancer. *Histopathology* **1997**, *30*, 556–562. [CrossRef] [PubMed]

12. Boorjian, S.; Ugras, S.; Mongan, N.P.; Gudas, L.J.; You, X.; Tickoo, S.K.; Scherr, D.S. Androgen receptor expression is inversely correlated with pathologic tumor stage in bladder cancer. *Urology* **2004**, *64*, 383–388. [CrossRef] [PubMed]

13. Boorjian, S.A.; Heemers, H.V.; Frank, I.; Farmer, S.A.; Schmidt, L.J.; Sebo, T.J.; Tindall, D.J. Expression and significance of androgen receptor coactivators in urothelial carcinoma of the bladder. *Endocr.-Relat. Cancer* **2009**, *16*, 123–137. [CrossRef] [PubMed]

14. Miyamoto, H.; Yang, Z.; Chen, Y.-T.; Ishiguro, H.; Uemura, H.; Kubota, Y.; Nagashima, Y.; Chang, Y.-J.; Hu, Y.-C.; Tsai, M.-Y.; et al. Promotion of Bladder Cancer Development and Progression by Androgen Receptor Signals. *JNCI J. Natl. Cancer Inst.* **2007**, *99*, 558–568. [CrossRef] [PubMed]

15. Hsu, J.-W.; Hsu, I.; Xu, D.; Miyamoto, H.; Liang, L.; Wu, X.-R.; Shyr, C.-R.; Chang, C. Decreased Tumorigenesis and Mortality from Bladder Cancer in Mice Lacking Urothelial Androgen Receptor. *Am. J. Pathol.* **2013**, *182*, 1811–1820. [CrossRef]

16. Kawahara, T.; Ide, H.; Kashiwagi, E.; El-Shishtawy, K.A.; Li, Y.; Reis, L.O.; Zheng, Y.; Miyamoto, H. Enzalutamide inhibits androgen receptor-positive bladder cancer cell growth. *Urol. Oncol.* **2016**, *34*, e15–e23. [CrossRef]

17. Kameyama, K.; Horie, K.; Mizutani, K.; Kato, T.; Fujita, Y.; Kawakami, K.; Kojima, T.; Miyazaki, T.; Deguchi, T.; Ito, M. Enzalutamide inhibits proliferation of gemcitabine-resistant bladder cancer cells with increased androgen receptor expression. *Int. J. Oncol.* **2017**, *50*, 75–84. [CrossRef]

18. Kawahara, T.; Inoue, S.; Kashiwagi, E.; Chen, J.; Ide, H.; Mizushima, T.; Li, Y.; Zheng, Y.; Miyamoto, H. Enzalutamide as an androgen receptor inhibitor prevents urothelial tumorigenesis. *Am. J. Cancer Res.* **2017**, *7*, 2041–2050. [CrossRef]

19. Kashiwagi, E.; Ide, H.; Inoue, S.; Kawahara, T.; Zheng, Y.; Reis, L.O.; Baras, A.S.; Miyamoto, H. Androgen receptor activity modulates responses to cisplatin treatment in bladder cancer. *Oncotarget* **2016**, *7*, 49169–49179. [CrossRef]

20. Baylin, S.B. DNA methylation and gene silencing in cancer. *Nat. Clin. Pract. Oncol.* **2005**, *2*, S4–S11. [CrossRef]

21. Dompe, C.; Janowicz, K.; Hutchings, G.; Moncrieff, L.; Jankowski, M.; Nawrocki, M.J.; Józkowiak, M.; Mozdziak, P.; Petitte, J.; Shibli, J.A.; et al. Epigenetic Research in Stem Cell Bioengineering-Anti-Cancer Therapy, Regenerative and Reconstructive Medicine in Human Clinical Trials. *Cancers* **2020**, *12*, 1016. [CrossRef] [PubMed]

22. Black, J.C.; Van Rechem, C.; Whetstine, J.R. Histone lysine methylation dynamics: Establishment, regulation, and biological impact. *Mol. Cell* **2012**, *48*, 491–507. [CrossRef] [PubMed]

23. Greer, E.L.; Shi, Y. Histone methylation: A dynamic mark in health, disease and inheritance. *Nat. Rev. Genet.* **2012**, *13*, 343–357. [CrossRef] [PubMed]

24. Kooistra, S.M.; Helin, K. Molecular mechanisms and potential functions of histone demethylases. *Nat. Rev. Mol. Cell Biol.* **2012**, *13*, 297–311. [CrossRef]

25. Baumgart, S.J.; Haendler, B. Exploiting Epigenetic Alterations in Prostate Cancer. *Int. J. Mol. Sci.* **2017**, *18*, 1017. [CrossRef]

26. Kahl, P.; Gullotti, L.; Heukamp, L.C.; Wolf, S.; Friedrichs, N.; Vorreuther, R.; Solleder, G.; Bastian, P.J.; Ellinger, J.; Metzger, E.; et al. Androgen receptor coactivators lysine-specific histone demethylase 1 and four and a half LIM domain protein 2 predict risk of prostate cancer recurrence. *Cancer Res.* **2006**, *66*, 11341–11347. [CrossRef]

27. Coffey, K.; Rogerson, L.; Ryan-Munden, C.; Alkharaif, D.; Stockley, J.; Heer, R.; Sahadevan, K.; O'Neill, D.; Jones, D.; Darby, S.; et al. The lysine demethylase, KDM4B, is a key molecule in androgen receptor signalling and turnover. *Nucleic Acids Res.* **2013**, *41*, 4433–4446. [CrossRef]

28. Han, M.; Xu, W.; Cheng, P.; Jin, H.; Wang, X. Histone demethylase lysine demethylase 5B in development and cancer. *Oncotarget* **2017**, *8*, 8980–8991. [CrossRef]

29. Deb, G.; Thakur, V.S.; Gupta, S. Multifaceted role of EZH2 in breast and prostate tumorigenesis. *Epigenetics* **2013**, *8*, 464–476. [CrossRef]

30. Liu, C.; Wang, C.; Wang, K.; Liu, L.; Shen, Q.; Yan, K.; Sun, X.; Chen, J.; Liu, J.; Ren, H.; et al. SMYD3 as an oncogenic driver in prostate cancer by stimulation of androgen receptor transcription. *J. Natl. Cancer Inst.* **2013**, *105*, 1719–1728. [CrossRef]

31. Mounir, Z.; Korn, J.M.; Westerling, T.; Lin, F.; Kirby, C.A.; Schirle, M.; McAllister, G.; Hoffman, G.; Ramadan, N.; Hartung, A.; et al. ERG signaling in prostate cancer is driven through PRMT5-dependent methylation of the Androgen Receptor. *Elife* **2016**, *5*, e13964. [CrossRef] [PubMed]

32. Lee, K.H.; Hong, S.; Kang, M.; Jeong, C.W.; Ku, J.H.; Kim, H.H.; Kwak, C. Histone demethylase KDM7A controls androgen receptor activity and tumor growth in prostate cancer. *Int. J. Cancer* **2018**, *143*, 2849–2861. [CrossRef] [PubMed]

33. Tsukada, Y.; Fang, J.; Erdjument-Bromage, H.; Warren, M.E.; Borchers, C.H.; Tempst, P.; Zhang, Y. Histone demethylation by a family of JmjC domain-containing proteins. *Nature* **2006**, *439*, 811–816. [CrossRef] [PubMed]

34. Meng, Z.; Liu, Y.; Wang, J.; Fan, H.; Fang, H.; Li, S.; Yuan, L.; Liu, C.; Peng, Y.; Zhao, W.; et al. Histone demethylase KDM7A is required for stem cell maintenance and apoptosis inhibition in breast cancer. *J. Cell. Physiol.* **2020**, *235*, 932–943. [CrossRef] [PubMed]

35. Yang, X.; Wang, G.; Wang, Y.; Zhou, J.; Yuan, H.; Li, X.; Liu, Y.; Wang, B. Histone demethylase KDM7A reciprocally regulates adipogenic and osteogenic differentiation via regulation of C/EBPalpha and canonical Wnt signalling. *J. Cell. Mol. Med.* **2019**, *23*, 2149–2162. [CrossRef]

36. Higashijima, Y.; Matsui, Y.; Shimamura, T.; Nakaki, R.; Nagai, N.; Tsutsumi, S.; Abe, Y.; Link, V.M.; Osaka, M.; Yoshida, M.; et al. Coordinated demethylation of H3K9 and H3K27 is required for rapid inflammatory responses of endothelial cells. *EMBO J.* **2020**, *39*, e103949. [CrossRef] [PubMed]

37. Grad, J.M.; Le Dai, J.; Wu, S.; Burnstein, K.L. Multiple Androgen Response Elements and a Myc Consensus Site in the Androgen Receptor (AR) Coding Region Are Involved in Androgen-Mediated Up-Regulation of AR Messenger RNA. *Mol. Endocrinol.* **1999**, *13*, 1896–1911. [CrossRef]

38. Blackburn, J.; Vecchiarelli, S.; Heyer, E.E.; Patrick, S.M.; Lyons, R.J.; Jaratlerdsiri, W.; van Zyl, S.; Bornman, M.S.R.; Mercer, T.R.; Hayes, V.M. TMPRSS2-ERG fusions linked to prostate cancer racial health disparities: A focus on Africa. *Prostate* **2019**, *79*, 1191–1196. [CrossRef]

39. Kim, J.; Coetzee, G.A. Prostate specific antigen gene regulation by androgen receptor. *J. Cell. Biochem.* **2004**, *93*, 233–241. [CrossRef]

40. Lai, J.; Myers, S.A.; Lawrence, M.G.; Odorico, D.M.; Clements, J.A. Direct Progesterone Receptor and Indirect Androgen Receptor Interactions with the Kallikrein-Related Peptidase 4 Gene Promoter in Breast and Prostate Cancer. *Mol. Cancer Res.* **2009**, *7*, 129. [CrossRef]

41. Schayek, H.; Seti, H.; Greenberg, N.M.; Sun, S.; Werner, H.; Plymate, S.R. Differential regulation of insulin-like growth factor-I receptor gene expression by wild type and mutant androgen receptor in prostate cancer cells. *Mol. Cell. Endocrinol.* **2010**, *323*, 239–245. [CrossRef] [PubMed]

42. Eisermann, K.; Broderick, C.J.; Bazarov, A.; Moazam, M.M.; Fraizer, G.C. Androgen up-regulates vascular endothelial growth factor expression in prostate cancer cells via an Sp1 binding site. *Mol. Cancer* **2013**, *12*, 7. [CrossRef] [PubMed]

43. Gao, L.; Schwartzman, J.; Gibbs, A.; Lisac, R.; Kleinschmidt, R.; Wilmot, B.; Bottomly, D.; Coleman, I.; Nelson, P.; McWeeney, S.; et al. Androgen receptor promotes ligand-independent prostate cancer progression through c-Myc upregulation. *PLoS ONE* **2013**, *8*, e63563. [CrossRef]

44. Xu, Y.; Chen, S.Y.; Ross, K.N.; Balk, S.P. Androgens induce prostate cancer cell proliferation through mammalian target of rapamycin activation and post-transcriptional increases in cyclin D proteins. *Cancer Res.* **2006**, *66*, 7783–7792. [CrossRef]

45. Li, Y.; Zhang, D.Y.; Ren, Q.; Ye, F.; Zhao, X.; Daniels, G.; Wu, X.; Dynlacht, B.; Lee, P. Regulation of a novel androgen receptor target gene, the cyclin B1 gene, through androgen-dependent E2F family member switching. *Mol. Cell. Biol.* **2012**, *32*, 2454–2466. [CrossRef] [PubMed]

46. Frezza, M.; Yang, H.; Dou, Q.P. Modulation of the tumor cell death pathway by androgen receptor in response to cytotoxic stimuli. *J. Cell. Physiol.* **2011**, *226*, 2731–2739. [CrossRef]

47. Kauffman, E.C.; Robinson, B.D.; Downes, M.J.; Powell, L.G.; Lee, M.M.; Scherr, D.S.; Gudas, L.J.; Mongan, N.P. Role of androgen receptor and associated lysine-demethylase coregulators, LSD1 and JMJD2A, in localized and advanced human bladder cancer. *Mol. Carcinog.* **2011**, *50*, 931–944. [CrossRef]

48. Shen, B.; Tan, M.; Mu, X.; Qin, Y.; Zhang, F.; Liu, Y.; Fan, Y. Upregulated SMYD3 promotes bladder cancer progression by targeting BCLAF1 and activating autophagy. *Tumour Biol. J. Int. Soc. Oncodev. Biol. Med.* **2016**, *37*, 7371–7381. [CrossRef]

49. Song, Y.; Wu, F.; Wu, J. Targeting histone methylation for cancer therapy: Enzymes, inhibitors, biological activity and perspectives. *J. Hematol. Oncol.* **2016**, *9*, 49. [CrossRef]

5

TERT Promoter Mutation as a Potential Predictive Biomarker in BCG-Treated Bladder Cancer Patients

Rui Batista [1,2,3,†], Luís Lima [4,†], João Vinagre [1,2,3,†], Vasco Pinto [2,3], Joana Lyra [2,3], Valdemar Máximo [1,2,3], Lúcio Santos [4] and Paula Soares [1,2,3,*]

[1] Instituto de Investigação e Inovação em Saúde (i3S), 4200-135 Porto, Portugal; rbatista@ipatimup.pt (R.B.); jvinagre@ipatimup.pt (J.V.); vmaximo@ipatimup.pt (V.M.)
[2] Instituto de Patologia e Imunologia Molecular da Universidade do Porto (IPATIMUP), 4200-135 Porto, Portugal; vasco.sa.pinto@gmail.com (V.P.); joanaritalyra@gmail.com (J.L.)
[3] Faculdade de Medicina da Universidade do Porto (FMUP), 4200-319 Porto, Portugal
[4] Grupo de Patologia e Terapêutica Experimental, Instituto Português de Oncologia do Porto FG, EPE (IPO-Porto), 4200-072 Porto, Portugal; luis14lima@gmail.com (L.L.); llarasantos@gmail.com (L.S.)
* Correspondence: psoares@ipatimup.pt
† These authors contributed equally to this work.

Abstract: Telomerase reverse transcriptase gene promoter (*TERTp*) mutations are recognized as one of the most frequent genetic events in bladder cancer (BC). No studies have focused on the relevance of TERTp mutations in the specific group of tumors treated with Bacillus Calmette–Guérin (BCG) intravesical therapy. Methods — 125 non muscle invasive BC treated with BCG therapy (BCG-NMIBC) were screened for *TERTp* mutations, *TERT* rs2853669 single nucleotide polymorphism, and Fibroblast Growth Factor Receptor 3 (*FGFR3*) hotspot mutations. Results — *TERTp* mutations were found in 56.0% of BCG-NMIBC and were not associated with tumor stage or grade. *FGFR3* mutations were found in 44.9% of the cases and were not associated with tumor stage or grade nor with *TERTp* mutations. The *TERT* rs2853669 single nucleotide polymorphism was associated with tumors of higher grade. The specific c.1-146G>A *TERTp* mutation was an independent predictor of nonrecurrence after BCG therapy (hazard ratio—0.382; 95% confidence interval—0.150–0.971, $p = 0.048$). Conclusions—*TERTp* mutations are frequent in BCG-NMIBC and -146G>A appears to be an independent predictive marker of response to BCG treatment with an impact in recurrence-free survival.

Keywords: *TERT* promoter mutations; *FGFR3*; non muscle invasive bladder cancer; BCG therapy

1. Introduction

Bladder cancer (BC) ranks as the fifth most common cancer in western society and the sixth most prevalent in the world, with an increasing incidence in the past years [1]. The increased incidence, along with the high costs in surveillance per BC patient, results in a high burden for public health systems [2,3]. BC can be divided in non muscle invasive (NMI) and muscle invasive (MI) tumors. NMI bladder cancer (NMIBC) accounts for 70% to 80% of all BC and is present as superficial and recurrent lesions that only seldom progress to an MI phenotype. Prompt treatment, usually with complete transurethral tumor resection, grants a 5-year survival rate that can surpass 90%. However, up to 70%-80% of them may relapse, making recurrence the main challenge in clinical management [3,4]. Present in approximately 70% of cases, Fibroblast Growth Factor Receptor 3 (FGFR3) activating mutations are the most frequent genetic event in the NMI phenotype [4]. MI bladder cancer (MIBC) accounts for the remaining 20%

to 30% of BC cases and presents as an invasive tumor at diagnosis. Characterized by a high risk of distant metastasis, MIBC prognosis is considerably worse, with 5-year survival rates often described as lower than 40% [5]. MI tumors are genetically more heterogeneous than NMI tumours; present in approximately half of the cases, *TP53* mutations are identified as the most frequent genetic alteration in these tumors [4].

Cell immortalization is a classic hallmark of cancer cells and telomerase reactivation is proposed to be involved in the underlying process. In a large part of cancer models, the intervening mechanisms remained elusive, until in 2013, mutations of the promoter of the telomerase (*TERT*) were described in melanoma [6,7]. We and others reported for the first time the presence of recurrent somatic mutations in the *TERT* promoter (*TERTp*) in numerous types of cancer, including BC [8–15]. Studies focusing on BC have described a prevalence of *TERTp* mutations ranging from 52% to 85% of the cases [10,13,14,16–19]. Conflicting results have been obtained on the association between *TERTp* mutations and BC clinical outcome [13,14]. A common polymorphism in *TERTp* (rs2853669 single nucleotide polymorphism) is also accountable to act as a modifier of the promoter mutations' effect on survival and tumor recurrence in several cancers, such as glioblastoma, liver, and bladder cancer [18,20,21].

Clinicopathological features are the central determinants of recurrence, and according to the European Organization for Research and Treatment of Cancer (EORTC), the NMIBC high-risk group includes high-grade papillary tumors, carcinoma in situ, and those with multifocal or recurrent lesions [22]. Tumor resection followed by a schedule of intravesical instillations with Bacillus Calmette–Guérin (BCG) is the standard adjuvant therapy for this high-risk group (henceforth referred to as BCG-NMIBC) [22,23]. Nonetheless, 30% to 40% of patients present either intolerance or recurrence following BCG treatment, demanding a life-long follow-up and repeated courses of treatment [24]. This clinical relevance is recognized and there is a shortage of dedicated genetic markers predicting BCG-NMIBC subgroup outcomes, in particular, the now recognized two most common genetic events in NMIBC—*TERT* promoter and *FGFR3* mutations.

In this study, we screened a series comprising 125 BCG-NMIBCs resected before BCG therapy initiation for *TERTp* mutations, *FGFR3* mutations, and for the *TERTp* rs2853669 polymorphism. This represents a unique report of *TERTp* and *FGFR3* mutation genotyping dedicated to the BCG-NMI group of BC. To investigate the significance of *TERTp* mutations in the BCG-treated tumor response, we compared the obtained results with the available clinicopathological data, including recurrence-free survival following BCG therapy.

2. Results

2.1. TERTp and FGFR3 Mutation Analysis

In the 125 BCG-treated NMIBC (BCG-NMIBC) tumors screened for *TERTp* mutations, 56.0% (70/125) of the cases were mutated. The c.1-124G>A mutation was detected in 36.8% (46/125) and the c.1-146G>A in 17.6% (22/125). In two cases (1.6%), both c.-124G>A and c.1-146 G>A mutations were observed (Table 1). *FGFR3* mutations (exons 7, 10 and 15) were evaluated in 107 cases. In the tumors screened for *FGFR3* mutations, 44.9% (48/107) of the cases were mutated (Table 1). The large majority was mutated in exon 7 and less frequently in exons 10 and 15 (Table 1). When analyzing *FGFR3* cases with only mutations in exon 7 (45 cases), 42.2% (19/45) presented the p.R248C mutation whereas the p.S249C mutation was present in 55.6% (25/45). One case harbored both mutations (2.2%). A comparison between *TERTp* mutation status and *FGFR3* status revealed no significant association between the two genetic events in the BCG-NMI tumors. The rs2853669 SNP was evaluated in 98 cases; rs2853669 AA genotype accounted for 39.8% (39/98) of the cases, AG genotype for 48.0% (47/98) and GG genotype for 12.2% (12/98) (Table 1).

Table 1. Telomerase reverse transcriptase gene promoter (*TERTp*) mutations, Fibroblast Growth Factor Receptor 3 (*FGFR3*) mutations, and rs2853669 prevalence across BCG-treated cases of nonmuscle invasive bladder cancers (BCG-NMIBC).

	BCG-NMIBC, *n* (%)
TERTp	
Wild type	55 (44.0)
Mutated	70 (56.0)
Specific mutations	
c.1-124G>A	46 (36.8)
c.1-146G>A	22 (17.6)
c.1-124G>A/c.1-146G>A	2 (1.6)
FGFR3	
Wild type	59 (55.1)
Mutated	48 (44.9)
Specific mutations	
Exon 7 p.R248C	19 (39.6)
Exon 7 p.S249C	25 (52.0)
Exon 10 p.Y375C	1 (2.1)
Exon 7 p.R248C + p.S249C	1 (2.1)
Exon 7 p.R248C + Exon 10 p.Y375C	1 (2.1)
Exon 7 p.R248C + Exon 15 p.K652E	1 (2.1)
rs2853669	
AA	39 (39.8)
AG	47 (48.0)
GG	12 (12.2)

2.2. Clinicopathological Characteristics and Genetic Alterations

A comparison between the clinicopathological characteristics of *TERTp* wild type and mutated cases was performed (Table 2). An association was found between *TERTp* mutations and recurrence status prior to BCG therapy, where an over-representation of *TERTp* mutations in primary tumors when compared with recurrent tumors can be detected (61.4% vs. 38.6%, $p = 0.048$).

In the BCG-NMIBC cases a statistically significant association between tumor size and *FGFR3* p.R248C mutations was found ($p = 0.048$). There was an over-representation of the mutation presence among tumors larger than 3 cm in comparison with the smaller ones (27.9% vs. 11.5%), Table S2. However, multivariate analysis revealed that FGFR3 p.R248C is not independently associated with tumor size.

The stratification of tumors in two groups, those wild type for both *TERTp* and *FGFR3* and those mutated for any, did not present statistically significant differences in the clinicopathological characteristics. Regarding the relationship of the studied polymorphism and clinicopathological features, an over-representation of the rs2853669 AA genotype was found in high-grade tumors when compared with low-grade tumors (77.4% vs. 22.6%, $p = 0.018$) (Table 3).

Table 2. Relation between clinicopathological data and *TERTp* mutation status in BCG-NMIBC.

	TERTp		
	Wild Type, *n* (%)	Mutated, *n* (%)	*p*-value
Age group			
<65 years	21 (38.2)	33 (47.1)	0.315
≥65 years	34 (61.8)	37 (52.9)	
Gender			
Female	11 (20.0)	8 (11.4)	0.185
Male	44 (80.0)	62 (88.6)	
Stage			
Ta	23 (41.8)	28 (40.0)	0.837
T1	32 (58.2)	42 (60.0)	
Grade			
Low	15 (27.3)	25 (35.7)	0.315
High	40 (72.7)	45 (64.3)	
Tumour size			
<3 cm	34 (63.0)	41 (58.6)	0.620
≥3 cm	20 (37.0)	29 (41.4)	
Multifocality			
No	28 (50.9)	32 (45.7)	0.564
Yes	27 (49.1)	38 (54.3)	
Recurrence status			
Primary	24 (43.6)	43 (61.4)	**0.048**
Recurrent	31 (56.4)	27 (38.6)	

p-Values obtained from Pearson's Chi-Square test for gender, stage, grade, tumor size, and multifocality and recurrence, bold values indicate $p < 0.05$.

Table 3. Relation between clinicopathological data and *rs2853669* single nucleotide polymorphism (SNP) status in BCG-NMIBC.

	rs2853669		
	AA, *n* (%)	G Carrier, *n* (%)	*p*-value
Age group			
<65 years	17 (41.5)	22 (38.6)	0.775
≥65 years	24 (58.5)	35 (61.4)	
Gender			
Female	5 (37.5)	34 (40.5)	0.736
Male	9 (64.3)	50 (59.5)	
Stage			
Ta	15 (39.5)	24 (40.0)	0.959
T1	23 (60.5)	36 (60.0)	
Grade			
Low	7 (22.6)	32 (47.8)	**0.018**
High	24 (77.4)	35 (52.2)	
Tumour size			
<3 cm	22 (34.9)	17 (50.0)	0.148
≥3 cm	41 (65.1)	17 (50.0)	
Multifocality			
No	19 (43.2)	20 (37.0)	0.536
Yes	25 (56.8)	34 (63.0)	
Recurrence status			
Primary	22 (43.1)	17 (36.2)	0.481
Recurrent	29 (56.9)	30 (63.8)	

p-Values obtained from Pearson's Chi-Square test for gender, stage, grade, tumor size, and multifocality and recurrence, bold values indicate $p < 0.05$.

2.3. Clinicopathological and Molecular Characteristics with BCG Therapy Success

Prior to tumor sampling, the BCG-NMIBC patients were treated with a scheme of BCG intravesical therapy. We evaluated how the clinicopathological characteristics affected BCG therapy outcome. Success was defined as no recurrence detected until the last surveillance check-up. Failure was defined as any recurrence after BCG treatment. After a univariate analysis, the age group $\geq$65 years (hazard ratio (HR): 2.827; 95% CI: 1.481–5.398; $p = 0.002$), multifocality (HR: 2.000; 95% CI: 1.096-3.649; $p = 0.024$) and maintenance BCG (mBCG) schedule (HR: 0.505; 95% CI: 0.282-0.902; $p = 0.021$) were the only variables significantly associated with the outcome, Table S1.

Next, we evaluated if the molecular characteristics have an effect on BCG therapy success. We performed a univariate analysis considering *TERTp* and *FGFR3* mutations and BCG therapy success. No statistically significant association was found on univariate analysis. To adjust for the effect of age group, multifocality, and BCG schedule on treatment success, we then performed a multivariate Cox regression analysis. When adjusted, the effect of status (wild type vs. mutated) for *TERTp* and *FGFR3* remained nonsignificant (Tables 4 and 5). However, when we considered *TERTp* c.1-146G>A carriers against *TERTp* non c.1-146G>A carriers (either *TERTp* wild type or c.1-124G>A), the c.1-146G>A mutation was significantly associated with therapy success (HR: 0.382; 95% CI: 0.150-0.971; $p = 0.043$) (Tables 4 and 5). In our series, the *TERTp* mutation c.1-146G>A was an independent predictor of therapy sucess following BCG intravesical therapy.

We further investigated the possible role of *TERTp* genetic events in predicting BCG therapy success by evaluating the presence of the single nucleotide polymorphism rs2853669 in the BCG-NMIBC series. We characterized cases as either carrier or noncarrier. No significant association was found for rs2853669 *per se*, or for *TERTp* mutation effect after splitting for rs2853669.

Table 4. Univariate analysis of the relation between *TERTp* and *FGFR3* mutations and recurrence after BCG treatment.

	BCG Therapy			
	Success, *n* (%)	Failure, *n* (%)	HR (95% CI)	*p*-value
TERTp				
Wild type	34 (43.0)	21 (45.7)	1.0	0.580
Mutated	45 (57.0)	25 (54.3)	0.848 (0.473–1.520)	
TERTp genotype				
Wild type	34 (43.0)	21 (45.6)	1.0	
c.1-124G > A	26 (32.9)	20 (43.5)	1.158 (0.626–2.143)	0.639
c.1-146G > A	17 (21.5)	5 (10.9)	0.410 (0.152–1.108)	0.079
c.1-124G>A/c.1-146G>A	2 (2.5)	0 (0.0)	0.464 (0.040–5.327)	0.464
TERTp c.1-146G>A status				
c.1-146G>A carriers	60 (75.9)	41 (89.1)	1.0	**0.043**
non c.1-146G>A carriers	19 (24.1)	5 (10.9)	0.382 (0.150–0.971)	
FGFR3				
Wild type	39 (60.0)	20 (51.3)	1.0	0.367
Mutated	26 (40.0)	19 (48.7)	1.336 (0.712–2.507)	
FGFR3 status				
Wild type	39 (60.0)	20 (51.3)	1.0	
p.R248C	12 (18.5)	7 (17.9)	1.158 (0.524–3.015)	0.608
p.S249C	14 (21.5)	11 (28.2)	0.410 (0.650–2.842)	0.415
p.R248C/p.S249C	0 (0.0)	1 (2.6)	1.584 (0.804–3.120)	0.184

p-values obtained from Wald test; bold values indicate $p < 0.05$. HR, Hazard Ratio; CI, Confidence Interval.

Table 5. Multivariate analysis and risk estimation of TERT c.1-146G>A mutation influence on BCG therapy outcome.

TERTp c.1-146G>A Status	HR [a]	95% CI	p-value
c.1-146G>A carriers	1.0	Referent	
non c.1-146G>A carriers	0.256	0.098-0.667	0.005
Age ≥ 65 years	2.370	1.206-4.661	0.012
Multifocality	1.883	0.964-3.677	0.064
Recurrent tumor	1.352	0.703-2.600	0.367
iBCG schedule	2.225	1.211-4.088	0.010

HR, Hazard Ratio; CI, Confidence Interval. [a] adjusted for age, multifocality, recurrence status, and BCG schedule.

2.4. TERTp Mutations and Recurrence-Free Survival

The recurrence-free survival function of all 125 BCG-treated NMIBC patients, grouped according to the existence of a *TERTp* mutation, was evaluated and log-rank testing revealed no statistically significant difference for either group (Figure S1). When considering *TERTp* c.1-146G>A carriers against *TERTp* non c.1-146G>A carriers (either *TERTp* wild type or c.1-124G>A), the *TERTp* c.1-146G>A patients presented a longer recurrence-free survival in comparison with the noncarriers (mean 126 months vs. mean 100 months, log rank $p = 0.035$) (Figure 1).

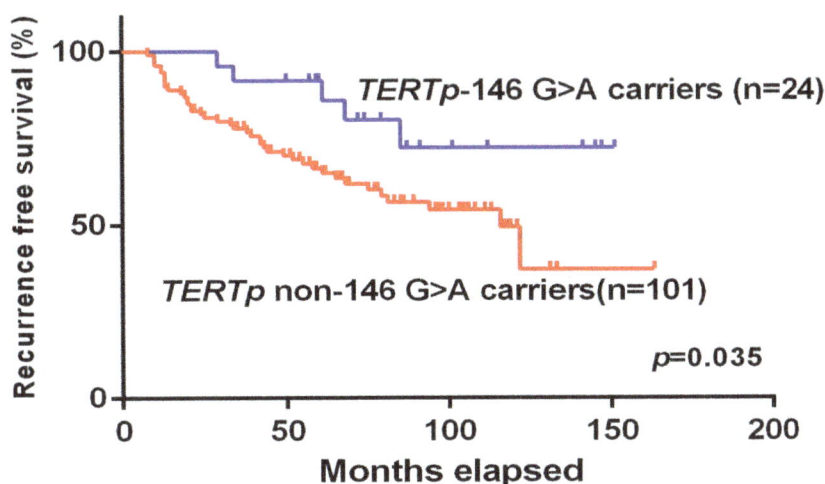

Figure 1. Kaplan–Meier recurrence-free survival function of BCG-NMIBC patients, grouped according to *TERTp* c.1-146G>A carriers against *TERTp* non c.1-146G>A carriers (either *TERTp* wild type or c.1-124G>A). Overall comparison of recurrence-free survival rates was performed using the log-rank test.

3. Discussion

TERTp mutations were reported in 52% to 85% of bladder cancer (BC) cases, depending on the series [10,13,14,16–19]. These results rank *TERTp* mutations as one of the most common genomic events observed in BC and possibly as the most frequent. Of all the *TERTp* mutations, c.1-124G>A has been consistently reported as the most frequent, detected in 88% to 95% of the positive cases [10,13,14,16–19]. In this study composed of BCG-treated NMIBC tumors, we report an overall *TERTp* mutation prevalence of 56.0%, in accordance with previously reported studies [10,13,14,16–19]. Conflicting results have been reported on the association between *TERTp* mutations and clinical stage and/or grade of bladder tumors. Wu et al. [19] found that *TERTp* mutations were more prevalent in MI tumors than in NMI tumors and in patients with advanced tumor stages. On the other hand, other studies reported no association between mutation status and stage or grade [13,14]. The results we present here support that *TERTp* mutations rates are not significantly different across grades or stages in this subset of BCG-treated NMIBC. However, it should be taken into account that this subset represents a group of particularly aggressive NMI tumors (BCG-NMIBC), and comparisons with NMIBC subseries in other studies must be made with caution.

Found in approximately 70% of tumors, *FGFR3* activating mutations are regarded as important genetic events in the NMI phenotype [4]. We found that 44.9% of the BCG-NMIBC cases were mutated for *FGFR3*. As *FGFR3* mutations are associated with low-grade and low-stage tumors and seem to predict a more favorable clinical outcome among patients with NMI tumors [3,25], it was expectable that the more aggressive BCG-NMIBC tumors presented lower mutation rates than those reported in other series [4]. Analyzing the specific *FGFR3* mutation distribution, a novel pattern emerges; previously, in NMIBC series, the most frequent mutations were at the exon 7 p.S249C (66.6% overall, 87.3% of the exon 7 mutations) and p.R248C (9.7% overall, 12.0% of the exon 7 mutations), and mutations in exon 10 and 15 were infrequent [26]. The *FGFR3* mutations detected in this study were mostly present on exon 7 (91.7%), but we observed a different prevalence of the specific mutations, with p.S249C accounting for 52.0%, and an enrichment for p.R248C, with 39.6%. In the BCG-NMIBC cases wild type and mutated for FGFR3, a statistically significant association between tumor size and FGFR3 p.R248C mutation was found ($p = 0.048$). However, multivariate analysis revealed that FGFR3 p.R248C is not independently associated with tumor size. One can discuss if FGFR3 p.R248C mutations are associated with more aggressive tumors, since it is particularly enriched in this subset of tumors and associated with larger tumor size in a univariate analysis. Loss of association in multivariate analysis may indicate that this association may be due to the influence of other clinicopathological features or, more likely, the analyzed cohort is too low to robustly perform this analysis. Further studies are required to elucidate these assumptions and findings. Finally, no significant association was found between the presence of *TERTp* and *FGFR3* mutations.

Intravesical BCG therapy is used as prophylaxis against NMIBC recurrences after tumor resection and it is in fact regarded as one of the first and most successful of all oncological immunotherapies [27,28]. BCG intravesical instillation results in multiple immune reactions. Although the precise immunological mechanism of BCG therapy is not clear, it appears to act through three main actions—infection of urothelial cells or bladder cancer cells, induction of immune responses, and induction of anti-tumour effects [27]. Although effective, 30% to 40% of the cases still show either intolerance or recurrence after BCG treatment, demanding life-long follow-up and repeated courses of treatment [24]. This results in extreme discomfort for the patients and exceedingly high financial costs, and ranks BC as the most expensive cancer per patient [3]. Biomarkers that could help identify which patients were more likely to respond to BCG versus those with risk of recurrence — those who would benefit the most from either a tighter surveillance or a different treatment — would be very useful in optimizing the clinical care offered to BC patients. In this study, we report the effects of *TERTp* and *FGFR3* mutations in BCG therapy success (recurrence or nonrecurrence) and recurrence-free survival. Age at BCG treatment, multifocality, and BCG schedule were independent predictors of BCG therapy success (defined as no recurrence), with the age group ≥65 years and multifocal tumours associated with a higher risk of recurrence, whereas mBCG schedule was associated with a lower risk of recurrence. These results are concordant with previous reports [29]. After adjusting for age, multifocality, and BCG schedule, we found no association between *FGFR3* mutations and BGC therapy success. Similarly, *TERTp*-mutated cases as a whole showed no difference when compared to wild type cases. However, when we compared carriers of the *TERTp* c.1-146G > A mutation against those without this mutation, we observed that this specific mutation was an independent predictor of better outcome (delayed or nonrecurrence).

Recently, Rachakonda et al. reported that a common polymorphism within a pre-existing Ets2 binding site in *TERTp*, rs2853669, acts as a modifier of the mutations' effect on survival and tumor recurrence [18]. The patients with the *TERTp* mutations presented a poorer survival in the absence, but not in the presence of the variant allele (G) of the polymorphism [18]. TERTp mutations in the absence of the variant allele were highly associated with disease recurrence in patients with Tis, Ta, and T1 tumors [18]. To further investigate this, we screened BCG-NMIBC tumors for this common

SNP. We found that rs2853669 carrier status did not modulate *TERTp* effect on BCG therapy success in our series, however, there was an association of rs2853669 AA carriers with tumors of higher grade. This association is in accordance with what Rachakonda and others described. In patients that harbor the germline rs2853669 AA genotype, the TERTp mutation effect is not reverted in the BC tumor. As Rachakonda described, patients with this combination (germline rs2853669 G absence, TERTp tumor positive) present poorer survival and increased disease recurrence, which are features compatible with the presence of more aggressive tumors, such as higher grade.

Finally, we analyzed recurrence-free survival after BCG treatment, comparing *TERTp* and *FGFR3* mutation status and specific mutations and rs2853669 carrier status. Kaplan–Meier survival analysis showed a promising recurrence-free survival advantage for those c.1-146G>A mutation carriers. Our results demonstrate that BCG-NMIBC c.1-146G>A mutation carriers are three time less likely to recur after BCG therapy and may have more favorable recurrence-free survival rates when compared to both *TERTp* wild type and c.1-124G>A cases. To interpret these findings, it is important to note that what we are evaluating is how *TERTp* mutations modulate the tumor response after BCG therapy. It has previously been suggested that the mechanism of BCG therapeutic effects on BC is related to its ability to reduce telomerase (*TERT*) activity [30] — we may speculate that c.1-146G>A mutated tumors might be more susceptible to the reduction of telomerase activity by BCG. As reported by Huang et al., *TERTp* mutations are associated with higher *TERT* transcription levels compared to wild type promoters but *TERTp* c.1-146G>A carriers have lower transcriptional capacity than those with the c.1-124G>A mutation [7]. We can speculate that the higher *TERT* expression induced by the c.1-124G>A mutation partially impairs BCG capability to sufficiently reduce telomeric activity to a therapeutic level — a level that could be achieved in a c.1-146G>A setting. Also, the lower frequency of *TERTp* mutations in BCG-treated recurrent tumors when compared to primary tumors could be explained by the enhanced BCG action on tumor cells harboring *TERTp* mutations, leading to clonal selection pressure towards cells harboring other alterations (such as *FGFR3* mutations) in recurrent tumors, hence shifting the prevalence of recurrent tumors towards TERTp-negative tumors. More studies comparing *TERT* expression and telomerase activity before and after BCG therapy with the different *TERTp* mutations are required to further interpret our results. To our knowledge, this study is one of the first studies addressing *TERTp* and *FGFR3* mutations in a BCG-NMI series of BC patients. We found no association between *TERTp* mutations, as a whole, and tumor grade or stage. However, we observed that the specific *TERTp* c.1-146G>A mutation was an independent predictor of nonrecurrence after BCG therapy in the BCG-NMI tumors. Our results suggest that it might be relevant to further study the role of *TERTp* mutations in tumor recurrence and as predictive markers of response to BCG therapy.

4. Materials and Methods

4.1. Human Cancer Samples and Clinicopathological Data

Formalin-fixed, paraffin-embedded (FFPE) tissues were obtained from 125 patients with NMI bladder urothelial cell carcinoma treated with intravesical BCG therapy, with samples being collected at the time of transurethral resection before any BCG therapy administration. Patients underwent resection of the tumors in the Portuguese Institute of Oncology — Francisco Gentil (IPO) Porto. Hematoxylin-eosin-stained sections were reviewed according to the standard histopathological examination by two independent pathologists. Staging and grading were conducted according to the American Joint Committee on Cancer [31], and the 2004 WHO classification system [32]. Clinicopathological and follow-up data were retrieved from the files of IPO databases. Age refers to age at BCG treatment initiation in the BCG-NMIBC group. Recurrence status characterizes the BCG-NMIBC cases as either a primary newly diagnosed tumor selected for BCG therapy or, alternatively, as a recurrence of a previously resected NMI tumor (that did not fill the criteria for being included in the BCG-NMIBC group before) that is only now selected for BCG therapy. BCG therapy selection was performed according to the EORTC criteria previously described [22]. BCG schedule characterizes the treatment regimen used as maintenance (mBCG) or induction-only (iBCG) intravesical BCG instillation. BCG therapy success was defined as no recurrence and failure was defined as any recurrence after BCG treatment. Analysis of patients' age by age groups (<65 years and ≥65 years) was recognized as an informative analysis and has been used previously [33]. All the procedures described in this study were in accordance with national and institutional ethical standards and previously approved by Local Ethical Review Committees (Ethics Committee of the Portuguese Institute of Oncology of Porto with the number CES IPOPFG-EPE 586/08 in 25 of September of 2008). According to Portuguese law, informed consent is not required for retrospective studies.

4.2. DNA Extraction, PCR, and Sanger Sequencing

DNA was obtained from FFPE (10-micron sections) after careful microdissection. DNA extraction was performed using an Ultraprep Tissue DNA Kit (AHN Biotechnologie, Nordhaussen, Germany) following manufacturer's instructions.

To screen for *TERTp* mutations, we analyzed by PCR followed by Sanger sequencing of the hotspots previously identified [10]. *TERTp* mutation analysis was performed with the pair of primers Fw *TERT*—5′-CAGCGCTGCCTGAAACTC-3′ and Rv *TERT*—5′-GTCCTGCCCCTTCACCTT-3′. Amplification of genomic DNA (25–100ng) was performed by PCR using the Qiagen Multiplex PCR kit (Qiagen, Hilden, Germany) according to the manufacturer's instructions. Sequencing reaction was performed with the ABI Prism BigDye Terminator Kit (Perkin Elmer, Foster City, CA, USA), and the fragments were run in an ABI prism 3100 Genetic Analyzer (Perkin-Elmer). The sequencing reaction was performed in a forward direction, and an independent PCR amplification/sequencing, both in a forward and reverse direction, was performed in positive samples or samples that were inconclusive. To screen for *FGFR3*, we analyzed the hotspots previously identified in exon 7, 10, and 15 in 107 BCG-NMIBC cases (18 cases have been excluded due to insufficient DNA for the analysis) by PCR followed by Sanger sequencing. *FGFR3* exon 7, 10, and 15 mutation analysis was performed with the respective pairs of primers Fw Exon 7—5′-AGTGGCGGTGGTGGTGAGGGAG-3′ and Rv Exon 7—5′-GCACCGCCGTCTGGTTGG-3′; Fw Exon 10—5′-CAACGCCCATGTCTTTGCAG-3′ and Rv Exon 10—5′-AGGCGGCAGAGCGTCACAG-3′; Fw Exon 15—5′-GACCGAGGACAACGTGATG-3′ and Rv Exon 15—5′-GTGTGGGAAGGCGGTGTTG-3′. Subsequent steps followed the same methodology as outlined for the *TERT* promoter mutation screening.

4.3. Single Nucleotide Polymorphism Assay

Screening for the rs2853669 polymorphism was performed in 98 BCG-NMIBC cases (27 cases were excluded due to insufficient DNA for the analysis) using the rs2853669 TaqMan® SNP Genotyping Assay (Applied Biosystems, Foster City, USA). Peripheral blood DNA was extracted using a genomic DNA extraction kit (Qiagen). The purified genomic DNA was used for the assay. The procedure was performed according to manufacturer's instructions.

4.4. Uromonitor Real-Time PCR screening Assay

Screening of 125 nonmuscle invasive BC tumors treated with BCG therapy (BCG-NMIBC) for *TERTp* mutations and *FGFR3* hotspot mutations were confirmed by using a specific IVD commercial kit Uromonitor®—Real-Time PCR kit for the amplification and detection of *TERTp* and *FGFR3* hotspot mutations (U-Monitor, Porto, Portugal), according to manufacturer's instructions.

4.5. Statistical Analysis

The statistical analysis was performed using IBM SPSS statistics software version 25.0. For the analysis of the relationship between patients' age, we used the independent-samples *t*-test. Pearson's Chi-square and Fisher's exact test were used in the statistical analysis of the other parameters, according to sample size. Cox proportional hazard ratios were estimated to obtain risks of recurrence for cases in each molecular factor stratum before and after adjusting for other confounding variables. Kaplan–Meier survival curves were computed by each category of the potential prognostic factors and the log-rank and Breslow tests were applied to compare curves. Means were used instead of medians because some survival curves did not fall under 50%. Results were considered statistically significant if $p < 0.05$.

Author Contributions: Conceptualization, R.B., J.V., V.M., L.S. and P.S.; data curation, L.L.; formal analysis, R.B. and L.L.; funding acquisition, J.V., V.M., L.S. and P.S.; investigation, R.B., L.L., J.V., V.P., J.L. and P.S.; methodology, R.B., V.P. and J.L.; project administration, L.S. and P.S.; resources, J.V. and P.S.; supervision, V.M., L.S. and P.S.; validation, R.B. and J.V.; writing—original draft, R.B., L.L., J.V., V.P. and J.L.; writing—review and editing, R.B., L.L., J.V., V.M., L.S. and P.S. All authors have read and agreed to the published version of the manuscript.

Abbreviations

BC	Bladder cancer
BCG	Bacillus Calmette–Guérin
BCG-NMI	BCG-treated nonmuscle invasive
NMI	Nonmuscle invasive

References

1. Ferlay, J.; Colombet, M.; Soerjomataram, I.; Mathers, C.; Parkin, D.M.; Pineros, M.; Znaor, A.; Bray, F. Estimating the global cancer incidence and mortality in 2018: GLOBOCAN sources and methods. *J. Int. Cancer* **2019**, *144*, 1941–1953. [CrossRef]

2. Ploeg, M.; Aben, K.K.; Kiemeney, L.A. The present and future burden of urinary bladder cancer in the world. *World J. Urol.* **2009**, *27*, 289–293. [CrossRef] [PubMed]

3. van Rhijn, B.W.; Burger, M.; Lotan, Y.; Solsona, E.; Stief, C.G.; Sylvester, R.J.; Witjes, J.A.; Zlotta, A.R. Recurrence and progression of disease in non-muscle-invasive bladder cancer: from epidemiology to treatment strategy. *Eur. Urol.* **2009**, *56*, 430–442. [CrossRef] [PubMed]

4. Netto, G.J. Molecular biomarkers in urothelial carcinoma of the bladder: are we there yet? *Nat. Rev. Urol.* **2011**, *9*, 41–51. [CrossRef] [PubMed]

5. Northrup, H.; Krueger, D.A.; International Tuberous Sclerosis Complex Consensus, G. Tuberous sclerosis complex diagnostic criteria update: recommendations of the 2012 Iinternational Tuberous Sclerosis Complex Consensus Conference. *Pediatr. Neurol.* **2013**, *49*, 243–254. [CrossRef]

6. Horn, S.; Figl, A.; Rachakonda, P.S.; Fischer, C.; Sucker, A.; Gast, A.; Kadel, S.; Moll, I.; Nagore, E.; Hemminki, K.; et al. TERT promoter mutations in familial and sporadic melanoma. *Science* **2013**, *339*, 959–961. [CrossRef]

7. Huang, F.W.; Hodis, E.; Xu, M.J.; Kryukov, G.V.; Chin, L.; Garraway, L.A. Highly recurrent TERT promoter mutations in human melanoma. *Science* **2013**, *339*, 957–959. [CrossRef]

8. Killela, P.J.; Reitman, Z.J.; Jiao, Y.; Bettegowda, C.; Agrawal, N.; Diaz, L.A., Jr.; Friedman, A.H.; Friedman, H.; Gallia, G.L.; Giovanella, B.C.; et al. TERT promoter mutations occur frequently in gliomas and a subset of tumors derived from cells with low rates of self-renewal. *Proc. Natl. Acad. Sci. USA* **2013**, *110*, 6021–6026. [CrossRef]

9. Liu, X.; Bishop, J.; Shan, Y.; Pai, S.; Liu, D.; Murugan, A.K.; Sun, H.; El-Naggar, A.K.; Xing, M. Highly prevalent TERT promoter mutations in aggressive thyroid cancers. *Endocr. Relat. Cancer* **2013**, *20*, 603–610. [CrossRef]

10. Vinagre, J.; Almeida, A.; Populo, H.; Batista, R.; Lyra, J.; Pinto, V.; Coelho, R.; Celestino, R.; Prazeres, H.; Lima, L.; et al. Frequency of TERT promoter mutations in human cancers. *Nat. Commun.* **2013**, *4*, 2185. [CrossRef]

11. Nault, J.C.; Mallet, M.; Pilati, C.; Calderaro, J.; Bioulac-Sage, P.; Laurent, C.; Laurent, A.; Cherqui, D.; Balabaud, C.; Zucman-Rossi, J. High frequency of telomerase reverse-transcriptase promoter somatic mutations in hepatocellular carcinoma and preneoplastic lesions. *Nat. Commun.* **2013**, *4*, 2218. [CrossRef] [PubMed]

12. Griewank, K.G.; Schilling, B.; Murali, R.; Bielefeld, N.; Schwamborn, M.; Sucker, A.; Zimmer, L.; Hillen, U.; Schaller, J.; Brenn, T.; et al. TERT promoter mutations are frequent in atypical fibroxanthomas and pleomorphic dermal sarcomas. *Mod. Pathol.: Off. J. US Can. Acad. Pathol. Inc.* **2014**, *27*, 502–508. [CrossRef] [PubMed]

13. Allory, Y.; Beukers, W.; Sagrera, A.; Flandez, M.; Marques, M.; Marquez, M.; van der Keur, K.A.; Dyrskjot, L.; Lurkin, I.; Vermeij, M.; et al. Telomerase reverse transcriptase promoter mutations in bladder cancer: high frequency across stages, detection in urine, and lack of association with outcome. *Eur. Urol.* **2014**, *65*, 360–366. [CrossRef] [PubMed]

14. Hurst, C.D.; Platt, F.M.; Knowles, M.A. Comprehensive mutation analysis of the TERT promoter in bladder cancer and detection of mutations in voided urine. *Eur. Urol.* **2014**, *65*, 367–369. [CrossRef]

15. Scott, G.A.; Laughlin, T.S.; Rothberg, P.G. Mutations of the TERT promoter are common in basal cell carcinoma and squamous cell carcinoma. *Mod. Pathol.: Off. J. US Can. Acad. Pathol. Inc.* **2014**, *27*, 516–523. [CrossRef]

16. Liu, X.; Wu, G.; Shan, Y.; Hartmann, C.; von Deimling, A.; Xing, M. Highly prevalent TERT promoter mutations in bladder cancer and glioblastoma. *Cell Cycle* **2013**, *12*, 1637–1638. [CrossRef]

17. Kinde, I.; Munari, E.; Faraj, S.F.; Hruban, R.H.; Schoenberg, M.; Bivalacqua, T.; Allaf, M.; Springer, S.; Wang, Y.; Diaz, L.A., Jr.; et al. TERT promoter mutations occur early in urothelial neoplasia and are biomarkers of early disease and disease recurrence in urine. *Cancer Res.* **2013**, *73*, 7162–7167. [CrossRef]

18. Rachakonda, P.S.; Hosen, I.; de Verdier, P.J.; Fallah, M.; Heidenreich, B.; Ryk, C.; Wiklund, N.P.; Steineck, G.; Schadendorf, D.; Hemminki, K.; et al. TERT promoter mutations in bladder cancer affect patient survival and disease recurrence through modification by a common polymorphism. *Proc. Natl. Acad. Sci. USA* **2013**, *110*, 17426–17431. [CrossRef]

19. Wu, S.; Huang, P.; Li, C.; Huang, Y.; Li, X.; Wang, Y.; Chen, C.; Lv, Z.; Tang, A.; Sun, X.; et al. Telomerase reverse transcriptase gene promoter mutations help discern the origin of urogenital tumors: a genomic and molecular study. *Eur. Urol.* **2014**, *65*, 274–277. [CrossRef]

20. Ko, E.; Seo, H.W.; Jung, E.S.; Kim, B.H.; Jung, G. The TERT promoter SNP rs2853669 decreases E2F1 transcription factor binding and increases mortality and recurrence risks in liver cancer. *Oncotarget* **2016**, *7*, 684–699. [CrossRef]

21. Batista, R.; Cruvinel-Carloni, A.; Vinagre, J.; Peixoto, J.; Catarino, T.A.; Campanella, N.C.; Menezes, W.; Becker, A.P.; de Almeida, G.C.; Matsushita, M.M.; et al. The prognostic impact of TERT promoter mutations in glioblastomas is modified by the rs2853669 single nucleotide polymorphism. *Int. J. Cancer* **2016**, *139*, 414–423. [CrossRef] [PubMed]

22. Babjuk, M.; Oosterlinck, W.; Sylvester, R.; Kaasinen, E.; Bohle, A.; Palou-Redorta, J.; Roupret, M.; European Association of U. EAU guidelines on non-muscle-invasive urothelial carcinoma of the bladder, the 2011 update. *Eur. Urol.* **2011**, *59*, 997–1008. [CrossRef] [PubMed]

23. Askeland, E.J.; Newton, M.R.; O'Donnell, M.A.; Luo, Y. Bladder Cancer Immunotherapy: BCG and Beyond. *Adv. Urol.* **2012**, *2012*, 181987. [CrossRef] [PubMed]

24. Yates, D.R.; Roupret, M. Contemporary management of patients with high-risk non-muscle-invasive bladder cancer who fail intravesical BCG therapy. *World J. Urol.* **2011**, *29*, 415–422. [CrossRef] [PubMed]

25. Billerey, C.; Chopin, D.; Aubriot-Lorton, M.H.; Ricol, D.; Gil Diez de Medina, S.; Van Rhijn, B.; Bralet, M.P.; Lefrere-Belda, M.A.; Lahaye, J.B.; Abbou, C.C.; et al. Frequent FGFR3 mutations in papillary non-invasive bladder (pTa) tumors. *Am. J. Pathol.* **2001**, *158*, 1955–1959. [CrossRef]

26. Roe, J.S.; Kim, H.; Lee, S.M.; Kim, S.T.; Cho, E.J.; Youn, H.D. p53 Stabilization and Transactivation by a von Hippel-Lindau Protein. *Mol. Cell* **2006**, *22*, 395–405. [CrossRef]

27. Kawai, K.; Miyazaki, J.; Joraku, A.; Nishiyama, H.; Akaza, H. Bacillus Calmette-Guerin (BCG) immunotherapy for bladder cancer: current understanding and perspectives on engineered BCG vaccine. *Cancer Sci.* **2013**, *104*, 22–27. [CrossRef]

28. Herr, H.W.; Morales, A. History of bacillus Calmette-Guerin and bladder cancer: an immunotherapy success story. *J. Urol.* **2008**, *179*, 53–56. [CrossRef]

29. Dabora, S.L.; Jozwiak, S.; Franz, D.N.; Roberts, P.S.; Nieto, A.; Chung, J.; Choy, Y.-S.; Reeve, M.P.; Thiele, E.; Egelhoff, J.C.; et al. Mutational Analysis in a Cohort of 224 Tuberous Sclerosis Patients Indicates Increased Severity of TSC2, Compared with TSC1, Disease in Multiple Organs. *Am. J. Hum. Genet.* **2001**, *68*, 64–80. [CrossRef]

30. Saitoh, H.; Mori, K.; Kudoh, S.; Itoh, H.; Takahashi, N.; Suzuki, T. BCG effects on telomerase activity in bladder cancer cell lines. *Int. J. Clin. Oncol.* **2002**, *7*, 165–170. [CrossRef]

31. Edge, S.B.; Compton, C.C. The American Joint Committee on Cancer: the 7th edition of the AJCC cancer staging manual and the future of TNM. *Ann. Surg. Oncol.* **2010**, *17*, 1471–1474. [CrossRef] [PubMed]

32. Davis, C.J.; Woodward, P.J.; Dehner, L.P.; Eble, J.N.; Sauter, G.; Epstein, J.I. WHO Classification of Tumors. Pathology and Genetics of Tumors of the Urinary System and Male Genital Organs. *IARC Press* **2004**, 267–276.

33. Lima, L.; Oliveira, D.; Tavares, A.; Amaro, T.; Cruz, R.; Oliveira, M.J.; Ferreira, J.A.; Santos, L. The predominance of M2-polarized macrophages in the stroma of low-hypoxic bladder tumors is associated with BCG immunotherapy failure. *Urol. Oncol.* **2014**, *32*, 449–457. [CrossRef] [PubMed]

6

Diagnostic and Prognostic Potential of MicroRNA Maturation Regulators Drosha, AGO1 and AGO2 in Urothelial Carcinomas of the Bladder

Anja Rabien [1,2,*], Nadine Ratert [1,2], Anica Högner [3], Andreas Erbersdobler [4], Klaus Jung [1,2], Thorsten H. Ecke [5,†] and Ergin Kilic [3,6,†]

[1] Department of Urology, Charité—Universitätsmedizin Berlin, Corporate Member of Freie Universität Berlin, Humboldt-Universität zu Berlin, and Berlin Institute of Health, 10117 Berlin, Germany; n.ratert@gmx.de (N.R.); klaus.jung@charite.de (K.J.)

[2] Berlin Institute for Urologic Research, 10117 Berlin, Germany

[3] Institute of Pathology, Charité—Universitätsmedizin Berlin, Corporate Member of Freie Universität Berlin, Humboldt-Universität zu Berlin, and Berlin Institute of Health, 10117 Berlin, Germany; anica.hoegner@charite.de (A.H.); e.kilic@pathologie-leverkusen.de (E.K.)

[4] Institute of Pathology, University Medicine Rostock, 18055 Rostock, Germany; andreas.erbersdobler@med.uni-rostock.de

[5] Department of Urology, HELIOS Hospital Bad Saarow, 15526 Bad Saarow, Germany; thorsten.ecke@helios-kliniken.de

[6] Institute of Pathology, Hospital Leverkusen, 51375 Leverkusen, Germany

*   Correspondence: anja.rabien@charite.de

†   These authors contributed equally to this work.

Abstract: Bladder cancer still requires improvements in diagnosis and prognosis, because many of the cases will recur and/or metastasize with bad outcomes. Despite ongoing research on bladder biomarkers, the clinicopathological impact and diagnostic function of miRNA maturation regulators Drosha and Argonaute proteins AGO1 and AGO2 in urothelial bladder carcinoma remain unclear. Therefore, we conducted immunohistochemical investigations of a tissue microarray composed of 112 urothelial bladder carcinomas from therapy-naïve patients who underwent radical cystectomy or transurethral resection and compared the staining signal with adjacent normal bladder tissue. The correlations of protein expression of Drosha, AGO1 and AGO2 with sex, age, tumor stage, histological grading and overall survival were evaluated in order to identify their diagnostic and prognostic potential in urothelial cancer. Our results show an upregulation of AGO1, AGO2 and Drosha in non-muscle-invasive bladder carcinomas, while there was increased protein expression of only AGO2 in muscle-invasive bladder carcinomas. Moreover, we were able to differentiate between non-muscle-invasive and muscle-invasive bladder carcinoma according to AGO1 and Drosha expression. Finally, despite Drosha being a discriminating factor that can predict the probability of overall survival in the Kaplan–Meier analysis, AGO1 turned out to be independent of all clinicopathological parameters according to Cox regression. In conclusion, we assumed that the miRNA processing factors have clinical relevance as potential diagnostic and prognostic tools for bladder cancer.

Keywords: bladder cancer; Drosha; AGO1; AGO2; biomarkers; immunohistochemistry

1. Introduction

In 2012, 430,000 new cases of bladder cancer were diagnosed worldwide. Thus, bladder cancer is the ninth most common cancer in the world with the highest incidence in Northern America,

Europe and some countries in Northern Africa and Western Asia [1]. Despite their heterogeneity, several characteristics have been found, which distinguish the subgroups of less aggressive, but often recurring non-muscle-invasive bladder cancer (NMIBC) and the more progressive muscle-invasive bladder cancer (MIBC). The latter holds an overall survival rate of 60% at most [2]. NMIBC develops from urothelial hyperplasia to low-grade carcinoma, with up to 15% proceeding to high-grade tumors. These cancers show characteristic alterations in the Ras-MAPK and PI3K-Akt pathways. The pathway leading to MIBC often includes dysplasia/carcinoma in situ and high-grade non-invasive carcinoma that accumulates common defects, e.g., in tumor suppressors, such as p53 or pRb, or in matrix metalloproteinases [2,3]. Although several potential biomarkers have been tested for their diagnostic and prognostic potential, targets for routine use are still needed.

A recent field of biomarker research has focused on microRNAs (miRNAs), which are involved in various biological processes, including tumorigenesis [4,5]. Several studies profiled the miRNA expression patterns in bladder cancer tissue and indicated some interesting findings regarding its diagnostic and/or prognostic potential [6,7]. The biogenesis of miRNAs is a multistep process involving a couple of protein complexes [8]. In the nucleus, miRNA genes are transcribed by RNA polymerase II/III into a long single or multiple primary miRNA, which is subsequently processed by the "Drosha microprocessor" into hairpin precursor miRNA (pre-miRNA). This "Drosha microprocessor" is a complex of the RNase III enzyme Drosha, its cofactor DiGeorge syndrome critical region gene 8 (DGCR8/Pasha) and other components. The pre miRNA is actively exported by exportin 5/Ras-related nuclear protein-guanosine triphosphate (Ran-GTP) to the cytoplasm. In this cellular compartment, RNase III enzyme Dicer converts pre miRNA to a mature double-stranded miRNA duplex that contains both the mature and its complementary strand and consists of about 20 nucleotides. The mature miRNA is subsequently loaded onto the miRNA Induced Silencing Complex (miRISC). The Argonaute (AGO) family proteins AGO1–AGO4 are the central components of the miRISC complex, which stabilize the mature miRNA strand. The other strand is degraded. AGO2 is the only protein with endonucleolytic activity that mediates the inhibition of target mRNA expression. The subsequent rate of miRNA complementarity and target mRNA affects the repression of translation or cleavage of mRNA. Additionally, there is some evidence indicating an alternative biogenesis pathway in which pre miRNAs are directly loaded onto the miRISC complex after Drosha processing, omitting Dicer processing [9].

As mentioned above, AGO1 and AGO2 are needed for the process of degrading mRNAs or impairing their translation, while Drosha plays a role in initial miRNA maturation. Consequently, it is postulated that they also play a key role in tumor behavior. Some studies have already reported a tumor specific expression of AGO1, AGO2, Dicer and Drosha in the urogenital tract. For example, the Argonautes have been implicated in clear cell renal cell carcinoma [10] and prostate cancer [11]. Meanwhile, the data for Argonautes and Drosha also exist for bladder carcinoma [12,13], but these are contradictory to our findings in major points and require discussion. The aim of our comprehensive immunohistochemical study was to investigate AGO1, AGO2 and Drosha expression in normal bladder urothelium and malignant bladder cancer tissue (NMIBC and MIBC) using a tissue microarray (TMA) as well as to correlate the expression of these proteins with clinicopathological parameters. We believe that our findings will support the potential of these three targets to become bladder carcinoma biomarkers but they will have to be carefully investigated further to avoid inaccurate conclusions indicated by the contradictory results in the literature.

2. Results

2.1. Immunostaining Pattern of AGO1, AGO2, and Drosha Expression in Bladder Tissue

All three targets appeared with a granular pattern in malignant and non-malignant tissue, while they were also often expressed in endothelial cells (Figures 1 and 2). AGO1 staining was found in the cytoplasm and partly in the nuclei of normal and tumor tissue (Figure 1A–C). AGO2 was mainly expressed in the cytoplasm and particularly in the pseudoluminal areas of tumors and adjacent normal tissue (Figure 1D–F). Furthermore, AGO2 was also found in lymphocytes (Figure 1F). Drosha staining was located in the cytoplasm and partly in the nucleus in normal and tumor tissue (Figure 2).

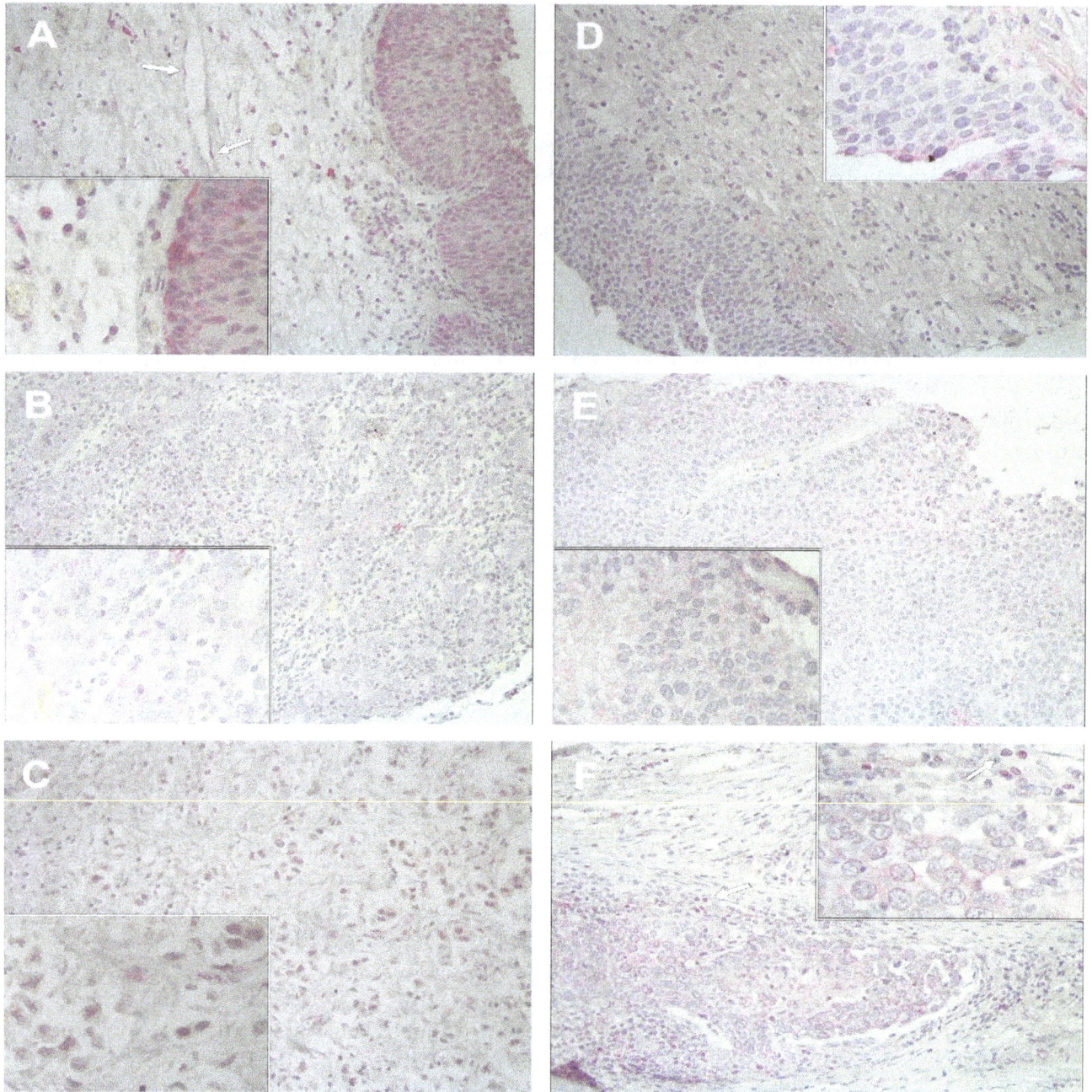

Figure 1. Immunohistochemical staining of AGO1 and AGO2 in bladder tissue. Representative images show the expression of AGO1 in non-malignant bladder tissue (**A**), in non-muscle-invasive pT1 tumor (**B**) and muscle-invasive pT3b tumor tissue (**C**); as well as the expression of AGO2 in normal bladder tissue (**D**), in non-muscle-invasive pTa tumor (**E**) and muscle-invasive pT3b tumor tissue (**F**). The arrows indicate the staining in endothelial cells (**A**) and AGO2 staining of lymphocytes (**F**). Pseudoluminal expression of AGO2 can be seen in (**D**). Magnification: 200×, inserts 400×.

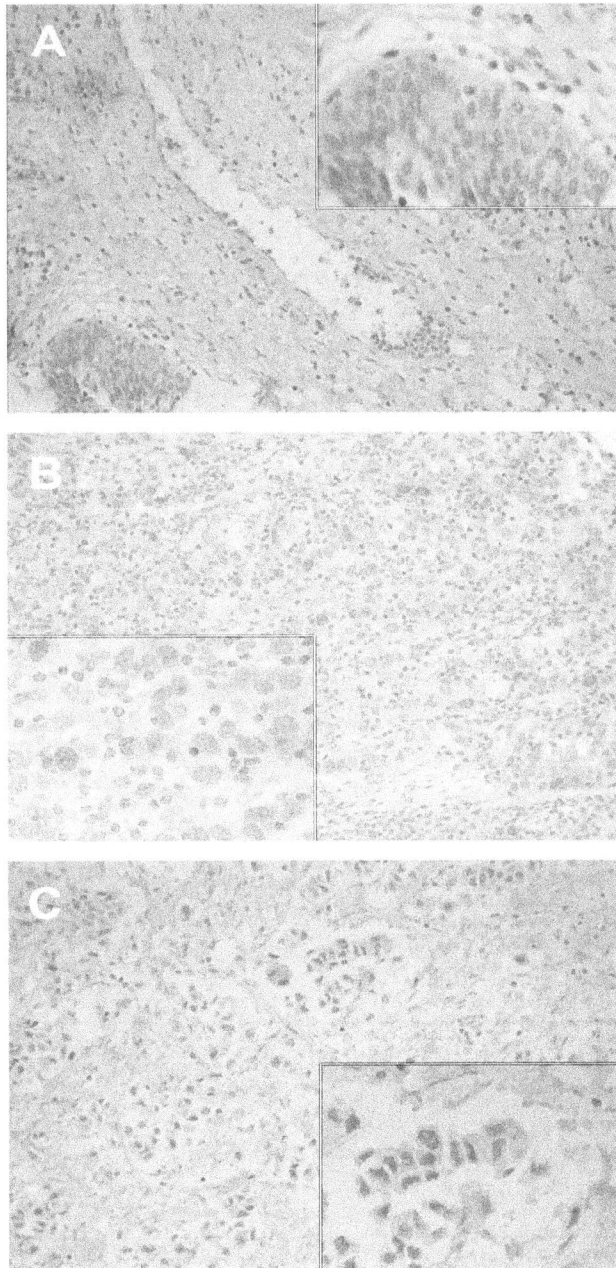

Figure 2. Immunohistochemical staining of Drosha in bladder tissue. Representative images show the expression of Drosha in non-malignant bladder tissue (**A**), in non-muscle-invasive pT1 tumor (**B**) and muscle-invasive pT3b tumor tissue (**C**). The staining of endothelial cells can be seen in (**A**). Magnification: 200×, inserts 400×.

2.2. AGO1, AGO2 and Drosha Expression in Bladder Carcinomas Compared to Non-Malignant Tissue and Association with Clinicopathological Parameters

The clinicopathological parameters of the bladder cancer cases are shown in Table 1. AGO1, AGO2 and Drosha were markedly upregulated in NMIBC compared to adjacent normal tissue. However, only AGO2 was significantly upregulated in MIBC (Table 2). Positive AGO2 staining identified 73/109 tumors (67%) without any difference between NMIBC and MIBC when calculating a Fisher's exact test (Table 3). However, AGO1 and Drosha expression was decreased in NMIBC compared to MIBC ($p < 0.001$, Table 3).

Table 1. Clinicopathological characteristics of the patients undergoing transurethral resection of the bladder or radical cystectomy.

Patient Characteristics (n = 112)	n (%)
Age, years [A]	
<69	52 (46.4)
≥69	60 (53.6)
Sex	
female	31 (27.7)
male	81 (72.3)
Tumor characteristics	
pT stage [B]	
pTa	42 (37.5)
pT1	20 (17.9)
pT2	26 (23.2)
pT3	18 (16.1)
pT4	6 (5.4)
WHO grade [B]	
low	37 (33.0)
high	75 (67.0)
Operative method	
TUR-B	85 (75.9)
RTX	27 (24.1)
Follow up, months [C]	
Mean	56
Median	53
Range	3–200
Status after follow-up time [C]	
alive	67 (60.9)
dead	43 (39.1)

[A] Age was dichotomized according to median; [B] WHO/ISUP criteria of 2016; [C] 110 cases available. WHO: World Health Organization; ISUP: International Society of Uropathology; TUR-B: transurethral resection of the bladder; RTX: radical cystectomy.

Table 2. Comparison of AGO1, AGO2, and Drosha expression in adjacent normal tissue to NMIBC as well as MIBC in valid cases.

Characteristics	Nonmalignant n (%)	NMIBC n (%)	MIBC n (%)
Argonaute 1	30 (100)	60 (100)	38 (100)
negative	22 (73.3)	23 (38.3)	30 (78.9)
positive	8 (26.7)	37 (61.7)	8 (21.1)
p value [A]		0.003	0.774
Argonaute 2	34 (100)	61 (100)	48 (100)
negative	27 (79.4)	21 (34.4)	15 (31.3)
positive	7 (20.6)	40 (65.6)	33 (68.8)
p value [A]		<0.001	<0.001
Drosha	35 (100)	61 (100)	45 (100)
negative	23 (65.7)	8 (13.1)	23 (51.1)
positive	12 (34.3)	53 (86.9)	22 (48.9)
p value [A]		<0.001	0.255

[A] Fisher's exact test. (N)MIBC: (non-)muscle-invasive bladder cancer.

None of the three targets was associated with the clinicopathological parameters of age and sex (Table 3). However, decreased expression of AGO1 (Chi-square test, p = 0.001) and Drosha (Chi-square test, p < 0.001) was associated with advanced pathological tumor stage and with MIBC compared to NMIBC (Fisher's exact test, $p < 0.001$) as mentioned above. Drosha levels were also associated with World Health Organization (WHO) grade (Fisher's exact test, $p = 0.045$). In order to assess the consistency between AGO1, AGO2 and Drosha expression, the McNemar test was utilized. We obtained significant differences between AGO1/AGO2 and AGO1/Drosha expression in bladder tumor tissue samples ($p < 0.001$; Table 3).

Table 3. Immunostaining of AGO1, AGO2 and Drosha associated with clinicopathological parameters of bladder cancer patients.

Para-meters n (%)	AGO1 $n = 98$			AGO2 $n = 109$			Drosha $n = 106$		
	neg 53 (54.1)	pos 45 (45.9)	p value	neg 36 (33.0)	pos 73 (67.0)	p value	neg 31 (29.2)	pos 75 (70.8)	p value
Age, years [A]									
<69	23 (23.5)	21 (21.4)	0.839 [B]	17 (15.6)	33 (30.3)	1.000 [B]	15 (14.2)	36 (34.0)	1.000 [B]
≥69	30 (30.6)	24 (24.5)		19 (17.4)	40 (36.7)		16 (15.1)	39 (36.8)	
Sex									
female	14 (14.3)	12 (12.2)	1.000 [B]	10 (9.2)	20 (18.3)	1.000 [B]	8 (7.5)	22 (20.8)	0.815 [B]
male	39 (39.8)	33 (33.7)		26 (23.9)	53 (48.6)		23 (21.7)	53 (50.0)	
pT stage									
pTa	18 (18.4)	23 (23.5)	0.001 [C]	17 (15.6)	24 (22.0)	0.437 [C]	3 (2.8)	38 (35.8)	<0.001 [C]
pT1	5 (5.1)	14 (14.3)		4 (3.7)	16 (14.7)		5 (4.7)	15 (14.2)	
pT2	15 (15.3)	5 (5.1)		9 (8.3)	16 (14.7)		10 (9.4)	13 (12.3)	
pT3	13 (13.3)	1 (1.0)		5 (4.6)	12 (11.0)		12 (11.3)	6 (5.7)	
pT4	2 (2.0)	2 (2.0)		1 (0.9)	5 (4.6)		1 (0.9)	3 (2.8)	
NMIBC	23 (23.5)	37 (37.8)	<0.001 [B]	21 (19.3)	40 (36.7)	0.838 [B]	8 (7.5)	53 (50.0)	<0.001 [B]
MIBC	30 (30.6)	8 (8.2)		15 (13.8)	33 (30.3)		23 (21.7)	22 (20.8)	
WHO grade [D]									
low	15 (15.3)	20 (20.4)	0.138 [B]	14 (12.8)	22 (20.2)	0.392 [B]	6 (5.7)	30 (28.3)	0.045 [B]
high	38 (38.8)	25 (25.5)		22 (20.2)	51 (46.8)		25 (23.6)	45 (42.5)	
AGO1 [E]									
neg	-	-	-	21 (21.9)	31 (32.3)	0.025 [B]	22 (23.7)	27 (29.0)	<0.001 [B]
pos	-	-	-	8 (8.3)	36 (37.5)		5 (5.4)	39 (41.9)	
AGO2 [E]									
neg	21 (21.9)	8 (8.3)	<0.001 [F]	-	-	-	11 (10.7)	23 (22.3)	0.649 [B]
pos	31 (32.3)	36 (37.5)		-	-	-	19 (18.4)	50 (48.5)	
Drosha [E]									
neg	22 (23.7)	5 (5.4)	<0.001 [F]	11 (10.7)	19 (18.4)	0.644 [F]	-	-	-
pos	27 (29.0)	39 (41.9)		23 (22.3)	50 (48.5)		-	-	-

[A] Age was dichotomized according to median; [B] Fisher's exact test ($p < 0.05$); [C] Chi-square test according to Pearson ($p < 0.05$); [D] WHO/ISUP criteria of 2016; [E] number of valid cases: Ago1/Ago2 $n = 96$, Ago1/Drosha $n = 93$, Ago2/Drosha $n = 103$; [F] McNemar test ($p < 0.05$). AGO: Argonaute; neg: negative, pos: positive staining; (N)MIBC: (non-)muscle-invasive bladder cancer; WHO: World Health Organization; ISUP: International Society of Uropathology.

2.3. Association of AGO1, AGO2 and Drosha Expression with Patient Survival

The overall survival times available for 110 cases were used in Kaplan–Meier survival analyses, and different subgroups were compared using Chi-square and the log-rank tests. As expected, higher pT stages and tumor grade were significantly associated with reduced patient survival time ($p < 0.001$). We also obtained significant associations by performing separate Kaplan–Meier analyses according to pTa and ≥pT1 tumors ($p < 0.001$) as well as for NMIBC and MIBC ($p = 0.001$). In order to assess the clinical relevance of AGO1, AGO2 and Drosha as prognostic markers in bladder cancer patients, the Kaplan–Meier analyses of dichotomized immunoreactivity data were conducted. AGO1 and AGO2 expression levels that were divided into negative and positive values did not show any significant differences for the available 96 cases and 107 cases, respectively (Figure 3A,B). However, Drosha had a significant correlation with the overall survival time, with a higher probability of survival associated with positive Drosha expression (73 cases, 20 events; 5-year survival of 73%) compared with negative expression (31 cases, 18 events; 5-year survival of 57%) (Figure 3C). Multivariate Cox regression analysis including the clinicopathological parameters of age, sex, pT stage and tumor grade combined with the three targets of AGO1, AGO2 and Drosha (alone or together) did not reveal any statistical significances, while AGO1 turned out to be independent of all patient parameters (Table S1).

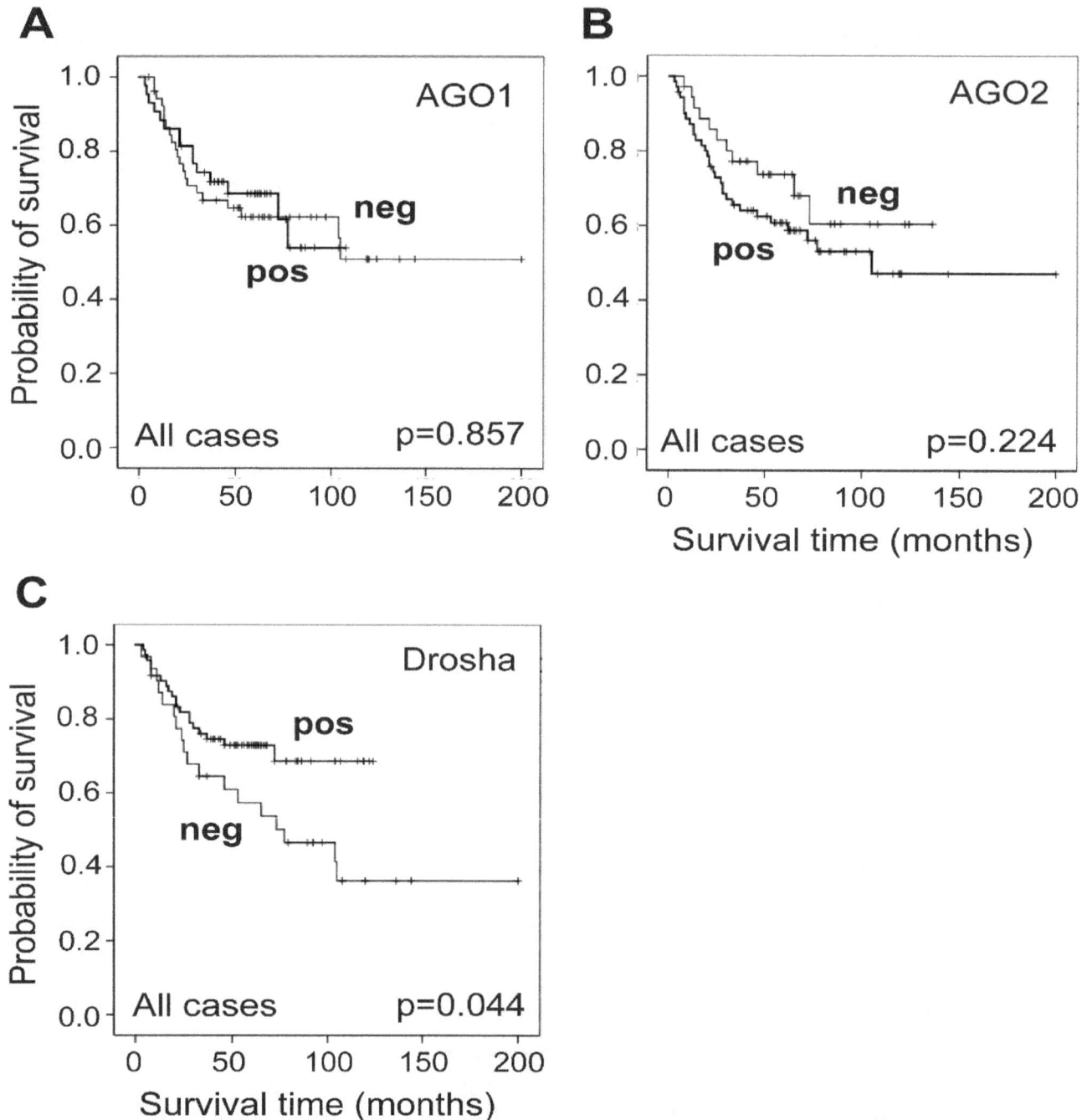

Figure 3. Kaplan–Meier analysis showing overall survival time of bladder cancer patients as a function of AGO1, AGO2 and Drosha levels. Dichotomized expression was not associated with overall survival for 96 cases of AGO1 (**A**) and 107 cases of AGO2 staining (**B**), but Drosha significantly indicated a higher probability of survival with positive expression regarding the 104 available cases (**C**). The overall survival time was defined as the months elapsed between transurethral resection or radical cystectomy and death or the last follow-up date. Censored cases were marked (+). Statistical significance was given as *p* < 0.05. Pos: positive, neg: negative.

3. Discussion

Nuclear cleavage of the primary miRNA by Drosha is an essential function in early miRNA maturation. The proteins of the Argonaute family, AGO1 and AGO2, define the next step in miRNA maturation in the cytoplasm and play a key role in post-transcriptional regulation, such as degrading mRNA or impairing its translation. There is an increasing number of studies examining the implication of miRNA maturation regulators in cancer pathobiology, whereas the contribution of Drosha and Argonautes to the diagnosis and clinicopathological behavior of bladder cancer still needs to be clarified. In this study, we investigated the immunohistochemical expression of Drosha, AGO1 and AGO2 proteins in bladder cancer and their association with clinicopathological parameters and overall survival in order to define the diagnostic and prognostic potentials of these miRNA processors for bladder carcinoma.

Higher expression levels of AGO1 and AGO2 associated with tumor progression have been found in different cancer entities, such as in epithelial skin cancer and ovarian cancer [14,15]. There was an upregulation of AGO2 expression in an estrogen receptor α-negative breast cancer cell line, in prostate cancer as well as in esophageal squamous cell carcinoma tissue, which indicates that AGO2 plays a key role in tumorigenesis [16,17]. Furthermore, in hematological cancers, such as multiple myeloma, high AGO2 levels have been reported as a marker of high-risk disease [18]. With regard to bladder carcinoma, previous studies have described the overexpression of Drosha, AGO1 and AGO2 compared to non-malignant bladder tissue [12,13], which we could attribute to NMIBC. In the case of AGO2, this overexpression was found both in NMIBC and MIBC. The differentiation of NMIBC and MIBC cases has not been considered in the earlier studies [12,13].

The association of AGO1 with AGO2 and Drosha according to our McNemar test hints at similar processes and changes of miRNA machinery in bladder cancer, although AGO2 and Drosha were different. With respect to clinicopathological parameters, we found decreased protein expression of AGO1 and Drosha to be significantly associated with higher tumor stage and with MIBC in comparison to NMIBC, although there were no differences for AGO2. In striking contrast, Yang et al. [12] detected a significant association of increased AGO2 levels with higher histological grade, lymph node metastasis and distant metastasis of bladder carcinoma. However, grade and statistical test were not further defined in this study. Zhang et al. [13] claimed that higher AGO2 and Drosha expression was associated with higher histological grade, pT stage ($\geq$T1) and recurrence of bladder carcinoma, although their table data indicated an association with lower grade. These results were inconsistent and the grade was not further defined but we could confirm an association of higher Drosha levels with the lower WHO grade according to criteria of 2016 if applicable to the study above. The decreased expression of AGO1 and Drosha in MIBC compared with NMIBC could suggest a shift from more active miRNA machinery to decreased activity. For bladder cancer, some increased oncogenic miRNAs and many decreased tumor-suppressive miRNAs have been described [19] and thus, a connection could be possible.

Higher Drosha [13] and AGO2 expressions [12,13] have been reported to correspond to shorter overall survival [12] or to shorter recurrence-free and cancer-specific survival [13] in Kaplan–Meier analysis although we only found Drosha to be significantly correlated with prolonged overall survival. Yang et al. [12] contains very few cases in the Kaplan–Meier curves so that the results, especially those indicating that AGO2 is an independent factor, are questionable. However, the other study [13] presents enough cases for sound results and stresses AGO2 as an independent prognostic factor in a reduced model with grade and pT stage only. We could not confirm the prognostic value of AGO2 in our analyses, which had a median observation time of 53 months in contrast to the 36 months [12] and 35 months [13] of the other studies. In contrast, our calculations just proved that AGO1 was independent of clinicopathological parameters, although AGO1 alone in univariate analysis was not of any prognostic value, which was in contrast with Drosha. The significance in the univariate analysis means that the variable can differentiate the lower and higher probability of survival on its own, but the multivariate Cox regression will provide the quality of the variable compared with other (known) patient parameters. According to the Reporting Recommendations for Tumor Marker Prognostic Studies (REMARK), which have been further explained in 2012 [20], we included all variables available in multivariate analysis. Frequently, significant univariate variables lack independence in the multivariate analysis, such as Drosha in our analysis, but there also are variables which only show their quality in multivariate comparison, such as AGO1 in our study. We could confirm the significance of AGO1 in the inclusion model in a backward Likelihood model with the same parameters as in Table S1 ($p = 0.018$). We believe that the value of AGO1 as a prognostic marker should be further evaluated.

Interestingly, in bladder tissue, we found that Drosha was not only present in nuclei, but also in the cytoplasm, which seems contrary to its functional role in nuclear miRNA maturation regulation. However, there are several reports on other tumor entities in which Drosha was observed in both compartments, such as smooth muscle tumors, melanoma, esophageal and breast cancer [21–24]. The data on localization of Drosha and AGO1 in bladder tissue have been lacking until now because Zhang et al. [13] did not present any in their study. We could confirm mainly the cytoplasmic expression of AGO2 described by Yang et al. [12] but added some details on staining for all three targets, such as the expression in endothelial cells or for AGO2 in lymphocytes, which should be taken into consideration by certain measures, such as Western blot analyses.

As the antibodies used were different from ours (AGO2, [12]), or were not exactly described [13], the difference in the results could have risen from different affinities or specificities, which accentuate the limitations of immunohistochemical studies. Our antibodies were selected according to the literature and were evaluated by an experienced pathologist (E.K.) to avoid artifacts. Another aspect is the difference between our tissue and scoring system (tissue microarray, scoring by intensity) and those of the other groups (full section per case, scoring by intensity and area) [12,13]; both have advantages and disadvantages. For our microarray, we wanted to avoid any bias in an area score for little spots. In histological tissue analysis, the quality of processed formalin-fixed and paraffin-embedded archival material may also influence the staining intensity. In our explorative study, the number of events analyzed was limited because of the limited number of investigated patients for whom comprehensive data were available. This seems to be the main restriction of our work. Further studies are necessary to elucidate the role of Drosha and AGOs in bladder cancer due to the shortcomings of the existing contradictory data.

4. Materials and Methods

4.1. Tissue Sample Selection

A TMA composed of 112 human urothelial carcinomas of the bladder was used for our retrospective study. Appropriate tissue was selected in accordance to availability and follow-up data of the cases. The study was approved by the Ethics Committee of the HELIOS Hospital in Bad Saarow, Germany (HRC-006913, 21, March, 2012), where all bladder cancer patients underwent radical cystectomy (RTX) or transurethral resection (TUR-B) between 1999 and 2010. Written informed consent was given according to the Declaration of Helsinki. In total, 85 TUR-B and 27 RTX were carried out and none of the patients received any chemotherapy or radiation prior to surgery. For each patient, the following clinical and pathological information was recorded: sex, age, tumor staging according to the International Union Against Cancer, histological grading in accordance with the WHO/ISUP criteria of 2016 and overall survival time in the months after surgery. An overview of patient clinicopathological characteristics is given in Table 1.

The surgical specimens of normal adjacent urothelial and urothelial tumor tissue were fixed in 4% buffered formaldehyde and embedded in paraffin. Histological diagnosis was established on standard hematoxylin and eosin-stained sections by a pathologist. Tumor tissue samples were subdivided into 62 NMIBC (pTa = 42 and pT1 = 20) and 50 MIBC tissue samples (pT2 = 26, pT3 = 18 and pT4 = 6) according to the European Association of Urology guidelines, 2011 [25] (Table 1). Additionally, the adjacent normal bladder tissues of 35 bladder tumor cases without any evidence for reactive histology were included. Patients with carcinoma in situ or metastasis were excluded.

4.2. Construction of Tissue Microarray

The areas of bladder carcinoma and adjacent normal tissue were marked on 3-μm hematoxylin/eosin (HE) stained sections of formalin-fixed paraffin-embedded tissue by a pathologist (A.E.) at Charité-Universitätsmedizin Berlin, Germany. Of the corresponding blocks, cores were punched out with a tissue arrayer (1.0 mm diameter; Beecher Instruments, Woodland, CA, USA) according to the previously marked areas, which were subsequently embedded into a new paraffin block as a TMA with maximal 125 cores per block and a tissue of at least 2 mm diameter. Histological conformation was established on HE stained sections (A.E.) according to tumor staging and WHO grading system of 2016.

4.3. Immunohistochemistry

Immunostaining was done as described previously [26]. The optimal concentration of the primary antibody was determined in a dilution series on test sections of larger urothelial cancer and corresponding adjacent normal tissue. Finally, the primary antibody against AGO1 (rabbit monoclonal antibody, cat. no. 5053 [clone D84G10]; Cell Signaling Technology, Inc.; Boston, MA, USA) was used at a dilution of 1:50 and incubated overnight at 4 °C. AGO2 (rabbit polyclonal antibody, cat. no. ab32381; Abcam, Cambridge, UK) was used at a dilution of 1:50 and incubated for 1 h at room temperature, while Drosha (rabbit polyclonal antibody, cat. no. ab12286, Abcam) was used at a dilution of 1:250 and incubated for 1 h at room temperature in a humid chamber. Detection was performed by conventional labeled streptavidin-biotin method with alkaline phosphatase as the reporting enzyme. Fast-Red TR/Naphthol AS-MX (cat. no. F4648; Sigma-Aldrich, Munich, Germany) was used as the chromogen. Finally, the TMA was counterstained with hematoxylin and fixed in an aqueous embedding medium. Antibody diluent solution without the application of respective primary antibodies was used as the negative control. Antibodies were checked by Western blotting using the human urinary bladder carcinoma cell lines RT-4 and RT-112 (Figure S1). Immunostainings were evaluated by a pathologist (E.K.) of Charité–Universitätsmedizin Berlin, who was blinded to the clinicopathological data. Immunohistochemical expression of AGO1, AGO2 and Drosha was classified in a binary manner from 0 to 1 according to the following assessment: 0 being no immunoreactivity; and 1 being positive immunoreactivity with staining intensities including cytoplasmic and nuclear staining. The number of assessable cases differed slightly between the three targets, because a few tissue spots disappeared during the staining procedure.

4.4. Statistics

Statistical analyses were carried out with SPSS 21.0 (IBM Corp., Somers, NY, USA). Fisher's exact test, Chi-square test according to Pearson and McNemar test were applied to determine the relationship between AGO1, AGO2 or Drosha immunostaining and clinicopathological characteristics. Univariate analyses for the overall survival time as a function of AGO1, AGO2 or Drosha expression were executed as Kaplan-Meier analyses using the log-rank test. The overall survival time as the primary clinical endpoint was defined as the months elapsed between TUR-B or RTX and either death or the last follow-up date. Multivariate analyses were calculated according to Cox regression. Two-sided p-values < 0.05 were considered to be statistically significant in all cases.

5. Conclusions

In our study, the altered expressions of AGO1, AGO2, and Drosha were investigated immunohistochemically in bladder cancer to evaluate their diagnostic and prognostic potential in non-invasive and invasive bladder carcinoma. The upregulation of the targets and differentiation of NMIBC and MIBC cases could improve diagnostics; additionally, AGO1 seems to hold prognostic potential for bladder cancer. However, our results stress the need for further research to bridge the gap of prognostic markers in urothelial carcinomas of the bladder. Based on our results, we suggest that Drosha and AGOs are important factors in the tumor biology of bladder cancer.

Author Contributions: N.R., K.J. and T.H.E. contributed to conception and design of the study. Acquisition of data was done by A.R., N.R., A.E., T.H.E. and E.K., A.R., N.R. and K.J. analyzed and interpreted data. A.R., N.R. and A.H. wrote the manuscript. A.R. and K.J. revised the manuscript. All authors read and approved the final manuscript.

Acknowledgments: A.R., N.R. and K.J. were supported by the Foundation for Urologic Research. We acknowledge support from the German Research Foundation (DFG) and the Open Access Publication Fund of Charité-Universitätsmedizin Berlin. The authors thank Siegrun Blauhut and Bettina Ergün for excellent technical assistance.

References

1. Antoni, S.; Ferlay, J.; Soerjomataram, I.; Znaor, A.; Jemal, A.; Bray, F. Bladder Cancer Incidence and Mortality: A Global Overview and Recent Trends. *Eur. Urol.* **2017**, *71*, 96–108. [CrossRef] [PubMed]

2. Zhao, M.; He, X.L.; Teng, X.D. Understanding the molecular pathogenesis and prognostics of bladder cancer: An overview. *Chin. J. Cancer Res.* **2016**, *28*, 92–98. [PubMed]

3. Mohammed, A.A.; El-Tanni, H.; El-Khatib, H.M.; Mirza, A.A.; Mirza, A.A.; Alturaifi, T.H. Urinary Bladder Cancer: Biomarkers and Target Therapy, New Era for More Attention. *Oncol. Rev.* **2016**, *10*. [CrossRef] [PubMed]

4. Bartel, D.P. MicroRNAs: Genomics, biogenesis, mechanism, and function. *Cell* **2004**, *116*, 281–297. [CrossRef]

5. Calin, G.A.; Croce, C.M. MicroRNA signatures in human cancers. *Nat. Rev. Cancer* **2006**, *6*, 857–866. [CrossRef] [PubMed]

6. Dong, F.; Xu, T.; Shen, Y.; Zhong, S.; Chen, S.; Ding, Q.; Shen, Z. Dysregulation of miRNAs in bladder cancer: Altered expression with aberrant biogenesis procedure. *Oncotarget* **2017**, *8*, 27547–27568. [CrossRef] [PubMed]

7. Mitash, N.; Tiwari, S.; Agnihotri, S.; Mandhani, A. Bladder cancer: Micro RNAs as biomolecules for prognostication and surveillance. *Indian J. Urol.* **2017**, *33*, 127–133. [PubMed]

8. Hata, A.; Kashima, R. Dysregulation of microRNA biogenesis machinery in cancer. *Crit. Rev. Biochem. Mol. Biol.* **2016**, *51*, 121–134. [CrossRef] [PubMed]

9. Cheloufi, S.; Dos Santos, C.O.; Chong, M.M.; Hannon, G.J. A dicer-independent miRNA biogenesis pathway that requires Ago catalysis. *Nature* **2010**, *465*, 584–589. [CrossRef] [PubMed]

10. Li, W.; Liu, M.; Feng, Y.; Xu, Y.F.; Che, J.P.; Wang, G.C.; Zheng, J.H.; Gao, H.J. Evaluation of Argonaute protein as a predictive marker for human clear cell renal cell carcinoma. *Int. J. Clin. Exp. Pathol.* **2013**, *6*, 1086–1094. [PubMed]

11. Bian, X.J.; Zhang, G.M.; Gu, C.Y.; Cai, Y.; Wang, C.F.; Shen, Y.J.; Zhu, Y.; Zhang, H.L.; Dai, B.; Ye, D.W. Down-regulation of Dicer and Ago2 is associated with cell proliferation and apoptosis in prostate cancer. *Tumor Biol.* **2014**, *35*, 11571–11578. [CrossRef] [PubMed]

12. Yang, F.Q.; Huang, J.H.; Liu, M.; Yang, F.P.; Li, W.; Wang, G.C.; Che, J.P.; Zheng, J.H. Argonaute 2 is up-regulated in tissues of urothelial carcinoma of bladder. *Int. J. Clin. Exp. Pathol.* **2014**, *7*, 340–347. [PubMed]

13. Zhang, Z.; Zhang, G.; Kong, C.; Bi, J.; Gong, D.; Yu, X.; Shi, D.; Zhan, B.; Ye, P. EIF2C, Dicer, and Drosha are up-regulated along tumor progression and associated with poor prognosis in bladder carcinoma. *Tumor Biol.* **2015**, *36*, 5071–5079. [CrossRef] [PubMed]

14. Sand, M.; Skrygan, M.; Georgas, D.; Arenz, C.; Gambichler, T.; Sand, D.; Altmeyer, P.; Bechara, F.G. Expression levels of the microRNA maturing microprocessor complex component DGCR8 and the RNA-induced silencing complex (RISC) components argonaute-1, argonaute-2, PACT, TARBP1, and TARBP2 in epithelial skin cancer. *Mol. Carcinog.* **2012**, *51*, 916–922. [CrossRef] [PubMed]

15. Vaksman, O.; Hetland, T.E.; Trope, C.G.; Reich, R.; Davidson, B. Argonaute, Dicer, and Drosha are up-regulated along tumor progression in serous ovarian carcinoma. *Hum. Pathol.* **2012**, *43*, 2062–2069. [CrossRef] [PubMed]

16. Adams, B.D.; Claffey, K.P.; White, B.A. Argonaute-2 expression is regulated by epidermal growth factor receptor and mitogen-activated protein kinase signaling and correlates with a transformed phenotype in breast cancer cells. *Endocrinology* **2009**, *150*, 14–23. [CrossRef] [PubMed]

17. Yoo, N.J.; Hur, S.Y.; Kim, M.S.; Lee, J.Y.; Lee, S.H. Immunohistochemical analysis of RNA-induced silencing complex-related proteins AGO2 and TNRC6A in prostate and esophageal cancers. *APMIS* **2010**, *118*, 271–276. [CrossRef] [PubMed]

18. Zhou, Y.; Chen, L.; Barlogie, B.; Stephens, O.; Wu, X.; Williams, D.R.; Cartron, M.A.; van, R.F.; Nair, B.; Waheed, S.; et al. High-risk myeloma is associated with global elevation of miRNAs and overexpression of EIF2C2/AGO2. *Proc. Natl. Acad. Sci. USA* **2010**, *107*, 7904–7909. [CrossRef] [PubMed]

19. Pop-Bica, C.; Gulei, D.; Cojocneanu-Petric, R.; Braicu, C.; Petrut, B.; Berindan-Neagoe, I. Understanding the Role of Non-Coding RNAs in Bladder Cancer: From Dark Matter to Valuable Therapeutic Targets. *Int. J. Mol. Sci.* **2017**, *18*, 1514. [CrossRef] [PubMed]

20. Altman, D.G.; McShane, L.M.; Sauerbrei, W.; Taube, S.E. Reporting Recommendations for Tumor Marker Prognostic Studies (REMARK): Explanation and elaboration. *PLoS. Med.* **2012**, *9*, e1001216. [CrossRef] [PubMed]

21. Jafarnejad, S.M.; Sjoestroem, C.; Martinka, M.; Li, G. Expression of the RNase III enzyme DROSHA is reduced during progression of human cutaneous melanoma. *Mod. Pathol.* **2013**, *26*, 902–910. [CrossRef] [PubMed]

22. Papachristou, D.J.; Sklirou, E.; Corradi, D.; Grassani, C.; Kontogeorgakos, V.; Rao, U.N. Immunohistochemical analysis of the endoribonucleases Drosha, Dicer and Ago2 in smooth muscle tumours of soft tissues. *Histopathology* **2012**, *60*, E28–E36. [CrossRef] [PubMed]

23. Passon, N.; Gerometta, A.; Puppin, C.; Lavarone, E.; Puglisi, F.; Tell, G.; Di, L.C.; Damante, G. Expression of Dicer and Drosha in triple-negative breast cancer. *J. Clin. Pathol.* **2012**, *65*, 320–326. [CrossRef] [PubMed]

24. Sugito, N.; Ishiguro, H.; Kuwabara, Y.; Kimura, M.; Mitsui, A.; Kurehara, H.; Ando, T.; Mori, R.; Takashima, N.; Ogawa, R.; et al. RNASEN regulates cell proliferation and affects survival in esophageal cancer patients. *Clin. Cancer Res.* **2006**, *12*, 7322–7328. [CrossRef] [PubMed]

25. Babjuk, M.; Oosterlinck, W.; Sylvester, R.; Kaasinen, E.; Bohle, A.; Palou-Redorta, J.; Roupret, M. EAU guidelines on non-muscle-invasive urothelial carcinoma of the bladder, the 2011 update. *Eur. Urol.* **2011**, *59*, 997–1008. [CrossRef] [PubMed]

26. Xu, C.; Jung, M.; Burkhardt, M.; Stephan, C.; Schnorr, D.; Loening, S.; Jung, K.; Dietel, M.; Kristiansen, G. Increased CD59 protein expression predicts a PSA relapse in patients after radical prostatectomy. *Prostate* **2005**, *62*, 224–232. [CrossRef] [PubMed]

7

Prognostic Role of Survivin and Macrophage Infiltration Quantified on Protein and mRNA Level in Molecular Subtypes Determined by RT-qPCR of *KRT5, KRT20* and *ERBB2* in Muscle-Invasive Bladder Cancer Treated by Adjuvant Chemotherapy

Thorsten H. Ecke [1,2,*], Adisch Kiani [3], Thorsten Schlomm [3], Frank Friedersdorff [3], Anja Rabien [3,4], Klaus Jung [3,4], Ergin Kilic [5], Peter Boström [6], Minna Tervahartiala [7], Pekka Taimen [8], Jan Gleichenhagen [9], Georg Johnen [9], Thomas Brüning [9], Stefan Koch [2,10], Jenny Roggisch [10] and Ralph M. Wirtz [11]

[1] Department of Urology, HELIOS Hospital Bad Saarow, DE-15526 Bad Sarrow, Germany
[2] Brandenburg Medical School, DE-14770 Brandenburg, Germany; stefan.koch@helios-gesundheit.de
[3] Department of Urology, Charité—Universitätsmedizin, Corporate Member of Freie Universität Berlin, Humboldt-Universität zu Berlin, and Berlin Institute of Health, DE-10098 Berlin, Germany; adisch.kiani@charite.de (A.K.); thorsten.schlomm@charite.de (T.S.); frank.friedersdorff@charite.de (F.F.); Anja.Rabien@charite.de (A.R.); klaus.jung@charite.de (K.J.)
[4] Berlin Institute for Urological Research, DE-10098 Berlin, Germany
[5] Institute of Pathology, DE-51375 Leverkusen, Germany; e.kilic@pathologie-leverkusen.de
[6] Department of Urology, Turku University Hospital, FI-20521 Turku, Finland; peter.j.bostrom@gmail.com
[7] MediCity Research Laboratory, Department of Medical Microbiology and Immunology, University of Turku, FI-20520 Turku, Finland; mmbost@utu.fi
[8] Institute of Pathology, Turku University Hospital, FI-20521 Turku, Finland; pepeta@utu.fi
[9] Institute for Prevention and Occupational Medicine of the German Social Accident Insurance (IPA), Institute of the Ruhr University Bochum, DE-44789 Bochum, Germany; Gleichenhagen@ipa-dguv.de (J.G.); johnen@ipa-dguv.de (G.J.); bruening@ipa-dguv.de (T.B.)
[10] Institute of Pathology, HELIOS Hospital Bad Saarow, DE-15526 Bad Sarrow, Germany; jenny.roggisch@helios-gesundheit.de
[11] STRATIFYER Molecular Pathology GmbH, DE-50935 Cologne, Germany; ralph.wirtz@stratifyer.de
* Correspondence: thorsten.ecke@helios-gesundheit.de

Abstract: Objectives: Bladder cancer is a heterogeneous malignancy. Therefore, it is difficult to find single predictive markers. Moreover, most studies focus on either the immunohistochemical or molecular assessment of tumor tissues by next-generation sequencing (NGS) or PCR, while a combination of immunohistochemistry (IHC) and PCR for tumor marker assessment might have the strongest impact to predict outcome and select optimal therapies in real-world application. We investigated the role of proliferation survivin/*BIRC5* and macrophage infiltration (CD68, MAC387, CLEVER-1) on the basis of molecular subtypes of bladder cancer (KRT5, KRT20, ERBB2) to predict outcomes of adjuvant treated muscle-invasive bladder cancer patients with regard to progression-free survival (PFS) and disease-specific survival (DSS). Materials and Methods: We used tissue microarrays (TMA) from n = 50 patients (38 males, 12 female) with muscle-invasive bladder cancer. All patients had been treated with radical cystectomy followed by adjuvant triple chemotherapy. Median follow-up time was 60.5 months. CD68, CLEVER-1, MAC387, and survivin protein were detected by immunostaining and subsequent visual inspection. *BIRC5, KRT5, KRT20, ERBB2,* and *CD68* mRNAs were detected by standardized RT-qPCR after tissue dot RNA extraction using a novel stamp technology. All these markers were evaluated in three different centers of excellence. Results: Nuclear staining rather than cytoplasmic staining of survivin predicted DSS as a single marker with high levels of survivin being associated with better PFS and DSS upon adjuvant chemotherapy (p = 0.0138 and p = 0.001, respectively). These results were validated by the quantitation of *BIRC5* mRNA by PCR (p = 0.0004 and p = 0.0508, respectively). Interestingly, nuclear staining of survivin protein was positively associated with *BIRC5* mRNA, while cytoplasmic staining was inversely related, indicating that the translocation of survivin protein into the nucleus occurred at a discrete, higher level of its mRNA. Combining survivin/*BIRC5* levels based on molecular subtype being assessed by *KRT20* expression improved the predictive value, with tumors having low survivin/*BIRC5* and *KRT20* mRNA levels having the best survival (75% vs. 20% vs. 10% 5-year DSS, p = 0.0005), and these values were independent of grading, node status, and tumor stage in multivariate analysis (p = 0.0167). Macrophage infiltration dominated in basal tumors and was inversely related with the luminal subtype marker gene expression. The presence of macrophages in survivin-positive or *ERBB2*-positive tumors was associated with worse DSS. Conclusions: For muscle-invasive bladder cancer patients, the proliferative activity as determined by the nuclear staining of survivin or RT-qPCR on the basis of molecular subtype characteristics outperforms single marker detections and single technology approaches. Infiltration by macrophages detected by IHC or PCR is associated with worse outcome in defined subsets of tumors. The limitations of this study are the retrospective nature and the limited number of patients. However, the number of molecular markers has been restricted and based on predefined assumptions, which resulted in the dissection of muscle-invasive disease into tumor–biological axes of high prognostic relevance, which warrant further investigation and validation.

Keywords: survivin; BIRC5; macrophage; KRT20; ERBB2; MIBC; prediction; RT-qPCR; adjuvant chemotherapy; survival; bladder cancer

---

1. Introduction

Bladder cancer is the fifth most frequent cancer in Europe. In 2018, its incidence and annual mortality rate were estimated to reach 197,105 and 64,966 cases, respectively [1]. Approximately 30% of these patients suffered from muscle-invasive bladder cancer (MIBC) at the time of initial diagnosis [2]. Radical cystectomy (RC) is the gold standard to treat these patients. Compared to patients with non-muscle-invasive bladder cancer (NMIBC), MIBC patients are subject to a high risk of cancer-related death.

In order to remedy this unsatisfactory situation, serious efforts have recently focused on new therapeutic strategies regarding the application of neoadjuvant and adjuvant chemotherapies [3]. A better risk assessment of patients has been recommended by developing novel predictive/prognostic models [4]. In clinical practice, the therapeutic management of these patients has so far been performed almost exclusively on the basis of clinical data and classical pathological TNM criteria but with few reliable results [4]. It is hoped that the identification of new molecular tissue biomarkers could help to stratify risk groups and determine patients who could have a benefit from adjuvant strategies after surgery [5]. In the last decades, many different markers (nucleic acid or protein based) have been identified to add more information on risk assessment. A subset of different markers was selected and further investigated in this study.

Survivin, also known as baculoviral IAP repeat containing 5 (BIRC5), is a member of the inhibitor of apoptosis family and has an important role in cell cycle regulation [6]. The protein survivin is present in different tumor tissues; it occurs in cytoplasm, but also in nuclei [7,8]. The protein is very rarely present in normal tissue [9]. Survivin acts as an apoptosis suppressor in cytoplasm and nuclei and influences cell division [8]. If the stress signal is high enough, survivin is released into cytoplasm, which leads to the inhibition of different caspases [10]. The relevance of *BIRC5* mRNA expression has been less studied in detail. However, its high prognostic impact for certain bladder cancer stages has been shown in the prospective UROMOL trial, wherein it belongs to a 12 gene signature with an adverse effect on survival for NMIBC [11].

CD68 is the most frequently used pan-macrophage marker. Its function is still unknown, but it has been considered to play a role in the phagocytic activities of tissue macrophages [12]. Common lymphatic endothelial and vascular endothelial receptor-1 (CLEVER-1, also known as stabilin-1 or STAB1) is a multifunctional immunosuppressive scavenger receptor expressed by lymphatic and vascular endothelial cells and tissue macrophages [13]. Its prognostic significance in bladder cancer is not clear, but there is evidence that high CLEVER-1-positive macrophage count associates with chemoresistance [14] in neoadjuvant-treated bladder cancer patients. The monoclonal antibody MAC387 detects an epitope on the calcium-binding protein MRP14/S100A9 present in the cytosol of monocytes and granulocytes [15]. It is the exclusive arachidonic acid-binding protein in human neutrophils and is thereby involved in the calcium-dependent cellular signal of lipid second messengers during inflammatory and metabolic changes of tumor-associated macrophages [16].

The molecular subtyping of bladder cancer has been well accepted after its initial introduction in 2014 [17–19]. Therein, the quantitation of *KRT5* and *KRT20* on mRNA level and/or their recapitulation on protein level by immunohistochemistry (IHC) have been identified as exemplary biomarkers for the molecular subtyping of basal and luminal tumors, respectively. In our previous work, we could show that *KRT20* is strongly associated with adverse outcome for pT1 NMIBC [20].

ERBB2 belongs to the key bladder cancer genes as recently defined in an international consensus paper [21]. Belonging to the EGFR-related receptor tyrosine kinase family, it is a key driver and well-established drug target in breast and gastric cancer. In our previous work, we showed that *ERBB2* mRNA expression is superior to the WHO grading of 1973 when dissecting the remaining risk in pT1 NMIBC exhibiting centrally confirmed grade 3 [22], with high *ERBB2* mRNA levels indicating inferior outcome (90% vs. 50% 5-year PFS, $p < 0.0001$). Higher levels are also associated with worse outcome in MIBC not being treated by adjuvant or neoadjuvant chemotherapy [23], with *ERBB2*-positive tumors above median mRNA expression having worse prognosis (20% vs. 60% 4-year DSS, $p = 0.009$). *ERBB2* mRNA is associated with luminal subtypes of bladder cancer [17–19].

However, the prognostic role of these markers in MIBC patients receiving adjuvant chemotherapy is unknown. The aim of the present study was to evaluate the prognostic role of the above-mentioned fundamental bladder cancer markers in the adjuvant situation and to test their clinical usefulness when assessed by IHC or PCR in context with clinical parameters to provide real-world evidence for the respective tumor biological motifs. The herein presented work served as a pilot study for validation of the above-mentioned biomarker assessment and moreover allowing the formulation of a working hypothesis for subsequent prospective non-interventional validation studies in the future. These studies are currently being planned and ultimately may lead to prospective interventional study designs.

2. Results

2.1. Patient Population

Clinical characteristics are presented in Table 1. The total study cohort consisted of 50 MIBC tumor patients diagnosed from 1996 to 2006 at a single institution. Median age was 65 years, with 76% male patients and 34% female patients; 50% of patients had ECOG status 0, while 34% and 16% were ECOG1 and ECOG2, respectively. Forty-two percent of patients were N0 at initial diagnosis, while 14% were N1 and 44% were N2. Median follow-up was 60.5 months with 54% of patients suffering from disease-specific deaths. Similar clinical characteristics were found in the analysis cohorts as defined in the cohort diagram (Table 1).

Table 1. Clinical characteristics of patients in the total cohort (n = 50), and the PCR (n = 39) and combined IHC and PCR subcohorts (n = 28). IHC: immunohistochemistry.

Cohort	Total Cohort	PCR Cohort	IHC & PCR Cohort
Size (n)	50	39	28
Age (years)			
Average	65	67	68.5
Range	49-80	48–80	48–80
Gender			
Male	38 (76%)	27 (69%)	18 (64%)
Female	12 (24%)	12 (31%)	10 (36%)
ECOG Performance Status			
0	25 (50%)	19 (49%)	11 (39%)
1	17 (34%)	13 (33%)	11 (39%)
2	8 (16%)	7 (18%)	6 (21%)
Lymph Node Metastases before Chemotherapy			
N0	21 (42%)	16 (41%)	10 (36%)
N1	7 (14%)	4 (10%)	2 (7%)
N2	22 (44%)	(19 (49%)	16 (57%)
Clinical outcome after Chemotherapy			
Progression	27 (54%)	21 (54%)	18 (64%)
Overall death	36 (72%)	29 (74%)	23 (82%)
Disease specific death	27 (54%)	21 (54%)	19 (68%)
Overall survival	14 (28%)	10 (26%)	5 (18%)
Response to Chemotherapy			
Complete response	20 (40%)	15 (38%)	8 (29%)
Partial response	3 (6%)	2 (5%)	1 (4%)
No change	25 (50%)	20 (51%)	18 (64%)

2.2. Distribution of Assessed Protein Markers across the Study Cohort

All investigated experimental markers could be determined by IHC or PCR in the same tissue microarray (TMA) samples of urinary bladder cancer transurethral resection of bladder (TURB) biopsies.

2.3. Distribution of Assessed mRNA Markers across the Study Cohort

As depicted in the remark diagram (Figure 1), TURB biopsies from 39 patients could be analyzed, while IHC data were available from 28 TURB biopsies.

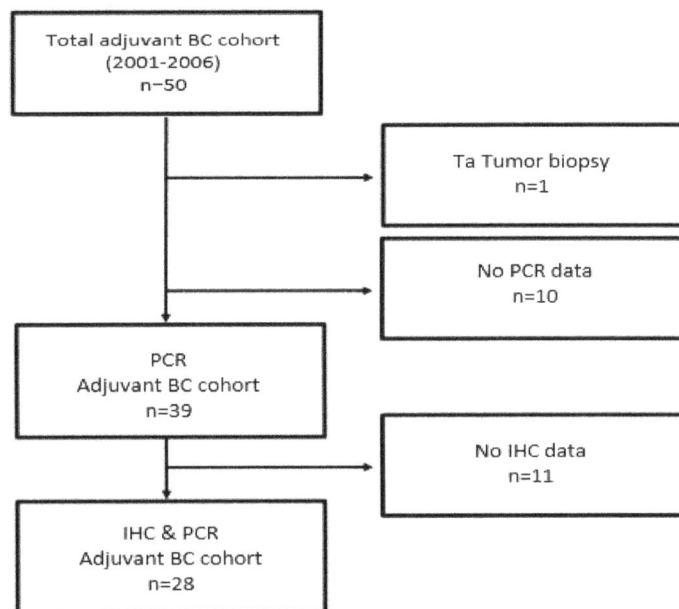

Figure 1. Remark diagram.

Data distribution of immunohistochemical staining of CD68, CLEVER-1, MAC387, and survivin by digital image analysis, visual inspection, or semi-quantitative assessment of cytoplasmic versus nuclear staining indicated a substantial infiltration of macrophages into the TURB biopsies of tumor specimens, while visual inspection reached higher sensitivity than image analysis. The numbers of CD68+ macrophages and CLEVER-1 positive macrophages and vessels were scored from three hotspots (areas with the most macrophages by eye) intratumorally and peritumorally with a 0.0625 mm² grid using 40× magnification when scoring macrophages and 20× when scoring lymphatic/blood vessels. The scoring was performed independently by two observers blinded to the clinical information. Cases with an inadequate quality of immunohistochemical staining or tumor morphology were excluded from further statistical analyses. Survivin protein expression could be observed in almost all TURB biopsies with varying extent, while the nuclear staining of survivin could be detected in only 60% of cases (Figure 2a).

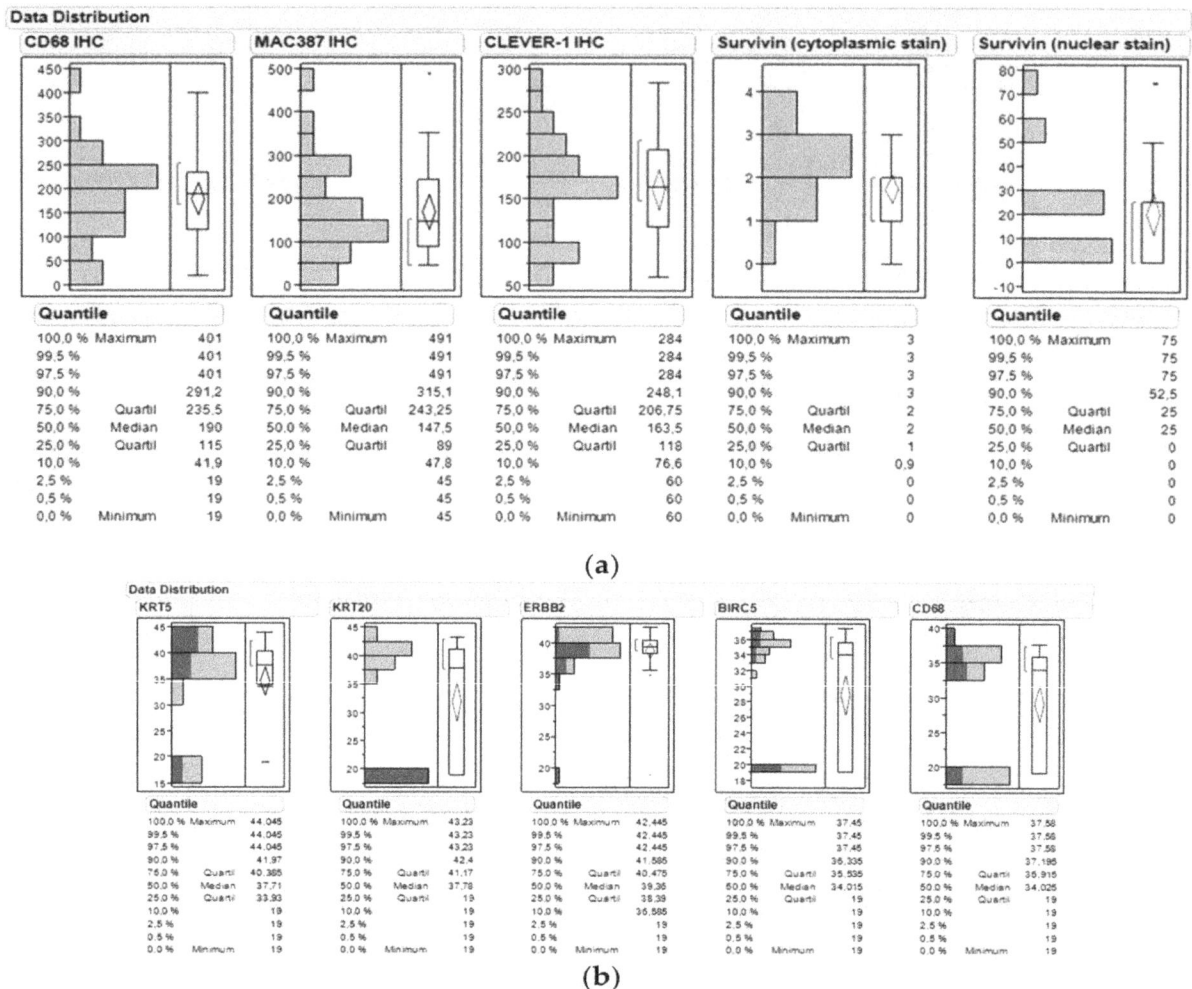

(a)

(b)

Figure 2. (**a**) Data distribution of immunohistochemical staining of CD68, MAC387, and common lymphatic endothelial and vascular endothelial receptor-1 (CLEVER-1) by visual analysis and survivin by semi-quantitative assessment of cytoplasmic versus nuclear stain; (**b**) Data distribution and box and whisker plot of *KRT5*, *KRT20*, *ERBB2*, *BIRC5*, and *CD68* mRNA levels in the bladder cancer study cohort treated by adjuvant chemotherapy (*n* = 39). Normalized gene expression (40-DCT method) as well as quantile values are depicted in the y-axis. DCT: Delta Cycle Threshold.

RNA expression of the candidate genes *KRT5*, *KRT20*, *ERBB2*, *BIRC5*, and *CD68* could also be detected to a varying extent. While *ERBB2* mRNA levels could be determined in almost all cases (38 of 39 samples), *KRT5* and *KRT20* mRNA were detected in fewer biopsies (31 of 39 and 24 of 39 samples, respectively). Similarly, *BIRC5* and *CD68* were detected in subsets of the TURB tissue dots (24 of 39 samples, each). A comparison of NMIBC and MIBC was possible for only four patients. Marker gene expression was comparable. However, with regard to *KRT20* expression, one MIBC did exhibit a significantly increased expression of the luminal marker *KRT20*.

2.4. Correlation of Protein and mRNA Markers on Basis of Molecular Subtyping and Clinical Variables

A comparison of survivin protein expression in cytoplasm versus nucleus compared to its respective mRNA level revealed that higher mRNA is positively associated to nuclear expression (Spearman rho 0.2949) and negatively associated with cytoplasmic stain (Spearman rho −0.3026), while both associations did not yet reach statistical significance due to small sample size (Figure 3).

Spearman Correlation

Variable	Covariable	Spearman ρ	p-value	-,8 -,6 -,4 -,2 0 ,2 ,4 ,6 ,8
Survivin (nuclear stain)	Survivin (cytoplasmic stain)	0,1620	0,4102	
BIRC5	Survivin (cytoplasmic stain)	-0,3026	0,1176	
BIRC5	Survivin (nuclear stain)	0,2949	0,1276	

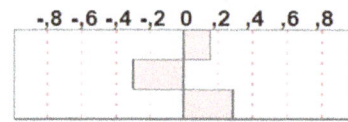

Figure 3. Spearman correlation of IHC staining and semi-quantitative assessment of survivin protein located in cytoplasmic versus nuclear localization with quantitative *BIRC5* (survivin) mRNA levels in the combined PCR and IHC cohort (*n* = 28). Graphical display of Spearman rho values and respective *p*-values are depicted.

As depicted in Figure 4a, Spearman correlation of the intergene RNA expression relations revealed a strong positive association between the two luminal cancer markers *KRT20* and *ERBB2* (Spearman rho 0.6811, *p* < 0.0001) and inverse relation between the luminal *KRT20* and basal *KRT5* marker (Spearman rho −0.3588, *p* = 0.0249) as expected. The negative association between *ERBB2* and *KRT5* was less prominent and not significant (Spearman rho −0.1473, *p* = 0.3709), indicating that several basal-like tumors harbor elevated *ERBB2* expression to some extent. Of note, the proliferation/apoptosis marker *BIRC5* was positively associated with *CD68* mRNA levels (Spearman rho 0.3484, *p* = 0.0156).

Non parametric Spearman correlation

Variable	Covariable	Spearman ρ	p.value	-,8 -,6 -,4 -,2 0 ,2 ,4 ,6 ,8
KRT20	KRT5	-0,3588	0,0249*	
ERBB2	KRT5	-0,1473	0,3709	
ERBB2	KRT20	0,6811	<,0001*	
BIRC5	KRT5	0,1095	0,5071	
BIRC5	KRT20	0,0092	0,9555	
BIRC5	ERBB2	-0,0481	0,7710	
CD68	KRT5	-0,0064	0,9692	
CD68	KRT20	-0,0674	0,6836	
CD68	ERBB2	-0,1582	0,3361	
CD68	BIRC5	0,3848	0,0156*	

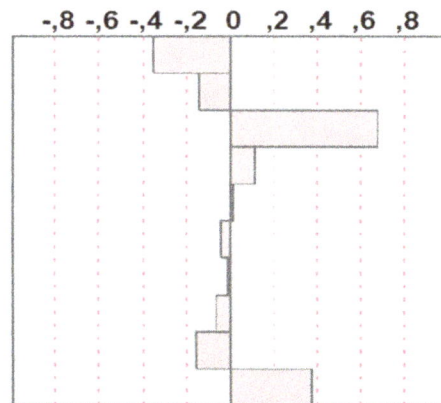

(a)

Figure 4. *Cont.*

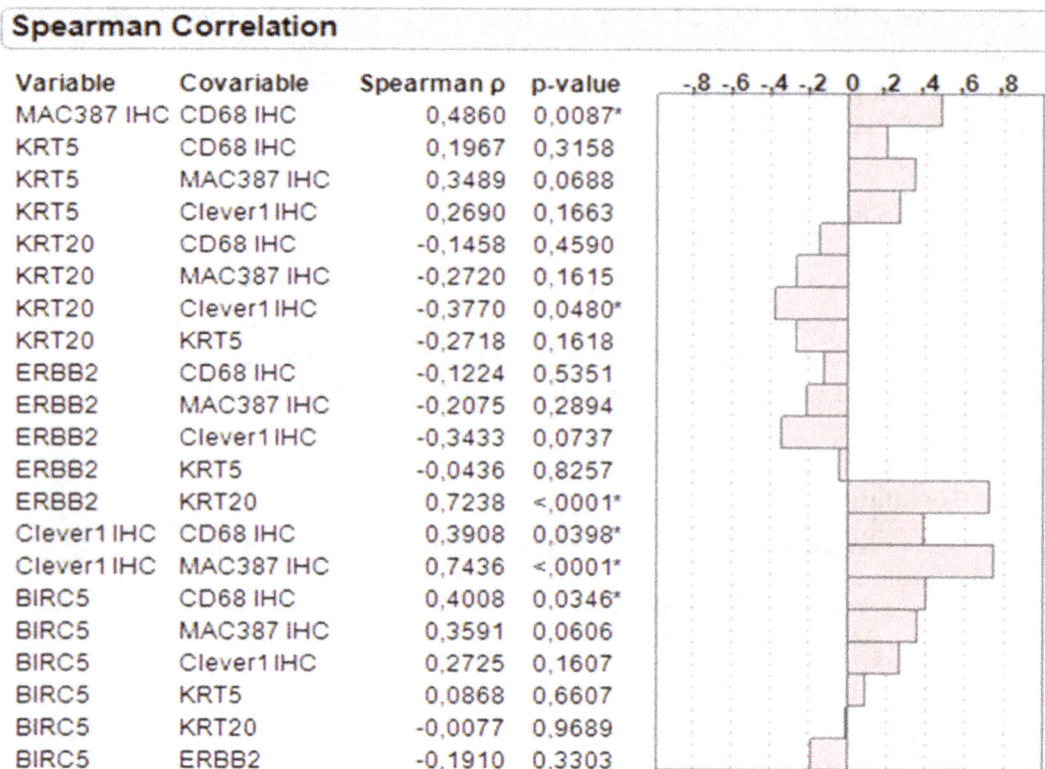

Spearman Correlation

Variable	Covariable	Spearman ρ	p-value	-,8 -,6 -,4 -,2 0 ,2 ,4 ,6 ,8
MAC387 IHC	CD68 IHC	0,4860	0,0087*	
KRT5	CD68 IHC	0,1967	0,3158	
KRT5	MAC387 IHC	0,3489	0,0688	
KRT5	Clever1 IHC	0,2690	0,1663	
KRT20	CD68 IHC	-0,1458	0,4590	
KRT20	MAC387 IHC	-0,2720	0,1615	
KRT20	Clever1 IHC	-0,3770	0,0480*	
KRT20	KRT5	-0,2718	0,1618	
ERBB2	CD68 IHC	-0,1224	0,5351	
ERBB2	MAC387 IHC	-0,2075	0,2894	
ERBB2	Clever1 IHC	-0,3433	0,0737	
ERBB2	KRT5	-0,0436	0,8257	
ERBB2	KRT20	0,7238	<,0001*	
Clever1 IHC	CD68 IHC	0,3908	0,0398*	
Clever1 IHC	MAC387 IHC	0,7436	<,0001*	
BIRC5	CD68 IHC	0,4008	0,0346*	
BIRC5	MAC387 IHC	0,3591	0,0606	
BIRC5	Clever1 IHC	0,2725	0,1607	
BIRC5	KRT5	0,0868	0,6607	
BIRC5	KRT20	-0,0077	0,9689	
BIRC5	ERBB2	-0,1910	0,3303	

(b)

Figure 4. (a) Correlation of normalized *KRT5, KRT20, ERBB2, BIRC5,* and *CD68* mRNA levels in the PCR cohort (*n* = 39) of bladder cancer patients treated with adjuvant chemotherapy. Graphical display of Spearman rho values and respective p-values are depicted. * indicates statistically significant results; **(b)** Correlation of *KRT5, KRT20, ERBB2,* and *BIRC5* mRNA levels with protein levels of CD68, MAC387, and CLEVER-1 determined by IHC in the combined PCR and IHC cohort (*n* = 28) of bladder cancer patients treated with adjuvant chemotherapy. Graphical display of Spearman rho values and respective p-values are depicted. * indicates statistically significant results.

In line with this, *BIRC5* mRNA was also positively associated with CD68 levels determined by IHC (Spearman rho 0.4008, *p* = 0.0346; Figure 4b). Interestingly, infiltration by macrophages as determined by IHC of CD68 and MAC387 tended to be negatively associated with luminal tumors as determined by *KRT20* (Spearman rho −0.2720 and −0.1458) and positively with basal tumors as determined by *KRT5* (Spearman rho 0.1967 and 0.3489).

Pearson correlation of *KRT5, KRT20, ERBB2, BIRC5,* and *CD68* mRNA levels with clinical variables such as performance status (PS), age, sex, body mass index (BMI), presence of carcinoma in situ (Cis), tumor stage (T-prim), and WHO Grade 1973 (G-prim) levels in the larger PCR cohort (Figure 5a) revealed that luminal tumors determined by *KRT20* mRNA were negatively associated with the presence of Cis and positively associated with higher age and male gender. In contrast, basal tumors determined by *KRT5* were negatively associated with BMI. Interestingly, macrophage infiltration was positively associated with age and Cis, while being negatively associated with grade. *BIRC5* mRNA was comparably associated with Cis. Similar associations were obtained by doing Spearman correlations (Table 2).

(a)

(b)

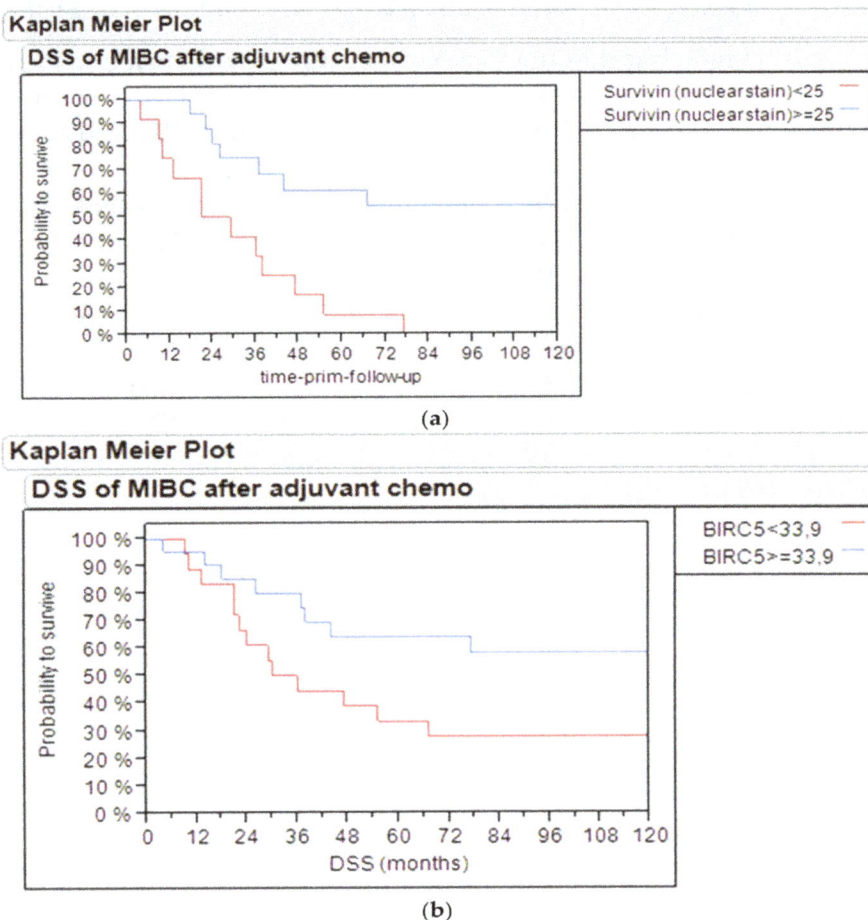

Figure 5. (a) Disease-specific survival (DSS) of bladder cancer patients treated with adjuvant chemotherapy based on survivin nuclear stain in the PCR and IHC cohort. (b) DSS of bladder cancer patients treated with adjuvant chemotherapy based on *BIRC5* mRNA expression in the PCR cohort.

Table 2. Pearson correlation of *KRT5, KRT20, ERBB2, BIRC5,* and *CD68* mRNA levels with performance status (PS), age, sex, body mass index (BMI), presence of carcinoma in situ (Cis), tumor size (T-prim), and WHO Grade 1973 (G-prim) levels in the PCR cohort of bladder cancer patients treated with adjuvant chemotherapy. Blue values indicate positive associations of significance, red values indicate negative associations of significance, and black values indicate insignificant trends.

	KRT5	KRT20	ERBB2	BIRC5	CD68	PS	Age	Sex	BMI	Cis	T-Prim	G-Prim
KRT5	1.0000	−0.1522	−0.0286	0.1052	0.0028	−0.0493	−0.0477	0.1678	−0.2302	−0.0040	−0.1413	0.0691
KRT20	−0.01522	1.0000	0.4266	0.0763	−0.1783	−0.0443	0.2165	0.2627	0.0498	−0.3599	−0.0544	0.1547
ERBB2	−0.0296	0.4266	1.0000	0.1019	0.0507	−0.2721	0.0280	0.3259	−0.0149	−0.0934	−0.1754	−0.0563
BIRC5	0.1052	0.0763	0.1019	1.0000	0.5390	−0.0578	0.2019	0.1273	−0.0553	0.2807	0.1831	0.0858
CD68	0.0028	−0.1783	0.0507	0.5390	1.0000	0.1646	0.3190	−0.0525	−0.1784	0.2361	0.1812	−0.2662
PS	−0.0493	−0.0443	−0.2721	−0.0578	0.1646	1.0000	0.3352	−0.1978	0.0978	−0.1370	0.1196	−0.0217
Age	−0.0477	0.2185	0.0280	0.2019	0.3190	0.3352	1.0000	0.1101	−0.3689	0.1915	−0.1977	−0.0184
Sex	0.1678	0.2827	0.3259	0.1273	−0.0625	−0.1978	0.1101	1.0000	0.0990	−0.0160	−0.1514	−0.0358
BMI	−0.2302	0.0498	−0.0149	−0.0553	−0.1784	0.0978	−0.3689	0.0990	1.0000	−0.2538	0.2724	−0.0904
Cis	−0.0040	−0.3599	−0.0934	0.2007	0.2361	−0.1370	0.1915	−0.0160	−0.2538	1.0000	−0.1852	0.0154
T-prim	−0.1413	−0.0544	−0.1754	0.1831	0.1612	0.1196	−0.1977	−0.1514	0.2724	−0.1852	1.0000	0.2200
G-prim	0.0691	0.1547	−0.0563	0.0858	−0.2662	−0.0217	−0.0184	−0.0356	−0.0904	0.0154	0.2200	1.0000

2.5. Disease-Specific Survival Analysis by Survivin and Macrophage Infiltration in Subtypes

Kaplan–Meier analysis revealed that high levels of survivin protein above the median expression (>25% positive nuclei) in the IHC cohort ($n = 28$) identified patients with improved disease-specific survival (DSS, 60% vs. 10% 5-year DSS, $p = 0.001$; Figure 5a) and PFS (60% vs. 10% 5-year PFS, $p = 0.0138$; Figure S1).

Similarly, in the enlarged PCR cohort (n = 39), high levels of *BIRC5* mRNA (DCT >33.9) identified patients with better outcome (60% vs. 30% 5-year DSS, $p = 0.0507$; Figure 5b) and progression-free survival (75% vs. 10% 5-year PFS, $p = 0.0042$; Figure S2).

Combining survivin expression and *KRT20* mRNA for outcome prediction revealed that *KRT20*-positive tumors as well as *BIRC5*-negative tumors had worse outcomes compared to survivin-positive tumors both on the protein level (20% and 10% vs. 75% 5-year DSS, $p = 0.0005$; Figure 6a) and mRNA level (30% each vs. 75% 5-year DSS, $p = 0.0358$; Figure 6b). Similarly, the combination of *KRT20* mRNA with *BIRC5* mRNA or survivin protein stain was significant for PFS ($p = 0.0181$ Figure S3 and $p = 0.0209$ Figure S4).

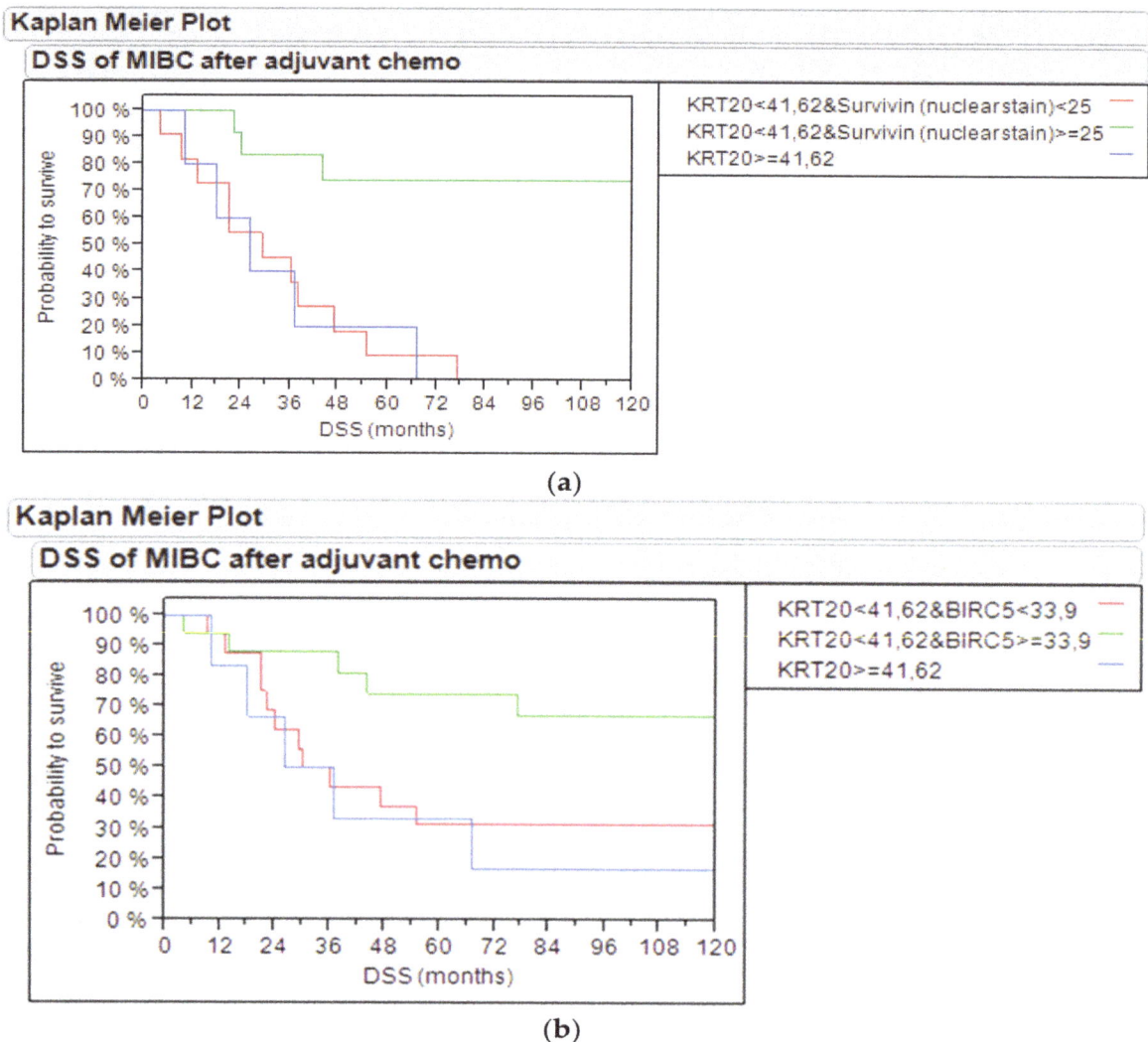

(a)

(b)

Figure 6. (a) DSS of bladder cancer patients treated with adjuvant chemotherapy based on *KRT20* mRNA and survivin nuclear protein stain in the PCR and IHC cohort; (b) DSS of bladder cancer patients treated with adjuvant chemotherapy based on *KRT20* and *BIRC5* mRNA expression in the PCR cohort.

Multivariate cox proportional hazard analysis of DSS revealed that the combination of *BIRC5* and *KRT20* mRNA to predict outcome was an independent prognostic factor, when age, sex, BMI, tumor stage, grade, and node status were included in the analysis ($p = 0.0167$, Table 3).

BMI and node status were also independent prognostic factors in multivariate cox regression. Similarly, multivariate cox proportional hazard analysis revealed that the combination of *BIRC5* and *KRT20* mRNA tended to be an independent prognostic factor for PFS ($p = 0.0816$; Table 4).

Table 3. Cox regression analysis for DSS by *BIRC5* × *KRT20* mRNA expression and clinicopathological features in the PCR cohort of bladder cancer patients treated with adjuvant chemotherapy. Statistically significant values are highlighted in boldface.

Parameter	Hazard Ratio	95% CI	*p*-Value
Age	1.07	0.99–1.14	0.0518
Sex	0.89	0.27–2.98	0.8329
BMI	1.16	1.00–1.24	**0.0499**
Node status	1.95	1.15–3.53	**0.0127**
Stage	1.13	0.42–3.16	0.8038
Grade	0.86	0.33–2.29	0.7638
KRT20 × BIRC5 Groups			
KRT20 low & BIRC5 high vs. KRT20 low & BIRC5 low	0.22	0.06–0.75	**0.0144**
KRT20 low & BIRC5 high vs. KRT20 high	0.24	0.06–0.94	**0.0407**
KRT20 low & BIRC5 low vs. KRT20 high	1.09	0.28–4.39	0.8988

Table 4. Cox regression analysis for progression-free survival (PFS) by *BIRC5* × *KRT20* mRNA expression and clinicopathological features in the PCR cohort of bladder cancer patients treated with adjuvant chemotherapy. Statistically significant values are highlighted in boldface.

Parameter	Hazard Ratio	95% CI	*p*-Value
Age	1.08	0.94–1.25	0.2911
Sex	1.25	0.23–7.45	0.7979
BMI	1.19	0.97–1.47	0.0985
Node status	1.75	0.89–3.87	0.1045
Stage	0.65	0.19–2.11	0.4750
Grade	0.86	0.33–2.29	0.4989
KRT20 × BIRC5 Groups			
KRT20 low & BIRC5 high vs. KRT20 low & BIRC5 low	0.15	0.02–0.79	**0.0252**
KRT20 low & BIRC5 high vs. KRT20 high	0.26	0.02–1.93	0.1908
KRT20 low & BIRC5 low vs. KRT20 high	1.77	0.41–8.92	0.4489

Combining survivin protein with the quantitation of macrophage infiltration based on protein or mRNA level revealed that the presence of macrophages in MIBC treated with adjuvant chemotherapy had an adverse effect on DSS. Tumors with high levels of nuclear survivin protein levels but low *CD68* mRNA levels had the best survival (70% vs. 40% vs. 10% 5-year DSS, $p = 0.0083$; Figure 7a). Similar results were found for PFS ($p = 0.0169$, Figure S5).

In line with this, tumors with high levels of nuclear survivin protein levels but low MAC387 protein levels had the best survival (100% vs. 30% vs. 10% 5-year DSS, $p = 0.0011$; Figure 7b). Similar results were found for PFS ($p = 0.0259$, Figure S6). Additionally, Figure S7 shows DSS of bladder cancer patients treated with adjuvant chemotherapy based on survivin nuclear protein stain and CLEVER-1 protein in the PCR and IHC cohort. Figure S8 shows PFS of bladder cancer patients treated with adjuvant chemotherapy based on survivin nuclear protein stain and CLEVER-1 protein in the PCR and IHC cohort.

Importantly and in contrast to previous publications, in pT1 NMIBC [22] and MIBC [23] not treated with chemotherapy, the overexpression of *ERBB2* was not related to adverse outcome (data not shown). However, within *ERBB2*-positive tumors (median mRNA expression), the presence of macrophages as determined by RT-qPCR of *CD68* had an adverse effect on the DSS of adjuvant-treated MIBC patients

(70% vs. 20% 5-year DSS, $p = 0.0280$; Figure 8). Similarly, the combination of *ERBB2* and *CD68* tended to predict PFS ($p = 0.0537$, Figure S9).

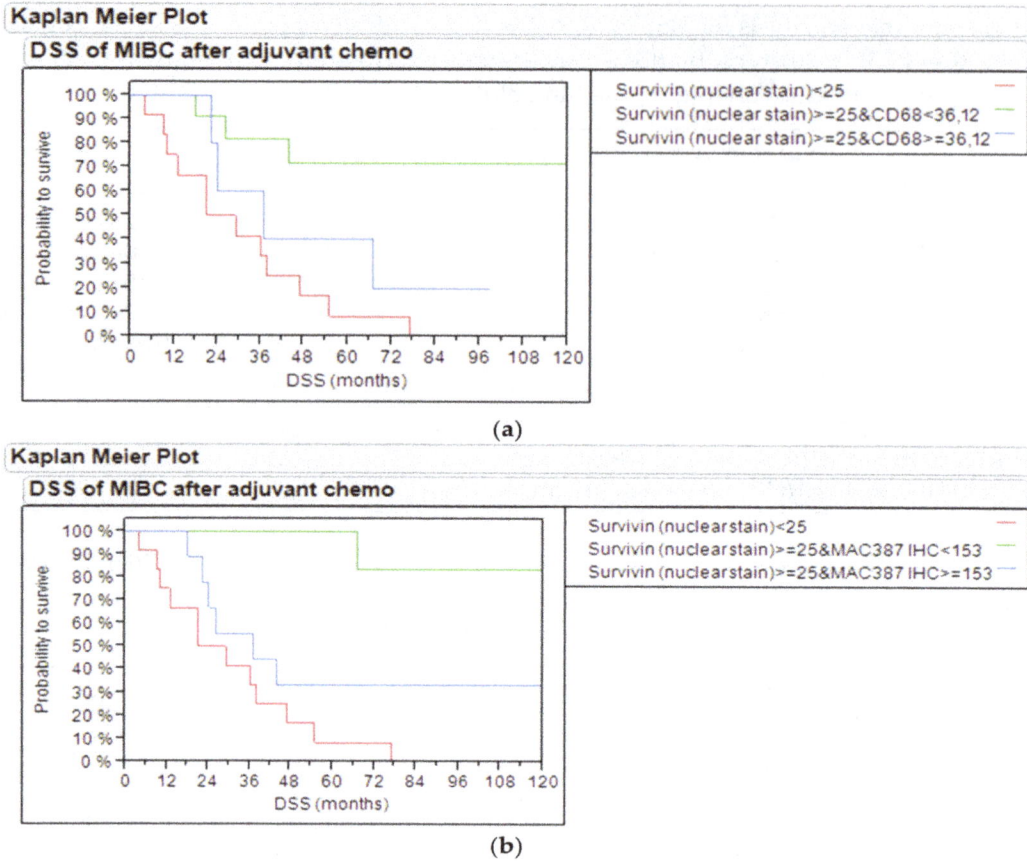

(a)

(b)

Figure 7. (a) DSS of bladder cancer patients treated with adjuvant chemotherapy based on survivin nuclear protein staining and *CD68* mRNA in the PCR and IHC cohort. (b) DSS of bladder cancer patients treated with adjuvant chemotherapy based on survivin nuclear protein staining and MAC387 protein in the PCR and IHC cohort.

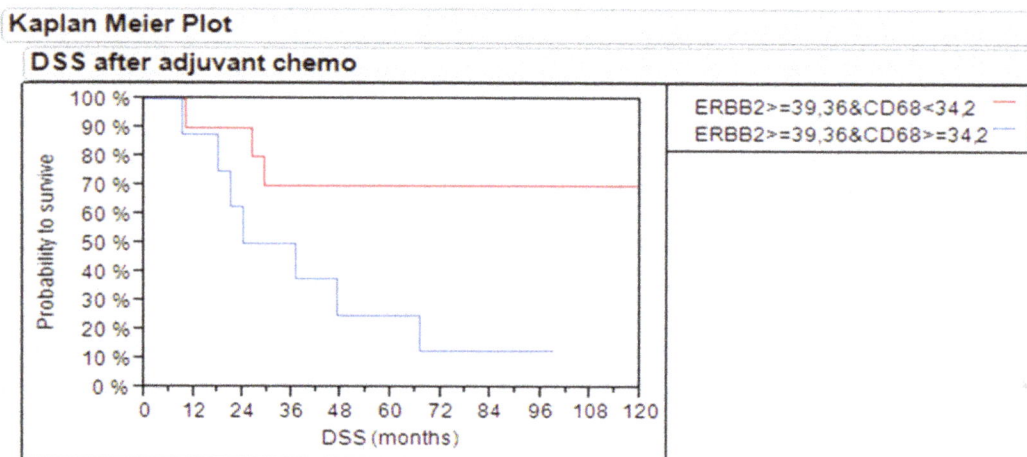

Figure 8. DSS of bladder cancer patients treated with adjuvant chemotherapy based on *ERBB2*-positive tumors in relation to *CD68* mRNA levels in the PCR and IHC cohort.

3. Discussion

High levels of survivin have been associated with poor prognosis in bladder cancer [24]. Survivin has also been described to be a predictor of cisplatin-resistance in gastric cancer, as well as in different cell lines [25,26]. A higher proliferative activity determined by *BIRC5* mRNA expression has been associated with worse outcome in NMIBC [11]. In line with this, a higher WHO 1973 grade was associated with *MKI67* and *ERBB2* mRNA levels [20]. Similarly, *FOXM1* mRNA expression was associated with a higher grade and stage as well as a 6 to 8-fold higher risk of progression in multivariable analysis ($p < 0.03$) of the UROMOL study (n = 488), which could be validated in independent NMIBC cohorts (n = 277) in silico [27]. Further analysis revealed that proliferation as determined by *FOXM1* mRNA expression was predictive for chemotherapy benefit in T1 NMIBC (n = 296) with patients having low *FOXM1* expression having better outcomes, irrespective of instillation therapy, while patients with high *FOXM1* expression benefitted from intravesical chemotherapy with mitomycin C [28]. In addition, meta-analysis revealed survivin protein and RNA to be associated with adverse outcome in NMIBC [29]. However, the predictive or prognostic role of proliferation and particularly of survivin is less clear for MIBC, particularly upon chemotherapeutic intervention targeting proliferative tissues. We showed that a high expression of survivin both on protein and RNA level was associated with good outcome in MIBC patients treated with adjuvant chemotherapy. It has to be noted that the triple chemotherapeutic regimen investigated within this study including taxol in addition to platinum-based chemotherapy is no standard regimen, which has to be taken into account when interpreting the results. However, it is reasonable that highly proliferative tissues do exhibit better response to chemotherapeutic regimen. Moreover, it has to be assumed that adding taxol to the standard chemotherapeutic regimen does not diminish the non-response of tumor tissues with low proliferative activity reflected by low survivin expression. This indicates that survivin might be a good predictive marker for chemotherapy benefit, which should be further investigated in randomized clinical trials. In contrast, low levels of nuclear staining of survivin were associated with the DSS of only 10% of patients after 5 years ($p = 0.001$), which indicates that tumors with low proliferation and apoptotic activity as indicated by survivin expression do require alternative treatment approaches.

In contrast, Als et al. identified survivin as a molecular marker for survival in locally advanced and/or metastatic bladder cancer following cisplatin-based chemotherapy [30]. In their study, multivariate analysis revealed that survivin expression was an independent marker for poor outcome, together with the presence of visceral metastases. In the group of patients without visceral metastases, both markers showed significant discriminating power as supplemental risk factors ($p < 0.0001$). Protein expression assessed by IHC was strongly correlated to response to chemotherapy. Another study on survivin was published by Pollard et al. [31]. This group evaluated an approach that combines genomic, proteomic, and therapeutic outcome datasets to identify novel putative urinary biomarkers of clinical outcome after neoadjuvant application of methotrexate, vinblastine, adriamycin, and cisplatin (MVAC). Using disease-free survival as a marker for clinical outcome, this group evaluated the ability of GGH, emmprin, survivin, and DBI expression in tumor tissue to stratify 27 patients treated with neoadjuvant MVAC. Interestingly, DBI ($p = 0.046$) but not GGH ($p = 0.190$), emmprin ($p = 0.066$), or survivin ($p = 0.393$) successfully stratified patients [31]. Our study revealed an inverse relation of survivin protein in cytoplasmic versus nuclear localization particularly when compared to its mRNA levels. This indicates the need of careful subcellular quantitation and may in part explain conflicting study results with regard to the prognostic and or predictive value of survivin expression, as discussed above.

Importantly, in our study, the proliferative subset of MIBC patients having better survival (i.e., 60% DSS after 5 years) could be further dissected by macrophage infiltration. Tervahartiala et al. [14] found that MAC387+ cells as well as CLEVER-1+ macrophages and vessels are associated with the response after neoadjuvant chemotherapy in bladder cancer patients. High MAC387+ tumor cell density was associated with disease progression after neoadjuvant chemotherapy, whereas the majority of patients with a lower amount of MAC387+ tumor cells exhibited a complete response. Patients with high amounts of CLEVER-1+ macrophages were associated with a poorer response to neoadjuvant chemotherapy, while higher amounts of CLEVER-1+ vessels were associated with a more favorable response [14]. The results of Tervahartiala et al. [14] verified also their previous studies where they could demonstrate that CD68 and MAC387 are associated with poorer survival in bladder cancer patients, whereas CLEVER-1-positive vessels act more as a protective marker [32].

In our study, we could validate that the presence of macrophages as determined by immunohistochemistry of CD68, CLEVER-1, and MAC387 or PCR of *CD68* was associated with worse disease-specific survival, particularly in tumors of high proliferative activity or elevated *ERBB2* mRNA expression.

Macrophages are challenging to investigate by immunohistochemistry due to their nature to cluster. This may lead to variations in results, especially when using TMAs and would require sufficient tissue sampling in routine clinical practice. TMAs are an efficient method in immunohistochemistry, but the results should be interpreted with care when studying clustering particles, e.g., macrophages. RNA quantitation may offer advantages by a more objective and standardized assessment of macrophage infiltration and the opportunity to embed the results in the context of immune infiltrates of diverse sets of T-cells with specified functions such as natural killer cells, helper cells, and regulatory T-cells.

The potential limitations of our study relate to its retrospective design and the impact of factors such as age and comorbidity on the indication of cystectomy and, consequently, on cancer-specific mortality in the elderly patients. The number of patients was limited, but the study included consecutive bladder cancer patients, who received adjuvant chemotherapy after radical cystectomy. Since retrospective designs do not guarantee causality, further prospective studies and the use of an independent series are warranted to prove the prognostic and predictive value of the analyzed marker combinations to robustly stratify the clinical outcome in real-world assessments.

4. Materials and Methods

4.1. Patients

4.1.1. Patient Population

From August 1996 to June 2006, a total of 50 patients diagnosed with bladder cancer were included in the trial. Together, 38 male patients and 12 female patients (average age 65 years, range 49–80 years) were included. Pathohistological T-category and grade for the primary tumors are as follows. The study included for the primary tumors pTaG2 (n = 1), pT1G2 (n = 9), pT1G3 (n = 7), pT2G1 (n = 1), pT2G2 (n = 10), and pT2G3 (n = 22) obtained by transurethral resection under institutional review board-approved protocols. Three patients showed carcinoma in situ (6%). All non-muscle invasive urothelial carcinomas included in the study progressed to muscle-invasive tumors under the follow-up. All patients were treated with radical surgery before chemotherapy. Patient characteristics, including lymph node status before chemotherapy as well as ECOG performance status at the point of starting chemotherapy, are summarized in Table 1. The study population had its origin in one single institution. The analysis of the different markers has been performed at different study sites.

4.1.2. Eligibility

Eligible patients for this trial were required to have either metastatic or locally advanced histologically confirmed transitional cell carcinoma of the urothelial tract. Patients who had received a previous systemic chemotherapy regimen were excluded. Previous radiation therapy was also an exclusion criterion.

Additional eligibility requirements included the following: an ECOG performance status of 0 to 2, a leukocyte count ≥3000/µL, a platelet count ≥100,000/µL, serum bilirubin <1.5 mg/dL, serum creatinine ≤2.5 mg/dL, and age >18 years. Patients with other active malignancies or any other serious or active medical conditions were excluded. Pregnant or lactating females were ineligible. The study protocol was approved by the Research Ethical Board of the Landesärztekammer Brandenburg (AS 25(bB)/2017;

AS 147(bB)/2013) for the German part of the study. For the Finnish part, there was an ethical approval from the Hospital District of Southwestern Finland. All methods in this study were carried out in accordance with relevant guidelines and regulations. The study was conducted in compliance with the current revision of the Declaration of Helsinki, guiding physicians and medical research involving human subjects. All patients were required to provide written informed consent prior to the study enrolment. The study did not affect the patients or their further treatment of follow-up in any way. All the sample collections were done on already existing tissue specimens received during the diagnosis and treatment of these patients.

4.2. Pretreatment Evaluation

Prior to enrollment in this trial, all patients were required to have a complete history, physical examination, complete blood counts, chemistry profile, and urine analysis. In addition, patients underwent computed tomography scans of the chest, abdomen, and pelvis with appropriate tumor measurements.

4.3. Assessment of Treatment Efficacy

All fifty patients received treatment with the following regimen: gemcitabine at a dose of 1000 mg/m^2 as a 30 min intravenous infusion followed by paclitaxel at a dose of 80 mg/m^2 as a 1 h intravenous infusion on days 1 and 8. On day 2, cisplatin at a dose of 50 mg/m^2 was administered as an intravenous infusion and hydration with 2000 mL NaCl 0.9%. The regimen was repeated every 21 days. Patients received standard paclitaxel premedication and antiemetic prophylaxis. Patients were evaluated for response to treatment after the completion of 4 courses (12 weeks). Reevaluation included a repeat of all previously abnormal radiologic studies with a repeat of objective tumor measurement. Patients who achieved an objective response (complete or partial) or stable disease after the completion of four courses of therapy continued treatment with this regimen. Treatment was continued for a total of six courses. None of the patients received neoadjuvant therapy before cystectomy.

Thirty-four patients who completed 6 courses and remained in remission were followed with further treatment of a single dose of gemcitabine at a dose of 1000 mg/m^2 as a 30 min intravenous infusion repeating every 28 days. This following treatment was continued for at least two years.

Two patients received the second-line chemotherapy (methotrexate, epirubicin and cisplatin chemotherapy (MEC)) because of rapid progression after a three-drug regimen with gemcitabine, paclitaxel, and cisplatin or during gemcitabine monotherapy.

4.4. Dose Modifications

All patients received full doses of all 3 agents on day 1 of the first course of treatment. Subsequent doses were based on hematologic and non-hematologic toxicity observed. Dose modifications for myelosuppression were determined by the blood counts measured on the day of scheduled treatment. Nadir blood counts were not used as a basis for dose reduction.

On day 1 of each course, full doses of all drugs were administered if the leukocyte count was ≥3000/µL and the platelet count was >100,000/µL. If the leukocyte count was <3000/µL or the platelet count was <100,000/µL, treatment was delayed for one or two days.

All patients with an ECOG performance status of 2 or with renal insufficiency in the stage of compensated retention received reduced doses of 50% to 70%. In case of good tolerance of the therapy, we applicated higher doses for following cycles.

4.5. Criteria for Follow-Up

The follow-up consisted of clinical examination, ultrasound of abdomen, and computed tomography scans of the chest, abdomen, and pelvis with appropriate tumor measurements every 6 months. Progression was defined as new metastatic disease or local progress during follow-up. Chemotherapy response was defined as absence of recurrence, progression, or death from the disease during follow-up. Responses were defined using the Response Evaluation criteria in Solid Tumors (RECIST). A complete response (CR) required the total disappearance of all clinically and radiographically detected tumors for at least 4 weeks. Patients had partial response (PR) if treatment produced a reduction of at least 30% in the sum of the longest diameter, with no evidence of new disease. No change (NC) was defined as patients who showed no visible reduction or even progress less than 20%. Patients who had the appearance of any new lesions or who had an increase of at least 20% in the size of any existing lesions had progressive disease (PD).

4.6. Clinical Follow-Up and Treatment Efficacy

Among the 50 cases analyzed, 26 progressed (52%), and 34 patients died (68%). Tumor-related death is 27 in total (54%). Twenty-one patients (42%) achieved complete response, three patients achieved partial response (6%), and for twenty-five patients (50%), no change was documented (Table 1).

The median time interval from diagnosis at the point of the first transurethral resection of the primary tumor and the date of death (or last follow-up) of all patients was 36.5 months (range: 8.0–221.0). The median time interval between the point of radical operation of the muscle-invasive tumor and the date of death (or last follow-up) of all patients was 49.0 months (range: 7.0–175.0). The median time interval between the point of chemotherapy and the date of death (or last follow-up) of all patients was 23.0 months (range: 3.0–171.0). The median time between primary resection and muscle-invasive tumor at the point of radical operation of all patients was 8.0 months (range: 6.0–58.0). The median time to progress between radical operation and the progressive disease of all patients was 13 months (range: 6.0–32.0).

4.7. Procedure

For each case, the most representative formalin-fixed, paraffin-embedded tissue block was selected for analysis. Sections (5 μm thickness) were deparaffinized with xylene and rehydrated with a graded alcohol series.

4.8. Immunostaining for CD68, MAC387, and CLEVER-1

The primary antibodies used were mouse monoclonal IgG1 antiCD68 (KP1) (concentration 1:5; ab845, Abcam, U.K.) and mouse monoclonal IgG1 antiMAC387 (concentration 1:500; ab22506, Abcam, U.K.), which detects the myelomonocytic L1 molecule calprotectin. CLEVER-1 (common lymphatic endothelial and vascular endothelial receptor-1, also known as STAB1 and FEEL-1) positive type 2 macrophages and vessels were detected with the rat IgG 2-7 antibody (concentration 1:5) [33,34]. The antibodies 3G6 (mouse IgG1 antibody against chicken T cells) [35] and MEL-14 [rat IgG2a antibody against mouse L-selectin (CD62L)] (Exbio, Czech Republic) were used as negative controls. The primary immunoreaction was performed with using the mouse/rat Vectastain Elite ABC Kit (Vector Laboratories). Sections for CD68 and MAC387 staining were heat pre-treated in citric acid (0.01 M, pH 6.0) in a 97 °C water bath for 20 min. Antigen retrieval for CLEVER-1-stained sections was performed with proteinase K (Dako, Glostrup, Denmark) (10 min at 37 °C), and the slides were washed three times with PBS after the pre-treatment. Endogenous peroxidase was blocked with 0.1% H_2O_2 for 30 min. Non-specific sites were blocked with horse (CD68 and MAC387) or rabbit (CLEVER-1) normal serum at room temperature for 20 min. Sections were incubated with primary antibodies overnight at 4 °C and then treated with biotinylated secondary antibody solution according to the manufacturer's instructions. After washing with PBS, Vectastain Elite ABC Reagent was added (30 min at room temperature), the slides were washed, and immunoreactions were detected using 3,3'-diaminobenzidine as a substrate. Slides were counterstained with hematoxylin, dehydrated, re-fixed in xylene, mounted with distyrene plasticizer xylene (DPX). The whole tumor and surrounding peritumoral area were screened by light microscopy. A detailed description of that scoring process has already been published by Boström et al. [32]. These experiments have been performed at University Hospital Turku (Finland).

4.9. Immunostaining for Survivin

Survivin antibody was provided by the Department of Molecular Medicine at the Institute for Prevention and Occupational Medicine of the German Social Accident Insurance in Bochum, Germany. A detailed description of recombinant survivin and antibody production as well as the analytical specificity of the survivin antibody can be found at Gleichenhagen et al. [36]. We used this method for survivin in a regular immunohistochemistry procedure. In this study, we are one of the first centers who evaluated this survivin antibody by immunohistochemistry. Reproducibility of the new survivin antibody as a component of an ELISA was investigated and published by Gleichenhagen et al. [36]. The experiments for immunostaining for survivin have been performed and evaluated at University Hospital Charité Berlin (Germany). Examples of immunohistochemical stainings are visible in Figures S10–S13.

4.10. Isolation of Tumor RNA

For RNA extraction from FFPE tissue, tissue dots (1.5 mm diameter, 5 μm cuts) from tissue microarray material were picked by stamp technology and further processed according to a commercially available bead-based extraction method (XTRACT kit; STRATIFYER Molecular Pathology GmbH, Cologne, Germany). RNA was eluted with 100 μL elution buffer, and then, RNA eluates were stored at −80 °C until use.

4.11. Gene Expression by RT-qPCR

The mRNA expression levels of KRT5, KRT20, ERBB2, BIRC5 and CD68 as well as one reference gene (REF), namely CALM2, were determined by RT-qPCR, which involves the reverse transcription of RNA and subsequent amplification of cDNA executed successively as a 1-step reaction using inventoried validated TaqMan Gene Expression Assays (MP002, MP015, MP452, MP089, MP120 and MP501, STRATIFYER Molecular Pathology GmbH, Köln, Germany). The robustness and usefulness of CALM2 as a housekeeping gene for diverse candidate genes as well as comparability to diverse IHC assessments such as CK20/KRT20, MKI67/Ki67, and PDL1, when used as a single reference gene, have been demonstrated in several of our own publications [20,37,38] and resulted in the introduction of CALM2 as a housekeeping gene in CE-certified IVD products such as Endopredict [39] and MammaTyper [40]. Each patient sample or control was analyzed with each assay mix in triplicate. The experiments were run on a Siemens Versant (Siemens, Germany) according to the following protocol: 5 min at 50 °C, 20 Sec at 95 °C, followed by 40 cycles of 15 Sec at 95 °C and 60 Sec at 60 °C. Forty amplification cycles were applied, and the cycle quantification threshold (Cq) values of three markers and one reference gene for each sample (S) were estimated as the median of the triplicate measurements. The final values were generated using ΔCT from the total number of cycles (40-DCT) to ensure that the normalized gene expression obtained by the test was proportional to the corresponding mRNA expression levels. This part of the work has been measured and analyzed at STRATIFYER Molecular Pathology, Cologne (Germany). Examples of immunostaining for survivin, CD68, CLEVER-1, and MAC387 are shown in Figures S11–S13.

4.12. Statistical Analysis

The Kaplan–Meier method, log-rank testing, and Cox proportional hazards regression models were used to analyze the associations between IHC and outcome. Partitioning tests were used to identify appropriate cut-off values for dichotomization of the continuous variables for Kaplan–Meier analysis. In the Cox proportional hazards regression models, the markers were evaluated as continuous variables. Outcome measures included DSS and OS. The survival time was calculated from the date of surgery to the date of the last follow-up or death. Any death due to bladder cancer (BC) or with metastatic BC was defined as cancer-specific mortality. All statistical tests were two-sided, and p-values <0.05 were considered statistically significant. All tests and calculations were performed using the software R, version 3.1.2 (R Development Core Team 2014) or JMP 9.0.0 (SAS Institute Inc, 100 SAS Campus Drive Cary, NC 27513-2414, USA).

5. Conclusions

Markers that are validated to predict poor prognosis in NMIBC and MIBC not being treated with chemotherapy, such as survivin and potentially *ERBB2*, exhibit inverse outcome relation upon adjuvant chemotherapeutic treatment, indicating their potential as being predictive for chemotherapy benefit. In addition, macrophage infiltration seems to have a key role in high-risk tumors that could be attributed to its potential of modulating the activity of infiltrating T-cells particularly under circumstances of the chemotherapeutic destruction of tumor cells and subsequent antigen presentation. The findings of the study are limited by the small size of the stud group and its retrospective character, but based on its results, we could demonstrate that further prospective studies with a higher number of patients might be worth pursuing. The combination of immunohistochemical and robust molecular methods being applicable in clinical routine situation harbors the promise of predicting the outcome of patients and serving as valuable pathological tools to better select patients for specific therapeutic interventions.

Supplementary Materials:

Figure S1: PFS of bladder cancer patients treated with adjuvant chemotherapy based on survivin nuclear stain in the PCR and IHC cohort. Figure S2: PFS of bladder cancer patients treated with adjuvant chemotherapy based on *BIRC5* mRNA expression in the PCR cohort. Figure S3: PFS of bladder cancer patients treated with adjuvant chemotherapy based on *KRT20* mRNA and survivin nuclear protein stain in the PCR and IHC cohort. Figure S4: PFS of bladder cancer patients treated with adjuvant chemotherapy based on *KRT20* and *BIRC5* mRNA expression in the PCR cohort. Figure S5: PFS of bladder cancer patients treated with adjuvant chemotherapy based on survivin nuclear protein stain and *CD68* mRNA in the PCR and IHC cohort. Figure S6: PFS of bladder cancer patients treated with adjuvant chemotherapy based on survivin nuclear protein stain and MAC387 protein in the PCR and IHC cohort. Figure S7: DSS of bladder cancer patients treated with adjuvant chemotherapy based on survivin nuclear protein stain and CLEVER-1 protein in the PCR and IHC cohort. Figure S8: PFS of bladder cancer patients treated with adjuvant chemotherapy based on survivin nuclear protein stain and CLEVER-1 protein in the PCR and IHC cohort. Figure S9: PFS of bladder cancer patients treated with adjuvant chemotherapy based on ERBB2 positive tumors in relation to *CD68* mRNA levels in the PCR and IHC cohort. Figure S10: Immunohistochemical staining of survivin. Figure S11: immunohistochemical staining of CD68. Figure S12: Immunohistochemical staining of CLEVER-1. Figure S13: immunohistochemical staining of MAC387.

Author Contributions: T.H.E. designed and performed study and cooperation, data collection, and drafted the manuscript. A.K., E.K., F.F., T.S., A.R., and K.J. performed and supervised experiments for survivin. P.B., M.T., and P.T. performed and supervised experiments for CLEVER-1, CD68 and MAC387. J.G., G.J. and T.B. performed survivin experiments. S.K. and J.R. helped collect the samples and supervised clinical data collection. R.M.W. defined candidate genes, performed and supervised experiments for nucleic acid extraction from tissue microarray dots and subsequent RT-qPCR of *KRT5, KRT20, ERBB2, CD68, BIRC5*. All authors have read and agreed to the published version of the manuscript.

Abbreviations

BC	bladder cancer
BIRC5	baculoviral IAP repeat containing 5 (BIRC5)
BMI	body mass index
BRCA1	breast cancer 1
Cis	carcinoma in situ
CLEVER-1	common lymphatic endothelial and vascular endothelial receptor-1
CR	complete response
DCT	Delta Cycle Threshold (gene expression based on difference of thereshold passing of individual genes when using qPCR)
DPX	distyrene plasticizer xylene
DSS	disease-specific survival
GC	gemcitabine and cisplatin chemotherapy
IHC	immunohistochemistry

N	lymph node status
MEC	methotrexate, epirubicin and cisplatin chemotherapy
MIBC	muscle-invasive bladder cancer
M	metastases status
MVAC	methotrexate, vinblastine, adriamycin and cisplatin chemotherapy
MVEC	methotrexate, vinblastine, epirubicin and cisplatin chemotherapy
NC	no change
NGS	next generation sequencing
NMIBC	non-muscle invasive bladder cancer
OS	overall survival
PCG	paclitaxel, cisplatin and gemcitabine chemotherapy
PCR	polymerase chain reaction
PD	progressive disease
PFS	progression-free survival
PR	partial response
RC	radical cystectomy
RECIST	Response Evaluation criteria in Solid Tumors
TMA	tissue microarray
TURB	transurethral resection of bladder

References

1. Ferlay, J.; Colombet, M.; Soerjomataram, I.; Mathers, C.; Parkin, D.M.; Piñeros, M.; Znaor, A.; Bray, F. Estimating the global cancer incidence and mortality in 2018: GLOBOCAN sources and methods. *Int. J. Cancer* **2018**, *144*, 1941–1953. [CrossRef]

2. Witjes, J.A.; Compérat, E.; Cowan, N.C.; De Santis, M.; Gakis, G.; Lebret, T.; Ribal, M.J.; Van Der Heijden, A.G.; Sherif, A. EAU Guidelines on Muscle-invasive and Metastatic Bladder Cancer: Summary of the 2013 Guidelines. *Eur. Urol.* **2014**, *65*, 778–792. [CrossRef]

3. Alfred Witjes, J.; Lebret, T.; Comperat, E.M.; De Santis, M.; Gakis, G.; Lebret, T.; Ribal, M.J.; Van der Heiden, M.J.; Sherif, A. Updated 2016 EAU Guidelines on Muscle-invasive and Metastatic Bladder Cancer. *Eur. Urol.* **2017**, *71*, 462–475. [CrossRef]

4. Kluth, L.A.; Black, P.C.; Bochner, B.H.; Catto, J.; Lerner, S.P.; Stenzl, A.; Sylvester, R.; Vickers, A.J.; Xylinas, E.; Shariat, S.F. Prognostic and Prediction Tools in Bladder Cancer: A Comprehensive Review of the Literature. *Eur. Urol.* **2015**, *68*, 238–253. [CrossRef] [PubMed]

5. Hoffmann, A.-C.; Wild, P.; Leicht, C.; Bertz, S.; Danenberg, K.D.; Danenberg, P.V.; Stöhr, R.; Stöckle, M.; Lehmann, J.; Schuler, M.; et al. MDR1 and ERCC1 Expression Predict Outcome of Patients with Locally Advanced Bladder Cancer Receiving Adjuvant Chemotherapy. *Neoplasia* **2010**, *12*, 628–636. [CrossRef] [PubMed]

6. Garg, H.; Suri, P.; Gupta, J.C.; Talwar, G.; Dubey, S. Survivin: A unique target for tumor therapy. *Cancer Cell Int.* **2016**, *16*, 49. [CrossRef] [PubMed]

7. Engels, K.; Knauer, S.; Metzler, D.; Simf, C.; Struschka, O.; Bier, C.; Mann, W.; Kovács, A.; Stauber, R.; Knauer, S.; et al. Dynamic intracellular survivin in oral squamous cell carcinoma: Underlying molecular mechanism and potential as an early prognostic marker. *J. Pathol.* **2007**, *211*, 532–540. [CrossRef] [PubMed]

8. Li, F.; Yang, J.; Ramnath, N.; Javle, M.M.; Tan, N. Nuclear or cytoplasmic expression of survivin: What is the significance? *Int. J. Cancer* **2005**, *114*, 509–512. [CrossRef]

9. Uren, A.G.; Wong, L.; Pakusch, M.; Fowler, K.J.; Burrows, F.J.; Vaux, D.L.; Choo, K. Survivin and the inner centromere protein INCENP show similar cell-cycle localization and gene knockout phenotype. *Curr. Boil.* **2000**, *10*, 1319–1328. [CrossRef]

10. Dohi, T.; Beltrami, E.; Wall, N.R.; Plescia, J.; Altieri, D.C. Mitochondrial survivin inhibits apoptosis and promotes tumorigenesis. *J. Clin. Investig.* **2004**, *114*, 1117–1127. [CrossRef]

11. Dyrskjøt, L.; Reinert, T.; Algaba, F.; Christensen, E.; Nieboer, D.; Hermann, G.G.; Mogensen, K.; Beukers, W.; Marquez, M.; Segersten, U.; et al. Prognostic Impact of a 12-gene Progression Score in Non-muscle-invasive Bladder Cancer: A Prospective Multicentre Validation Study. *Eur. Urol.* **2017**, *72*, 461–469. [CrossRef] [PubMed]

12. Holness, C.L.; Simmons, D.L. Molecular cloning of CD68, a human macrophage marker related to lysosomal glycoproteins. *Blood* **1993**, *81*, 1607–1613. [CrossRef] [PubMed]

13. Kzhyshkowska, J.; Gratchev, A.; Goerdt, S. Stabilin-1, a homeostatic scavenger receptor with multiple functions. *J. Cell Mol. Med.* **2006**, *10*, 635–649. [CrossRef] [PubMed]

14. Tervahartiala, M.; Taimen, P.; Mirtti, T.; Koskinen, I.; Ecke, T.; Jalkanen, S.; Boström, P.J. Immunological tumor status may predict response to neoadjuvant chemotherapy and outcome after radical cystectomy in bladder cancer. *Sci. Rep.* **2017**, *7*, 12682. [CrossRef]

15. Goebeler, M.; Roth, J.; Teigelkamp, S.; Sorg, C. The monoclonal antibody MAC387 detects an epitope on the calcium-binding protein MRP14. *J. Leukoc. Boil.* **1994**, *55*, 259–261. [CrossRef]

16. Netea-Maier, R.T.; Smit, J.; Netea, M.G. Metabolic changes in tumor cells and tumor-associated macrophages: A mutual relationship. *Cancer Lett.* **2018**, *413*, 102–109. [CrossRef]

17. The Cancer Genome Atlas Research Network; Cancer Genome Atlas Research Network Comprehensive molecular characterization of urothelial bladder carcinoma. *Nature* **2014**, *507*, 315–322. [CrossRef]

18. Choi, W.; Porten, S.; Kim, S.; Willis, D.; Plimack, E.R.; Hoffman-Censits, J.; Roth, B.; Cheng, T.; Tran, M.; Lee, I.-L.; et al. Identification of distinct basal and luminal subtypes of muscle-invasive bladder cancer with different sensitivities to frontline chemotherapy. *Cancer Cell* **2014**, *25*, 152–165. [CrossRef]

19. Damrauer, J.S.; Hoadley, K.A.; Chism, D.D.; Fan, C.; Tignanelli, C.; Wobker, S.E.; Yeh, J.J.; Milowsky, M.I.; Iyer, G.; Parker, J.S.; et al. Intrinsic subtypes of high-grade bladder cancer reflect the hallmarks of breast cancer biology. *Proc. Natl. Acad. Sci. USA* **2014**, *111*, 3110–3115. [CrossRef]

20. Breyer, J.; Wirtz, R.M.; Otto, W.; Erben, P.; Kriegmair, M.C.; Stoehr, R.; Eckstein, M.; Eidt, S.; Denzinger, S. In stage pT1 non-muscle-invasive bladder cancer (NMIBC), high KRT20 and low KRT5 mRNA expression identify the luminal subtype and predict recurrence and survival. *Virchows Arch.* **2017**, *470*, 267–274. [CrossRef]

21. Kamoun, A.; De Reyniès, A.; Allory, Y.; Sjödahl, G.; Robertson, A.G.; Seiler, R.; Hoadley, K.A.; Groeneveld, C.S.; Al-Ahmadie, H.; Choi, W.; et al. A Consensus Molecular Classification of Muscle-invasive Bladder Cancer. *Eur. Urol.* **2020**, *77*, 420–433. [CrossRef] [PubMed]

22. Breyer, J.; Wirtz, R.M.; Otto, W.; Laible, M.; Schlombs, K.; Erben, P.; Kriegmair, M.C.; Stoehr, R.; Eidt, S.; Denzinger, S.; et al. Predictive value of molecular subtyping in NMIBC by RT-qPCR of ERBB2, ESR1, PGR and MKI67 from formalin fixed TUR biopsies. *Oncotarget* **2017**, *8*, 67684–67695. [CrossRef] [PubMed]

23. Kriegmair, M.; Wirtz, R.; Worst, T.; Breyer, J.; Ritter, M.; Keck, B.; Boehmer, C.; Otto, W.; Eckstein, M.; Weis, C.; et al. Prognostic Value of Molecular Breast Cancer Subtypes based on Her2, ESR1, PGR and Ki67 mRNA-Expression in Muscle Invasive Bladder Cancer. *Transl. Oncol.* **2018**, *11*, 467–476. [CrossRef] [PubMed]

24. Akhtar, M.; Gallagher, L.; Rohan, S. Survivin: Role in Diagnosis, Prognosis, and Treatment of Bladder Cancer. *Adv. Anat. Pathol.* **2006**, *13*, 122–126. [CrossRef] [PubMed]

25. Tran, J.; Master, Z.; Yu, J.L.; Rak, J.; Dumont, D.J.; Kerbel, R.S. A role for survivin in chemoresistance of endothelial cells mediated by VEGF. *Proc. Natl. Acad. Sci. USA* **2002**, *99*, 4349–4354. [CrossRef]

26. Nakamura, M.; Tsuji, N.; Asanuma, K.; Kobayashi, D.; Yagihashi, A.; Hirata, K.; Torigoe, T.; Sato, N.; Watanabe, N. Survivin as a predictor of cis-diamminedichloroplatinum sensitivity in gastric cancer patients. *Cancer Sci.* **2004**, *95*, 44–51. [CrossRef]

27. Rinaldetti, S.; Wirtz, R.; Worst, T.S.; Hartmann, A.; Breyer, J.; Dyrskjøt, L.; Erben, P. FOXM1 predicts disease progression in non-muscle invasive bladder cancer. *J. Cancer Res. Clin. Oncol.* **2018**, *144*, 1701–1709. [CrossRef]

28. Breyer, J.; Wirtz, R.M.; Erben, P.; Rinaldetti, S.; Worst, T.S.; Stoehr, R.; Eckstein, M.; Sikic, D.; Denzinger, S.; Burger, M.; et al. FOXM1 overexpression is associated with adverse outcome and predicts response to intravesical instillation therapy in stage pT1 non-muscle-invasive bladder cancer. *BJU Int.* **2018**, *123*, 187–196. [CrossRef]

29. Jeon, C.; Kim, M.; Kwak, C.; Kim, H.H.; Ku, J.H. Prognostic Role of Survivin in Bladder Cancer: A Systematic Review and Meta-Analysis. *PLoS ONE* **2013**, *8*, e76719. [CrossRef]

30. Als, A.B.; Von Der Maase, H.; Koed, K.; Mansilla, F.; Toldbod, H.E.; Jensen, J.L.; Jensen, K.M.; Dyrskjøt, L.; Ulhøi, B.P.; Sengeløv, L.; et al. Emmprin and Survivin Predict Response and Survival following Cisplatin-Containing Chemotherapy in Patients with Advanced Bladder Cancer. *Clin. Cancer Res.* **2007**, *13*, 4407–4414. [CrossRef]

31. Pollard, C.; Nitz, M.; Baras, A..; Williams, P.; Moskaluk, C.; Theodorescu, D. Genoproteomic mining of urothelial cancer suggests {gamma}-glutamyl hydrolase and diazepam-binding inhibitor as putative urinary markers of outcome after chemotherapy. *Am. J. Pathol.* **2009**, *175*, 1824–1830. [CrossRef] [PubMed]

32. Boström, M.M.; Irjala, H.; Mirtti, T.; Taimen, P.; Kauko, T.; Ålgars, A.; Jalkanen, S.; Boström, P.J. Tumor-Associated Macrophages Provide Significant Prognostic Information in Urothelial Bladder Cancer. *PLoS ONE* **2015**, *10*, e0133552. [CrossRef] [PubMed]

33. Palani, S.; Maksimow, M.; Miiluniemi, M.; Auvinen, K.; Jalkanen, S.; Salmi, M. Stabilin-1/CLEVER-1, a type 2 macrophage marker, is an adhesion and scavenging molecule on human placental macrophages. *Eur. J. Immunol.* **2011**, *41*, 2052–2063. [CrossRef] [PubMed]

34. Irjala, H.; Elima, K.; Johansson, E.-L.; Merinen, M.; Kontula, K.; Alanen, K.; Grénman, R.; Salmi, M.; Jalkanen, S. The same endothelial receptor controls lymphocyte traffic both in vascular and lymphatic vessels. *Eur. J. Immunol.* **2003**, *33*, 815–824. [CrossRef]

35. Salmi, M.; Jalkanen, S. A 90-kilodalton endothelial cell molecule mediating lymphocyte binding in humans. *Science* **1992**, *257*, 1407–1409. [CrossRef]

36. Gleichenhagen, J.; Arndt, C.; Casjens, S.; Meinig, C.; Gerullis, H.; Raiko, I.; Bruning, T.; Ecke, T.; Johnen, G. Evaluation of a New Survivin ELISA and UBC((R)) Rapid for the Detection of Bladder Cancer in Urine. *Int. J. Mol. Sci.* **2018**, *19*, 226. [CrossRef]

37. Eckstein, M.; Wirtz, R.M.; Pfannstil, C.; Wach, S.; Stoehr, R.; Breyer, J.; Erlmeier, F.; Gunes, C.; Nitschke, K.; Weichert, W.; et al. A multicenter round robin test of PD-L1 expression assessment in urothelial bladder cancer by immunohistochemistry and RT-qPCR with emphasis on prognosis prediction after radical cystectomy. *Oncotarget* **2018**, *9*, 15001–15014. [CrossRef]

38. Eckstein, M.; Strissel, P.; Strick, R.; Weyerer, V.; Wirtz, R.; Pfannstiel, C.; Wullweber, A.; Lange, F.; Erben, P.; Stoehr, R.; et al. Cytotoxic T-cell-related gene expression signature predicts improved survival in muscle-invasive urothelial bladder cancer patients after radical cystectomy and adjuvant chemotherapy. *J. Immunother. Cancer* **2020**, *8*, e000162. [CrossRef]

39. Filipits, M.; Dafni, U.; Gnant, M.; Polydoropoulou, V.; Hills, M.; Kiermaier, A.; De Azambuja, E.; Larsimont, D.P.; Rojo, F.; Viale, G.; et al. Association of p27 and Cyclin D1 Expression and Benefit from Adjuvant Trastuzumab Treatment in HER2-Positive Early Breast Cancer: A TransHERA Study. *Clin. Cancer Res.* **2018**, *24*, 3079–3086. [CrossRef]

40. Sinn, H.-P.; Schneeweiss, A.; Keller, M.; Schlombs, K.; Laible, M.; Seitz, J.; Lakis, S.; Veltrup, E.; Altevogt, P.; Eidt, S.; et al. Comparison of immunohistochemistry with PCR for assessment of ER, PR, and Ki-67 and prediction of pathological complete response in breast cancer. *BMC Cancer* **2017**, *17*, 124. [CrossRef]

8

Diagnostic and Prognostic Potential of Biomarkers CYFRA 21.1, ERCC1, p53, FGFR3 and TATI in Bladder Cancers

Milena Matuszczak and Maciej Salagierski *

Department of Urology, Collegium Medicum, University of Zielona Góra, 65-046 Zielona Góra, Poland;
matuszczakmilena@gmail.com
* Correspondence: m.salagierski@cm.uz.zgora.pl

Abstract: The high occurrence of bladder cancer and its tendency to recur in combination with a lifelong surveillance make the treatment of superficial bladder cancer one of the most expensive and time-consuming. Moreover, carcinoma in situ often leads to muscle invasion with an unfavorable prognosis. Currently, invasive methods including cystoscopy and cytology remain a gold standard. The aim of this study was to explore urine-based biomarkers to find the one with the best specificity and sensitivity, which would allow optimizing the treatment plan. In this review, we sum up the current knowledge about Cytokeratin fragments (CYFRA 21.1), Excision Repair Cross-Complementation 1 (ERCC1), Tumour Protein p53 (Tp53), Fibroblast Growth Factor Receptor 3 (FGFR3), Tumor-Associated Trypsin Inhibitor (TATI) and their potential applications in clinical practice.

Keywords: biomarkers; bladder cancer; tumor markers; prognosis

---

1. Introduction: Bladder Cancer Issues and Biomarkers

Bladder cancer is the most common urinary site of malignancy and the second most common reason of cancer deaths from the genitourinary tract after prostate cancer in the United States, with 81,400 new cases and 17,980 deaths in the year 2020 [1]. Globally there are about 430,000 new cases diagnosed each year [2].

Favorably, non-invasive lesions constitute approximately 75–80% of newly diagnosed urothelial bladder cancers (UBC). More than 50% of UBCs are caused by smoking. Other important factors include occupational exposure to aromatic amines and polycyclic hydrocarbons. Less evident is the impact of diet and environmental pollution. Increasing data indicate that genetic predisposition plays a role in UBC pathogenesis [2–4].

There are two major groups of patients with distinct prognosis and molecular features.

Carcinoma in situ (CIS) and tumors staged as Ta, T1 are grouped as non-muscle-invasive bladder cancers (NMIBC) [5]. NMIBC patients generally have a significant risk of recurrence and potential clinical course for progression [6] but their life expectancy is long and the cancer rarely progresses to muscle invasion. For NMIBC, the major problem is that after the initial transurethral resection of the bladder (TURB), they characteristically recur in 50–70% of cases, with only approximately 10–20% of cases progressing to muscle-invasive bladder cancer (MIBC) [7].

Muscle-invasive tumors very often metastasize and are usually diagnosed de novo, the prognosis is unfavorable and for decades there has been made no major innovation in therapy. Papillary non-invasive cancers (pTa) grow up from carcinoma in situ (CIS) of the urothelium (frequently TP53-mutated, a high-grade lesion) and often metastasize and evolve into muscle invasion [8]. Robertson et al. demonstrated that MIBC shows high overall mutation rates but fortunately most of them seem to be passenger variation without any functional meaning, or repeated genetic alterations including the *TP53, FGFR3, PIK3CA* and *RB1* genes' mutations [4,9].

Muscle-invasive bladder cancer (MIBC) is a high risk but potentially curable disease. Unfortunately, still nearly half of patients die from MIBC despite getting the appropriate treatment [10,11]. The major problem in the management of superficial bladder cancer is its tendency to recur. Lifelong surveillance with a relatively long-life expectancy (5-year survival rate > 90%) makes it the most expensive and time-consuming malignancy to treat.

In recent years, a great effort has been put in the search for new potential biomarkers such as protein 53 (p53), ERCC1, CYFRA 21.1, FGFR3 and TATI in the prognosis and prediction of bladder cancer. The *FGFR3* mutations could be a marker of low-grade and early stage tumors, while the changes in p53 appear better in detecting high-grade or advanced cancers.

2. Diagnostic and Prognostic Potential of Bladder Cancer Biomarkers

2.1. Cytokeratin Fragment 21.1 (CYFRA 21.1)

Cytokeratin fragments (CYFRA 21.1) is an ELISA-based assay that detects the concentration of a soluble fragment of cytokeratin 19 by using two monoclonal antibodies [12]. The studies have shown that the differentiation between liquid biopsies of healthy (non-cancer) individuals and BC patients may be done using this biomarker.

Authors [13] concluded that both serum and urine CYFRA 21.1 present decisive indexes for bladder cancer diagnosis. They made a systematic analysis which indicated the pooled sensitivities and specificities for the serum and urine CYFRA 21.1 were of 42%, 82%, 94% and 80%, respectively. The areas under the receiver operating characteristic curves (AUC) for the serum and urine CYFRA 21.1 were in sequence 0.88 and 0.87 (Table 1).

In an extensive meta-analysis of three case–control studies Kuang [14] confirmed that urinary or serum samples containing CYFRA21.1 can be used as diagnostic biomarkers and for the distinction between local and metastatic bladder cancer. In this meta-analysis, all healthy individuals had a lower CYFRA21.1 level than patients with bladder cancer. The locally invasive disease showed also lower CYFRA 21.1 levels than the subgroup with metastatic bladder cancer. Notwithstanding, between patients with bladder cancer stage I and stage II, and among the group of patients with local stage II and III were no significant differences in the CYFRA21.1 level. Therefore, CYFRA 21.1 cannot be useful in differentiating grades I–III of local bladder cancer but may be used as a diagnostic biomarker and to detect metastases.

Nisman [15] evaluated that for detecting transitional cell tumors that were grade 1 with CYFRA 21.1 measured in urine samples gave a three-times higher sensitivity compared with the sensitivity of cytology.

CYFRA 21.1 has a high sensitivity for identifying high-grade and CIS tumors and a greater accuracy for the detection of primary tumors than for the recurrence, but it cannot be used for an early detection of BC. The specificity of this test is between 73% and 86% and the sensitivity is between 70% and 90% [12,15,16].

Andreadis and colleagues [17] analyzed a group of 142 patients with invasive bladder cell carcinoma, including 56 patients with stage T1-4 N0 M0 and 86 with involved lymph nodes or distant metastases. The control group contained 33 healthy volunteers. Seven per cent of patients with the locally advanced disease and 66% of patients with the metastatic disease had an elevated level of this biomarker. CYFRA 21.1 may also be a useful tool in indicating the response to chemotherapy.

Importantly, Nisman and colleagues [15] showed that CYFRA 21.1 detected 100% of CIS, 92.8% of invasive bladder tumors (T2 or higher classification) and 91.9% of grade 3 tumors. The CYFRA 21.1 assay identified almost all tumors (with the exception of only one) that had a positive cytology. Moreover, the assay detected 65% of recurrent tumors and 71% of primary tumors that were omitted by cytopathology.

Unfortunately, CYFRA 21.1 is a false positive in the group of patients with urinary tract infections, stones, history of pelvic radiotherapy, urethral catheterization or BCG intravesical instillation within the three previous months. Even years following intravesical immunotherapy with the BCG level of urinary CYFRA 21.1 may be elevated.

Importantly, the abnormal serum level of CYFRA 21.1 [18] corresponds with a worse response.
In conclusion, Washino [19] observed that serum CYFRA 21.1 might be a marker of high-grade and advanced urothelial carcinoma. On the contrary, CEA and CA19-9 were not demonstrated as potential tumor markers.

The centrifugation step in the methodology is the very important one to improve the precision of this assay by removing cells' debris that contains a large amount of CYFRA 21.1, i.e., after this process, a significant decrease in the number of true positive and false positive results can be observed [20].

CYFRA 21.1 is considered as one of the best urinary markers for bladder cancer. Jeong and colleagues noticed that CYFRA 21.1 and NMP22 are the most effective at predicting bladder cancer [21]. However, there is a disadvantage being that the concentrations of both markers are strongly influenced by benign urological diseases, intravesical instillations and also a disappointing performance in low-stage bladder cancer.

Table 1. Predictive capacity of bladder cancer biomarkers.

Protein Name	Gene Symbol	Purpose	Diagnostic Value	Prognostic Value	FDA Approved	Method	Samples Used (No. Patients)	Predicitive Capacity	Reference
CYFRA 21.1	KRT19	Diagnostic and surveillance	Both serum and urine CYFRA 21.1 levels provide an effective index for the diagnosis of BC.	High risk of malignancy- significantly higher serum level of CYFRA 21.1 according to tumour stage ($p < 0.01$) and grade ($p < 0.05$). Patients with increased CYFRA 21.1 level had significantly worse disease-specific survival ($p < 0.0001$, log rank test) [19]. Moreover, patients with metastases had a higher CYFRA 21.1 level than those with locally invasive BC [14].	No	Meta-analysis performed using STATA 12.0 on the base of studies had published before 2 November 2014 in EMBASE, Web of Science and Medline databases. Quality of the studies was assessed by revised QUADAS tools, all of selected studies were English language publications and evaluate diagnostic accuracy of CYFRA 21.1 in patients with BC. Systematic review included 13 studies and 1,262 BC and 1,233 non-bladder cancer patients. 8 studies measured urine and 5 serum level of CYFRA 21.1. In serum detection of CYFRA 21.1 471 BC and 296 non- bladder cancer patients were analyzed. Urine CYFRA 21.1 studies included 538 BC and 678 non-bladder cancer patients.	Urine ($n = 538$ BC/678 control) Serum ($n = 471$ BC/296 control)	Sensitivity = 82% Specificity = 80% AUC = 0.87 Sensitivity = 42% Specificity = 94% AUC = 0.88	[12–14,19]
DNA EXCISION REPAIR PROTEIN ERCC-1	ERCC1	Diagnostic and surveillance	71.3% (308/432) of cases was ERCC1 positive. Ta = 3.2% T1 = 11.7% T2 = 21.4% T3 = 45.1% T4 = 18.5% CIS = 8.1% LG = 20.8% HG = 79.2%	ERCC positive tumour had significantly better disease-free survival (HR 0.7, $p = 0.028$) than ERCC1 negative tumours. ERCC1 positive tumours has significantly reduced risk of recurrences (HR 0.71, $p = 0.021$). The 5-year DFS and CSS were better for ERCC1 positive than negative, and were respectively 62% vs 49% and 70% vs 59%. However, there was no important outcomes of adjuvant cisplatin-based chemotherapy by ERCC1 status.	No	Study cohort had 432 patients and 308 of tumours expressed ERCC1. Staining was conducted using Abcam® mouse monoclonal antibody and expression of ERCC1was evaluated by 2 pathologists. Chi-square test was made to assessed differences between ERCC1 expression. All analyses were performed with STATA®, version 13.1. Primary tumour samples collected at RC, cells were lysed and total RNA was extracted with Qiagen® kit. ERCC1 mRNA expression was measured by RNA sequencing and confirmed by qPCR using TaqMan® gene expression assays.	UCB cell lines in vitro ($n = 432$)	No data	[22]
TUMOR SUPPRESSOR P53	TP53 gene	Diagnostic (as a complementary tool) and surveillance	54% (56/103) of cases had TP53 mutations. Ta = 40% T1 = 52% T2 = 80% CIS = 55% LG = 34% HG = 62%	High risk of malignancy-significant difference of TP53 mutations according to tumour stage ($p = 0.005$) and to cellular grade ($p < 0.001$).	No	Sample collection of urine and tumours from 103 patients. Extraction of mRNA was made by Micro mRNA Purification Kit. Then Verso Kit® were used to reverse transcription, amplification was performed by PCR PrimeStar®. FASAY assay was used to detect TP53 mutations in tumour tissues and urinary cells. Statistical test was performed using SPSS software®, version 17.	Primary bladder tumours and associated urine ($n = 103$)	Sensitivity = 34% Specificity = 87% PPV = 0.76 NPV = 0.53	[23]

Table 1. *Cont.*

Protein Name	Gene Symbol	Purpose	Diagnostic Value	Prognostic Value	FDA Approved	Method	Samples Used (No. Patients)	Predicitive Capacity	Reference
FIBROBLAST GROWTH FACTOR RECEPTOR 3	FGFR3 gene	Diagnostic (as a complementary tool) and surveillance	36% (37/103) of cases had FGFR3 mutations. Ta = 55% T1 = 29% T2 = 19% CIS = 10% LG = 62% HG = 26%	Low risk of malignancy-negative association of FGFR3 mutations based on tumour stage (p = 0.002) and cellular grade (p < 0.001) [23]. Low level of FGFR3 expression is an independent predictor of cancer progression and is associated with HG tumours [24].	No*	Sample collection of urine and tumours from 103 patients. Extraction of genomic DNA was performed by QIAamp Viral RNA® Mini kit. Multiplex PCR Kit were used to amplification. Snapshot® kit was used to detect FGFR3 eight most frequent mutations hotspots in tumour tissues and urinary cells (two independent analysis were carried out). Statistical test was performed using SPSS software®, version 17.	Primary bladder tumours and associated urine (n = 103)	Sensitivity = 43% Specificity = 98% PPV = 0.94 NPV = 0.76	[23]
								Sensitivity = 97.6% Specificity = 84.8% AUC = 0.96 NPV = 0.996 (1)	[25]
TUMOR-ASSOCIATED TRYPSIN INHIBITOR	SPINK1 gene	Diagnostic and surveillance	49.1% (54/110) of cases had TATI expression. Stage <T2 = 66.7% Stage ≥T2 = 44.9% LG = 76.2% HG = 44.9%	Low risk of malignancy- negative association of TATI expression was positively correlated based on tumour stage (p = 0.048) and poor differentiation (p = 0.013). Significant differences were observed between TATI-positive and negative specimens in PFS and OS (Log-rank test, p = 0.003, 0.003). In a group of patients with BC undergoing RC TATI expression was independent protective factor. Moreover, TATI expression could enhance prognostic value of p53.	No	Study cohort had 110 patients and 54 of tumours, undergone RC, expressed TATI. Staining was conducted using Abcam® anti-TATI monoclonal antibody and expression of TATI was evaluated by 2 pathologists. Proportion of immune-positive cells and their staining intensity was scored in two scales and used to evaluation of TATI expression. All analyses were performed with SPSS software, version 21.	Tissue microarrays from UCB (n = 110)	No data	[26]
						Study cohort consisted of 160 patients, divided into 3 groups. Group 1 had 80 primary HG UBC. Group 2 of 40 healthy volunteers and group 3 of 40 benign UBC. TATI was measured using a radioimmunoassay according to the manufacturer's instructions (Orion Diagnostica). Analyses were performer with STATA®, statistical software, version 6.0	Urine (n = 160)	Sensitivity = 85.7% Specificity = 77.5%	[27]

(1) Using a logistic regression analysis with a model consisting of the 3 markers' methylation values, FGFR3 status, age and known smoker status at the diagnosis time. * It is available THERASCREEN® FGFR RGQ RT-PCR KIT. Abbreviations: HR—Hazard Ratio, n—number of patients participating in study, p—calculated probability, CIS—carcinoma in situ, HG—high grade, LG—low grade, FASAY—Functional Analysis of Separated Allele in Yeast, ELISA—enzyme-linked immunosorbent assay, IHC—immunohistochemistry, RC—radical cystectomy, BC—bladder cancer, CCS—cancer specific survival, DFS—disease-free survival, UCB—urothelial carcinoma of bladder, qPCR—quantitative polymerase chain reaction, PPV—positive predictive value, NPV—negative predictive value.

2.2. Excision Repair Cross-Complementation 1 (ERCC1)

The nucleotide excision repair (NER) pathway is important for the protection of genomic stability and for the removal of platinum-induced DNA adducts and cisplatin resistance [28,29]. The key molecules in this pathway belong to the excision repair cross-complementing group 1 (ERCC1) [30].

The ERCC1 role is detecting, repairing and rate-limiting the interstrand cross-links in DNA [31]. Therefore, this enzyme may be representative for the crucial DNA damage repair ability of the cell [32,33]. In a group of patients treated with a surgical resection, ERCC1 as the DNA repair protein may also be engaged in weakening the malignancy of tumors by reducing the amount of mutations. Moreover, genetic testing of ERCC1 expression levels could personalize the chemotherapy by selecting the patients who would benefit from platinum-based chemotherapy. A variety of tumors, including bladder tumors, show that the ERCC1 level is strongly associated with cisplatin resistance [34].

One of the first reports in the literature presenting the impact of ERCC1 expression on the survival of oncologically treated patients was the study of George R. Simon. In 2005, Simon's analysis included 51 patients who were operated on for non-small cell lung cancer and determined their ERCC1 expression. The median survival in the ERCC1 positive expression group was found to be significantly longer—94.9 months compared with 35.5 months in the negative ERCC1 group. The conclusions were that the ERCC1 expression might be an independent prognostic factor for survival in lung cancer [32].

In 2006, Olaussen's work on a large group of patients was published, which included the results of a study of 761 patients after radical lung cancer surgery. The goal was to identify a group of patients who might take an advantage from adjuvant treatment. The study showed that the benefit of adjuvant chemotherapy concerned the patients with a negative ERCC1 expression. An interesting finding was that in the group that did not receive chemotherapy but was only treated surgically, patients with a positive ERCC1 expression had a longer survival compared with those with a negative ERCC1 expression [31].

In advanced non-small cell lung cancer, the ERCC1 expression has a significant prognostic value and its high level is associated with a longer survival in patients who do not receive chemotherapy after a complete resection [31,32]. Piljić et al. indicated that the ERCC1 expression in all stages of lung carcinoma has a great value in monitoring patients receiving chemotherapy based on platinum [35]. Li et al. indicated that in a group of patients with advanced non-small cell lung cancer, ERCC1-negative had better progression-free survival (PFS) ($p = 0.016$) and overall survival (OS) ($p = 0.030$) in comparison with positive patients [36].

The value of ERCC1 has also been confirmed in other cancers. ERCC1 is one of the most frequent in 84% or even more of colon cancers, and reductions of a DNA repair gene has been observed [37,38]. In 40% of the crypts within 10 cm on each side of colonic adenocarcinomas, ERCC1 was found to be deficient [37]. The literature data presented above show a significant relationship between the ERCC1 expression and survival in different types of cancer.

In 2012, Sun [39] analyzed 93 patients with BC who underwent radical cystectomy and they demonstrated that ERCC1 can be used as a prognostic and predictive biomarker in this group. An ERCC1-positive expression was found in 58% of patients, and the study group was divided into those who received additional adjuvant chemotherapy and those without chemotherapy. It was found that patients after radical cystectomy without adjuvant chemotherapy with a high ERCC1 expression have a significantly longer five-year survival than those with a low expression, 84% to 49%, respectively. It has also been reported that ERCC1-negative patients potentially may benefit from adjuvant chemotherapy.

Klatte and colleagues [22] presented the work assessing ERCC1 as a prognostic and predictive biomarker of bladder cancer after cystectomy. In a group of 432 patients, a positive expression was found in 71% of patients. Patients with an ERCC1-positive expression had a significantly better five-year disease-free survival (DFS) than those with an ERCC1-negative expression, 62% to 49%, and cancer-specific survival (CSS), 70% to 59%, respectively. In the ERCC1-positive group, the risk of bladder cancer (BC) recurrence and death due to BC was 30% lower. Patients undergoing radical cystectomy with an ERCC1-positive expression had better survival values than those with a negative expression. Therefore, ERCC1 may be an independent prognostic marker for bladder cancer.

Similar conclusions were made in Hemdan's report. They evaluated a group of 244 patients who underwent radical cystectomy or neoadjuvant chemotherapy and radical cystectomy. Negative ERCC1 correlated with a worse overall survival in the group with only surgical treatment. It was noted that neoadjuvant chemotherapy would benefit mainly patients with an ERCC1-negative expression, while for those who were ERCC1-positive, the influence was minimal [40].

Another meta-analysis was published by Urun [41], performed on 1425 patients from 13 studies, and patients with an ERCC1-positive expression constituted 24–76% of the examined populations. The role of ERCC1 as a prognostic factor of survival was assessed in patients with advanced bladder cancer treated with platinum-based chemotherapy. The conclusions were that a positive ERCC1 expression is not significantly related to overall survival, but has a significant impact on worse progression-free survival, and may be an indicator of worse survival in patients with advanced bladder cancer, but large prospective studies are needed to consider ERCC1 as a prognostic marker in patients with advanced bladder cancer.

Sakano [42] suggested that, in the group of patients with bladder cancer undergoing a combined trimodality approach, the disease-specific survival might be predicted by the expression of ERCC1 and XRCC1. A positive expression of these molecules was connected with better disease-specific survival rates but further research is needed to confirm these results.

Analyzing the previous studies, gives controversial information about predicting the prognostic role of ERCC1 in the treatment of advanced bladder cancer. In 2018, Eldehna [34] conducted a descriptive study on 80 patients with muscle-invasive bladder cancer (stages T2–T4a) who received platinum-based chemotherapy. The results of their research showed a significant relationship between a platinum-based treatment response and the ERCC1 expression in bladder cancer tissue samples ($p = 0.013$). It was an indicative association between a negative immuno-expression and more favorable outcome but no difference between the ERCC1 expression and mean overall survival or progression-free survival in different immune-expression levels in patients was apparent. Therefore, ERCC1 may be a potential predictive but not prognostic marker and for this reason, genetic testing could personalize chemotherapy by selecting the patients who would benefit from a platinum-based treatment in bladder cancer.

In summary, ERCC1-positive tumors were associated with better prognosis in cases without chemotherapies. However, in cases with chemotherapies, ERCC1-negative tumors were associated with a better outcome.

The most possible explanation for the above scenario seems related to the function of this enzyme, which appears crucial in the DNA damage repair ability of the cell. The above DNA repair, related to the ERCC1 activity, is, however, non-beneficial for patients treated with chemotherapy, potentially leading to an "antichemotherapeutic" activity.

2.3. Tumour Protein p53 (TP53)

The common oncosuppressor gene mutated in all human cancers and the most frequently mutated gene in MIBC is the tumor protein p53 (*TP53*) [43]. Genomic integrity and stability are maintained by *TP53* via triggering a cell-cycle arrest, apoptosis, autophagy and DNA repair. Mutant p53 proteins silence the autophagy related gene (ATG) which affects the autophagic flow, and therefore suppresses regulation to the autophagic vesicles formation and their fusion with lysosomes [44]. Additionally, p53 preferentially binds to the AMPKα subunit and inhibits the AMPK activation. Mutp53s become oncogenic via the activation of AMPK [45].

Bladder carcinogenesis is closely associated with tumor suppressor dysfunction and the inactivation of *TP53* [46]. Therefore, p53 has been studied as a marker of urothelial cell carcinoma recurrence and progression.

Cheap and simple methods to detect the abnormal function of p53 is immunohistochemistry staining (IHC). The short half-life of wild-type p53 prevents its intra-nuclear accumulation [47].

Increased p53 accumulation in the cell nucleus is a result of *TP53* mutations.

Immunohistochemical patterns of *TP53* mutations are strongly associated with the progression of urothelial cell carcinoma. Plenty of data illustrate that from non-missense mutations (i.e., nonsense, insertion and deletion) to wild-type *TP53*, the expression of p53's IHC increases. That promotes the grow up of an invasive phenotype of bladder cancer [48]. The high expression of p53 has been associated with features of tumor aggressiveness and correlated with poor oncological outcomes [43,49]. Therefore, this protein level was higher in more advanced bladder cancer [50,51]. Plenty of studies have indicated that p53 can be useful to assess the level of progress and to prognose urothelial cell carcinoma [49,51].

However, Ciccasese and colleagues [52] published a study with a contradictory opinion. In their opinion, the single p53 marker is not good enough as a prognostic marker of MIBC.

Moreover, the most aggressive T1 high-grade cancers appear to be also associated with the expression of this protein. The progression from T1 NMIBC to T1HG can be predicted by a p53 overexpression [53].

Authors [51] collected data from 70 patients and showed that 16% of patients with low-grade and 91% of patients with high-grade lesions were p53-positive. There was 33% positivity in Tis, 55% in T1, 72% in T2 and 100% in T3a and T3b. These results indicated a strong intensification of p53 staining—94.6% of high-grade and 5.4% of low-grade tumors. Moreover, the p53 accumulation in the nucleus, in a group treated with radical cystectomy and in other MIBCs, has a prognostic value [54].

Another study showed that an aggressive tumor phenotype is strongly associated with the overexpression of p53 [43]. MIBC and CIS correlated with a high level of *TP53* deletion and mutation [55]. According to the TCGA cohort data [4], 89% of MIBCs have an inactivated TP53 cell-cycle pathway, with *TP53* mutations in 48%. Bladder epithelial cells become malignant by the TP53/RB1 pathway or the FGFR3/RAS pathway [55].

2.4. Fibroblast Growth Factor Receptor 3 (FGFR3)

Fibroblast growth factor receptor 3 (FGFR3) alternations are associated with urothelial cell carcinoma pathogenesis [56,57]. FGFR3 is activated by the mutation or overexpression in many bladder tumors at any stage, but is predominantly active in low-grade NMIBCs [58,59]. Higher levels of FGFR3 expression were observed in low-grade, non-invasive tumors and recurrent non-invasive tumors than in invasive and non-invasive high-grade carcinoma [57].

This marker is associated with a lower chance of progression to a muscle-invasive disease and it is like a hallmark of the low-grade pathway. FGFR3 alternations occur mainly in non-invasive tumors [59,60], specifically in the luminal-papillary subtype (35%), which has the best overall survival and is characterized by a papillary morphology [59,61]. Moreover, many studies indicated that *FGFR3* mutation and the risk of progression are an inverse interaction. Therefore, patients with MIBC and the *FGFR3* mutation have better survival rates [62]. Another study suggests that also the progression in pT1 tumors is in negative correlation with the *FGFR3* mutation [63]. Many studies confirm that *FGFR3* mutations correlate with an overall benign effect [59,63,64]. Moreover, in the risk stratification, surveillance and diagnosis of low- or high-risk NMIBC patients, *FGFR3* mutations combined with the promoter hyper-methylation of *HS3ST2*, *SEPTIN9* and *SLIT2* have shown 97.6% sensitivity and 84.8% specificity (Table 1) [25]. The presence of the *FGFR3* mutation in urine is observed not only in low-grade tumors but it also seems to be associated with future recurrence [65,66].

FGFR3 is involved in tumorigenesis in ~40% of invasive bladder cancer and in the majority (~80%) of low-grade non-invasive (stage Ta) bladder cancers [59]. Tomlinson et al. observed an FGFR3 overexpression in nearly 40% of MIBC, whereas mutations occurred in 21% of MIBC [67]. Sung [56] observed that an FGFR3 overexpression results in the worst overall survival and disease-free survival in a group of patients with adjuvant chemotherapy. In a group without this treatment, no prognostic significance was observed.

High levels of FGFR3- and PIK3CA-mutated DNA in urine can be useful in predicting later metastasis and progression in NMIBC [68]. Choi et al. indicated that *FGFR3* mutations are characteristic for the luminal type of MIBC [69]. In conclusion, FGFR3 may be an important therapeutic target in both non-invasive and invasive BC [58,59].

In the results of their research, Beukers [60] confirmed that mutations in *FGFR3* were more often observed in low-grade tumors and the papillary urothelial neoplasm of low malignant potential (PUNLMP) + G1 (61.9%) than in high-grade tumors G2 + G3, at 17.2%. It was also observed that *FGFR3* mutations were more frequent in non-invasive tumors' Tis and Ta stages, at 53.4%, than in the invasive stages of T1 and T2, at 12.5%. Mutations correlated with a better survival rate and occurred in a higher level in non-invasive than in advanced diseases, and these values for TaG1, TaG2, TaG3 + T1 and T2 were 67.3%, 43.3%, 20.3% and 6.3% respectively. It was also noticed, but with no statistically significant correlation, that *FGFR3* mutations increase the possibility of disease recurrence [70]. Hosen et al. showed that *FGFR3* mutations have no significant influence on patient survival and that in the Ta, T1, TaG1 and TaG2 diseases, it did not significantly predict the recurrence rate [70].

Knowles et al. also demonstrated that the *FGFR3/HRAS* mutation was often present in the development of urothelial hyperplasia, which can progress to non-invasive papillary tumors with high recurrence rates via the FGFR3/RAS pathway [8].

Van Rhijn [63] conducted a study on a group of 132 patients with primary pT1 bladder cancer. The diagnosis was confirmed after a uropathologist review of the slides. *FGFR3* mutations were identified by a SNaPshot® analysis in 37 of 132 pT1 bladder cancer cases (28%) and an altered P53 expression was determined by standard immunohistochemistry in 71 of them (54%). Both molecular alternations were observed in 8% of patients. In predicting progression, carcinoma in situ and the status of the *FGFR3* mutation were significant but *TP53* was not. It was also mentioned that the presence of *FGFR3* mutations helps to identify patients who have a better disease prognosis because the *FGFR3* mutation occurs with lower grade and altered *TP53* with high-grade pT1 bladder cancer.

Hernández and colleagues [64] analyzed 772 samples from patients with bladder tumors reviewed by expert pathologists. Their results indicated that *FGFR3* mutations were more frequently observed in neoplasms with low malignant potential, at 77%, and in tumors TaG1, at 61%, and TaG2, at 58%, than in tumors TaG3, at 34%, and T1G3, at 17%. They also confirm the association between superficial tumors and a high presence of recurrence. Nevertheless, a significant increase risk was observed only in the group of patients with TaG1 tumors. In this study, another positive correlation of good prognosis and occupancy of FGFR3 was confirmed.

Kompier [71] performed a study on 118 patients with primary and recurrent NMI-BC. They analyzed the *FGFR3* mutation status in the disease process. The analyzed group had 2133 cystoscopies done within the median follow-up of 8.8 years and 414 tumor recurrences developed in 80 patients. *FGFR3* mutations were equally distributed in the recurrences and the primary tumors (63%). Different tumors may have a variety of *FGFR3* mutations types. Mutant or wild-type primary tumors had a similar risk of recurrence but in 81% of recurrences, a mutation was found. In this group, recurrences developed after 10 years and, in comparison with the wild-type primary tumor, occurred in a lower grade and stage.

Therefore, a follow-up surveillance based on the presence of the *FGFR3* mutation analysis with the reduction in the number of cystoscopies may be considered [71].

In another study, Kompier and colleagues [72] confirmed the correlations between a low risk of progression and better disease-specific survival in the primary mutant FGFR3 tumor and worse prognosis in the group of patients with an overexpression of p53.

Williams et al. found that in the selection of patients for the FGFR-targeted therapy, the existence of a fusion protein, which indicates other classes of mutations in a group with a high FGFR3 expression, may be helpful [58].

The study [73] shows that *FGFR3* mutations may influence tumorigenesis by regulating an acute inflammatory response which via the immune cells destroys the tumor cells. Therefore, there may be potential treatment strategy for the early stage of FGFR3-mutated or overexpressed BC based on the synchronal inhibition of FGFR3 and the immune modulators.

Noel [23] conducted a pilot study to assess the *TP53* and *FGFR3* mutations in urine and tumoral tissues samples that had been collected from 103 BC patients. Mutations in *TP53* were detected in 54% of the 103 bladder tumors and the distribution increased with the cellular grade ($p < 0.001$). The *TP53* mutation presented 34% of low- grade (LG) and 62% of high- grade (HG) tumors. The potential prognostic value of *TP53* may indicate a significant difference in the tumor stage ($p = 0.005$). The specificity was 87%, with the positive predictive value (PPV) 76% and with the negative predictive value (NPV) 53%. However, the sensitivity in the urine test was only 34% (Table 1).

In 36% of analyzed tumors, *FRFG3* mutations were identified and their distribution decreased with the cellular grade ($p < 0.001$). They occurred in 62% of LG tumors versus 26% in HG. A negative correlation was also between the *FGFR3* mutations and tumor stage ($p = 0.002$). All predictive capacities were better for the *FGFR3* than for the *TP53* mutations measured in this study, the sensitivity was 43% and the specificity was 98%, with the PPV 94% and the NPV 76% (Table 1) [23].

The results showed that TP53/FGFR3 could be useful as a complementary tool in diagnosis but could not replace urine cytology. The tumor stage and grade are strongly correlated with the *FGFR3* and *TP53* mutations, which are in "mirror distribution" [23].

Kang [24] enrolled 120 patients with primary pT1 BC and examined in this subgroup the utility of expression levels and mutation status of *FGFR3* as a prognostic marker. In this study, 40% of patients had *FGFR3* mutations and those patients also had significantly higher levels of the FGFR3 expression compared with the FGFR3 wild-type BC ($p < 0.001$). The mutation status was not associated with cancer progression, but a low level of FGFR3 correlated with cancer progression and HG tumors ($p = 0.001$ and $p = 0.006$). Therefore, the FGFR3 expression level was, in the multivariate analysis, identified as an independent predictor of cancer progression (Table 1). Significant was also the correlation between the *FGFR3* mutation and a low tumor grade. In tumor recurrence, both the *FGFR3* mutation status and mRNA expression level revealed no significant differences ($p = 0.264$ and $p = 0.856$, respectively).

In conclusion, FGFR3 may be used as a urine-based assay in the detection of primary tumors, recurrences, for prognosis and targeted therapies.

2.5. Tumor-Associated Trypsin Inhibitor (TATI)

TATI is a peptide produced at lower concentrations in many healthy tissues, especially in the gastrointestinal and urogenital tracts but also in the gall bladder, kidney and breast.

It occurs in high concentrations by several tumors such as gynecologic, gastrointestinal, urologic, lung, breast, head and neck cancers [74–79]. An increased level of TATI is also observed in renal failure and in dialysis patients because this peptide is cleared from the circulation by renal excretion. Therefore, a low glomerular filtration rate correlates with an increase in TATI [80].

TATI is connected with tumor aggression because it appears in the co-expression with tumor-associated trypsin, which participates in moderating tumor-associated protease cascades [81].

TATI is produced at high concentrations by mucinous ovarian tumors, and was initially isolated from the urine of a patient with ovarian cancer. The most useful clinical application of this peptide is observed in the detection of ovarian tumors: benign and malignant [82].

TATI occurs in a high level also in other benign and malignant diseases. Pancreatitis and strong acute phase reactions (when serum CRP is clearly increased (>90 mg/L)) such as severe injury or inflammatory diseases trigger a TATI expression. This fact is a limiting factor of the use of TATI as a tumor marker but it does not invalidate this peptide [83]. In cancers, an increased TATI concentration is associated not only with tumor production but also acute phase reactions caused by tissue destruction during cancer invasion [81].

Serum values of TATI have also been used in patients with muscle-invasive and metastatic transitional cell carcinoma, to monitor the response to therapy. In 1996, Pectasides [74] suggested that TATI might be potentially useful in monitoring the efficacy of treatment in transitional cell carcinoma of the bladder. Significantly modified values of TATI were observed in metastatic diseases, in patients with complete or partial remission and non-responders. An important increase in TATI in T2-T4-N0M0 tumors were in the non-responders.

Kelloniemi et al. showed that for the identification group of patients with adverse prognosis in transitional cell carcinoma serum, TATI might be an independent prognostic factor [84].

Shariat [85] indicated that TATI is more specific than NMP22 for the detection of bladder transitional cell carcinoma (TCC). They showed also that higher levels of TATI were in TCC patients and in more invasive stages.

In 2006, Hotakainen [86] reported that a TATI expression was observed in all non-invasive tumors and benign tissues, but the expression was lower in the muscle-invasive tumors. Therefore, they concluded that the TATI expression decreases with the rising stage and grade of the tumor in bladder cancer. Therefore, as for TATI, Shariat [85] showed that higher levels of TATI were associated with more invasive TCC but Hotakainen [86] revealed that the TATI expression decreases with the rising stage. The discrepancy between the results of the studies is most probably related to the different populations of bladder cancer patients. The study by Shariat [85], comprised of 153 consecutive patients who had a history of previous, histologically confirmed bladder cancer, without evidence of muscle invasion (stages Ta, T1 and/or CIS). In the Hotakainen ($n = 28$) group, the individuals were affected with both non-invasive and invasive BC.

Gkialas [27] showed that TATI was significantly more sensitive in stage Ta (80%) than was CYFRA 21-1 (32%), UBC (12%) and cytology (20%). TATI was different also between stages and was more sensitive compared with other tumor markers for stage T1.

Patschan and colleagues [87] confirmed that the TATI level shows a positive correlation with low-stage tumors and the favorable differentiation of bladder cancer. They also showed in univariate analyses, that a decreased level of TATI was associated with high recurrences and cancer-specific mortality.

Liu [26] made a similar conclusion that a decrease in the TATI expression correlated with a more advanced disease. Moreover, in the progression of bladder cancer, the prognostic value of a p53 overexpression can be enhanced by TATI.

Bladder cancer management is one of the most complex and expensive in uro-oncology. An ideal biomarker of the future should be potentially able to detect the disease before its clinical manifestation. The BC mortality rate is another major reason to obtain a similar screening method to that available in other cancers, i.e., prostate and colon.

Currently, flexible cystoscopy remains a mainstay in BC diagnosis and it appears unlikely that available biomarkers would quickly rule out this standard approach in clinical practice. On the other hand, developing markers showing a correlation with cancer aggressiveness and being able to distinguish between aggressive and non-aggressive tumors appears of utmost clinical importance. Hopefully, one of the discussed markers might become helpful in patients' selection for an appropriate treatment plan and personalized cancer medicine. The prospective studies on a larger group of individuals are still needed in order to obtain additional prognostic information that will improve results, reduce adverse effects and in future allow us to individualize bladder cancer treatments.

Author Contributions: All authors made substantial contributions to this work; acquisition and interpretation of data by online search, M.S., M.M.; draft and supervision of the work, M.S.; revision of the work, M.S. All authors have approved the final version and agree to be personally accountable for the author's own contributions.

Abbreviations

AUC	Area under the curve
BC	Bladder cancer
BCG	Bacille Calmette–Guérin
CIS	Carcinoma in situ
CK	Cytokeratin
CSS	Cancer-specific survival
CYFRA 21.1	Cytokeratin fragment 21.1
DFS	Disease-free survival
ERCC1	Excision repair cross-complementing group 1
HG	High grade
IHC	Immunohistochemistry staining
LG	Low grade
MIBC	Muscle-invasive bladder cancer
NMIBC	Non-muscle invasive bladder cancer
NPV	Negative predictive value
OS	Overall survival
PFS	Progression-free survival
PPV	Positive predictive value
PUNLMP	Papillary urothelial neoplasm of low malignant potential
TURBT	Transurethral resection of bladder tumor
UBC	Urothelial bladder cancer
UC	Urothelial carcinoma

References

1. Siegel, R.L.; Miller, K.D.; Jemal, A. Cancer statistics, 2020. *CA A Cancer J. Clin.* **2020**, *70*, 7–30. [CrossRef]
2. Antoni, S.; Ferlay, J.; Soerjomataram, I.; Znaor, A.; Jemal, A.; Bray, F. Bladder cancer incidence and mortality: A global overview and recent trends. *Eur. Urol.* **2017**, *71*, 96–108. [CrossRef] [PubMed]
3. Sanli, O.; Dobruch, J.; Knowles, M.A.; Burger, M.; Alemozaffar, M.; Nielsen, M.E.; Lotan, Y. Bladder cancer. *Nat. Rev. Dis. Primers* **2017**, *3*, 1–19. [CrossRef] [PubMed]
4. Robertson, A.G.; Kim, J.; Al-Ahmadie, H.; Bellmunt, J.; Guo, G.; Cherniack, A.D.; Hinoue, T.; Laird, P.W.; Hoadley, K.A.; Akbani, R.; et al. Comprehensive molecular characterization of muscle-invasive bladder cancer. *Cell* **2017**, *171*, 540–556. [CrossRef] [PubMed]
5. Humphrey, P.A.; Moch, H.; Cubilla, A.L.; Ulbright, T.M.; Reuter, V.E. The 2016 WHO classification of tumours of the urinary system and male genital organs—Part B: Prostate and bladder tumours. *Eur. Urol.* **2016**, *70*, 106–119. [CrossRef]
6. Czerniak, B.; Dinney, C.; McConkey, D. Origins of bladder cancer. *Annu. Rev. Pathol. Mech. Dis.* **2016**, *11*, 149–174. [CrossRef]
7. Babjuk, M.; Burger, M.; Zigeuner, R.; Shariat, S.F.; van Rhijn, B.W.G.; Compérat, E.; Sylvester, R.J.; Kaasinen, E.; Böhle, A.; Redorta, J.P.; et al. EAU Guidelines on Non–Muscle-invasive urothelial carcinoma of the bladder: Update 2013. *Eur. Urol.* **2013**, *64*, 639–653. [CrossRef]
8. Knowles, M.A.; Hurst, C.D. Molecular biology of bladder cancer: New insights into pathogenesis and clinical diversity. *Nat. Rev. Cancer* **2014**, *15*, 25–41. [CrossRef]
9. Inamura, K. Bladder cancer: New insights into its molecular pathology. *Cancers* **2018**, *10*, 100. [CrossRef]
10. Burger, M.; Catto, J.W.F.; Dalbagni, G.; Grossman, H.B.; Herr, H.; Karakiewicz, P.; Kassouf, W.; Kiemeney, L.A.; Vecchia, C.L.; Shariat, S.; et al. Epidemiology and risk factors of urothelial bladder cancer. *Eur. Urol.* **2013**, *63*, 234–241. [CrossRef]
11. Woldu, S.L.; Bagrodia, A.; Lotan, Y. Guideline of guidelines: Non-muscle-invasive bladder cancer. *BJU Int.* **2017**, *119*, 371–380. [CrossRef] [PubMed]
12. Huang, Y.-L.; Chen, J.; Yan, W.; Zang, D.; Qin, Q.; Deng, A.-M. Diagnostic accuracy of cytokeratin-19 fragment (CYFRA 21–1) for bladder cancer: a systematic review and meta-analysis. *Tumor Biol.* **2015**, *36*, 3137–3145. [CrossRef] [PubMed]

13. Guo, X.-G.; Long, J.-J. Cytokeratin-19 fragment in the diagnosis of bladder carcinoma. *Tumor Biol.* **2016**, *37*, 14329–14330. [CrossRef] [PubMed]

14. Kuang, L.I.; Song, W.J.; Qing, H.M.; Yan, S.; Song, F.L. CYFRA21-1 levels could be a biomarker for bladder cancer: A meta-analysis. *Genet. Mol. Res.* **2015**, *14*, 3921–3931. [CrossRef]

15. Nisman, B.; Barak, V.; Shapiro, A.; Golijanin, D.; Peretz, T.; Pode, D. Evaluation of urine CYFRA 21-1 for the detection of primary and recurrent bladder carcinoma. *Cancer* **2002**, *94*, 2914–2922. [CrossRef]

16. D'Costa, J.J.; Goldsmith, J.C.; Wilson, J.S.; Bryan, R.T.; Ward, D.G. A systematic review of the diagnostic and prognostic value of urinary protein biomarkers in urothelial bladder cancer. *Bladder Cancer* **2016**, *2*, 301–317. [CrossRef]

17. Andreadis, C.; Touloupidis, S.; Galaktidou, G.; Kortsaris, A.H.; Boutis, A.; Mouratidou, D. Serum CYFRA 21–1 in patients with invasive bladder cancer and its relevance as a tumor marker during chemotherapy. *J. Urol.* **2005**, *174*, 1771–1776. [CrossRef]

18. Nisman, B.; Yutkin, V.; Peretz, T.; Shapiro, A.; Barak, V.; Pode, D. The follow-up of patients with non-muscle-invasive bladder cancer by urine cytology, abdominal ultrasound and urine CYFRA 21-1: A pilot study. *Anticancer Res.* **2009**, *29*, 4281–4285.

19. Washino, S.; Hirai, M.; Matsuzaki, A.; Kobayashi, Y. Clinical usefulness of CEA, CA19-9, and CYFRA 21-1 as tumor markers for urothelial bladder carcinoma. *Urol. Int.* **2011**, *87*, 420–428. [CrossRef]

20. Dittadi, R.; Barioli, P.; Gion, M.; Mione, R.; Barichello, M.; Capitanio, G.; Cocco, G.; Cazzolato, G.; De Biasi, F.; Praturlon, S.; et al. Standardization of assay for cytokeratin-related tumor marker CYFRA21.1 in urine samples. *Clin. Chem.* **1996**, *42*, 1634–1638. [CrossRef]

21. Jeong, S.; Park, Y.; Cho, Y.; Kim, Y.R.; Kim, H.-S. Diagnostic values of urine CYFRA21-1, NMP22, UBC, and FDP for the detection of bladder cancer. *Clin. Chim. Acta* **2012**, *414*, 93–100. [CrossRef] [PubMed]

22. Klatte, T.; Seitz, C.; Rink, M.; Rouprêt, M.; Xylinas, E.; Karakiewicz, P.; Susani, M.; Shariat, S.F. ERCC1 as a prognostic and predictive biomarker for urothelial carcinoma of the bladder following radical cystectomy. *J. Urol.* **2015**, *194*, 1456–1462. [CrossRef] [PubMed]

23. Noel, N.; Couteau, J.; Maillet, G.; Gobet, F.; D'Aloisio, F.; Minier, C.; Pfister, C. TP53 and FGFR3 Gene mutation assessment in urine: Pilot study for bladder cancer diagnosis. *Anticancer Res.* **2015**, *35*, 4915–4921. [PubMed]

24. Kang, H.W.; Kim, Y.-H.; Jeong, P.; Park, C.; Kim, W.T.; Ryu, D.H.; Cha, E.-J.; Ha, Y.-S.; Kim, T.-H.; Kwon, T.G.; et al. Expression levels of FGFR3 as a prognostic marker for the progression of primary pT1 bladder cancer and its association with mutation status. *Oncol. Lett.* **2017**, *14*, 3817–3824. [CrossRef] [PubMed]

25. Roperch, J.-P.; Grandchamp, B.; Desgrandchamps, F.; Mongiat-Artus, P.; Ravery, V.; Ouzaid, I.; Roupret, M.; Phe, V.; Ciofu, C.; Tubach, F.; et al. Promoter hypermethylation of HS3ST2, SEPTIN9 and SLIT2 combined with FGFR3 mutations as a sensitive/specific urinary assay for diagnosis and surveillance in patients with low or high-risk non-muscle-invasive bladder cancer. *BMC Cancer* **2016**, *16*, 704. [CrossRef]

26. Liu, A.; Xue, Y.; Liu, F.; Tan, H.; Xiong, Q.; Zeng, S.; Zhang, Z.; Gao, X.; Sun, Y.; Xu, C. Prognostic value of the combined expression of tumor-associated trypsin inhibitor (TATI) and p53 in patients with bladder cancer undergoing radical cystectomy. *Cancer Biomark.* **2019**, *26*, 281–289. [CrossRef]

27. Gkialas, I.; Papadopoulos, G.; Iordanidou, L.; Stathouros, G.; Tzavara, C.; Gregorakis, A.; Lykourinas, M. Evaluation of urine tumor-associated trypsin inhibitor, CYFRA 21-1, and urinary bladder cancer antigen for detection of high-grade bladder Carcinoma. *Urology* **2008**, *72*, 1159–1163. [CrossRef]

28. Rabik, C.A.; Dolan, M.E. Molecular mechanisms of resistance and toxicity associated with platinating agents. *Cancer Treat. Rev.* **2007**, *33*, 9–23. [CrossRef]

29. Martin, L.P.; Hamilton, T.C.; Schilder, R.J. Platinum resistance: The role of DNA repair pathways. *Clin. Cancer Res.* **2008**, *14*, 1291–1295. [CrossRef]

30. Metzger, R.; Bollschweiler, E.; Hölscher, A.H.; Warnecke-Eberz, U. ERCC1: Impact in multimodality treatment of upper gastrointestinal cancer. *Future Oncol.* **2010**, *6*, 1735–1749. [CrossRef]

31. Olaussen, K.A.; Dunant, A.; Fouret, P.; Brambilla, E.; André, F.; Haddad, V.; Taranchon, E.; Filipits, M.; Pirker, R.; Popper, H.H.; et al. DNA repair by ERCC1 in Non–Small-Cell Lung Cancer and Cisplatin-Based Adjuvant Chemotherapy. *N. Engl. J. Med.* **2006**, *355*, 983–991. [CrossRef] [PubMed]

32. Simon, G.R.; Sharma, S.; Cantor, A.; Smith, P.; Bepler, G. ERCC1 expression is a predictor of survival in resected patients with non-small cell lung cancer. *Chest* **2005**, *127*, 978–983. [CrossRef] [PubMed]

33. Rosell, R.; Pifarré, A.; Monzó, M.; Astudillo, J.; López-Cabrerizo, M.P.; Calvo, R.; Moreno, I.; Sánchez-Céspedes, M.; Font, A.; Navas-Palacios, J.J. Reduced survival in patients with stage-I non-small-cell lung cancer associated with DNA-replication errors. *Int. J. Cancer* **1997**, *74*, 330–334. [CrossRef]

34. Eldehna, W.M.; Fouda, M.M.; Eteba, S.M.; Abdelrahim, M.; Elashry, M.S. Gene expression of excision repair cross-complementation group 1 enzyme as a novel predictive marker in patients receiving platinum-based chemotherapy in advanced bladder cancer. *Benha Med. J.* **2018**, *35*, 42–48. [CrossRef]

35. Piljić Burazer, M.; Mladinov, S.; Matana, A.; Kuret, S.; Bezić, J.; Glavina Durdov, M. Low ERCC1 expression is a good predictive marker in lung adenocarcinoma patients receiving chemotherapy based on platinum in all TNM stages—A single-center study. *Diagn. Pathol.* **2019**, *14*, 105. [CrossRef]

36. Li, Z.; Qing, Y.; Guan, W.; Li, M.; Peng, Y.; Zhang, S.; Xiong, Y.; Wang, D. Predictive value of APE1, BRCA1, ERCC1 and TUBB3 expression in patients with advanced non-small cell lung cancer (NSCLC) receiving first-line platinum–paclitaxel chemotherapy. *Cancer Chemother. Pharmacol.* **2014**, *74*, 777–786. [CrossRef]

37. Facista, A.; Nguyen, H.; Lewis, C.; Prasad, A.R.; Ramsey, L.; Zaitlin, B.; Nfonsam, V.; Krouse, R.S.; Bernstein, H.; Payne, C.M.; et al. Deficient expression of DNA repair enzymes in early progression to sporadic colon cancer. *Genome Integr.* **2012**, *3*, 3. [CrossRef]

38. Smith, D.H.; Fiehn, A.-M.K.; Fogh, L.; Christensen, I.J.; Hansen, T.P.; Stenvang, J.; Nielsen, H.J.; Nielsen, K.V.; Hasselby, J.P.; Brünner, N.; et al. Measuring ERCC1 protein expression in cancer specimens: Validation of a novel antibody. *Sci. Rep.* **2014**, *4*, 4313. [CrossRef]

39. Sun, J.-M.; Sung, J.-Y.; Park, S.H.; Kwon, G.Y.; Jeong, B.C.; Seo, S.I.; Jeon, S.S.; Lee, H.M.; Jo, J.; Choi, H.Y.; et al. ERCC1 as a biomarker for bladder cancer patients likely to benefit from adjuvant chemotherapy. *BMC Cancer* **2012**, *12*, 187. [CrossRef]

40. Hemdan, T.; Segersten, U.; Malmström, P.-U. 122 ERCC1-negative tumors benefit from neoadjuvant cisplatin-based chemotherapy whereas patients with ERCC1-positive tumors do not—Results from a cystectomy trial database. *Eur. Urol. Suppl.* **2014**, *13*, e122. [CrossRef]

41. Urun, Y.; Leow, J.J.; Fay, A.P.; Albiges, L.; Choueiri, T.K.; Bellmunt, J. ERCC1 as a prognostic factor for survival in patients with advanced urothelial cancer treated with platinum based chemotherapy: A systematic review and meta-analysis. *Crit. Rev. Oncol. Hematol.* **2017**, *120*, 120–126. [CrossRef] [PubMed]

42. Sakano, S.; Ogawa, S.; Yamamoto, Y.; Nishijima, J.; Miyachika, Y.; Matsumoto, H.; Hara, T.; Matsuyama, H. ERCC1 and XRCC1 expression predicts survival in bladder cancer patients receiving combined trimodality therapy. *Mol. Clin. Oncol.* **2013**, *1*, 403–410. [CrossRef] [PubMed]

43. Chen, L.; Liu, Y.; Zhang, Q.; Zhang, M.; Han, X.; Li, Q.; Xie, T.; Wu, Q.; Sui, X. p53/PCDH17/Beclin-1 proteins as prognostic predictors for urinary bladder cancer. *J. Cancer* **2019**, *10*, 6207–6216. [CrossRef] [PubMed]

44. Choundhury, S.; Kolukula, V.; Preet, A.; Albanese, C.; Maria, A. Dissecting the pathways that destabilize mutant p53: The proteasome or autophagy? *Cell Cycle* **2013**, *12*, 1022–1029. [CrossRef]

45. Zhou, G.; Wang, J.; Zhao, M.; Xie, T.-X.; Tanaka, N.; Sano, D.; Patel, A.A.; Ward, A.M.; Sandulache, V.C.; Jasser, S.A.; et al. Gain-of-function mutant p53 promotes cell growth and cancer cell metabolism via inhibition of AMPK activation. *Mol. Cell* **2014**, *54*, 960–974. [CrossRef]

46. Mitra, A.P. Molecular substratification of bladder cancer: Moving towards individualized patient management. *Ther. Adv. Urol.* **2016**, *8*, 215–233. [CrossRef]

47. Ando, K.; Oki, E.; Saeki, H.; Yan, Z.; Tsuda, Y.; Hidaka, G.; Kasagi, Y.; Otsu, H.; Kawano, H.; Kitao, H.; et al. Discrimination of p53 immunohistochemistry-positive tumors by its staining pattern in gastric cancer. *Cancer Medicine* **2014**, *4*, 75–83. [CrossRef]

48. Puzio-Kuter, A.M.; Castillo-Martin, M.; Kinkade, C.W.; Wang, X.; Shen, T.H.; Matos, T.; Shen, M.M.; Cordon-Cardo, C.; Abate-Shen, C. Inactivation of p53 and Pten promotes invasive bladder cancer. *Genes Dev.* **2009**, *23*, 675–680. [CrossRef]

49. Shariat, S.F.; Chade, D.C.; Karakiewicz, P.I.; Ashfaq, R.; Isbarn, H.; Fradet, Y.; Bastian, P.J.; Nielsen, M.E.; Capitanio, U.; Jeldres, C. Combination of multiple molecular markers can improve prognostication in patients with locally advanced and lymph node positive bladder cancer. *J. Urol.* **2010**, *183*, 68–75. [CrossRef]

50. Daizumoto, K.; Yoshimaru, T.; Matsushita, Y.; Fukawa, T.; Uehara, H.; Ono, M.; Komatsu, M.; Kanayama, H.; Katagiri, T. A DDX31/Mutant–p53/EGFR axis promotes multistep progression of muscle-invasive bladder cancer. *Cancer Res.* **2018**, *78*, 2233–2247. [CrossRef]

51. Qamar, S.; Inam, Q.A.; Ashraf, S.; Khan, M.S.; Khokhar, M.A.; Awan, N. Prognostic Value of p53 expression intensity in urothelial cancers. *J. Coll. Physicians Surg. Pak.* **2017**, *27*, 232–236. [PubMed]

52. Ciccarese, C.; Massari, F.; Blanca, A.; Tortora, G.; Montironi, R.; Cheng, L.; Scarpelli, M.; Raspollini, M.R.; Vau, N.; Fonseca, J.; et al. Tp53 and its potential therapeutic role as a target in bladder cancer. *Expert Opin. Ther. Targets* **2017**, *21*, 401–414. [CrossRef] [PubMed]

53. Du, J.; Wang, S.; Yang, Q.; Chen, Q.; Yao, X. p53 status correlates with the risk of progression in stage T1 bladder cancer: A meta-analysis. *World J. Surg. Oncol.* **2016**, *14*, 137. [CrossRef] [PubMed]

54. Shariat, S.F.; Lotan, Y.; Karakiewicz, P.I.; Ashfaq, R.; Isbarn, H.; Fradet, Y.; Bastian, P.J.; Nielsen, M.E.; Capitanio, U.; Jeldres, C.; et al. p53 predictive value for pT1-2 N0 disease at radical cystectomy. *J. Urol.* **2009**, *182*, 907–913. [CrossRef] [PubMed]

55. Moch, H.; Cubilla, A.L.; Humphrey, P.A.; Reuter, V.E.; Ulbright, T.M. The 2016 WHO classification of tumours of the urinary system and male genital organs—Part A: Renal, penile, and testicular tumours. *Eur. Urol.* **2016**, *70*, 93–105. [CrossRef] [PubMed]

56. Sung, J.-Y.; Sun, J.-M.; Chang Jeong, B.; Il Seo, S.; Soo Jeon, S.; Moo Lee, H.; Choi, H.Y.; Kang, S.Y.; Choi, Y.-L.; Young Kwon, G. FGFR3 overexpression is prognostic of adverse outcome for muscle-invasive bladder carcinoma treated with adjuvant chemotherapy11This work was supported by Grant CB-2011-04-01 from Korean Foundation for Cancer Research grant and by a Global Frontier Project Grant (NRF-M1AXA002-2010-0029795) of the National Research Foundation funded by the Ministry of Education, Science and Technology of Korea. *Urol. Oncol. Semin. Orig. Investig.* **2014**, *32*, 49.e23–49.e31. [CrossRef]

57. Akanksha, M.; Sandhya, S. Role of FGFR3 in Urothelial Carcinoma. *Iran. J. Pathol.* **2019**, *14*, 148–155. [CrossRef]

58. Williams, S.V.; Hurst, C.D.; Knowles, M.A. Oncogenic FGFR3 gene fusions in bladder cancer. *Hum. Mol. Genet.* **2012**, *22*, 795–803. [CrossRef]

59. Di Martino, E.; Tomlinson, D.C.; Knowles, M.A. A decade of FGF receptor research in bladder cancer: Past, present, and future challenges. *Adv. Urol.* **2012**, *2012*, 1–10. [CrossRef]

60. Beukers, W.; van der Keur, K.A.; Kandimalla, R.; Vergouwe, Y.; Steyerberg, E.W.; Boormans, J.L.; Jensen, J.B.; Lorente, J.A.; Real, F.X.; Segersten, U.; et al. FGFR3, TERT and OTX1 as a urinary biomarker combination for surveillance of patients with bladder cancer in a large prospective multicenter study. *J. Urol.* **2017**, *197*, 1410–1418. [CrossRef]

61. Hurst, C.D.; Knowles, M.A. Multiomic profiling refines the molecular view. *Nat. Rev. Clin. Oncol.* **2017**, *15*, 203–204. [CrossRef] [PubMed]

62. Van Oers, J.M.M.; Zwarthoff, E.C.; Rehman, I.; Azzouzi, A.-R.; Cussenot, O.; Meuth, M.; Hamdy, F.C.; Catto, J.W.F. FGFR3 mutations indicate better survival in invasive upper urinary tract and bladder tumours. *Eur. Urol.* **2009**, *55*, 650–658. [CrossRef] [PubMed]

63. Van Rhijn, B.W.G.; van der Kwast, T.H.; Liu, L.; Fleshner, N.E.; Bostrom, P.J.; Vis, A.N.; Alkhateeb, S.S.; Bangma, C.H.; Jewett, M.A.S.; Zwarthoff, E.C.; et al. The FGFR3 mutation is related to favorable pT1 bladder cancer. *J. Urol.* **2012**, *187*, 310–314. [CrossRef] [PubMed]

64. Hernandez, S.; Lopez-Knowles, E.; Lloreta, J.; Kogevinas, M.; Amorós, A.; Tardón, A.; Carrato, A.; Serra, C.; Malats, N.; Real, F.X. Prospective study of fgfr3 mutations as a prognostic factor in nonmuscle invasive urothelial bladder carcinomas. *J. Clin. Oncol.* **2006**, *24*, 3664–3671. [CrossRef]

65. Critelli, R.; Fasanelli, F.; Oderda, M.; Polidoro, S.; Assumma, M.B.; Viberti, C.; Preto, M.; Gontero, P.; Cucchiarale, G.; Lurkin, I.; et al. Detection of multiple mutations in urinary exfoliated cells from male bladder cancer patients at diagnosis and during follow-up. *Oncotarget* **2016**, *7*, 67435. [CrossRef]

66. Frantzi, M.; Makridakis, M.; Vlahou, A. Biomarkers for bladder cancer aggressiveness. *Curr. Opin. Urol.* **2012**, *22*, 390–396. [CrossRef]

67. Tomlinson, D.; Baldo, O.; Harnden, P.; Knowles, M. FGFR3 protein expression and its relationship to mutation status and prognostic variables in bladder cancer. *J. Pathol.* **2007**, *213*, 91–98. [CrossRef]

68. Christensen, E.; Birkenkamp-Demtröder, K.; Nordentoft, I.; Høyer, S.; van der Keur, K.; van Kessel, K.; Dyrskjøt, L. Liquid biopsy analysis of FGFR3 and PIK3CA hotspot mutations for disease surveillance in bladder cancer. *Eur. Urol.* **2017**, *71*, 961–969. [CrossRef]

69. Choi, W.; Porten, S.; Kim, S.; Willis, D.; Plimack, E.R.; Hoffman-Censits, J.; McConkey, D.J. Identification of distinct basal and luminal subtypes of muscle-invasive bladder cancer with different sensitivities to frontline chemotherapy. *Cancer Cell* **2014**, *25*, 152–165. [CrossRef]

70. Hosen, I.; Rachakonda, P.S.; Heidenreich, B.; de Verdier, P.J.; Ryk, C.; Steineck, G.; Hemminki, K.; Kumar, R. Mutations inTERTpromoter andFGFR3and telomere length in bladder cancer. *Int. J. Cancer* **2015**, *137*, 1621–1629. [CrossRef]

71. Kompier, L.C.; van der Aa, M.N.; Lurkin, I.; Vermeij, M.; Kirkels, W.J.; Bangma, C.H.; van der Kwast, T.H.; Zwarthoff, E.C. The development of multiple bladder tumour recurrences in relation to the FGFR3mutation status of the primary tumour. *J. Pathol.* **2009**, *218*, 104–112. [CrossRef] [PubMed]

72. Kompier, L.C.; Lurkin, I.; van der Aa, M.N.M.; van Rhijn, B.W.G.; van der Kwast, T.H.; Zwarthoff, E.C. FGFR3, HRAS, KRAS, NRAS and PIK3CA mutations in bladder cancer and their potential as biomarkers for surveillance and therapy. *PLoS ONE* **2010**, *5*, e13821. [CrossRef] [PubMed]

73. Foth, M.; Ismail, N.F.B.; Kung, J.S.C.; Tomlinson, D.; Knowles, M.A.; Eriksson PIwata, T. FGFR3 mutation increases bladder tumourigenesis by suppressing acute inflammation. *J. Pathol.* **2018**, *246*, 331–343. [CrossRef] [PubMed]

74. Pectasides, D.; Bafaloucos, D.; Antoniou, F.; Gogou, L.; Economides, N.; Varthalitis, J.; Athanassiou, A. TPA, TATI, CEA, AFP, β-HCG, PSA, SCC, and CA 19-9 for monitoring transitional cell carcinoma of the bladder. *Am. J. Clin. Oncol.* **1996**, *19*, 271–277. [CrossRef]

75. Järvisalo, J.; Hakama, M.; Knekt, P.; Stenman, U.H.; Leino, A.; Teppo, L.; Maatela, J.; Aromaa, A. Serum tumor markers CEA, CA 50, TATI, and NSE in lung cancer screening. *Lung Cancer* **1993**, *10*, 276. [CrossRef]

76. Sjöström, J.; Alfthan, H.; Joensuu, H.; Stenman, U.; Lundin, J.; Blomqvist, C. Serum tumour markers CA 15-3, TPA, TPS, hCG β and TATI in the monitoring of chemotherapy response in metastatic breast cancer. *Scand. J. Clin. Lab. Investig.* **2001**, *61*, 431–441. [CrossRef]

77. Paavonen, J.; Lehtinen, M.; Lehto, M.; Laine, S.; Aine, R.; Räsänen, L.; Stenman, U.H. Concentrations of tumor-associated trypsin inhibitor and C-reactive protein in serum in acute pelvic inflammatory disease. *Clin. Chem.* **1989**, *35*, 869–871. [CrossRef]

78. Lasson, Å.; Borgström, A.; Ohlsson, K. Elevated pancreatic secretory trypsin inhibitor levels during severe inflammatory disease, renal insufficiency, and after various surgical procedures. *Scand. J. Gastroenterol.* **1986**, *21*, 1275–1280. [CrossRef]

79. Huhtala, M.-L.; Kahanpää, K.; Seppää, M.; Halila, H.; Stenman, U.-H. Excretion of a tumor-associated trypsin inhibitor (TATI) in urine of patients with gynecological malignancy. *Int. J. Cancer* **1983**, *31*, 711–714. [CrossRef]

80. Goumas, P.D.; Mastronikolis, N.S.; Mastorakou, A.N.; Vassilakos, P.J.; Nikiforidis, G.C. Evaluation of TATI and CYFRA 21-1 in patients with head and neck squamous cell carcinoma. *ORL* **1997**, *59*, 106–114. [CrossRef]

81. Tramonti, P.G.; Ferdeghini, M.; Donadio, C.; Annichiarico, C.; Norpoth, M.; Bianchi, R.; Bianchi, C. Serum levels of tumor associated trypsin inhibitor (TATT) and glomerular filtration rate. *Ren. Fail.* **1998**, *20*, 295–302. [CrossRef] [PubMed]

82. Stenman, U.-H.; Koivunen, E.; Itkonen, O. Biology and function of tumor-associated trypsin inhibitor, tati. *Scand. J. Clin. Lab. Investig.* **1991**, *51*, 5–9. [CrossRef] [PubMed]

83. Stenman, U.-H. Tumor-associated trypsin inhibitor. *Clin. Chem.* **2002**, *48*, 1206–1209. [CrossRef] [PubMed]

84. Kelloniemi, E.; Rintala, E.; Finne, P.; Stenman, U.-H. Tumor-associated trypsin inhibitor as a prognostic factor during follow-up of bladder cancer. *Urology* **2003**, *62*, 249–253. [CrossRef]

85. Shariat, S.F.; Herman, M.P.; Casella, R.; Lotan, Y.; Karam, J.A.; Stenman, U.-H. Urinary levels of tumor-associated trypsin inhibitor (TATI) in the detection of transitional cell carcinoma of the urinary bladder. *Eur. Urol.* **2005**, *48*, 424–431. [CrossRef]

86. Hotakainen, K.; Bjartell, A.; Sankila, A.; Järvinen, R.; Paju, A.; Rintala, E.; Haglund, C.; Stenman, U.-H. Differential expression of trypsinogen and tumor-associated trypsin inhibitor (TATI) in bladder cancer. *Int. J. Oncol.* **2006**, *28*, 95–101. [CrossRef]

87. Patschan, O.; Shariat, S.F.; Chade, D.C.; Karakiewicz, P.I.; Ashfaq, R.; Lotan, Y.; Hotakainen, K.; Stenman, U.-H.; Bjartell, A. Association of tumor-associated trypsin inhibitor (TATI) expression with molecular markers, pathologic features and clinical outcomes of urothelial carcinoma of the urinary bladder. *World J. Urol.* **2011**, *30*, 785–794. [CrossRef]

9

Diagnostic and Prognostic Implications of FGFR3^{high}/Ki67^{high} Papillary Bladder Cancers

Mirja Geelvink [1], Armin Babmorad [1], Angela Maurer [1], Robert Stöhr [2], Tobias Grimm [3], Christian Bach [4], Ruth Knuechel [1], Michael Rose [1,†] and Nadine T. Gaisa [1,*,†]

1   Institute of Pathology, RWTH Aachen University, Pauwelsstrasse 30, 52074 Aachen, Germany; mirja.geelvink@rwth-aachen.de (M.G.); armin.babmorad@rwth-aachen.de (A.B.); amaurer@ukaachen.de (A.M.); rknuechel-clarke@ukaachen.de (R.K.); mrose@ukaachen.de (M.R.)

2   Institute of Pathology, University Hospital Erlangen, Friedrich-Alexander University Erlangen-Nürnberg (FAU), 91054 Erlangen, Germany; Robert.Stoehr@uk-erlangen.de

3   Department of Urology, Ludwig Maximilian University Munich, 81377 Munich, Germany; Tobias_Grimm@med.uni-muenchen.de

4   Department of Urology, RWTH Aachen University, 52074 Aachen, Germany; chbach@ukaachen.de

*   Correspondence: ngaisa@ukaachen.de

†   These authors are contributed equally.

Abstract: Prognostic/therapeutic stratification of papillary urothelial cancers is solely based upon histology, despite activated FGFR3-signaling was found to be associated with low grade tumors and favorable outcome. However, there are FGFR3-overexpressing tumors showing high proliferation—a paradox of coexisting favorable and adverse features. Therefore, our study aimed to decipher the relevance of FGFR3-overexpression/proliferation for histopathological grading and risk stratification. $N = 142$ ($n = 82$ pTa, $n = 42$ pT1, $n = 18$ pT2-4) morphologically G1–G3 tumors were analyzed for immunohistochemical expression of FGFR3 and Ki67. Mutation analysis of *FGFR3* and *TP53* and FISH for *FGFR3* amplification and rearrangement was performed. SPSS 23.0 was used for statistical analysis. Overall FGFR3^{high}/Ki67^{high} status ($n = 58$) resulted in a reduced Δmean progression-free survival (PFS) ($p < 0.01$) of 63.92 months, and shorter progression-free survival ($p < 0.01$; mean PFS: 55.89 months) in pTa tumors ($n = 50$). *FGFR3*^{mut}/*TP53*^{mut} double mutations led to a reduced Δmean PFS ($p < 0.01$) of 80.30 months in all tumors, and *FGFR3*^{mut}/*TP53*^{mut} pTa tumors presented a dramatically reduced PFS ($p < 0.001$; mean PFS: 5.00 months). Our results identified FGFR3^{high}/Ki67^{high} papillary pTa tumors as a subgroup with poor prognosis and encourage histological grading as high grade tumors. Tumor grading should possibly be augmented by immunohistochemical stainings and suitable clinical surveillance by endoscopy should be performed.

Keywords: FGFR3; Ki67; TP53; bladder cancer; prognosis

1. Introduction

Bladder cancer is the second most common genitourinary malignancy [1]. At primary diagnosis, most of the tumors are papillary non-invasive cancers (pTa) which are mostly well differentiated but show a high rate of recurrence. Those tumors are characterized by certain molecular alterations as for example FGFR3 activation [2–5]. Up to 30% of all patients have invasive disease at diagnosis. These tumors frequently derive from flat carcinoma in situ (CIS) of the urothelium (a high grade lesion, often *TP53*-mutated) and quickly develop muscle-invasion and metastasis [6,7]. Current prognostic and therapeutic stratification in urothelial cancers is therefore based on tumor staging and grading at histological examination. Staging criteria is the depth of invasion defined by the tumor node metastasis (TNM)-classification of the Union Internationale Contre le Cancer (UICC) [8]. The tumor grading is based upon architectural order and nuclear shape features, which have been thoroughly defined as diagnostic criteria in the 2004 WHO classification of bladder cancer in order to achieve reproducible and comparable diagnoses worldwide. Low grade (LG) tumors show uniform, slightly enlarged nuclei in an orderly, polarized architecture, sometimes with a prominent palisading of the basal layer. Mitotic figures are infrequent [9,10]. High grade (HG) tumors show more pleomorphic nuclei with multiple mitotic features and various extent of architectural disarray [10]. Based on previous genetic analyses and clinical observations, it has been proposed that the histological appearance (grading) of tumors correlates with the underlying genetic alterations, and low grade tumors were regarded genetically stable, whereas high grade tumors, harboring a high number of genetic alterations, were considered genetically "unstable" [7]. Proposed prognostic markers in papillary non-invasive tumors have been the Ki67 labeling index (marker for cell proliferation) and keratin 20 expression (marker for cell differentiation). Tumors with Ki67 $\geq$ 15% were regarded as highly proliferative [11–13] and aberrant expression of keratin 20 was linked to disease recurrence in pTa tumors [14]. Lately, Hurst et al. conducted a comprehensive molecular study on n = 141 papillary non-invasive bladder cancers (low grade, G1 and G2 according to WHO 1973) and found lower overall mutation rates, but more mutations in chromatin modifying genes than in muscle-invasive bladder cancer, and two distinct genomic subgroups of tumors (genomic subtype 1 and 2). The majority of tumors with genomic subtype 1 showed no or only few copy-number alterations. Genomic subtype 2 was characterized by loss of 9q (including the mTORC1 regulator TSC1), increased Ki67 labeling index, upregulated mTORC1 signaling (comprising the overrepresentation of genes in processes that are involved in the unfolded protein response, glycolysis, and cholesterol homeostasis) as well as enrichment for DNA repair and cell-cycle genes [15]. *FGFR3* mutations were not found to be significantly different in both subgroups (72% vs. 89%) and *TP53* mutations were absent [15]. The authors did not show a correlation of molecular profiles with specific histological features.

However, in routine histological diagnostics, pathologists often see papillary non-invasive tumors with quite uniform, relatively small nuclei, which give a "crowded" impression, but seem to be of "low nuclear grade". Interestingly, Ki67 labeling in these tumors is often enhanced and from this point of view a reconsideration of a possible "high grade"-biology is implicated. Opposite to the negative predictive impact of a high Ki67 index, these tumors often show a strong expression of FGFR3, which indicates an activation of the signaling pathway resulting in cellular proliferation, but is generally associated with a benign course of disease with higher recurrence rates but less progression [7]. Being aware of this diagnostic-biological "dilemma", we delineated in this study the immunohistochemical and genetic basis of such FGFR3[high]/Ki67[high] papillary bladder cancers in order to reveal their prognostic impact.

2. Results

2.1. Immunohistochemical Combination of Ki67-Index and FGFR3 Levels Defines Worse Patients' Outcome

Overall, FGFR3 and Ki67 protein expression was analyzed by immunohistochemistry (Figure 1A–I) in n = 142 primary bladder tumors comprising n = 82 papillary non-invasive tumors (for cohort characteristics, see Table S1). In this cohort, 87/142 patients (61.3%) showed a high Ki67-index ($\geq$15% positivity) and 100/142 bladder cancer patients (70.4%) were characterized by strong FGFR3 expression (Tomlinson Score 3) (Figure S1A,C). In papillary non-invasive pTa tumors, 82.9% showed strong FGFR3 and 54.9% increased Ki67 expression (Figure S1B,D).

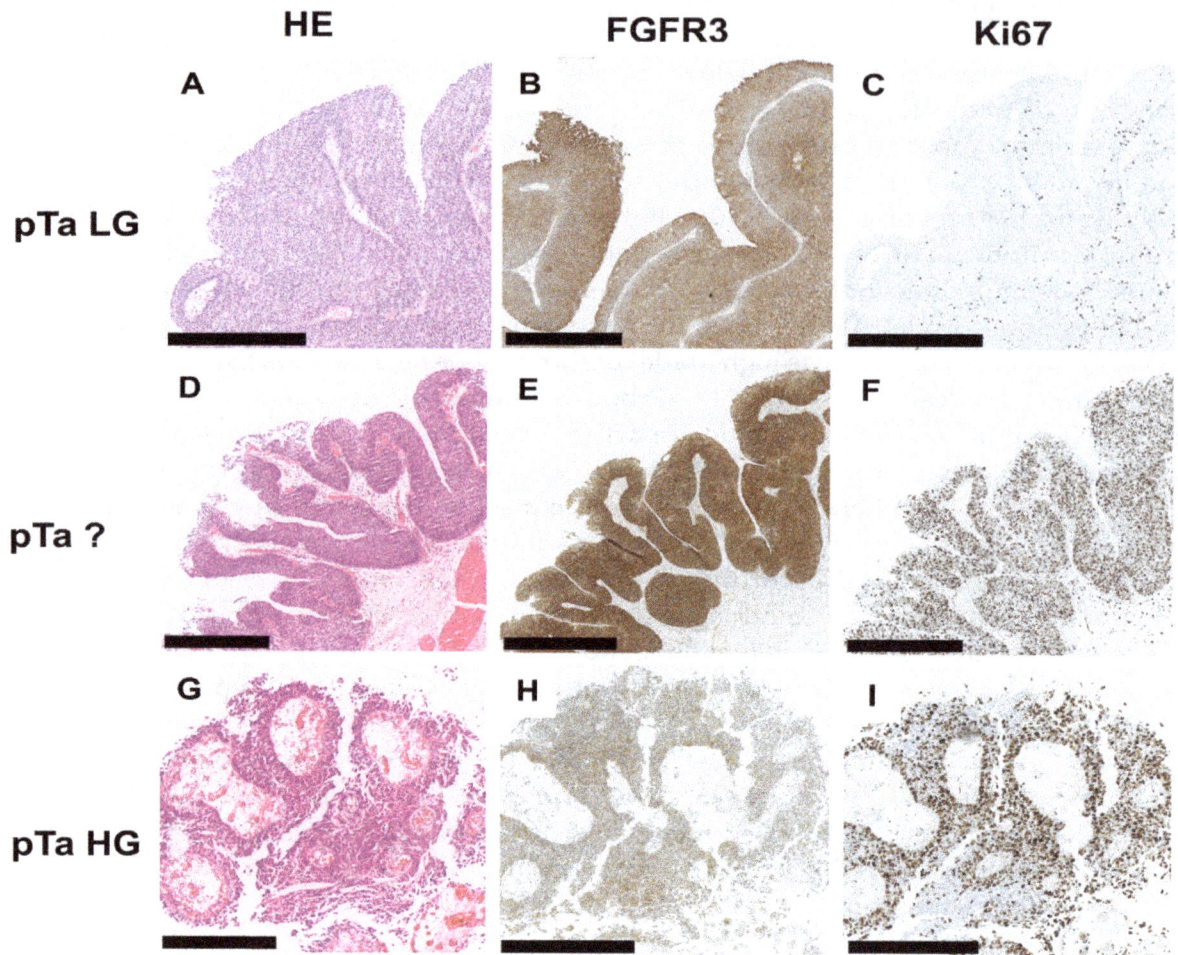

Figure 1. FGFR3 and Ki67 protein expression in papillary non-invasive (pTa) bladder tumors. Immunohistochemical staining for FGFR3 and Ki67 protein of representative tumors are shown. (**A–C**) pTa low grade (LG) tumor: (**A**) Hematoxylin and Eosin (HE) staining; (**B**) strong FGFR3 immunoreactivity; and (**C**) only a few cell nuclei are positive for Ki67 expression. (**D–F**) pTa tumor with "crowded low nuclear grade" (pTa?) morphology: (**D**) HE staining; (**E**) strong FGFR3 immunoreactivity; and (**F**) high nuclear Ki67 protein staining. (**G–I**) pTa high grade (HG) tumor: (**G**) HE staining; (**H**) moderate FGFR3 protein expression; and (**I**) high nuclear Ki67 staining. Scale bar: 500 μm; original digital magnifications vary from 5× to 7×.

Next, associations between clinico-pathological characteristics and both FGFR3 and Ki67 protein expression were tested. FGFR3 expression and Ki67 index correlated with tumor grading (FGFR3: $p < 0.001$, Ki67: $p < 0.001$), but only FGFR3 expression was significantly associated with tumor stage (FGFR3: $p < 0.001$) (Tables 1 and 2). No association was found between FGFR3/Ki67 and age at diagnosis or gender.

Table 1. Clinico-pathological parameters in correlation to FGFR3 protein expression.

		FGFR3 Expression [a]			
	n	0–2	3	*p*-Value [b]	Spearman ρ
Parameter:					
Age at diagnosis					
<70 years	67	20	47	0.946	0.006
≥70 years	75	22	53		
Gender					
female	31	10	21	0.372	0.031
male	111	32	79		
Histological tumor grade					
low grade	49	3	46	**<0.001**	−0.373
high grade	93	39	54		
Tumor stage					
pTa	82	14	68	**<0.001**	−0.320
pT1–pT4	60	28	32		

[a] Tomlinson score according to [16]; [b] Fisher's exact test; Significant *p*-values are marked in bold face.

Table 2. Clinico-pathological parameters in correlation to Ki67 protein expression.

		Ki67 Expression [a]			
	n	<15%	≥15%	*p*-Value [b]	Spearman ρ
Parameter:					
Age at diagnosis					
<70 years	67	31	36	0.083	0.146
≥70 years	75	24	51		
Gender					
female	31	14	17	0.408	0.070
male	111	41	70		
Histological tumor grade					
low grade	49	34	15	**<0.001**	0.457
high grade	93	21	72		
Tumor stage					
pTa	82	37	45	0.069	0.175
pT1–pT4	60	18	42		

[a] According to [11]; [b] Fisher's exact test; Significant *p*-values are marked in bold face.

To assess the clinical impact, Kaplan–Meier analyses were performed. FGFR3 expression had no significant impact on progression-free survival (PFS) (Figure 2A). In contrast, enhanced Ki67 expression (≥15%) significantly predicted shorter progression-free survival (Δmean PFS: 2.71 months, $p = 0.043$). Finally, we aimed to decipher the potential prognostic impact of combined FGFR3 expression and Ki67 index: FGFR3[high]/Ki67[high] status was found in $n = 58$ cases. A combined analysis of FGFR3/Ki67 positivity (Figure 2C and Figure S2A) resulted in a reduced Δmean PFS ($p < 0.01$) of 63.92 months when comparing FGFR3[high]/Ki67[high] tumors (mean PFS: 54.87 months ± 6.73; 95% CI: 41.78 to 68.05) with all other combinations (mean PFS: 118.78 months ± 6.95; 95% CI: 105.17 to 132.40). If, for example, both markers were expressed at low levels, bladder cancer patients showed no progressive disease at all (Figure S2A). Therefore, our results identify FGFR3[high]/Ki67[high] tumors as an aggressive subgroup.

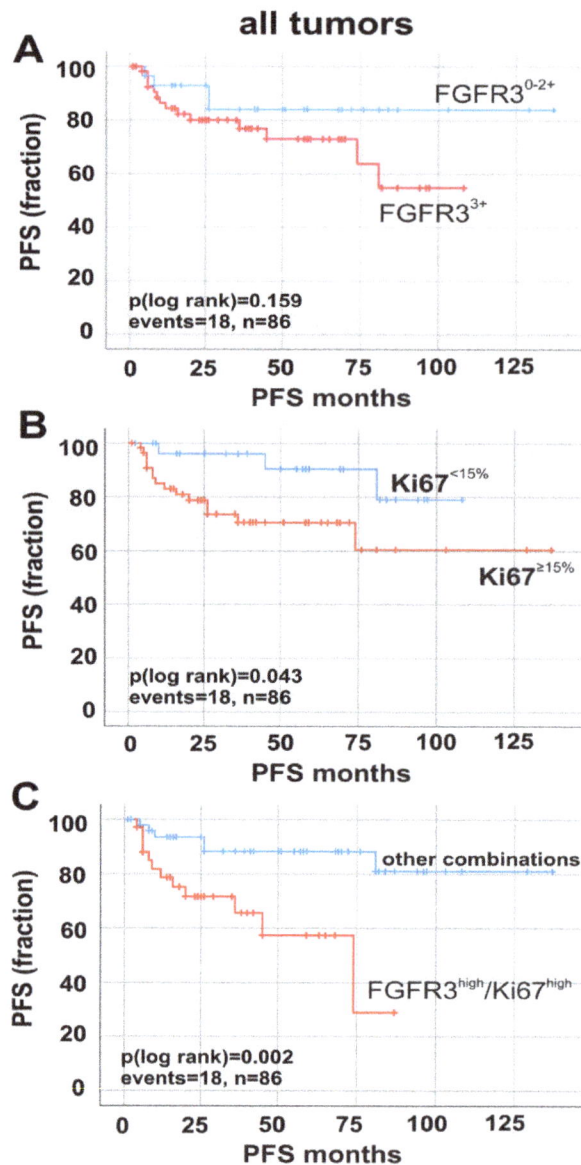

Figure 2. Prognostic impact of FGFR3 and Ki67 protein expression in all tumors (pTa, pT1 and pT2–4). Kaplan–Meier survival curves display progression-free survival (PFS). (**A**) Survival curves of patients with high FGFR3 expression (red curve, $n = 56$) compared to low FGFR3 expression (blue curve, $n = 30$). (**B**) Kaplan–Meier analysis of patients with high Ki67 expression (red curve, $n = 56$) compared to low Ki67 expression (blue curve, $n = 30$). (**C**) Survival curve analysis of FGFR3^{high}/Ki67^{high} expression (red curve, $n = 34$) compared to all other combinations of FGFR3 and Ki67 expression (blue curve, $n = 32$). n: overall number of cases; events: overall events of tumor progression.

The calculated Cox regression model (including the potentially prognostic parameters stage, grade, age, keratin 20 and keratin 5/6) confirmed independency of the clinical impact of a FGFR3^{high}/Ki67^{high} status on progression-free survival. Patients displaying a combined overexpression of FGFR3 and Ki67 showed an approximately four-fold higher risk for tumor progression (multivariate hazard ratio (HR): 3.943, 95% CI: 1.247 to 12.466, $p = 0.019$) (Table 3).

Table 3. Multivariate Cox regression analysis of immunohistochemical markers including all factors potentially influencing PFS.

Variable	HR	p-Value	95%CI	
			Lower	Upper
FGFR3 high/Ki67high	3.943	**0.019**	1.247	12.466
pT status	0.957	0.941	0.295	3.105
Tumor grade	0.846	0.823	0.196	3.653
Keratin 5/6	0.482	0.280	0.128	1.812
Keratin 20	0.424	0.115	0.146	1.232
Age	1.773	0.347	0.537	5.847

2.2. Prognostic Impact of Ki67-Index and FGFR3 Overexpression in Papillary Non-Invasive (pTa) Tumors

Stratifying our cohort by invasiveness, i.e., into papillary non-invasive (pTa) and invasive tumors (pT1–pT4), FGFR3 overexpression (Tomlinson Score 3) was not associated with tumor progression in pTa bladder cancer ($p > 0.05$ for PFS) (Figure 3A).

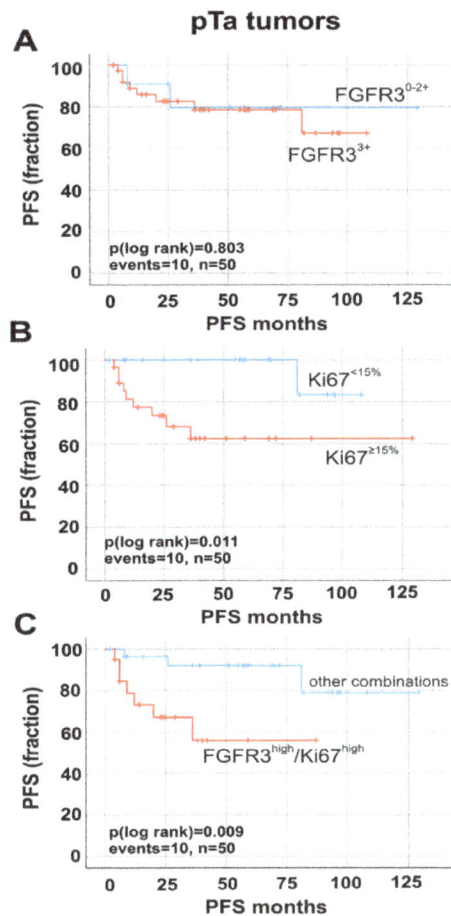

Figure 3. Prognostic impact of FGFR3 and Ki67 protein expression in papillary non-invasive (pTa) tumors. Kaplan–Meier survival curves demonstrate progression-free survival (PFS). (**A**) Survival curves of patients with high FGFR3 expression (red curve, $n = 39$) compared to low FGFR3 expression (blue curve, $n = 11$). (**B**) Kaplan–Meier analysis of patients with high Ki67 expression (red curve, $n = 28$) compared to low Ki67 expression (blue curve, $n = 22$). (**C**) Impact of combined markers on risk stratification of tumor progression is shown. Survival curve analysis of FGFR3high/Ki67high expression (red curve, $n = 20$) compared to all other combinations of FGFR3 and Ki67 expression (blue curve, $n = 30$) in pTa tumors. n, overall number of cases; events, overall events of tumor progression.

Single marker analysis of high Ki67-index correlated with progression-free survival (Δmean PFS: 17.06 months, $p = 0.011$) (Figure 3B). Now, combining the two immunohistochemical markers, univariate Kaplan–Meier curve revealed a significant impact of FGFR3^{high}/Ki67^{high} expression on patients' outcome only in pTa tumors. In fact, patients with high FGFR3^{high}/Ki67^{high} showed a significantly ($p < 0.01$) shorter progression-free survival (mean PFS: 55.89 months $\pm$ 9.23; 95% CI: 37.82 to 73.98) compared to those patients with all other combinations of FGFR3/Ki67 expression (mean PFS: 113.85 months $\pm$ 8.12; 95% CI: 97.94 to 129.77, $p = 0.009$) (Figure 3C).

2.3. Altered Molecular FGFR3/TP53 Status Predicts Worse Patients' Survival

Since we hypothesized that FGFR3-overexpression and high cell proliferation might indicate a higher risk for progression in papillary non-invasive tumors, we further investigated the molecular status of our cohort by studying both mutations for *FGFR3* as papillary and *TP53* as invasive markers (for detailed mutation data, see Table S2). In total, 48 out of 99 (48.5%) analyzed patients harbored mutations within the *FGFR3* gene (Figure 4A).

The most frequent mutation was p.S249C (pTa: 13/21, pT1: 10/22, pT2–4: 2/5). *FGFR3* mutations showed no significant association with clinico-pathological parameters like tumor stage or grade (Table S3). *TP53* mutations were present in $n = 23/98$ (23.5%) patients (Figure 4A). There were $n = 18/23$ (78.3%) tumors which solely showed missense mutations (pTa: 6/6, pT1: 7/11, pT2–4: 5/6) and $n = 5/23$ (21.7%) tumors with mutations leading to a premature transcription stop either due to the appearance of a stop codon or a frameshift (pTa: 0/6, pT1: 4/11, pT2–4: 1/6). *TP53* mutations correlated with tumor grade ($p < 0.05$) but not with stage (Table S4). Mutations in both genes (referred to as double mutations) were found in $n = 6/99$ (6.1%) patients.

Survival analysis revealed no significant association between single mutations, i.e., *FGFR3* or *TP53*, with patient's outcome for PFS (Figure 4B,C). However, mutations in both genes (*FGFR3*^{mut}/*TP53*^{mut}) predicted unfavorable prognosis for PFS. Double mutations led to a reduced Δmean PFS ($p < 0.01$) of 80.30 months: *FGFR3*^{mut}/*TP53*^{mut} tumors (mean PFS: 27.08 months $\pm$ 8.41; 95% CI: 10.59 to 43.57) showed shorter PFS in contrast with all other combinations (mean PFS: 107.83 months $\pm$ 8.62; 95% CI: 90.49.17 to 124.28) (Figure 4D and Figure S2B).

Multivariate analysis confirmed the prognostic impact of *FGFR3*^{mut}/*TP53*^{mut} tumors. Double mutated tumors exhibited a 6.6 times higher risk for tumor progression (multivariate hazard ratio (HR): 6.563, 95% CI: 1.694 to 25.425, $p = 0.006$) (Table 4).

2.4. Prognostic Impact of FGFR3 and TP53 Mutations in Papillary Non-Invasive (pTa) Tumors

Next, we focused on pTa tumors, in particular those with FGFR3-overexpression and high cell proliferation. In pTa tumors, the following distribution was found: $n = 17/42$ (40.5%) *FGFR3*^{wt}/*TP53*^{wt}, $n = 19/42$ (45.2%) *FGFR3*^{mut}/*TP53*^{wt}, $n = 4/42$ (9.5%) *FGFR3*^{wt}/*TP53*^{mut} and $n = 2/42$ (4.8%) *FGFR3*^{mut}/*TP53*^{mut}. On the contrary, pT1 tumors showed $n = 9/39$ (23.1%) *FGFR3*^{wt}/*TP53*^{wt}, $n = 19/39$ (48.7%) *FGFR3*^{mut}/*TP53*^{wt}, $n = 8/39$ (20.5%) *FGFR3*^{wt}/*TP53*^{mut} and $n = 3/39$ (7.7%) *FGFR3*^{mut}/*TP53*^{mut}. pT2–4 tumors represented with the following mutational pattern: $n = 8/18$ (44.4%) *FGFR3*^{wt}/*TP53*^{wt}, $n = 4/18$ (22.2%) *FGFR3*^{mut}/*TP53*^{wt}, $n = 5/18$ (27.8%) *FGFR3*^{wt}/*TP53*^{mut} and $n = 1/18$ (5.6%) *FGFR3*^{mut}/*TP53*^{mut}.

Survival analyses revealed a correlation between *FGFR3* mutations and shorter PFS ($p = 0.041$) in pTa tumors (Figure 5A). *TP53* mutations did not show any effects ($p > 0.05$) on PFS (Figure 5B). Interestingly, tumors exhibiting double mutation status *FGFR3*^{mut}/*TP53*^{mut} ($n = 6$) presented a dramatically reduced Δmean PFS ($p < 0.001$) of 102.52 months (mean PFS: 5.00 months $\pm$ 1.00; 95% CI: 3.04 to 6.96) in pTa tumors (Figure 5C) compared with all other combinations (mean PFS: 107.52 months $\pm$ 9.72; 95% CI: 88.46 to 126.57).

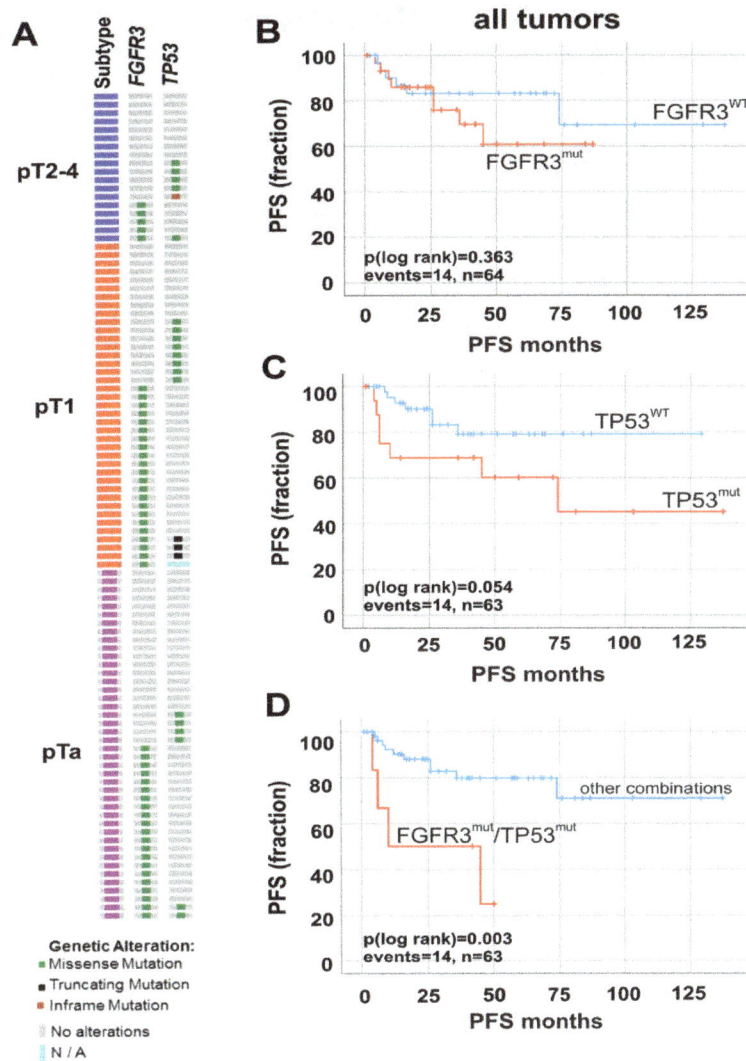

Figure 4. *FGFR3* and *TP53* mutation frequency and prognostic impact on tumor progression. (**A**) Oncoprint graph for *FGFR3* and *TP53* mutation analysis. (**B**–**D**) Kaplan–Meier survival curves display progression-free survival (PFS). (**B**) Survival curves of tumors with detected *FGFR3* mutations (red curve, $n = 30$) compared to non-mutated *FGFR3* gene status (blue curve, $n = 34$). (**C**) Kaplan–Meier analysis of tumors with mutated *TP53* (red curve, $n = 17$) compared to wildtype *TP53* (blue curve, $n = 46$). (**D**) Impact of double mutations on risk stratification of tumor progression is demonstrated. Univariate analysis of double mutations (red curve, $n = 6$) compared to all other combinations of mutated and non-mutated *FGFR3* and *TP53* genes (blue curve, $n = 57$). n, overall number of cases; events, overall events of tumor progression.

Table 4. Multivariate Cox regression analysis of molecular markers including all factors potentially influencing PFS.

Variable	HR	*p*-Value	95%CI	
			Lower	Upper
FGFR3^{mut}/*TP53*^{mut}	6.563	**0.006**	1.694	25.425
pT status	1.179	0.821	0.284	4.896
Tumor grade	0.241	0.138	0.037	1.580
Keratin 5/6	0.714	0.621	0.188	2.712
Keratin 20	0.872	0.814	0.279	2.730
Age	1.41	0.584	0.412	2.809

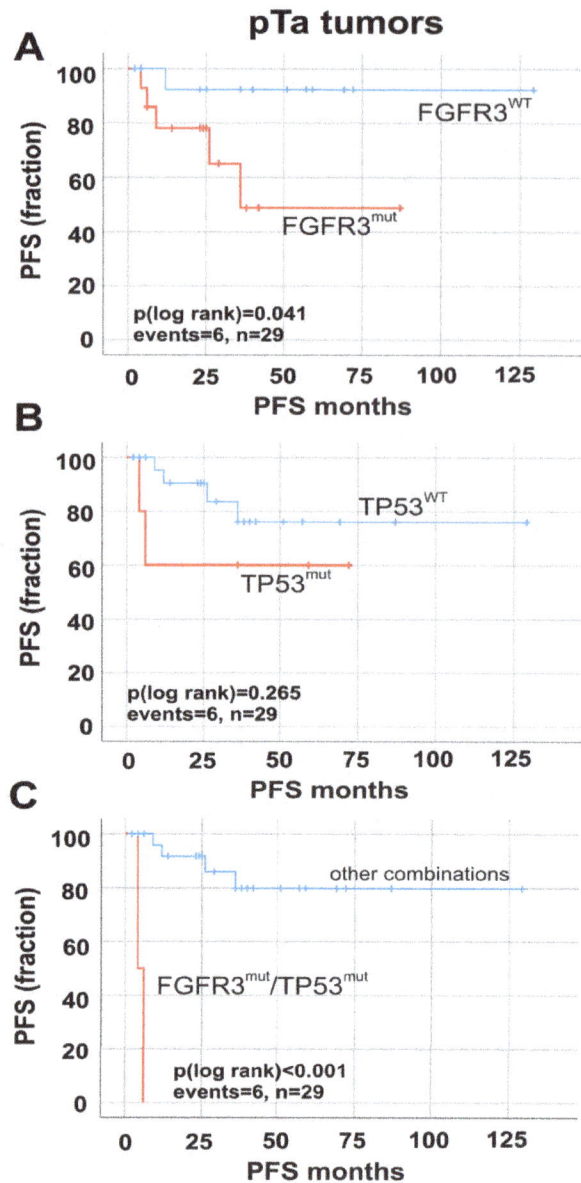

Figure 5. Prognostic impact of *FGFR3* and *TP53* mutations on tumor progression in papillary non-invasive (pTa) tumors. Progression-free survival (PFS) is shown. (**A**) Univariate survival analysis illustrates that detected *FGFR3* mutations (red curve, $n = 14$) predict shorter PFS compared to non-mutated *FGFR3* gene status (blue curve, $n = 15$). (**B**) Kaplan–Meier analysis of tumors with mutated *TP53* (red curve, $n = 5$) compared to wildtype *TP53* (blue curve, $n = 24$). (**C**) Impact of double mutations on risk stratification of tumor progression is shown. Survival analysis of double mutations (red curve, $n = 2$) compared to all other combinations of mutated and non-mutated *FGFR3* and *TP53* genes (blue curve, $n = 27$) in pTa tumors. n: overall number of cases; events: overall events of tumor progression.

Finally, we assessed the clinical impact of immunohistochemical and mutational status as a combined approach. Survival analysis displayed that $FGFR3^{mut}/TP53^{mut}$ double mutated tumors were significantly associated with worse patients' outcome only in FGFR3 and Ki67 overexpressing tumors: reduced PFS in $FGFR3^{high}/Ki67^{high}$ double mutated tumors compared with all other combinations of molecular status of *TP53* and *FGFR3* ($FGFR3^{wt}/TP53^{wt}$ $p = 0.001$; $FGFR3^{mut}/TP53^{wt}$ $p < 0.001$; $FGFR3^{wt}/TP53^{mut}$ $p = 0.116$) (data not shown). However, it has to be noted that the number of double mutations is very low, and, hence, statistical validity should be enhanced in future studies.

2.5. FGFR3^{high}/Ki67^{high} Tumors Define a Subset of pTa Tumors Including Lesions with Molecular FGFR3 Pathway Activation

Prognostic stratification of bladder cancer patients in routine histopathological diagnostics claims simple and cost-effective means, therefore, we evaluated the concordance of immunohistochemical staining results and molecular status.

The majority of FGFR3^{high}/Ki67^{high} tumors was characterized by conjunct FGFR3 mutations with a significant correlation only in papillary non-invasive tumors (pTa $n = 19/27$ (70.4%), $p < 0.001$) but not in pT1 and pT2–4 tumors (Table S5). There was no significant correlation between FGFR3^{high}/Ki67^{high} tumors and TP53 mutations independently of the given tumor stage (data not shown).

To evaluate the diagnostic potential of immunohistochemical markers covering the molecular FGFR3 pathway, we performed ROC (Receiver operating characteristics) curve statistics to calculate sensitivity and specificity. Accordingly, both immunohistochemical markers detect FGFR3 mutations with 90.5% sensitivity and 61.9% specificity (area under curve (AUC): 0.776, $p = 0.004$, positive predictive value (PPV): 70.4%, negative predictive value (NPV): 85.7%). These data show that FGFR3^{high}/Ki67^{high} tumors include papillary lesions with mutation-based altered FGFR3 signaling, but also tumors without molecular alterations (pTa $n = 8/27$ (29.6%)). Hence, our data give evidence that FGFR3^{high}/Ki67^{high} tumors define a subset of pTa tumors associated with poor prognosis potentially decoupled from the described protective effect of FGFR3 activation [7].

3. Discussion

In our study, we systematically analyzed papillary non-invasive and invasive tumors for distinct prognostic immunohistochemical and molecular markers. We focused on a subgroup of immunohistochemically FGFR3^{high}/Ki67^{high} tumors in order to reveal their prognostic impact on patient survival and re-evaluate their histological classification/grading.

Although, according to nuclear and architectural criteria, these papillary tumors appear to be orderly and more "nuclear low grade", we found them associated with worse PFS compared with FGFR3^{high}/Ki67^{low} tumors. This was especially evident in pTa tumors, where mean progression-free survival was reduced to 55 instead of 113 months. Therefore, we asked whether these tumors harbor a special molecular phenotype turning them into aggressive ones. In literature FGFR3 and TP53 mutations were initially thought to be mutually exclusive as FGFR3 mutations were associated with pTa and LG tumors ("papillary pathway"), whereas the TP53 mutations were often found in invasive and HG carcinomas ("CIS/invasive pathway") [17,18]. Notwithstanding, Hernandez et al. reported FGFR3 and TP53 mutations to be independently distributed in a large series of pT1G3 tumors, that were consequently interpreted as a particular group of bladder tumors that could not be classified into either one pathway or the other [4]. In our study, we saw a similar trend with well-known inverse relationships between FGFR3 and TP53 mutations for both stage and grade, while mutations in FGFR3 and TP53 revealed an independent but not mutually exclusive assignment (six tumors with double mutations). Biologically activated FGFR3 signaling promotes cell proliferation and tumor growth, however interestingly, highest numbers of FGFR3-alterations are found in benign papillary or low grade papillary tumors with usually low proliferation (Ki67) index [19–21]. TP53 inactivation results in reduced cellular apoptosis and thus maintains tumor growth via reduced cell death [22–25]. We hypothesized that a FGFR3^{high}/Ki67^{high} phenotype might be resulting from inactivated p53, however we found no sufficient molecular evidence for this theory in our cohort. Recent comprehensive sequencing data of papillary non-invasive bladder tumors revealed a genomic subtype 2, which is characterized by loss of 9q (including TSC1), increased Ki67 labeling index, upregulated mTORC1 signaling, glycolysis, features of the unfolded protein response, altered cholesterol homeostasis and DNA repair [15]. Therefore, high proliferation might be explained by mutations in DNA repair genes or the deletion/mutation of TSC1, which consequently leads towards an upregulation of mTORC1 and PIK3CA mutations. Further analyses to strengthen this theory have to be performed in the future.

Comprehensive molecular data of bladder cancer has been gained in the recent years [15,26,27], however, complex multigene analysis and RNA expression analysis are costly and laborious, and therefore cost-effective simple analyses for routine histological examination are needed. In our study, we analyzed whether fast and simple immunohistochemical analyses are suitable to detect a more aggressive molecular subtype. We found a highly significant correlation between strong FGFR3/Ki67 immunohistochemical staining and *FGFR3* mutation status, which indicates that FGFR3 protein expression is more frequent than mutational activation [16]. Moreover, our FGFR3^{high}/Ki67^{high} subgroup also comprises those neoplasms without any molecular (*FGFR3* and/or *TP53*) alterations defining in this combination a subset of pTa tumors with poor prognosis, i.e., FGFR3 overexpression was associated with unfavorable outcome as previously shown, for instance, for invasive bladder tumors treated with adjuvant chemotherapy [28]. Thus, our data support the proposed clinical significance of these two immunohistochemical markers for diagnostic and prognostic stratification of more aggressive papillary non-invasive bladder tumors.

Taken together, we found immunohistochemically FGFR3^{high}/Ki67^{high} pTa tumors associated with worse prognosis/survival, despite appearing histologically of "lower nuclear grade"/G2. Even if these tumors appear to be "low grade" (according to the 2004 WHO classification), we recommend classifying them as "high grade" pTa tumors. In light of our findings, we suggest immunohistochemical staining for FGFR3 and Ki67 in order to gain evidence for this more aggressive molecular subgroup with worse prognosis. These patients probably could profit from close endoscopic follow-up, as especially urine cytology might also be challenging/less sensitive due to their minimal nuclear changes.

4. Materials and Methods

4.1. Patient Samples, Tissue Microarrays and DNA

We retrospectively selected urothelial bladder cancer cases (mutational analysis: $n = 42$ pTa, $n = 39$ pT1, $n = 18$ pT2–4; immunohistochemical analysis: $n = 82$ pTa, $n = 42$ pT1, $n = 18$ pT2–4) from our pathology archive and from the archive of the Institute of Pathology in Erlangen. Formalin-fixed paraffin-embedded (FFPE) surgical specimens were used to construct tissue microarrays (all samples) and extract DNA ($n = 99$ samples) using Qiagen kits (Qiagen, Hilden, Germany) as previously described [29–31]. Patient information was obtained by the Department of Urology and the local ethics committee approved a retrospective, pseudonymized study of archival tissues (RWTH EK 009/12). Histological tumor grade and stage was classified according to WHO 2004 classification [8].

4.2. Immunohistochemistry

For immunohistochemical stainings, TMA sections were pretreated with DAKO PT-Link heat induced antigen retrieval with Low pH (pH 6) or High pH (pH 9) Target Retrieval Solution (DAKO, Hamburg, Germany) and incubated for 30 min at room temperature with respective antibodies in a DAKO Autostainer (DAKO). For stainings anti-FGFR3 (clone B9, PTlink pH6, dilution 1:25, Flex+M; Santa Cruz Biotechnology, Heidelberg, Germany), anti-Ki67 (clone MIB-1, PTlink pH 6, dilution 1:400, Flex+M; DAKO), anti-CK 20 (clone Ks20.8, PTlink pH 6, dilution 1:200, Flex+M; DAKO), and anti-CK5/6 (clone D5/16 B4, PTlink pH 9, dilution 1:100, Flex+M; DAKO) were used. Appropriate linker molecules EnVision^{TM}FLEX+ (mouse/rabbit), EnVision FLEX/HRP detection system and counterstaining with EnVision FLEX Hematoxylin were applied. Stainings were evaluated by an experienced uropathologist (NTG) who was blinded for patient identity, diagnosis and clinical follow-up results. FGFR3 positivity was reported according to a semiquantitative scoring system developed by Tomlinson et al. [16]. All other stainings were evaluated for staining intensities (0 = no staining, 1 = weak staining, 2 = moderate staining, 3 = strong staining) and percentages of positive stained tumor cells. Results were judged as follows: Keratin 20 positive $\geq$10% stained cells [14,32], Keratin 5/6 positive $\geq$10% [32], Ki67 positive $\geq$15% [11,13] stained cells.

4.3. Fluorescence In Situ Hybridization

ZytoLight Dual Color Probe SPEC FGFR3/*CEN* 4 and *ZytoLight* Dual Color Break Apart Probe SPEC FGFR3 (Zytovision, Bremerhaven, Germany) were hybridized onto 3 μm TMA sections according to the manufacturer's protocols. Slides were evaluated with a Zeiss Axiovert 135 fluorescence microscope (Carl Zeiss, Oberkochen, Germany), and Diskus Software (MIL 7.5, 4.80) (Büro Hilgers, Königswinter, Germany) using appropriate channels/filters (AHF ZyGreen F36-720, AHF ZyOrange F36-740, AHF DAPI, AHF F56-700). Signals of 60 nuclei of tumor cells were counted at high magnification ($\times$1000) and judged as described previously [33].

4.4. Sanger Sequencing

PCR-amplification of exons 7, 10 and 15 of the *FGFR3* gene and exons 5, 6, 7, 8 and 9 of *TP53* were carried out using routine protocols. Primers and annealing temperatures are given in Table S6. PCR products were purified by either ExoSAP-IT (Affymetrix, Lahr/Schwarzwald, Germany) or a PCR purification kit (PerkinElmer Chemagen, Baesweiler, Germany) according to the manufacturer's instructions. Sanger sequencing of both strands was run on an ABI PRISM 3500 Genetic Analyzer (Applied Biosystems, Weiterstadt, Germany) using the Big dye Terminator kit (Applied Biosystems), the same primer sets and the seq purification kit (PerkinElmer Chemagen).

4.5. Statistical Analysis

Statistical analysis was performed using SPSS (Statistical Package for the Social Sciences) software version 23.0 (SPSS Inc., Chicago, IL, USA). p-values < 0.05 were considered significant. Statistical associations between clinico-pathological and molecular factors were determined by Fisher's exact test. Correlation analysis was performed by calculating a Spearman's rank correlation coefficient. Survival (progression-free survival (PFS)) was calculated using the Kaplan–Meier method with log-rank statistics. Survival was measured from surgery until relapse, death or progression and was censored for patients alive without evidence of event at the last follow-up date. Multivariate Cox-regression analysis was performed to test for an independently prognostic value of FGFR3-Ki67 protein expression and *FGFR3-TP53* mutations. Receiver operating characteristics (ROC) curves were calculated to assess biomarker performance of immunohistochemical markers regarding molecular alterations.

Author Contributions: Conceptualization, R.K. and N.T.G; Methodology, M.G., A.B., A.M. and M.R.; Software, M.R.; Validation, R.S.; Resources, T.G. and C.B.; Writing—Original Draft Preparation, N.T.G., M.G. and M.R.; Writing—Review and Editing, A.M., A.B., R.S., T.G., and C.B.; Visualization, M.R.; and Supervision, R.K. and N.T.G.

Acknowledgments: The authors appreciate the excellent technical support of Ursula Schneider, Inge Losen, Patrick Kühl and Oliver Dohmen.

References

1. Siegel, R.L.; Miller, K.D.; Jemal, A. Cancer statistics. *CA Cancer J. Clin.* **2018**, *68*, 7–30. [CrossRef]
2. Van Rhijn, B.W.; Lurkin, I.; Radvanyi, F.; Kirkels, W.J.; Van der Kwast, T.H.; Zwarthoff, E.C. The fibroblast growth factor receptor 3 (FGFR3) mutation is a strong indicator of superficial bladder cancer with low recurrence rate. *Cancer Res.* **2001**, *61*, 1265–1268. [PubMed]
3. Billerey, C.; Chopin, D.; Aubriot-Lorton, M.H.; Ricol, D.; Gil Diez de Medina, S.; van Rhijn, B.; Bralet, M.P.; Lefrere-Belda, M.A.; Lahaye, J.B.; Abbou, C.C.; et al. Frequent FGFR3 mutations in papillary non-invasive bladder (pTa) tumors. *Am. J. Pathol.* **2001**, *158*, 1955–1959. [CrossRef]

4.   Hernandez, S.; Lopez-Knowles, E.; Lloreta, J.; Kogevinas, M.; Jaramillo, R.; Amoros, A.; Tardón, A.; García-Closas, R.; Serra, C.; Carrato, A.; et al. FGFR3 and Tp53 mutations in T1G3 transitional bladder carcinomas: Independent distribution and lack of association with prognosis. *Clin. Cancer. Res.* **2005**, *11*, 5444–5450. [CrossRef] [PubMed]

5.   Neuzillet, Y.; van Rhijn, B.W.; Prigoda, N.L.; Bapat, B.; Liu, L.; Bostrom, P.J.; Fleshner, N.E.; Gallie, B.L.; Zlotta, A.R.; Jewett, M.A.; et al. FGFR3 mutations, but not FGFR3 expression and FGFR3 copy-number variations, are associated with favourable non-muscle invasive bladder cancer. *Virchows. Arch.* **2014**, *465*, 207–213. [CrossRef] [PubMed]

6.   Wu, X.R. Urothelial tumorigenesis: A tale of divergent pathways. *Nat. Rev. Cancer.* **2005**, *5*, 713–725. [CrossRef] [PubMed]

7.   Knowles, M.A.; Hurst, C.D. Molecular biology of bladder cancer: New insights into pathogenesis and clinical diversity. *Nat. Rev. Cancer* **2015**, *15*, 25–41. [CrossRef] [PubMed]

8.   Brierley, J.; Gospodarowicz, M.K.; Wittekind, C. *TNM Classification of Malignant Tumours*, 8th ed.; John Wiley & Sons Inc.: Chichester, UK; Hoboken, NJ, USA, 2017; ISBN 9781119263579.

9.   Montironi, R.; Lopez-Beltran, A.; Scarpelli, M.; Mazzucchelli, R.; Cheng, L. Morphological classification and definition of benign, preneoplastic and non-invasive neoplastic lesions of the urinary bladder. *Histopathology* **2008**, *53*, 621–633. [CrossRef] [PubMed]

10. Moch, H.; Humphrey, P.A.; Ulbright, T.M.; Reuter, V.E. *International Agency for Research on Cancer. WHO Classification of Tumours of the Urinary System and Male Genital Organs*, 4th ed.; International Agency for Research on Cancer: Lyon, France, 2016; ISBN 9789283224372.

11. Cina, S.J.; Lancaster-Weiss, K.J.; Lecksell, K.; Epstein, J.I. Correlation of Ki-67 and p53 with the new World Health Organization/International Society of Urological Pathology Classification System for Urothelial Neoplasia. *Arch. Pathol. Lab. Med.* **2001**, *125*, 646–651. [CrossRef] [PubMed]

12. Hentic, O.; Couvelard, A.; Rebours, V.; Zappa, M.; Dokmak, S.; Hammel, P.; Maire, F.; O'Toole, D.; Lévy, P.; Sauvanet, A.; et al. Ki-67 index, tumor differentiation, and extent of liver involvement are independent prognostic factors in patients with liver metastases of digestive endocrine carcinomas. *Endocr. Relat. Cancer* **2011**, *18*, 51–59. [CrossRef] [PubMed]

13. Bertz, S.; Otto, W.; Denzinger, S.; Wieland, W.F.; Burger, M.; Stohr, R.; Link, S.; Hofstädter, F.; Hartmann, A. Combination of CK20 and Ki-67 immunostaining analysis predicts recurrence, progression, and cancer-specific survival in pT1 urothelial bladder cancer. *Eur. Urol.* **2014**, *65*, 218–226. [CrossRef] [PubMed]

14. Harnden, P.; Mahmood, N.; Southgate, J. Expression of cytokeratin 20 redefines urothelial papillomas of the bladder. *Lancet* **1999**, *353*, 974–977. [CrossRef]

15. Hurst, C.D.; Alder, O.; Platt, F.M.; Droop, A.; Stead, L.F.; Burns, J.E.; Burghel, G.J.; Jain, S.; Klimczak, L.J.; Lindsay, H.; et al. Genomic Subtypes of Non-invasive Bladder Cancer with Distinct Metabolic Profile and Female Gender Bias in KDM6A Mutation Frequency. *Cancer Cell* **2017**, *32*, 701–715. [CrossRef] [PubMed]

16. Tomlinson, D.C.; Baldo, O.; Harnden, P.; Knowles, M.A. FGFR3 protein expression and its relationship to mutation status and prognostic variables in bladder cancer. *J. Pathol.* **2007**, *213*, 91–98. [CrossRef] [PubMed]

17. Van Rhijn, B.W.; van der Kwast, T.H.; Vis, A.N.; Kirkels, W.J.; Boeve, E.R.; Jobsis, A.C.; Zwarthoff, E.C. FGFR3 and P53 characterize alternative genetic pathways in the pathogenesis of urothelial cell carcinoma. *Cancer. Res.* **2004**, *64*, 1911–1914. [CrossRef] [PubMed]

18. Bakkar, A.A.; Wallerand, H.; Radvanyi, F.; Lahaye, J.B.; Pissard, S.; Lecerf, L.; Kouyoumdjian, J.C.; Abbou, C.C.; Pairon, J.C.; Jaurand, M.C.; et al. FGFR3 and TP53 gene mutations define two distinct pathways in urothelial cell carcinoma of the bladder. *Cancer. Res.* **2003**, *63*, 8108–8112. [PubMed]

19. Hernandez, S.; Lopez-Knowles, E.; Lloreta, J.; Kogevinas, M.; Amoros, A.; Tardon, A.; Carrato, A.; Serra, C.; Malats, N.; Real, F.X. Prospective study of FGFR3 mutations as a prognostic factor in nonmuscle invasive urothelial bladder carcinomas. *J. Clin. Oncol.* **2006**, *24*, 3664–3671. [CrossRef] [PubMed]

20. Junker, K.; van Oers, J.M.; Zwarthoff, E.C.; Kania, I.; Schubert, J.; Hartmann, A. Fibroblast growth factor receptor 3 mutations in bladder tumors correlate with low frequency of chromosome alterations. *Neoplasia* **2008**, *10*, 1–7. [CrossRef] [PubMed]

21. Van Rhijn, B.W.; Zuiverloon, T.C.; Vis, A.N.; Radvanyi, F.; van Leenders, G.J.; Ooms, B.C.; Kirkels, W.J.; Lockwood, G.A.; Boevé, E.R.; Jöbsis, A.C.; et al. Molecular grade (FGFR3/MIB-1) and EORTC risk scores are predictive in primary non-muscle-invasive bladder cancer. *Eur. Urol.* **2010**, *58*, 433–441. [CrossRef] [PubMed]

22. Sigal, A.; Rotter, V. Oncogenic mutations of the p53 tumor suppressor: The demons of the guardian of the genome. *Cancer. Res.* **2000**, *60*, 6788–6793. [PubMed]

23. Zuckerman, V.; Wolyniec, K.; Sionov, R.V.; Haupt, S.; Haupt, Y. Tumour suppression by p53: The importance of apoptosis and cellular senescence. *J. Pathol.* **2009**, *219*, 3–15. [CrossRef] [PubMed]

24. Oren, M.; Rotter, V. Mutant p53 gain-of-function in cancer. *Cold Spring Harb. Perspect Biol.* **2010**, *2*, a001107. [CrossRef] [PubMed]

25. Rivlin, N.; Brosh, R.; Oren, M.; Rotter, V. Mutations in the p53 Tumor Suppressor Gene: Important Milestones at the Various Steps of Tumorigenesis. *Genes Cancer* **2011**, *2*, 466–474. [CrossRef] [PubMed]

26. Weinstein, J.N.; Akbani, R.; Broom, B.M.; Wang, W.; Verhaak, R.G.; McConkey, D.; Lerner, S.; Morgan, M.; Creighton, C.J.; Smith, C.; et al. Comprehensive molecular characterization of urothelial bladder carcinoma. *Nature* **2014**, *507*, 315–322. [CrossRef]

27. Hedegaard, J.; Lamy, P.; Nordentoft, I.; Algaba, F.; Hoyer, S.; Ulhoi, B.P.; Vang, S.; Reinert, T.; Hermann, G.G.; Mogensen, K.; et al. Comprehensive Transcriptional Analysis of Early-Stage Urothelial Carcinoma. *Cancer Cell* **2016**, *30*, 27–42. [CrossRef] [PubMed]

28. Sung, J.Y.; Sun, J.M.; Chang, J.B.; Seo, S.I.; Soo, J.S.; Moo, L.H.; Yong, C.H.; Young, K.S.; Choi, Y.L.; Young, K.G. FGFR3 overexpression is prognostic of adverse outcome for muscle-invasive bladder carcinoma treated with adjuvant chemotherapy. *Urol. Oncol.* **2014**, *32*, e23–e31. [CrossRef]

29. Gaisa, N.T.; Graham, T.A.; McDonald, S.A.; Canadillas-Lopez, S.; Poulsom, R.; Heidenreich, A.; Jakse, G.; Tadrous, P.J.; Knuechel, R.; Wright, N.A. The human urothelium consists of multiple clonal units, each maintained by a stem cell. *J Pathol.* **2011**, *225*, 163–171. [CrossRef] [PubMed]

30. Fischbach, A.; Rogler, A.; Erber, R.; Stoehr, R.; Poulsom, R.; Heidenreich, A.; Schneevoigt, B.S.; Hauke, S.; Hartmann, A.; Knuechel, R.; et al. Fibroblast growth factor receptor (FGFR) gene amplifications are rare events in bladder cancer. *Histopathology* **2015**, *66*, 639–649. [CrossRef] [PubMed]

31. Molitor, M.; Junker, K.; Eltze, E.; Toma, M.; Denzinger, S.; Siegert, S.; Knuechel, R.; Gaisa, N.T. Comparison of structural genetics of non-schistosoma-associated squamous cell carcinoma of the urinary bladder. *Int. J. Clin. Exp. Pathol.* **2015**, *8*, 8143–8158. [PubMed]

32. Gaisa, N.T.; Braunschweig, T.; Reimer, N.; Bornemann, J.; Eltze, E.; Siegert, S.; Toma, M.; Villa, L.; Hartmann, A.; Knuechel, R. Different immunohistochemical and ultrastructural phenotypes of squamous differentiation in bladder cancer. *Virchows. Arch.* **2011**, *458*, 301–312. [CrossRef] [PubMed]

33. Baldia, P.H.; Maurer, A.; Heide, T.; Rose, M.; Stoehr, R.; Hartmann, A.; Williams, S.V.; Knowles, M.A.; Knuechel, R.; Gaisa, N.T. Fibroblast growth factor receptor (FGFR) alterations in squamous differentiated bladder cancer: A putative therapeutic target for a small subgroup. *Oncotarget* **2016**, *7*, 71429–71439. [CrossRef] [PubMed]

10

Circulating Tumour DNA in Muscle-Invasive Bladder Cancer

Melissa P. Tan [1,2], Gerhardt Attard [3] and Robert A. Huddart [1,2,*]

[1] Division of Radiotherapy & Imaging, Institute of Cancer Research, 15 Cotswold Road, Sutton, Surrey SM2 5NG, UK; melissa.tan@icr.ac.uk

[2] Academic Urology Unit, The Royal Marsden NHS Foundation Trust, Downs Road, Sutton, Surrey SM2 5PT, UK

[3] Research Department of Oncology, UCL Cancer Institute, University College London, 72 Huntley Street, London WC1E 6DD, UK; g.attard@ucl.ac.uk

[*] Correspondence: robert.huddart@icr.ac.uk

Abstract: Circulating tumour DNA (ctDNA) is an attractive tool in cancer research, offering many advantages over tissue samples obtained using traditional biopsy methods. There has been increasing interest in its application to muscle-invasive bladder cancer (MIBC), which is recognised to be a heterogeneous disease with overall poor prognosis. Using a range of platforms, studies have shown that ctDNA is detectable in MIBC and may be a useful biomarker in monitoring disease status and guiding treatment decisions in MIBC patients. Currently, with no such predictive or prognostic biomarkers in clinical practice to guide treatment strategy, there is a real unmet need for a personalised medicine approach in MIBC, and ctDNA offers an exciting avenue through which to pursue this goal. In this article, we present an overview of work to date on ctDNA in MIBC, and discuss the inherent challenges present as well as the potential future clinical applications.

Keywords: circulating tumour DNA (ctDNA); muscle-invasive bladder cancer (MIBC); biomarker

1. Introduction

In the drive towards personalised medicine, circulating tumour DNA (ctDNA) is an invaluable tool in cancer research, offering unique advantages over tissue samples collected using traditional biopsy methods. Its collection via a simple blood draw allows serial samples to be conveniently and safely taken over a course of treatment, thus facilitating the study of tumour dynamics, treatment resistance, and disease progression. Furthermore, it has been suggested that ctDNA samples are likely to provide a more representative snapshot of an individual's cancer compared with biopsy samples as tumour clones from the primary, micro-, and macro-metastatic deposits are present in a single sample [1,2].

These advantages have been exploited in numerous studies across various cancers including colorectal, breast, prostate, and lung malignancies [3–6]. ctDNA levels have been shown to be associated with disease burden [7,8] and in an analysis of serial samples, increasing levels have been shown to pre-date radiological progression [4,9,10]. Analysis of sequential samples taken over a course of treatment have also demonstrated tumour evolution with the emergence of subclones documented at disease progression [11–13]. In addition to plasma, tumour DNA fragments have also been detected in other body fluids such as urine and cerebrospinal fluid [14].

There has been a surge of interest in recent years focusing on ctDNA in muscle-invasive bladder cancer (MIBC); a heterogeneous disease with an aggressive natural history and poor prognosis. With no predictive or prognostic biomarkers in current clinical practice to guide treatment strategy, there is a real need to develop a personalised medicine approach to optimise patient outcomes, and ctDNA offers an innovative approach to address this challenge.

In this review article, we provide a brief background on ctDNA before summarising research to date on ctDNA in MIBC, discussing the challenges present and future clinical applications.

2. Circulating Tumour DNA: Background

2.1. Biology of Circulating DNA

It has long been known that plasma contains nucleic acid fragments including those of DNA (genomic, mitochondrial, and viral), RNA, and micro-RNA; these have been collectively termed circulating nucleic acids. The mechanism by which nucleic acid fragments are released into the circulation remains under debate, but is thought to involve apoptosis, necrosis, and secretion [15]. Circulating DNA (cDNA) fragments are typically less than 200 bp in length. They are thought to undergo hepatic and renal excretion, and the reported half-life of cDNA fragments ranges between 16 min and 2.5 h [9,15,16]. While increased levels of cDNA are seen in malignancy and have been reported to be associated with tumour burden and prognosis in some cancer sites [17–19], raised levels are also seen in benign conditions such as pregnancy, trauma, or inflammation, meaning that cDNA levels alone are not necessarily a specific biomarker in the diagnosis or management of cancer [15].

In the majority of patients with malignancies, cDNA is mainly composed of wildtype, i.e., normal DNA, but may also contain fragments derived from the primary tumor, distant metastases, and micrometastases. The proportion of circulating tumour DNA (ctDNA) fragments (tumour fraction) has been shown to increase with disease burden [3,4,7], and also to vary between tumour types [7]. Although some patients with very advanced disease have demonstrated high tumour fractions above 50% [11], these are the minority and in numerous studies of metastatic disease, tumour fractions as low as 0.04% [4,20] have been reported. Indeed, a recent abstract reported an estimated median tumour fraction of 1.9% in metastatic urothelial cancer [21]. One of the challenges of working with ctDNA, therefore, is in detecting and quantifying the tumour fraction, particularly in the setting of early disease where levels may be in region of 0.01% [3].

2.2. Circulating DNA vs. Circulating Tumour DNA

In order to distinguish ctDNA from wildtype DNA, it is necessary to identify and detect somatic aberrations harboured by the tumour fragments. Quantification of fragments containing aberrations, which may include single nucleotide variants (SNVs), copy number alterations (CNAs), or structural variants, is used as a surrogate of tumour fraction.

There are various approaches to achieve this. One strategy is to first identify aberrations present in a patient's tumour tissue using either a broad de novo sequencing approach (e.g., whole exome or whole genome sequencing) or using a pre-determined set of assays or targeted sequencing panels encompassing known relevant aberrations in the cancer of interest. Aberrations identified in tumour tissue can then be detected in cDNA using polymerase chain reaction (PCR)-based specific assays or a focused next generation sequencing (NGS) approach. An alternative is to sequence the cDNA upfront using either of the approaches described above. However, in order to perform whole genome or whole exome sequencing on cDNA, a minimum tumour fraction is required, in the order of at least 10–20% [22,23], and so this approach is precluded in a significant proportion of cases where tumour fraction does not meet this threshold.

While employing a broad sequencing approach allows an overview of aberrations present, allows assessment of copy number alterations, and supports the design of patient-specific plasma assays, cost may often be a prohibitive factor, particularly if high levels of coverage are sought to identify low frequency aberrations with confidence.

A targeted panel or pre-determined set of assays is more cost-effective, but there is the risk that tumour fraction may be underestimated or ctDNA may not be detected if the individual's relevant mutations are not included in the panel. Furthermore, using specific assays means that mutations arising over time or under selective pressure from treatment will not be identified unless included on the panel. There is thus a balance to be achieved in selecting an approach with sufficient breadth and depth that allows the question being asked to be answered. In the context of MIBC, we shall see that both approaches have been employed, and we discuss this further in the next section of this review.

In trying to improve detection rates of ctDNA, it has been suggested that as tumour fragments are shorter than wildtype DNA fragments [24–26], fragment size selection will be enriched for ctDNA and thus allow very low frequency aberrations to be more readily detected [27]. This approach may be useful for increasing detection of ctDNA in patients with early disease or rare variants.

Whichever approach is employed, ultra-sensitive techniques are required to detect the low levels of ctDNA present. Digital PCR techniques such as BEAMing or droplet digital PCR (ddPCR) have allowed research in this area to progress with sensitivity thresholds of 0.01% [3,28]. However, these approaches only allow a few aberrations to be interrogated at a time, and thus require a priori knowledge regarding aberrations to be detected.

3. Muscle-Invasive Bladder Cancer

3.1. Overview

Muscle-invasive bladder cancer is a heterogeneous disease with an overall poor prognosis [29]. Several molecular profiling studies have identified a number of molecular subtypes that are suggested to have different spectrums of mutations and clinical behaviour [30–32]. Sequencing studies have demonstrated that it has a high mutational burden, third only to melanoma and lung [30], but yet, in contrast to other tumour types, there are currently no approved biomarkers to guide its management. Radical treatment options in MIBC include neoadjuvant platinum-based combination chemotherapy followed by surgery, or in patients where surgery is deemed unsuitable or a bladder preservation strategy is being pursued, chemoradiation may be offered as part of a trimodality approach. In the palliative setting, platinum-based chemotherapy remains the mainstay of treatment, with the recently approved immune checkpoint inhibitors offering a further line of treatment. There is a real unmet clinical need for predictive and prognostic biomarkers in MIBC in order to develop a personalised approach if outcomes are to be improved. ctDNA in MIBC thus promises to be an exciting avenue to enable researchers to better understand the molecular biology, study treatment resistance and disease progression, and identify potential therapeutic targets.

3.2. Potential Clinical Applications of ctDNA in MIBC

ctDNA has the potential to be clinically useful at every step of the treatment pathway in MIBC, from early diagnosis, monitoring or predicting response to treatment in both the radical and palliative settings, assessing the need for adjuvant treatment, and in monitoring for recurrence or progression. Currently, one area of particular interest is in predicting and monitoring response to neoadjuvant chemotherapy. International guidelines [33,34] currently recommend all patients with localised disease are offered neoadjuvant cisplatin-based chemotherapy. However, up to 60% of patients do not respond [35,36] and these patients have thus not only been subjected to unnecessary toxicity, but have also experienced a delay to their definitive treatment, with a potential detrimental effect on outcome [37]. A minimally invasive biomarker to predict response or more sensitively monitor response would thus be of huge clinical benefit, and ctDNA offers the potential to achieve this.

4. CtDNA in MIBC

4.1. Overview

Some of the first work on ctDNA in MIBC dates back to 1991 when Sidransky et al. demonstrated the presence of *p53* mutations in the urinary sediment of three patients with MIBC [38]. Over a decade later, cDNA and ctDNA levels in plasma were shown to be higher in bladder cancer patients than in healthy controls [39,40]. Then, there followed a hiatus in publications on ctDNA in MIBC until Bettegowda et al.'s landmark paper [7], where next generation sequencing was performed on tumour tissue from three patients with metastatic MIBC as part of a broader pan-cancer cohort. A *p53* mutation was identified in each of the patients and was successfully detected in plasma in all three cases. In this small subset of patients, clinical outcomes were not reported, although the paper overall reported increased ctDNA levels with advanced disease. In the last two years, there has been a surge of publications looking at ctDNA in MIBC. Table 1 summarises representative publications including select poster abstracts as of June 2018. Some of the earlier studies have included superficial, i.e., <T2 disease; non-muscle-invasive bladder cancer (NMIBC), and MIBC in a cohort. However, more recently, MIBC has been considered separately and this is in keeping with fact that NMIBC and MIBC have been shown to have different molecular profiles [41].

4.2. ctDNA Is Detectable Using Commercially Available Panels

In 2016, Sonpavde et al. [42] presented work showing that aberrations in cDNA could be detected in 25/29 (86.2%) patients with metastatic urothelial cancer using a commercially available panel composed of 68 cancer-related genes. Using the updated, now 73-gene panel (Guardant360), the group further went on to demonstrate aberrations in plasma from 265/294 (90%) patients with metastatic lower tract urothelial cancer [43]. *TP53* (48%), *ARID1A* (17%), and *PIK3CA* (14%) were the most commonly reported aberrations. They also compared these results from plasma with publically available data from previous NGS studies reporting aberrations in tumour tissue, and reported similar results in terms of the frequency of reported aberrations included on the panel.

Using an alternative 62-gene panel (FoundationACT), McGregor et al. [21] found at least one aberration in plasma of 48/66 (73%) patients with metastatic urothelial cancer. A proportion of their cohort also had sequencing data on baseline tumour tissue available, and the authors reported an example where plasma taken at the time of cisplatin resistance showed persistence of *ERBB2* and *TP53* mutations identified in baseline tumour tissue alongside a new *NF1* aberration. This demonstrates a potential application of ctDNA in furthering our understanding of disease progression and treatment resistance in MIBC, with the potential ability to monitor patients during treatment for evidence of response or the emergence of new potential targets.

Of note, both of these ctDNA panels that were used contained at most only 9 of the most frequent 23 gene mutations documented in the TCGA report [30], and omitted many of the chromatin-modifying gene alterations frequently seen in MIBC, for example, *KMT2D* and *KDM6A* (observed in 28% and 26% of TCGA MIBC cases, respectively). *ERCC2*, which has been put forward as a potential biomarker of sensitivity to cisplatin chemotherapy [44], is also absent. However, as the primary aim of these panels is to identify potential targeted therapy options in the clinical setting, it could be argued that these omissions do not have any clinical impact for MIBC patients, given that there are currently no associated therapies for these targets. However, in the research setting, the omission of these frequently mutated genes is a limitation of these panels in the exploration of potential targets and the study of disease biology.

Table 1. Representative publications including select poster abstracts as of June 2018.

Reference	Year	n	Cohort	Method	Key Findings
Bettegowda et al. [7]	2014	3	Metastatic MIBC	One-hundred-gene panel on tumour tissue; SafeSeq on plasma for patient-specific aberrations	TP53 mutations detected in tumour tissue of 3/3 patients, and detectable in plasma of all three patients
Sonpavde et al. $ [42]	2016	29	Advanced urothelial cancer (MIBC = 27/29)	Sixty-eight-gene commercially available panel to sequence a single plasma sample from each patient (Guardant360)	Aberrations detected in 86.2% patients
Birkenkamp-Demtröder et al. [45]	2016	12	NMIBC: six with recurrence and six with progression to MIBC	WES/WGS/mate-pair sequencing on tumour tissue; personalised ddPCR on sequential plasma samples	ctDNA detectable in 10/12; ctDNA detected several months before clinical diagnosis of progression to MIBC in 4/6 patients
Christensen et al. [46]	2017	1: 363; 2: 468	1: NMIBC 2: Cx (MIBC ≥ 363/468)	ddPCR assays to screen for PIK3CA and FGFR3 hotspots in tissue, urinary supernatant, and plasma	Eleven percent of Cx cohort had ≥1 mutation detected in tumour tissue. Analysis of 23 paired urine and plasma showed higher levels of ctDNA in urine. In 27 Cx plasma samples analysed, high levels of ctDNA in plasma associated with disease recurrence
Vandekerkhove et al. [47]	2017	51	MIBC: 14/51 N0M0 disease; 27/51 N+ve/M1 disease	Bladder cancer-specific targeted panel (50 genes) on plasma from 44 patients including sequential samples; WES on plasma from eight patients to assess mutational burden	ctDNA detected in 25/44 (56.8%) patients with tumour fractions ranging from 3.9–72.6%; All with tumour fraction >30% had distant metastatic disease. Mutational burden derived from targeted sequencing panel consistent with that from WES
Patel et al. [48]	2017	17	MIBC (starting NAC)	Eight-gene TAm-Seq panel (for SNVs) and shallow WGS for copy number assessment on tumour tissue, plasma, urinary cell pellet, and urinary supernatant	Aberration detected in plasma or urine of 10/17 patients pre-NAC. Greater levels of ctDNA detection in urine. Detection of plasma or urine ctDNA pre-cycle two NAC associated with disease recurrence
Birkenkamp-Demtröder et al. [49]	2017	60	MIBC: 50 NAC; 10 palliative chemotherapy	Three ddPCR assays to screen for PIK3CA and FGFR3 mutation in tumour tissue; WES on tumour tissue and germline in 24. Personalised ddPCR assays in plasma for 26 patients	PIK3CA/FGFR3 assays positive in 19/60; ctDNA detectable in patients prior to clinically detected recurrence with median lead time 101 days
McGregor et al. $ [21]	2018	66	Metastatic urothelial cancer	Commercially available 62-gene panel to sequence plasma (FoundationACT)	ctDNA aberrations detected in 48/66 (73%); Estimated median tumour fraction 1.9%
Barata et al. [50]	2017	22	Metastatic urothelial cancer	Compared sequencing results from tumour tissue and plasma sequenced using two different commercially available panels	Concordance between the two tests was 16.4%
Soave et al. [51]	2017	72	Radical Cx (>46/72 MIBC)	Tested 43 regions covering 37 genes for copy number variations (multiplex ligation dependent probe amplification)	cDNA had CNV in 48.6% samples; Overall CNV status not associated with clinical outcome; gain in KLF5, ZFHX3, and CDH1 associated with reduced cancer-specific survival

Table 1. *Cont.*

Reference	Year	n	Cohort	Method	Key Findings
Agarwal et al. [43]	2018	369	Metastatic urinary tract cancer (294/369—lower urinary tract cancer)	Commercially available 73-gene panel (Guardant360) used to sequence plasma	Similar aberrations seen when compared with publically available NGS data on tumour tissue
Cheng et al. $ [52]	2017	26	Metastatic urothelial cancer	Used a 341–468-gene NGS assay (MSK-IMPACT) to sequence plasma (n = 26) and archival tumour tissue (n = 15)	ctDNA detected in 69% patients. Interval between plasma sampling and tissue collection was 35 days to >4 years; Identical tissue and plasma profiles in 20% (3/15)

Abbreviations: MIBC: muscle-invasive bladder cancer; NMIBC: non-MIBC; ctDNA: circulating tumour DNA; NAC: neoadjuvant chemotherapy; WES: whole exome sequencing; WGS: whole genome sequencing; Cx: cystectomy; NGS: next generation sequencing; CNV: copy number variation; SNV: single nucleotide variation; ddPCR: droplet digital polymerase chain reaction; N+ve: node positive; M1: distant metastases; TAm-Seq: tagged amplicon sequencing. $: poster abstract.

The high aberration detection rates of up to 90%, however, are not to be ignored as other groups using custom, albeit much smaller panels/assays have reported lower ctDNA detection rates. Of note, the above cohorts were composed exclusively of patients with advanced disease where ctDNA levels would be expected to be higher and thus more readily detectable. As yet in the literature, there are no reports of using such commercially available panels to profile patients with non-metastatic disease.

4.3. Using Patient-Specific Assays to Detect ctDNA

4.3.1. In NMIBC Cohorts

In one of the first papers to apply a personalised approach to bladder cancer, Birkenkamp-Demtröder et al. [45] used whole exome sequencing (WES), whole genome sequencing (WGS) and/or matepair sequencing to identify mutations in fresh frozen tumour tissue before designing personalised ddPCR assays for use on urine and plasma in a cohort comprising of 12 patients with NMIBC with either disease recurrence or progression to MIBC. ctDNA was detectable in 10/12 (83.3%) patients, including those with non-invasive disease only. In 4/6 (66.7%) patients progressing to muscle-invasive disease, detection of ctDNA pre-dated clinical diagnosis of MIBC by several months.

Christensen et al. [46] also detected ctDNA in patients with NMIBC and MIBC, but used a targeted approach with ddPCR assays to detect three hotspot mutations in *PIK3CA* (E545K) and *FGFR3* (S249C, Y373C), first in tumour tissue and then in plasma and urinary supernatant. In 201 urine samples from patients with NMIBC taken during their disease course, they reported overall higher urinary ctDNA levels in those later progressing to MIBC when compared with those with no progression. Kaplan-Meier progression free survival estimates for a subset of 25 showed that those with ctDNA urinary levels above the median at initial visit had increased progression rates to MIBC (7/13; 54%) compared with those with ctDNA levels below the median (1/12; 8%; $p = 0.036$).

However, within their cystectomy cohort of 468 patients, of whom at least 363 had MIBC, only 44/403 (11%; 65 excluded as insufficient material) had at least one mutation detected in tissue using the *PIK3CA* and *FGFR3* assays. Of those, 27 urine and 27 plasma samples were analysed. A third of patients (9/27) had detectable ctDNA in plasma. Increased ctDNA levels in plasma were associated with lower recurrence-free survival and overall survival. ctDNA levels were overall found to be higher in urine than in plasma [46].

Using the TCGA data portal [53], it can be shown that 62/412 (15%) MIBC patients possess at least one of the three hotspot mutations tested by Christensen et al. [46], which is slightly higher than the detection rate of 11% reported. The authors suggest that the procurement of tissue from a tissue microarray contributed to a low yield of DNA at the tumour tissue screening step, which may have resulted in missed cases. The subsequent low detection rate (33%) in plasma, despite the use of ddPCR, likely reflects the fact that as a cystectomy cohort, patients had localised disease with very low ctDNA fractions. This study highlights the importance of selecting aberrations to capture as many patients as possible, especially when utilising techniques where only a few aberrations can be interrogated at one time.

However, despite small numbers and heterogeneous cohorts consisting mainly of NMIBC, these studies demonstrate proof-of-concept in using both broad and targeted approaches in screening tumour tissue for aberrations to subsequently detect in plasma and urine in patients with bladder cancer. The results raise the possibility of using ctDNA to monitor patients with NMIBC for progression to MIBC. However much work is needed before this can be explored in the setting of a prospective clinical trial, and one of the key steps will be in determining the optimal aberration panel with which to identify and quantify ctDNA.

4.3.2. In MIBC Cohorts

Building upon previous work, Birkenkamp-Demtröder et al. [49] used the same three ddPCR assays for *PIK3CA* and *FGFR3* hotspot mutations in combination with WES to screen diagnostic tumour tissue taken at transurethral resection (TUR) in 60 patients with MIBC, comprising of 50 commencing NAC and 10 commencing palliative chemotherapy. Using the three assays, at least one mutation was found in 19/60 patients (31.7%). WES was additionally performed on tissue from 24 patients and aberrations identified in 100%. The authors went on to design 84 personalised assays for 61 genes for a final cohort of 26 patients. Of note, only 2/26 (7.7%) had aberrations identified using only the PIK3CA/FGFR3 assays. Plasma and urine samples were tested although longitudinal results were available only for plasma. Blood was taken at pre-defined time points during treatment and follow-up.

Of the 24 patients proceeding to radical cystectomy following chemotherapy, 12/24 (50%) relapsed at a median of 275 days. In 6/12 (50%) of relapsing patients, ctDNA was detectable at a median of 137 days resulting in a median positive lead time of 101 days. However, ctDNA was also detected at some time point in 50% of patients who remained disease-free post-surgery, so the presence of ctDNA post-cystectomy is not specific for relapse [49]. However, the authors noted a significant association between high plasma ctDNA levels in samples taken at one week to four months post-cystectomy, and disease relapse, thus suggesting that ctDNA may allow more sensitive detection of disease recurrence post-surgery, and may be useful in the selection of patients for further treatment. Samples taken before, during, and after treatment for disease relapse were also analysed with an overall decrease in levels after 2–5 cycles of treatment correlating with radiological response, and subsequent increase in levels correlating with progression.

While this paper omits some technical details from its methodology, it sets the scene for the potential use of ctDNA in the post-operative setting to assess risk of recurrence and perhaps guide decisions on adjuvant treatment. Once again, the importance of selecting an appropriate panel of aberrations to target is highlighted, given that in 92.3%, personalised assay design was dependent upon data from whole exome sequencing.

The potential for ctDNA to detect recurrence before clinical or radiological confirmation was also demonstrated by Patel et al. [48]. In a cohort of 17 MIBC patients embarking on neoadjuvant platinum-based chemotherapy, the authors performed tagged amplicon sequencing (TAm-Seq) using a bladder cancer-specific panel of eight genes to detect mutant DNA in TUR tumour tissue, plasma, urinary cell pellet (UCP), and urinary supernatant (USN). The eight genes were BRAF, CTNNB1, FGFR3, HRAS, KRAS, NFE2L2, PIK3CA, and TP53, and were anticipated to encompass 72% of patients based upon TCGA data. A TERT promoter assay did not perform well and so was excluded. They also performed shallow whole genome sequencing in order to assess copy number alterations (CNAs). Samples were collected over a median period of 83 days from commencing NAC, with a median of 15 samples per patient. Patients were followed up for a median of 742 days from commencing NAC, and 588 days after completing definitive therapy.

On sequencing the available tumour tissue from 16 patients, single nucleotide variations (SNVs) were detected in 12/16 (75%) patients. The most frequent SNVs were in TP53, KRAS, and PIK3CA. Copy number alterations were identified in all 16 TUR samples, with the most frequent being CDKN2A loss, E2F3/SOX4 gain, and PPARG gain.

Subsequent testing in plasma, UCP, and USN in the 12 patients with tumour tissue SNVs showed detection of mutant DNA in 4/12 (33%), 5/12 (42%), and 5/12 (42%), respectively. CNAs were detected in 4/16 (33%), 8/15 (53%), and 8/16 (50%) of plasma, UCP, and USN samples, respectively. Of note, shallow WGS on serial samples from five patients showed evidence of tumour evolution under the selective pressure of NAC. Overall, aberrations were detected in 10/17 (59%) patients in plasma and urine samples taken prior to commencing NAC. Detection of aberrations at this point did not predict the response to treatment. However, upon analysing samples taken prior to cycle two NAC, the authors found that mutant DNA was present in 5/6 (83%) patients that relapsed, but was not detected in relapse-free patients (specificity 100%, sensitivity 83%). The median lead time over radiological diagnosis of progression was 243 days. Of note, of the five patients with mutant DNA present, only one patient had aberrations detected in plasma. Overall, higher levels of detection were noted in urine compared with plasma, although no single sample type captured all the aberrations present [48].

Although this was a relatively small cohort, the comprehensive assessment of plasma and urine shows great promise for ctDNA as a potential biomarker of response to treatment in the radical setting, and suggests that assessment of both plasma and urine is warranted at least in the neoadjuvant setting. In both these studies, it is again demonstrated that the optimal panel of genes and platform to interrogate MIBC remains unclear with PIK3CA and FGFR3 assays allowing ctDNA analysis in only 7.7%, and a combination of eight TAm-Seq assays and shallow WGS detecting ctDNA in 59%. However, with sequencing costs continuing to fall, it may be that broad approaches such as WES, which identified aberrations in 100% of tumour tissue samples, become more accessible. This strategy, however, would depend upon the availability of contemporary tissue samples and would thus likely necessitate repeat biopsies, particularly in those previously treated or with relapsed disease, which may be neither achievable on a practical level nor acceptable to patients.

Another question to consider is whether the identification of aberrations in tumour tissue first is necessary or indeed useful given potential intra-tumour heterogeneity and tumour evolution over time. Cheng et al. [52] used the 341–468 gene MSK IMPACT panel to profile plasma samples from 26 patients with metastatic urothelial cancer. At least one mutation was detected in 18/26 (69%). For 15 patients, archived tumour tissue was also sequenced using the same panel. The interval between tissue and plasma sampling ranged from 35 days to >4 years, and 11/15 patients had received treatment during this period. They reported that the tissue and plasma profiles were identical in only 3/15 (20%) of patients where the interval between samples ranged from 35 days to <1.5 years. Six out of fifteen (40%) had mutations identified in plasma, but not in tissue, and vice versa in 11/15 (73%). They concluded that the differences may reflect tumour evolution or intratumour heterogeneity. It may then be that sequencing archived tissue to detect aberrations of interest may not always identify the most appropriate targets in ctDNA, and may not be the ideal strategy particularly in patients who have received treatment or demonstrated a change in disease status in the intervening period. In these situations, upfront analysis of ctDNA is an attractive option, particularly when repeat up to date tissue biopsies are not possible.

4.4. Using a MIBC-Specific Panel to Sequence Plasma Upfront

Vandekerkhove et al. [47] designed a 50-gene bladder cancer-specific panel based upon published data on recurrent mutations and copy number changes in bladder cancer, including the TCGA report. In designing the panel, the authors noted that 98% of patients from the TCGA MIBC dataset (consisting primarily of subjects with non-metastatic disease) had a non-synonymous mutation in at least one of the 50 genes included on their panel. With target depth of 500–1000×, aberrations would be detected in those with tumour fraction of 5% or more.

Fifty-one patients with MIBC were recruited, including 37 with nodal or distant metastases. Plasma from all those with nodal or distant metastases, and seven with organ-confined disease were sequenced using the targeted panel. Overall, 25/44 (56.8%) patients demonstrated a ctDNA fraction above the 2% detection threshold set. The tumour fraction ranged from 3.9 to 72.6% with all samples demonstrating greater than 30% tumour fraction originating from patients with distant metastatic disease. In those with tumour fractions between 3.9–30%, 52% had distant metastatic disease. Only one of the seven patients with localised disease had detectable ctDNA [47]. This association of higher tumour content with higher disease burden is in keeping with previous work in other tumour types [7]. In three patients with metastatic disease where ctDNA was detected at more than one time-point over the course of chemotherapy, aberrations identified were consistent [47]. Frequently mutated genes included TP53, PIK3CA, and ARID1A; over 50% of patients had chromatin-modifying gene aberrations and this work has demonstrated that like the commercially available panels, upfront NGS analysis of plasma cDNA can identify potentially actionable aberrations. Of note, the only recurrent mutations seen were known hotspot regions in ERBB2, PIK3CA, and the TERT promoter. All other mutations were unique to individual patients and this highlights the incredible (and challenging) heterogeneity seen in MIBC.

Whole exome sequencing was also performed on 11 samples with tumour fraction over 25% from eight patients, with the primary aim of comparing mutation rates derived from the targeted sequencing data with that from WES data. The WES results correlated with targeted sequencing data, although the difference in sequencing depth meant that mutations seen on targeted panel were not always called on exome data [47]. Mutation rates derived from whole exome data and targeted sequencing data were also correlated, which is of interest given that mutational burden has been put forward as a predictor of response to immune checkpoint agents. The potential to assess mutational burden on a plasma sample rather than tissue biopsy is a potential advantage in the clinical trial setting, where patients may not otherwise be able or willing to undergo an invasive procedure as part of trial entry.

5. Conclusions

In the last two years, significant progress has been made in the field of ctDNA in MIBC and the knowledge base has grown rapidly. We have seen that ctDNA can be detected, with varying degrees of sensitivity, in the plasma and urine of patients with localised and metastatic MIBC. The levels detected have been demonstrated to be associated with tumour burden and while samples taken at one time-point are able to allow the identification of potentially actionable aberrations, the real value of ctDNA lies in the ease of obtaining sequential samples. By analysing samples taken over a course of treatment or during follow-up, early results in small trials suggest that the presence of ctDNA may indicate minimal residual disease following surgery, or predict for future disease recurrence with greater sensitivity than that offered by current standard radiological assessment. This is hugely exciting and the implications are potentially practice changing, but there is much work to be done before ctDNA can be applied in the clinical setting.

A key challenge is in refining the detection of ctDNA. MIBC is somewhat unique from other cancer types where ctDNA research is perhaps more established. Whereas a select few assays, for example, *APC* or *KRAS* mutations in colorectal cancer, *BRAF* in melanoma encompass a significant proportion of patients, and are thus reliable aberrations to use a surrogate for tumour fraction, the equivalent targets have yet to be demonstrated in MIBC. While this is in part because of the heterogeneity of the disease, it is also likely attributable to the fact that the molecular landscape of MIBC was only more recently explored when compared with other cancer subtypes. It has since been put forward that 90% MIBC patients have at least one mutation in hotspot regions of *PIK3CA, TP53*, or the *TERT* promoter, and so a panel encompassing these should be of relevance to the vast majority [23]. While these genes were included in the 50-gene bladder cancer specific panel by Vandekerkhove et al. [47], the detection threshold set of 2% for tumour fraction likely accounts for their plasma ctDNA detection rate of 56.8% falling short of the theoretical 90% described. It will be of great interest to see whether more sensitive methods, for example, ddPCR assays for this three-gene panel, will indeed encompass the majority of MIBC patients, including those with localised disease where low tumour fractions make detection more technically challenging. Furthermore, the use of so-called molecular barcodes, as recently explored in MIBC samples, offer another method to improve detection thresholds [54].

A unique feature of bladder cancer is the availability of ctDNA in urine. We have seen that ctDNA was more readily detectable in urine in a cohort of patients undergoing neoadjuvant treatment [48], and it seems reasonable to suggest that this is by virtue of the close proximity of the primary tumour to urine, i.e., the shedding of tumour DNA fragments directly into urine. It may well be that urinary ctDNA is most relevant in patients with localised disease, while plasma ctDNA reflects the systemic burden of disease.

While great promise is shown in the use of ctDNA to detect recurrence earlier than current standard approaches, an important consideration is also whether or not detecting recurrence earlier has any impact on clinical outcomes, and this can only be determined through prospective clinical trials.

MIBC is rapidly catching up with other more established tumour sites in the field of ctDNA research, and the clinical implications are huge in this poor prognosis disease where there are currently no biomarkers in everyday clinical use. By fully harnessing the potential of ctDNA, a truly personalised approach bypassing spatial and temporal barriers in cancer research appears possible and is key in furthering our understanding of MIBC and ultimately improving clinical outcomes.

Abbreviations

bp	Base pairs
cDNA	Circulating DNA
ctDNA	Circulating tumour DNA
CNA	Copy number alteration
MIBC	Muscle-invasive bladder cancer
NAC	Neoadjuvant chemotherapy
NGS	Next generation sequencing
PCR	Polymerase chain reaction
TUR	Transurethral resection
SNV	Single nucleotide variant
WES	Whole exome sequencing
WGS	Whole genome sequencing

References

1. Chan, K.C.; Jiang, P.; Zheng, Y.W.; Liao, G.J.; Sun, H.; Wong, J.; Siu, S.S.; Chan, W.C.; Chan, S.L.; Chan, A.T.; et al. Cancer genome scanning in plasma: Detection of tumor-associated copy number aberrations, single-nucleotide variants, and tumoral heterogeneity by massively parallel sequencing. *Clin. Chem.* **2013**, *59*, 211–224. [CrossRef] [PubMed]

2. Murtaza, M.; Dawson, S.J.; Pogrebniak, K.; Rueda, O.M.; Provenzano, E.; Grant, J.; Chin, S.F.; Tsui, D.W.; Marass, F.; Gale, D.; et al. Multifocal clonal evolution characterized using circulating tumour DNA in a case of metastatic breast cancer. *Nat. Commun.* **2015**, *6*, 8760. [CrossRef] [PubMed]

3. Diehl, F.; Li, M.; Dressman, D.; He, Y.; Shen, D.; Szabo, S.; Diaz, L.A., Jr.; Goodman, S.N.; David, K.A.; Juhl, H.; et al. Detection and quantification of mutations in the plasma of patients with colorectal tumors. *Proc. Natl. Acad. Sci. USA* **2005**, *102*, 16368–16373. [CrossRef] [PubMed]

4. Dawson, S.J.; Tsui, D.W.; Murtaza, M.; Biggs, H.; Rueda, O.M.; Chin, S.F.; Dunning, M.J.; Gale, D.; Forshew, T.; Mahler-Araujo, B.; et al. Analysis of circulating tumor DNA to monitor metastatic breast cancer. *N. Engl. J. Med.* **2013**, *368*, 1199–1209. [CrossRef] [PubMed]

5. Romanel, A.; Tandefelt, D.G.; Conteduca, V.; Jayaram, A.; Casiraghi, N.; Wetterskog, D.; Salvi, S.; Amadori, D.; Zafeiriou, Z.; Rescigno, P.; et al. Plasma AR abiraterone-resistant prostate cancer. *Sci. Transl. Med.* **2015**, *7*, 312. [CrossRef] [PubMed]

6. Jamal-Hanjani, M.; Wilson, G.A.; Horswell, S.; Mitter, R.; Sakarya, O.; Constantin, T.; Salari, R.; Kirkizlar, E.; Sigurjonsson, S.; Pelham, R.; et al. Detection of ubiquitous and heterogeneous mutations in cell-free DNA from patients with early-stage non-small-cell lung cancer. *Ann. Oncol.* **2016**, *27*, 862–867. [CrossRef] [PubMed]

7. Bettegowda, C.; Sausen, M.; Leary, R.J.; Kinde, I.; Wang, Y.; Agrawal, N.; Bartlett, B.R.; Wang, H.; Luber, B.; Alani, R.M.; et al. Detection of circulating tumor DNA in early- and late-stage human malignancies. *Sci. Transl. Med.* **2014**, *6*, 224. [CrossRef] [PubMed]

8. Parkinson, C.A.; Gale, D.; Piskorz, A.M.; Biggs, H.; Hodgkin, C.; Addley, H.; Freeman, S.; Moyle, P.; Sala, E.; Sayal, K.; et al. Exploratory analysis of tp53 mutations in circulating tumour DNA as biomarkers of treatment

response for patients with relapsed high-grade serous ovarian carcinoma: A retrospective study. *PLoS Med.* **2016**, *13*, e1002198. [CrossRef] [PubMed]

9. Diehl, F.; Schmidt, K.; Choti, M.A.; Romans, K.; Goodman, S.; Li, M.; Thornton, K.; Agrawal, N.; Sokoll, L.; Szabo, S.A.; et al. Circulating mutant DNA to assess tumor dynamics. *Nat. Med.* **2008**, *14*, 985–990. [CrossRef] [PubMed]

10. Garcia-Murillas, I.; Schiavon, G.; Weigelt, B.; Ng, C.; Hrebien, S.; Cutts, R.J.; Cheang, M.; Osin, P.; Nerurkar, A.; Kozarewa, I.; et al. Mutation tracking in circulating tumor DNA predicts relapse in early breast cancer. *Sci. Transl. Med.* **2015**, *7*, 302. [CrossRef] [PubMed]

11. Murtaza, M.; Dawson, S.J.; Tsui, D.W.; Gale, D.; Forshew, T.; Piskorz, A.M.; Parkinson, C.; Chin, S.F.; Kingsbury, Z.; Wong, A.S.; et al. Non-invasive analysis of acquired resistance to cancer therapy by sequencing of plasma DNA. *Nature* **2013**, *497*, 108–112. [CrossRef] [PubMed]

12. Carreira, S.; Romanel, A.; Goodall, J.; Grist, E.; Ferraldeschi, R.; Miranda, S.; Prandi, D.; Lorente, D.; Frenel, J.S.; Pezaro, C.; et al. Tumor clone dynamics in lethal prostate cancer. *Sci. Transl. Med.* **2014**, *6*, 254. [CrossRef] [PubMed]

13. Abbosh, C.; Birkbak, N.J.; Wilson, G.A.; Jamal-Hanjani, M.; Constantin, T.; Salari, R.; Quesne, J.L.; Moore, D.A.; Veeriah, S.; Rosenthal, R.; et al. Phylogenetic ctdna analysis depicts early stage lung cancer evolution. *Nature* **2017**, *545*, 446. [CrossRef] [PubMed]

14. Peng, M.; Chen, C.; Hulbert, A.; Brock, M.V.; Yu, F. Non-blood circulating tumor DNA detection in cancer. *Oncotarget* **2017**, *8*, 69162–69173. [CrossRef] [PubMed]

15. Schwarzenbach, H.; Hoon, D.S.; Pantel, K. Cell-free nucleic acids as biomarkers in cancer patients. *Nat. Rev. Cancer* **2011**, *11*, 426–437. [CrossRef] [PubMed]

16. Wan, J.C.M.; Massie, C.; Garcia-Corbacho, J.; Mouliere, F.; Brenton, J.D.; Caldas, C.; Pacey, S.; Baird, R.; Rosenfeld, N. Liquid biopsies come of age: Towards implementation of circulating tumour DNA. *Nat. Rev. Cancer* **2017**, *17*, 223–238. [CrossRef] [PubMed]

17. Ellinger, J.; Muller, S.C.; Stadler, T.C.; Jung, A.; von Ruecker, A.; Bastian, P.J. The role of cell-free circulating DNA in the diagnosis and prognosis of prostate cancer. *Urol. Oncol.* **2011**, *29*, 124–129. [CrossRef] [PubMed]

18. Cargnin, S.; Canonico, P.L.; Genazzani, A.A.; Terrazzino, S. Quantitative analysis of circulating cell-free DNA for correlation with lung cancer survival: A systematic review and meta-analysis. *J. Thorac. Oncol.* **2017**, *12*, 43–53. [CrossRef] [PubMed]

19. Valpione, S.; Gremel, G.; Mundra, P.; Middlehurst, P.; Galvani, E.; Girotti, M.R.; Lee, R.J.; Garner, G.; Dhomen, N.; Lorigan, P.C.; et al. Plasma total cell-free DNA (cfDNA) is a surrogate biomarker for tumour burden and a prognostic biomarker for survival in metastatic melanoma patients. *Eur. J. Cancer* **2018**, *88*, 1–9. [CrossRef] [PubMed]

20. Newman, A.M.; Bratman, S.V.; To, J.; Wynne, J.F.; Eclov, N.C.; Modlin, L.A.; Liu, C.L.; Neal, J.W.; Wakelee, H.A.; Merritt, R.E.; et al. An ultrasensitive method for quantitating circulating tumor DNA with broad patient coverage. *Nat. Med.* **2014**, *20*, 548–554. [CrossRef] [PubMed]

21. McGregor, B.A.; Chung, J.; Bergerot, P.G.; Forcier, B.; Grivas, P.; Choueiri, T.K.; Ross, J.S.; Ali, S.M.; Stephens, P.J.; Miller, V.A.; et al. Correlation of circulating tumor DNA (ctDNA) ssessment with tissue-based comprehensive genomic profiling (CGP) in metastatic urothelial cancer (MUC). *J. Clin. Oncol.* **2018**, *36*, 453. [CrossRef]

22. Adalsteinsson, V.A.; Ha, G.; Freeman, S.S.; Choudhury, A.D.; Stover, D.G.; Parsons, H.A.; Gydush, G.; Reed, S.C.; Rotem, D.; Rhoades, J.; et al. Scalable whole-exome sequencing of cell-free DNA reveals high concordance with metastatic tumors. *Nat. Commun.* **2017**, *8*, 1324. [CrossRef] [PubMed]

23. Todenhofer, T.; Struss, W.J.; Seiler, R.; Wyatt, A.W.; Black, P.C. Liquid biopsy-analysis of circulating tumor DNA (ctDNA) in bladder cancer. *Bladder Cancer* **2018**, *4*, 19–29. [CrossRef] [PubMed]

24. Mouliere, F.; Robert, B.; Arnau Peyrotte, E.; Del Rio, M.; Ychou, M.; Molina, F.; Gongora, C.; Thierry, A.R. High fragmentation characterizes tumour-derived circulating DNA. *PLoS ONE* **2011**, *6*, e23418. [CrossRef] [PubMed]

25. Volik, S.; Alcaide, M.; Morin, R.D.; Collins, C. Cell-free DNA (cfDNA): Clinical significance and utility in cancer shaped by emerging technologies. *Mol. Cancer Res.* **2016**, *14*, 898–908. [CrossRef] [PubMed]

26. Thierry, A.R.; El Messaoudi, S.; Gahan, P.B.; Anker, P.; Stroun, M. Origins, structures, and functions of circulating DNA in oncology. *Cancer Metastasis Rev.* **2016**, *35*, 347–376. [CrossRef] [PubMed]

27. Underhill, H.R.; Kitzman, J.O.; Hellwig, S.; Welker, N.C.; Daza, R.; Baker, D.N.; Gligorich, K.M.; Rostomily, R.C.; Bronner, M.P.; Shendure, J. Fragment length of circulating tumor DNA. *PLoS Genet.* **2016**, *12*, e1006162. [CrossRef] [PubMed]

28. Conteduca, V.; Wetterskog, D.; Sharabiani, M.T.A.; Grande, E.; Fernandez-Perez, M.P.; Jayaram, A.; Salvi, S.; Castellano, D.; Romanel, A.; Lolli, C.; et al. Androgen receptor gene status in plasma DNA associates with worse outcome on enzalutamide or abiraterone for castration-resistant prostate cancer: A multi-institution correlative biomarker study. *Ann. Oncol.* **2017**, *28*, 1508–1516. [CrossRef] [PubMed]

29. Stein, J.P.; Lieskovsky, G.; Cote, R.; Groshen, S.; Feng, A.C.; Boyd, S.; Skinner, E.; Bochner, B.; Thangathurai, D.; Mikhail, M.; et al. Radical cystectomy in the treatment of invasive bladder cancer: Long-term results in 1054 patients. *J. Clin. Oncol.* **2001**, *19*, 666–675. [CrossRef] [PubMed]

30. Robertson, A.G.; Kim, J.; Al-Ahmadie, H.; Bellmunt, J.; Guo, G.; Cherniack, A.D.; Hinoue, T.; Laird, P.W.; Hoadley, K.A.; Akbani, R.; et al. Comprehensive molecular characterization of muscle-invasive bladder cancer. *Cell* **2017**, *171*, 540–556. [CrossRef] [PubMed]

31. Choi, W.; Porten, S.; Kim, S.; Willis, D.; Plimack, E.R.; Hoffman-Censits, J.; Roth, B.; Cheng, T.; Tran, M.; Lee, I.L.; et al. Identification of distinct basal and luminal subtypes of muscle-invasive bladder cancer with different sensitivities to frontline chemotherapy. *Cancer Cell* **2014**, *25*, 152–165. [CrossRef] [PubMed]

32. Seiler, R.; Ashab, H.A.; Erho, N.; van Rhijn, B.W.; Winters, B.; Douglas, J.; Van Kessel, K.E.; Fransen van de Putte, E.E.; Sommerlad, M.; Wang, N.Q.; et al. Impact of molecular subtypes in muscle-invasive bladder cancer on predicting response and survival after neoadjuvant chemotherapy. *Eur. Urol.* **2017**, *72*, 544–554. [CrossRef] [PubMed]

33. Alfred Witjes, J.; Lebret, T.; Comperat, E.M.; Cowan, N.C.; De Santis, M.; Bruins, H.M.; Hernandez, V.; Espinos, E.L.; Dunn, J.; Rouanne, M.; et al. Updated 2016 eau guidelines on muscle-invasive and metastatic bladder cancer. *Eur. Urol.* **2017**, *71*, 462–475. [CrossRef] [PubMed]

34. Chang, S.S.; Bochner, B.H.; Chou, R.; Dreicer, R.; Kamat, A.M.; Lerner, S.P.; Lotan, Y.; Meeks, J.J.; Michalski, J.M.; Morgan, T.M.; et al. Treatment of non-metastatic muscle-invasive bladder cancer: Aua/asco/astro/suo guideline. *J. Urol.* **2017**, *198*, 552–559. [CrossRef] [PubMed]

35. Zargar, H.; Espiritu, P.N.; Fairey, A.S.; Mertens, L.S.; Dinney, C.P.; Mir, M.C.; Krabbe, L.M.; Cookson, M.S.; Jacobsen, N.E.; Gandhi, N.M.; et al. Multicenter assessment of neoadjuvant chemotherapy for muscle-invasive bladder cancer. *Eur. Urol.* **2015**, *67*, 241–249. [CrossRef] [PubMed]

36. Zargar, H.; Shah, J.B.; van Rhijn, B.W.; Daneshmand, S.; Bivalacqua, T.J.; Spiess, P.E.; Black, P.C.; Kassouf, W. Neoadjuvant dose dense mvac versus gemcitabine and cisplatin in patients with cT3-4aN0M0 bladder cancer treated with radical cystectomy. *J. Urol.* **2018**, *199*, 1452–1458. [CrossRef] [PubMed]

37. Lee, C.T.; Madii, R.; Daignault, S.; Dunn, R.L.; Zhang, Y.; Montie, J.E.; Wood, D.P. Cystectomy delay more than 3 months from initial bladder cancer diagnosis results in decreased disease specific and overall survival. *J. Urol.* **2006**, *175*, 1262–1267. [CrossRef]

38. Sidransky, D.; Voneschenbach, A.; Tsai, Y.C.; Jones, P.; Summerhayes, I.; Marshall, F.; Paul, M.; Green, P.; Hamilton, S.R.; Frost, P.; et al. Identification of p53 gene-mutations in bladder cancers and urine samples. *Science* **1991**, *252*, 706–709. [CrossRef] [PubMed]

39. Utting, M.; Werner, W.; Dahse, R.; Schubert, J.; Junker, K. Microsatellite analysis of free tumor DNA in urine, serum and plasma of patients: A minimally invasive method for the detection fo bladder cancer. *Clin. Cancer Res.* **2002**, *8*, 35–40. [PubMed]

40. Ellinger, J.; Bastian, P.J.; Ellinger, N.; Kahl, P.; Perabo, F.G.; Buttner, R.; Muller, S.C.; Ruecker, A. Apoptotic DNA fragments in serum of patients with muscle invasive bladder cancer: A prognostic entity. *Cancer Lett.* **2008**, *264*, 274–280. [CrossRef] [PubMed]

41. Knowles, M.A.; Hurst, C.D. Molecular biology of bladder cancer: New insights into pathogenesis and clinical diversity. *Nat. Rev. Cancer* **2015**, *15*, 25–41. [CrossRef] [PubMed]

42. Sonpavde, G.; Nagy, R.; Apolo, N.; Pal, S.; Grivas, P.; Vaishampayan, U.; Lanman, R.; Talasaz, A. Circulating cell-free DNA profiling of patients with advanced urothelial carcinoma. *J. Clin. Oncol.* **2016**, *34*, 358. [CrossRef]

43. Agarwal, N.; Pal, S.K.; Hahn, A.W.; Nussenzveig, R.H.; Pond, G.R.; Gupta, S.V.; Wang, J.; Bilen, M.A.; Naik, G.; Ghatalia, P.; et al. Characterization of metastatic urothelial carcinoma via comprehensive genomic profiling of circulating tumor DNA. *Cancer* **2018**, *124*, 2115–2124. [CrossRef] [PubMed]

44. Van Allen, E.M.; Mouw, K.W.; Kim, P.; Iyer, G.; Wagle, N.; Al-Ahmadie, H.; Zhu, C.; Ostrovnaya, I.; Kryukov, G.V.; O'Connor, K.W.; et al. Somatic *ERCC2* mutations correlate with cisplatin sensitivity in muscle-invasive urothelial carcinoma. *Cancer Discov.* **2014**, *4*, 1140–1153. [CrossRef] [PubMed]

45. Birkenkamp-Demtröder, K.; Nordentoft, I.; Christensen, E.; Hoyer, S.; Reinert, T.; Vang, S.; Borre, M.; Agerbaek, M.; Jensen, J.B.; Orntoft, T.F.; et al. Genomic alterations in liquid biopsies from patients with bladder cancer. *Eur. Urol.* **2016**, *70*, 75–82. [CrossRef] [PubMed]

46. Christensen, E.; Birkenkamp-Demtröder, K.; Nordentoft, I.; Hoyer, S.; van der Keur, K.; van Kessel, K.; Zwarthoff, E.; Agerbaek, M.; Orntoft, T.F.; Jensen, J.B.; et al. Liquid biopsy analysis of *FGFR3* and *PIK3CA* hotspot mutations for disease surveillance in bladder cancer. *Eur. Urol.* **2017**, *71*, 961–969. [CrossRef] [PubMed]

47. Vandekerkhove, G.; Todenhofer, T.; Annala, M.; Struss, W.J.; Wong, A.; Beja, K.; Ritch, E.; Brahmbhatt, S.; Volik, S.V.; Hennenlotter, J.; et al. Circulating tumor DNA reveals clinically actionable somatic genome of metastatic bladder cancer. *Clin. Cancer Res.* **2017**, *23*, 6487–6497. [CrossRef] [PubMed]

48. Patel, K.M.; van der Vos, K.E.; Smith, C.G.; Mouliere, F.; Tsui, D.; Morris, J.; Chandrananda, D.; Marass, F.; van den Broek, D.; Neal, D.E.; et al. Association of plasma and urinary mutant DNA with clinical outcomes in muscle invasive bladder cancer. *Sci. Rep.* **2017**, *7*, 5554. [CrossRef] [PubMed]

49. Birkenkamp-Demtröder, K.; Christensen, E.; Nordentoft, I.; Knudsen, M.; Taber, A.; Hoyer, S.; Lamy, P.; Agerbaek, M.; Jensen, J.B.; Dyrskjot, L. Monitoring treatment response and metastatic relapse in advanced bladder cancer by liquid biopsy analysis. *Eur. Urol.* **2017**, *73*, 535–540. [CrossRef] [PubMed]

50. Barata, P.C.; Koshkin, V.S.; Funchain, P.; Sohal, D.; Pritchard, A.; Klek, S.; Adamowicz, T.; Gopalakrishnan, D.; Garcia, J.; Rini, B.; et al. Next-generation sequencing (NGS) of cell-free circulating tumor DNA and tumor tissue in patients with advanced urothelial cancer: A pilot assessment of concordance. *Ann. Oncol.* **2017**, *28*, 2458–2463. [CrossRef] [PubMed]

51. Soave, A.; Chun, F.K.; Hillebrand, T.; Rink, M.; Weisbach, L.; Steinbach, B.; Fisch, M.; Pantel, K.; Schwarzenbach, H. Copy number variations of circulating, cell-free DNA in urothelial carcinoma of the bladder patients treated with radical cystectomy: A prospective study. *Oncotarget* **2017**, *8*, 56398–56407. [CrossRef] [PubMed]

52. Cheng, M.L.; Shady, M.; Cipolla, C.K.; Funt, S.; Arcila, M.E.; Al-Ahmadie, H.; Rosenberg, J.E.; Bajorin, D.F.; Berger, M.F.; Tsui, D.; et al. Comparison of somatic mutation profiles from cell free DNA (cfDNA) versus tissue in metastatic urothelial carcinoma (MUC). *J. Clin. Oncol.* **2017**, *35*, 4533.

53. National Cancer Institute GDC Data Portal. Available online: https://portal.gdc.cancer.gov/ (accessed on 15 July 2018).

54. Christensen, E.; Nordentoft, I.; Vang, S.; Birkenkamp-Demtröder, K.; Jensen, J.B.; Agerbaek, M.; Pedersen, J.S.; Dyrskjot, L. Optimized targeted sequencing of cell-free plasma DNA from bladder cancer patients. *Sci. Rep.* **2018**, *8*, 1917. [CrossRef] [PubMed]

mRNA-Expression of *KRT5* and *KRT20* Defines Distinct Prognostic Subgroups of Muscle-Invasive Urothelial Bladder Cancer Correlating with Histological Variants

Markus Eckstein [1,*,†], Ralph Markus Wirtz [2,3,†], Matthias Gross-Weege [4,†], Johannes Breyer [5,†], Wolfgang Otto [5,†], Robert Stoehr [1,†], Danijel Sikic [6,†], Bastian Keck [6,†], Sebastian Eidt [3,†], Maximilian Burger [5,†], Christian Bolenz [7,†], Katja Nitschke [4,†], Stefan Porubsky [8,†], Arndt Hartmann [1,†] and Philipp Erben [4,†]

[1] Institute of Pathology, University of Erlangen-Nuremberg, 91054 Erlangen, Germany; robert.stoehr@uk-erlangen.de (R.S.); arndt.hartmann@uk-erlangen.de (A.H.)
[2] STRATIFYER Molecular Pathology GmbH, 50935 Cologne, Germany; ralph.wirtz@stratifyer.de
[3] Institute of Pathology at the St Elisabeth Hospital Köln-Hohenlind, 50935 Cologne, Germany; Sebastian.eidt@stratifyer.de
[4] Department of Urology, University Medical Centre Mannheim, Medical Faculty Mannheim, University of Heidelberg, 68167 Mannheim, Germany; matthias.gross-weege@umm.de (M.G.-W.); katja.nitschke@medma.uni-heidelberg.de (K.N.); Philipp.Erben@medma.uni-heidelberg.de (P.E.)
[5] Department of Urology, University of Regensburg, 93053 Regensburg, Germany; Johannes.breyer@ukr.de (J.B.); wolfgang.otto@ukr.de (W.O.); maximilian.burger@ukr.de (M.B.)
[6] Department of Urology and Pediatric Urology, University Hospital Erlangen, 91058 Erlangen, Germany; danijel.sikic@uk-erlangen.de (D.S.); Bastian.keck@web.de (B.K.)
[7] Department of Urology, University of Ulm, 89081 Ulm, Germany; Christian.Bolenz@uniklinik-ulm.de
[8] Department of Pathology, University Medical Centre Mannheim, Medical Faculty Mannheim, University of Heidelberg, 68167 Mannheim, Germany; Stefan.porubsky@medma.uni-heidelberg.de
* Correspondence: markus.eckstein@uk-erlangen.de
† On behalf of the BRIDGE Consortium.

Abstract: Recently, muscle-invasive bladder cancer (MIBC) has been subclassified by gene expression profiling, with a substantial impact on therapy response and patient outcome. We tested whether these complex molecular subtypes of MIBC can be determined by mRNA detection of keratin 5 (*KRT5*) and keratin 20 (*KRT20*). Reverse transcriptase quantitative polymerase chain reaction (RT-qPCR) was applied to quantify gene expression of *KRT5* and *KRT20* using TaqMan®-based assays in 122 curatively treated MIBC patients (median age 68.0 years). Furthermore, in silico analysis of the MD Anderson Cancer Center (MDACC) cohort (GSE48277 + GSE47993) was performed. High expression of *KRT5* and low expression of *KRT20* were associated with significantly improved recurrence-free survival (RFS) and disease-specific survival disease specific survival (DSS: 5-year DSS for *KRT5* high: 58%; 5-year DSS for *KRT20* high: 29%). *KRT5* and *KRT20* were associated with rates of lymphovascular invasion and lymphonodal metastasis. The combination of *KRT5* and *KRT20* allowed identification of patients with a very poor prognosis (*KRT20*+/*KRT5*−, 5-year DSS 0%, $p < 0.0001$). In silico analysis of the independent MDACC cohorts revealed congruent results (5-year DSS for *KRT20* low vs. high: 84% vs. 40%, $p = 0.042$). High *KRT20*-expressing tumors as well as *KRT20*+/*KRT*− tumors were significantly enriched with aggressive urothelial carcinoma variants (micropapillary, plasmacytoid, nested).

Keywords: Bladder cancer; muscle-invasive bladder cancer; molecular diagnostics; molecular subtyping; *KRT5*; *KRT20*

1. Introduction

Urothelial bladder cancer (UBC) is one of the 10 most common malignancies worldwide, with nearly 386,000 new cases and nearly 150,200 deaths per year [1]. Non-muscle-invasive bladder cancer (NMIBC) variants (70%) are not immediately life-threatening but often progress, while muscle-invasive bladder cancer (MIBC) tumors account only for nearly 30%, but are responsible for most deaths [2]. Due to the high cost of treatment modalities and the often necessary lifelong surveillance, UBC is one of the most expensive tumor entities [3].

The current standard of care in MIBC is radical cystectomy with perioperative platinum-based chemotherapy in selected cases. At present, clinical management of MIBC suffers from two major problems: First, the therapy selection is heavily influenced by a limited clinicopathological staging system, resulting in high rates of inadequate treatment [4]. Second, due to limited insight into molecular variants, it is not yet possible to identify potential (chemo)therapy responders [2,5]. Therefore, several groups have started to characterize UBC by gene expression profiling, as was previously done for breast cancer [6,7], which identified highly prognostic molecular signatures [5,8–19]. The MD Anderson Cancer Center (MDACC) subtypes resembled those identified for breast cancer and showed typical mRNA expression profiles of basal and luminal markers, with keratin 5 (KRT5) expression being highly upregulated in basal and keratin 20 (KRT20) being upregulated in luminal tumors. The third subtype (p53-like) is characterized by either a luminal or basal expression profile and an activated p53 wild-type pathway, which might be caused by prominent immune cell infiltration [14,20]. Recently, we demonstrated the high prognostic relevance of assessing KRT5 and KRT20 expression in high-risk NMIBC [21]. High KRT5 mRNA expression identified a subgroup of nonluminal NMIBC that showed superior recurrence-free survival (RFS) and progression-free survival (PFS) despite being World Health Organization (WHO) grade 3 and stage pT1. In contrast, NMIBC with high KRT20 mRNA expression was accompanied by significantly increased rates of tumor progression.

Here, we tested whether molecular subtyping by KRT20 and KRT5 mRNA expression is also applicable in MIBC. The main aim of this study was to prove the possibility and feasibility of introducing those two markers into the clinicopathological routine.

2. Material and Methods

2.1. Patient Population, Specimen Collection, and Histopathological Evaluation

Formalin-fixed paraffin-embedded (FFPE) tumor tissue samples were obtained from 169 patients with histologically confirmed MIBC (pT2-4) who were treated with radical cystectomy in conjunction with bilateral lymphadenectomy at a single center between 1999 and 2007 by 2 oncological surgeons with substantial cystectomy experience. Thirty-two patients received adjuvant platinum-containing chemotherapy (in the final study cohort, 22 patients received adjuvant platinum-containing chemotherapy). None of the patients underwent neoadjuvant radiation or chemotherapy. Hematoxylin and Eosin stained HE sections were reevaluated according to the 2017 Union internationale contre le cancer (UICC) staging manual and graded according to the common grading systems (World Health Organization1973 and 2016) by 3 experienced uropathologists (A.H., S.P., M.E.) [22]. Primary squamous cell carcinomas, pure neuroendocrine carcinomas, tumors originating from other organs (metastases or arising from neighboring organs), samples with low calmodulin 2 (CALM2) housekeeping gene expression (Ct values $\geq$ 28.0) and cases with missing follow-up data were excluded (n = 47). The final cohort consisted of 122 patients. The median follow-up period was 26.5 months (range 0.7–180.8 months). Follow-up data were achieved from local tumor registries and clinical case files, and by telephone calls to last known treating private practices.

In total, 59 patients had a recurrence: 44 patients with distant metastases, 5 patients with isolated local recurrences with delayed distant metastases, and 10 patients with co-occurrence of local and distant recurrence. The date of recurrence was defined as first confirmation of local and/or distant metastasis. Most recurrences were confirmed by computed tomography, but due to the retrospective nature of this study, in several cases we did not know the modality of recurrence detection. None of the patients received local resection of local recurrences or distant metastases.

All patients gave informed consent, and the study was approved by the institutional review board under numbers 2013-517N-MA (approval date: 21.02.2013) and 2016-814R-MA (approval date: 05.04.2016). To validate RT-qPCR-data, array gene expression data (Illumina HumanHT-12 WG-DASL V4.0 R2 expression beadchip) of 44 MIBC patients from the MDACC cohort (GSE48276) were analyzed (median age 67.6, range 41–89.6 years) [14].

2.2. RNA Isolation from FFPE Tissue

RNA was extracted from FFPE tissue using 10 μm sections, which were processed in a fully automated manner by a commercially available bead-based extraction method (XTRACT kit; STRATIFYER Molecular Pathology GmbH, Cologne, Germany). RNA was eluted with 100 μL elution buffer and RNA eluates were analyzed. The section was taken from a paraffin block containing a tumor area of at least 5 × 5 mm with a total tumor content of at least 30% tumor cells.

2.3. mRNA Quantification by RT-qPCR

RT-qPCR was applied for relative quantification of *KRT5* and *KRT20* mRNA as well as *CALM2* (calmodulin 2; housekeeping gene) expression by using gene-specific TaqMan®-based assays as described previously [21,23]. *CALM2* is a stably expressed gene among breast cancer tumor tissue samples and has been applied successfully to bladder cancer specimens [21,24,25]. Each patient sample or control was analyzed in triplicate. Experiments were run on a Siemens Versant (Siemens, Germany) according to the following protocol: 5 min at 50 °C, 20 s at 95 °C, followed by 40 cycles of 15 s at 95 °C and 60 s at 60 °C. Forty amplification cycles were applied and the cycle quantification threshold (Ct) values of 3 markers and 1 reference gene for each sample were estimated as the mean of the 3 measurements. Ct values were normalized by subtracting the Ct value of the housekeeping gene CALM2 from the Ct value of the target gene (ΔCt).

2.4. Statistical Analysis

All *p*-values were calculated 2-sided, and values of <0.05 were considered to be significant. Survival analyses were performed by univariate Kaplan–Meier regressions and tested for significance with the log-rank. Results were considered to be significant if the test revealed significance levels <0.05. Multivariate analyses were performed by Cox proportional hazard regression model, including all relevant clinicopathological characteristics (pT-Stage, pN-Stage, lymphovascular invasion (L), blood vessel invasion (V), age, gender, receipt of adjuvant platinum-containing chemotherapy, status of resection margins, and tumor grading (WHO 2016 and WHO 1973)). Statistical analyses of numeric continuous variables were performed by nonparametric tests (Wilcoxon rank-sum test, Kruskal–Wallis test). Contingency analysis of nominal variables was performed by Pearson's chi-squared test. Correlation analysis of numeric continuous variables was performed using Spearman rank correlations. All statistical analyses were performed with GraphPad Prism 7.2 (GraphPad Software Inc., La Jolla, CA, USA) and JMP SAS 13.2 (SAS, Cary, NC, USA).

3. Results

3.1. Clinicopathological Data and Expression of KRT5 and KRT20 mRNA in MIBC

The distribution of clinicopathological data of the entire cohort and respective *KRT*-expression subgroups (*KRT5* high vs. low; *KRT20* high vs. low; Epi-Typer Class 1, Epi-Typer Class 2) including age, gender, pT-Stage, pN-Stage, and grading (WHO 1973, WHO 2004/2016) is depicted in Table 1.

Table 1. Clinicopathological characteristics of the Mannheim cohort (overall and respective subgroups). KRT, keratin; L, lymphovascular invasion; V, blood vessel invasion; R, resection margin; WHO, World Health Organization; n.s., not significant; G, Grade; T, Tumor. * p-Value a: $KRT5_{high}$ vs. $KRT5_{low}$; p-value b: $KRT20_{high}$ vs. $KRT20_{low}$.

Characteristic	Total	KRT5 High	KRT5 Low	KRT20 High	KRT20 Low	p-Value
Cohort size (n)	122	89	33	48	74	
Mean age (years)	67.9	67.9	68.4	67.5	67.9	a: n.s. b: n.s.
Gender (n)						
Male	89 (73%)	66 (74%)	23 (70%)	34 (71%)	55 (74%)	a: n.s.
Female	33 (27%)	23 (26%)	10 (30%)	14 (29%)	19 (26%)	b: n.s.
Adjuvant chemotherapy	22 (18%)	14 (16%)	8 (24%)	9 (19%)	13 (17%)	n.s.
Pathological characteristics						
pTis (concomitant)	43 (35%)	34 (38%)	9 (27%)	19 (40%)	24 (32%)	a: n.s. b: n.s.
pT2	33 (27%)	28 (31%)	5 (15%)	14 (29%)	19 (26%)	a: 0.027
pT3	62 (51%)	44 (50%)	18 (55%)	25 (52%)	37 (50%)	b: n.s.
pT4	27 (22%)	17 (19%)	10 (30%)	9 (19%)	18 (24%)	
pN0	74 (60%)	60 (67%)	14 (42%)	20 (42%)	54 (73%)	a: 0.0005
pN1-2	48 (37%)	29 (33%)	19 (57%)	28 (58%)	20 (27%)	b: 0.002
L0	62 (51%)	52 (58%)	10 (30%)	17 (35%)	45 (61%)	a: 0.005
L1	60 (49%)	37 (52%)	23 (70%)	31 (65%)	29 (39%)	b: 0.006
V0	104 (85%)	81 (91%)	23 (70%)	42 (87%)	61 (84%)	a: 0.005
V1	18 (15%)	8 (9%)	10 (30%)	6 (13%)	12 (16%)	b: n.s.
R0	105 (86%)	77 (86%)	28 (85%)	42 (88%)	63 (85%)	a: n.s.
R1	17 (14%)	12 (14%)	5 (15%)	6 (12%)	11 (15%)	b: n.s.
Grading						
WHO 1973						
G1	0 (0%)	0 (0%)	0 (0%)	0 (0%)	0 (0%)	
G2	27 (22%)	21 (24%)	6 (18%)	11 (23%)	16 (22%)	a: n.s.
G3	95 (78%)	68 (76%)	27 (82%)	37 (77%)	58 (78%)	b: n.s.
WHO 2004						
Low grade	0 (0%)	0 (0%)	0 (0%)	0 (0%)	0 (0%)	a: n.s.
High grade	122 (100%)	89 (100%)	33(100%)	48 (100%)	74 (100%)	b: n.s.

Characteristic	Epi-Typer Class 1	Epi-Typer Class 2		p-Value
Cohort size (n)	103	19		
Mean age (years)	67.9	71		n.s.
Gender (n)				
Male	75 (73%)	14 (74%)		n.s.
Female	28 (27%)	5 (26%)		
Adjuvant chemotherapy	17 (17%)	5 (26%)		n.s.
Pathological T stage				

Table 1. *Cont.*

Characteristic	Total	*KRT5* High	KRT5 Low	KRT20 High	KRT20 Low	*p*-Value
pTis (concomitant)		37 (36%)		6 (31%)		n.s.
pT2						
pT3						
pT4						
Pathological characteristics						
pN0		69 (67%)		5 (26%)		0.0009
pN1-2		34 (33%)		14 (74%)		
L0		58 (56%)		4 (21%)		0.004
L1		45 (44%)		15 (79%)		
V0		90 (87%)		14 (74%)		n.s.
V1		13 (13%)		5 (26%)		
R0		89 (86%)		16 (84%)		n.s.
R1		14 (14%)		3 (16%)		
Grading WHO 1973						
G1		0 (0%)		0 (0%)		n.s.
G2		22 (21%)		5 (26%)		n.s.
G3		81 (79%)		14 (74%)		n.s.
Grading WHO 2004						
Low grade		0 (0%)		0 (0%)		n.s.
High grade		103 (100%)		19 (100%)		n.s.

Distribution of clinic-pathological determinants across the entire cohort and respective subgroups. *p*-value a: $KRT5_{high}$ vs. $KRT5_{low}$; *p*-value b: $KRT20_{high}$ vs. $KRT20_{low}$.

Data distribution of normalized *KRT5* and *KRT20* expression levels had a broad dynamic range (Figure 1A). Expression of *KRT5* and *KRT20* correlated inversely ($r = -0.42$, $p < 0.0001$; Figure 1A). Consistent with previous studies, there was a significant association between high *KRT5* expression and squamous and sarcomatoid differentiation (Figure 1C) [14]. Tumors with variant histology (micropapillary, nested, plasmacytoid) showed an interesting keratin expression pattern: they showed high expression of *KRT20*, while the expression of *KRT5* was very low in these cases (Figure 1C,D). High expression of *KRT5* was associated with a lower rate of lymphovascular invasion (LVI) ($p = 0.0004$) and lymphonodal metastasis ($p = 0.002$; Figure 1B), while high *KRT20* expression correlated positively with LVI/nodal status (Figure 1B). Furthermore, luminal bladder cancer variants (micropapillary, plasmacytoid, nested) exhibited significantly lower levels of *KRT5* and significantly higher levels of *KRT20* expression than conventional UBC or basal variants (sarcomatoid, squamous; Figure 1E).

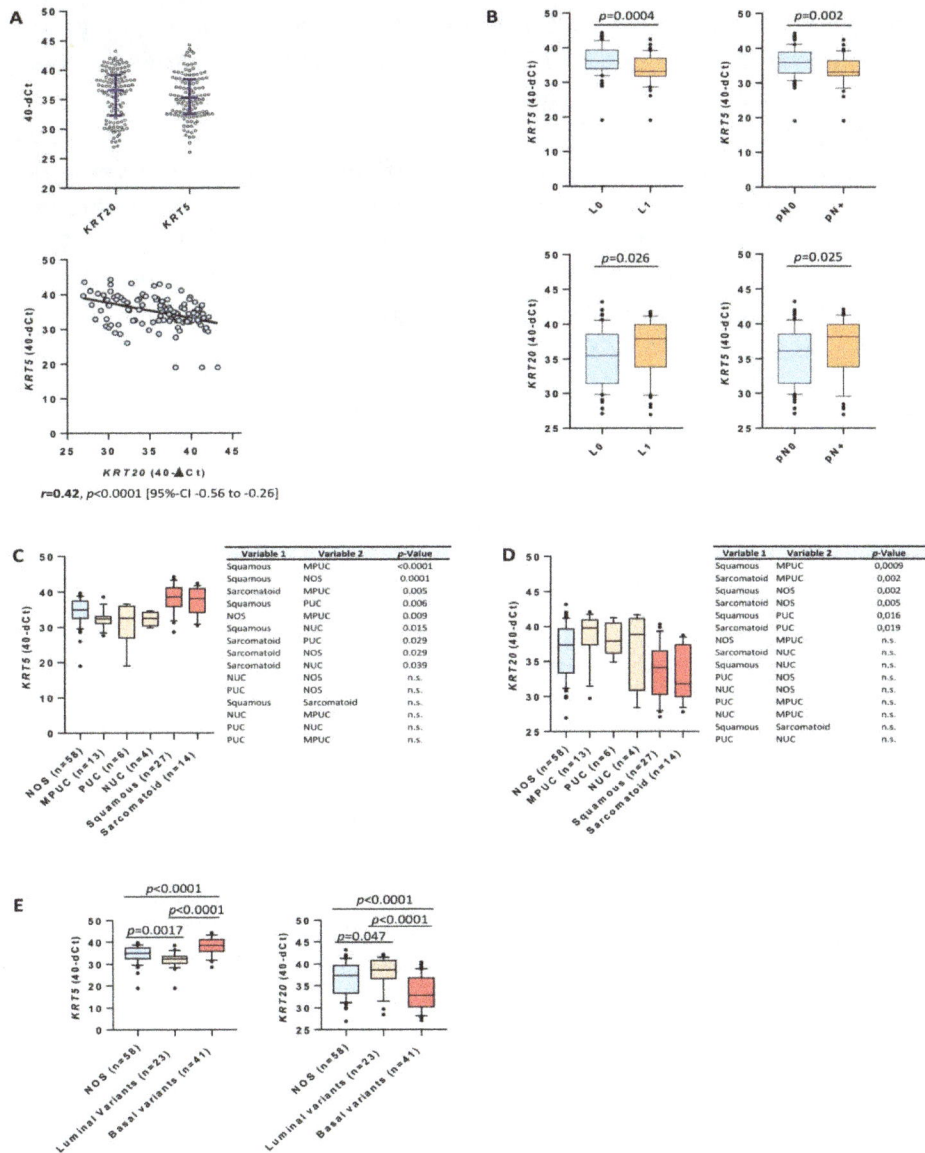

Figure 1. (**A**) Data distribution of *KRT5* and *KRT20* mRNA levels in patients with muscle-invasive bladder cancer (MIBC) treated with radical cystectomy and correlation of *KRT5* and *KRT20* mRNA levels. Blue bars within the boxplot indicate median value and 25%/75% quartiles. The black line in the correlation plot indicates the strength of correlation. (**B**) Correlation of *KRT5* mRNA expression levels with N-stage and lymphovascular invasion (L; L1 = lymphovascular invasion present; L0 = lymphovascular invasion absent; pN0 = no lymphnode metastasis present; pN+ = lymphnode metastasis present). High expression of *KRT5* mRNA is associated with significantly lower rates of LVI and nodal metastasis. (**C,D**) Distribution of *KRT5* and *KRT20* in conventional (not otherwise specified; NOS), micropapillary (MPUC), plasmacytoid (PUC), nested (NUC), squamous, and sarcomatoid differentiated urothelial carcinomas. (**E**) Distribution of *KRT20* and *KRT5* stratified by conventional urothelial carcinomas, luminal variants (including nested, plasmacytoid, and micropapillary carcinomas), and basal variants (including squamous and sarcomatoid carcinomas).

3.2. KRT5 and KRT20 mRNA Expression Defines Highly Prognostic Relevant Subgroups of MIBC

As shown in Figure 2A,B the differential expression of *KRT5* and *KRT20* clearly defines two distinct subgroups. High *KRT20* mRNA expression was significantly associated with worse RFS (multivariate hazard ratio (HR) = 2.33) and DSS (multivariate = HR 2.24; Figure 2A, Supplementary Table S1). Low *KRT5* expression level was associated with unfavorable RFS (multivariate HR = 1.47) and DSS (multivariate HR = 1.59; Figure 2B, Supplementary Table S1). Next, an algorithm (Epi-Typer) based on the above calculated cutoffs for *KRT5* and *KRT20* mRNA expression was used to further subclassify the tumors, as depicted in Figure 2C. *KRT5* and *KRT20* cutoffs were calculated by a predictive monoforest algorithm stratified by disease-specific survival status (disease-specific death vs. no disease-specific death). There was no statistically significant difference between the $KRT5^+/KRT20^-$ and $KRT5^+/KRT20^+$ subtypes with regard to RFS and DSS when these two groups were summarized to the $KRT5^+/KRT20^{+/-}$ phenotype (data not shown). The $KRT20^+/KRT5^-$ (class 2) subgroup showed a very poor prognosis with 5-year RFS (multivariate HR = 2.10; Figure 2C) and DSS of 0% (multivariate HR = 3.20; Figure 2C), whereas the $KRT5^+/KRT20^{+/-}$ (class 1) subgroup showed a favorable prognosis with 5-year RFS of 52% and 5-year DSS of 58% (Figure 2C).

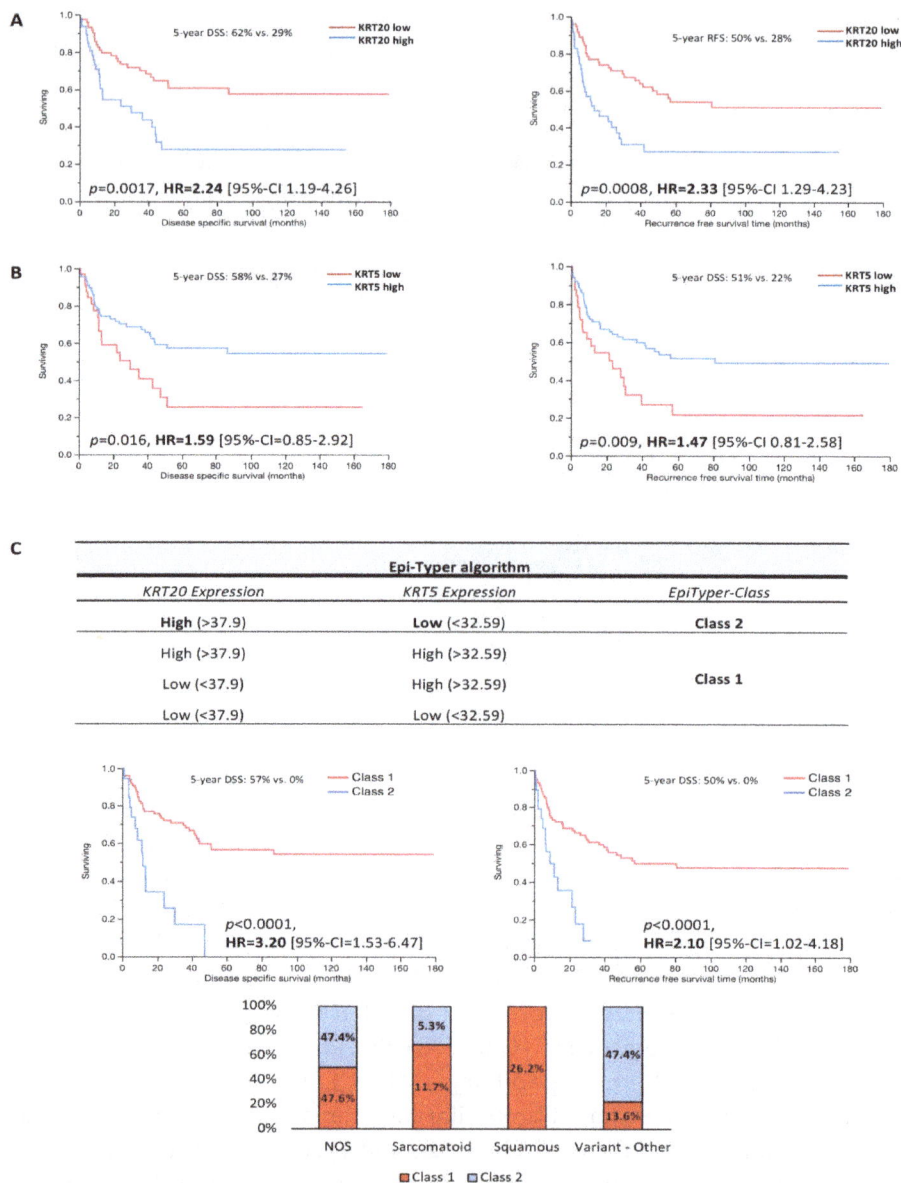

Figure 2. Kaplan–Meier analysis for recurrence-free survival (RFS) and disease-specific survival (DSS) based on (**A**) *KRT20* and (**B**) *KRT5* mRNA expression levels. (**C**) Epi-Typer algorithm and Kaplan–Meier analysis in the MIBC cohort for RFS and DSS based on marker combination (Epi-Typer) of *KRT5* and *KRT20* mRNA expression levels (red color: tumors within Epi-Typer Class 1; blue color: tumors within Epi-Typer Class 2).

3.3. Multivariate Data Analysis

Multivariate Cox–proportional hazard models were calculated including fixed clinicopathological variables: pT-Stage, pN-Stage, Grading WHO 1973, Grading WHO 2016 (no impact; all included tumors were high grade), lymphovascular invasion, blood vessel invasion, age at cystectomy, gender, resection margin status, receipt of adjuvant platinum-containing chemotherapy, and presence of urothelial carcinoma in situ. Models were calculated for each respective cutoff group (*KRT5* high vs. low, *KRT20* high vs. low, Epi-Typer classes). Detailed multivariate analyses are depicted in Supplementary Table S1, including multivariate hazard ratios, significance levels, and 95% confidence intervals.

3.4. KRT5 and KRT20 mRNA Expression in the MDACC Cohort

Data validation was performed using in silico MDACC data (GSE48276; GSE = gene set enrichment) [14]. The basal subtype was significantly enriched with *KRT5* ($p = 0.0002$), whereas the luminal subtype showed significant enrichment with *KRT20* ($p = 0.0005$) (Figure 3). High expression of *KRT20* mRNA was associated with significantly worse DSS, while *KRT5* mRNA expression had no prognostic impact ($p = 0.042$ for *KRT20* and $p = 0.075$ for *KRT5*; Figure 3). In addition, the Epi-Typer algorithm added no prognostic impact to the *KRT20/KRT5* cutoff (data not shown).

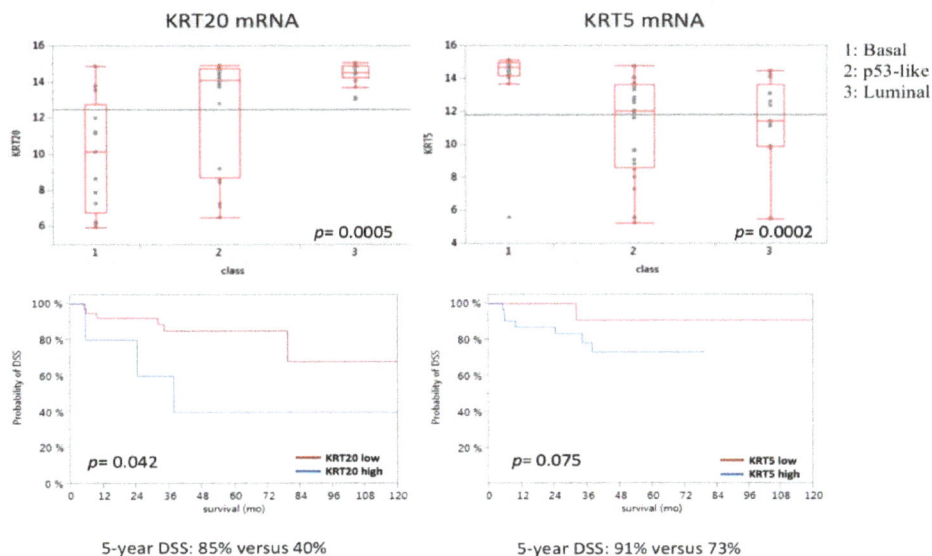

Figure 3. Association of *KRT5* and *KRT20* mRNA expression levels with MDACC molecular subtypes (MDACC cohort). Class 1 = basal, Class 2 = p53-like, Class 3 = luminal. As expected, luminal tumors were enriched with *KRT20* and basal tumors were enriched with *KRT5*. p53-like subtype shows a broad expression range of both genes. Basal tumors show a slightly higher proliferation rate. Kaplan–Meier regression analysis is unfavorable for highly *KRT20*-expressing tumors.

4. Discussion

Treatment options for UBC have evolved minimally over the last decades. Recent genome-wide mRNA expression analyses have revealed molecular subtypes with huge prognostic and predictive impact. Here, we show the possibility of stratifying MIBC into relevant subgroups by using two of the most prominent markers of the genome-wide approaches, the inversely related cytokeratins *KRT5* and *KRT20*, as surrogate markers for nonluminal and luminal differentiation. *KRT5* is a marker of stem or progenitor cells and can be found in basal-like carcinoma subtypes, often with squamous/sarcomatoid histological features, whereas *KRT20*, a marker of superficial umbrella cells, is enriched in luminal subtypes [8,9,12–15,17,20,26–28].

Most interestingly, the *KRT20* positive luminal subtype displayed worse RFS and DSS in MIBC, similar to previously published results in NMIBC [17,21]. This association between improved survival and keratin mRNA expression was also evident in the MDACC cohort (Figure 3) [14]. Furthermore, high expression of *KRT5* and low expression of *KRT20* were associated with a lower prevalence of lymphovascular invasion and lymphonodal metastasis, which is consistent with the favorable prognosis of *KRT5*-enriched MIBC in our cohort. At first glance, these results seem paradoxical, since the luminal subtype including *KRT20* was previously shown to be associated with a favorable prognosis [14], but are explainable due to characteristics of our cohort: (1) the *KRT20* high phenotype contains 23 cases with variant histology, of which are 13 micropapillary, 6 plasmacytoid, and 4 nested UBCs, which have been shown to be highly aggressive luminal variants with poor prognosis [29–33]; (2) many luminal tumors with and without variant histology are enriched with epithelial to mesenchymal transition (EMT) like gene expression pathways [18,29]. In a recent TCGA (=the cancer genome atlas) publication, Robertson et al. demonstrated that the luminal tumor family can be further subdivided into a luminal papillary cluster (no EMT-like pattern, favorable prognosis) and two luminal phenotypes with highly aggressive behavior (luminal, luminal infiltrated), which showed worse prognosis than basal differentiated tumors [18]. Luminal tumors with variant histology clustered into the aggressive luminal tumor families. Interestingly, Hedegaard et al. demonstrated that luminal NMIBC with poor PFS exhibited a strongly activated cancer-stem-cell-like and EMT signature and showed a huge parallel to the genomically unstable and infiltrated subtypes defined by the Lund group [13,17]. Additionally, in the past, several studies demonstrated the association between high *KRT20* expression and high tumor stage and grade [34]. High *KRT20* expression in lymph nodes after radical cystectomy is associated with a higher tumor stage, a higher rate of micrometastasis, and a worse outcome [35]. Moreover, high expression of *KRT20* in the bone marrow prior to radical cystectomy is associated with a worse outcome [36]. However, luminal tumors with favorable prognosis and *KRT20/KRT5* expression above the cutoff threshold are included in the favorable Epi-Typer class 1. This could mean that highly aggressive luminal tumors exhibit a strong *KRT20* polarized luminal-only phenotype with very low *KRT5* expression, while less aggressive luminal tumors show a mixed expression phenotype, reflecting differentiation that is still more closely related to the normal urothelial expression phenotype. Interestingly, we could prove that luminal variants exhibit significantly higher levels of *KRT20* and significantly lower levels of *KRT5* than conventional or basal variants (squamous/sarcomatoid). On the other hand, highly *KRT5*-expressing tumors are suggested to be of basal subtype and to respond better to neoadjuvant chemotherapy [5], which did not show worse survival than conventional luminal UBC in our cohort. However, the Epi-Typer algorithm is able to stratify class 1 basal and luminal tumors to identify patients who could benefit from neoadjuvant chemotherapy. Due to the lack of patients with neoadjuvant treatment in our cohort, the predictive potential of our RT-qPCR assay has to be investigated in an upcoming study.

As demonstrated previously in NMIBC, the assessment of cytokeratin (CK) 5 and CK20 protein expression by immunohistochemistry correlates well with *KRT5* and *KRT20* mRNA expression but lacks prognostic value [21], which is in line with previous breast cancer studies investigating *MKI67* (*marker of proliferation Ki-67*), *ER* (*estrogen receptor*), *ERBB2* (*Erb-B2 Receptor Tyrosine Kinase 2*), and *PR* (*progesterone receptor*) mRNA and protein expression [37]. Therefore, RT-qPCR has been considered as a possible alternative for immunohistochemistry, as it is objective and not affected by interobserver variability [37–40]. Furthermore, simple gene expression assays in a ready-to-use format are quite simple to establish and to perform on small devices (e.g., Cepheid approaches) compared to immunohistochemistry on expansive autostainers. Tests on such platforms are very cheap and highly standardized, and need little hands-on time. Furthermore, no big laboratory inventory is needed to perform these ready-to-use assays, and therefore they are also suitable for small centers, private practices, or labs that do not have the opportunity to establish the extremely expensive infrastructure for next-generation sequencing or immunohistochemistry. On the other hand, there are several disadvantages with such tests: Due to the increased treatment individualization, they tend to oversimplify biological backgrounds. Furthermore, important predictive genetic alterations—e.g., microsatellite instability for response to checkpoint inhibition [41], recombinant DNA mismatch repair deficiency status for neoadjuvant chemotherapy [42], and others—are not assessable with such simple tests. Taken together, simple tests may play a big role in initial risk stratification to stratify which patients could benefit from further large-scale analysis after initial curative treatment.

Taken together, our data suggest that RT-qPCR-based molecular subtyping of UBC by *KRT5* and *KRT20* mRNA expression is a suitable method to predict RFS and DSS of MIBC patients (Epi-Typer) and could be used in small centers without access to huge immunohistochemistry facilities. Since our study is limited by its retrospective nature, small study cohort, and data from a single center, our results have to be further investigated in upcoming prospective trials with regard to specific treatment modalities.

Author Contributions: Study conduction: B.K., C.B., M.B., A.H., P.E.; Study supervision: B.K., C.B., M.B., A.H., P.E.; Data acquisition—Follow-up data: M.G.W., K.N., P.E., C.B.; Pathological reevaluation: M.E., S.P., A.H.; qPCR assessments: R.M.W., R.S., D.S., S.E., K.N.; Data analysis: M.E., J.B., W.O., D.S., P.E.; Manuscript writing: M.E., P.E.; Critical revision of the manuscript: All contributing authors.

Abbreviations

UBC	urothelial bladder cancer
MIBC	muscle-invasive bladder cancer
CK	cytokeratin
KRT	keratin
MKI67	marker of proliferation Ki67
CALM2	calmodulin 2
FFPE	formalin-fixed paraffin-embedded
MDACC	MD Anderson Cancer Center
PFS	progression-free survival
RFS	recurrence-free survival
DSS	disease-specific survival
NMIBC	non-muscle-invasive bladder cancer
RT-qPCR	reverse-transcription quantitative polymerase chain reaction

References

1. Jemal, A.; Bray, F.; Center, M.M.; Ferlay, J.; Ward, E.; Forman, D. Global cancer statistics. *CA Cancer J. Clin.* **2011**, *61*, 69–90. [CrossRef] [PubMed]
2. Shah, J.B.; McConkey, D.J.; Dinney, C.P. New strategies in muscle-invasive bladder cancer: On the road to personalized medicine. *Clin. Cancer Res.* **2011**, *17*, 2608–2612. [CrossRef] [PubMed]
3. Svatek, R.S.; Hollenbeck, B.K.; Holmang, S.; Lee, R.; Kim, S.P.; Stenzl, A.; Lotan, Y. The economics of bladder cancer: Costs and considerations of caring for this disease. *Eur. Urol.* **2014**, *66*, 253–262. [CrossRef] [PubMed]
4. Svatek, R.S.; Shariat, S.F.; Novara, G.; Skinner, E.C.; Fradet, Y.; Bastian, P.J.; Kamat, A.M.; Kassouf, W.; Karakiewicz, P.I.; Fritsche, H.M.; et al. Discrepancy between clinical and pathological stage: External validation of the impact on prognosis in an international radical cystectomy cohort. *BJU Int.* **2011**, *107*, 898–904. [CrossRef] [PubMed]
5. Seiler, R.; Ashab, H.A.; Erho, N.; van Rhijn, B.W.; Winters, B.; Douglas, J.; Van Kessel, K.E.; Fransen van de Putte, E.E.; Sommerlad, M.; Wang, N.Q.; et al. Impact of Molecular Subtypes in Muscle-invasive Bladder Cancer on Predicting Response and Survival after Neoadjuvant Chemotherapy. *Eur. Urol.* **2017**, *72*, 544–554. [CrossRef] [PubMed]
6. Perou, C.M.; Sorlie, T.; Eisen, M.B.; van de Rijn, M.; Jeffrey, S.S.; Rees, C.A.; Pollack, J.R.; Ross, D.T.; Johnsen, H.; Akslen, L.A.; et al. Molecular portraits of human breast tumours. *Nature* **2000**, *406*, 747–752. [CrossRef] [PubMed]

7. Cancer Genome Atlas Network. Comprehensive molecular portraits of human breast tumours. *Nature* **2012**, *490*, 61–70. [CrossRef] [PubMed]

8. Blaveri, E.; Simko, J.P.; Korkola, J.E.; Brewer, J.L.; Baehner, F.; Mehta, K.; Devries, S.; Koppie, T.; Pejavar, S.; Carroll, P.; et al. Bladder cancer outcome and subtype classification by gene expression. *Clin. Cancer Res.* **2005**, *11*, 4044–4055. [CrossRef] [PubMed]

9. Dyrskjot, L.; Thykjaer, T.; Kruhoffer, M.; Jensen, J.L.; Marcussen, N.; Hamilton-Dutoit, S.; Wolf, H.; Orntoft, T.F. Identifying distinct classes of bladder carcinoma using microarrays. *Nat. Genet.* **2003**, *33*, 90–96. [CrossRef] [PubMed]

10. Kim, W.J.; Kim, E.J.; Kim, S.K.; Kim, Y.J.; Ha, Y.S.; Jeong, P.; Kim, M.J.; Yun, S.J.; Lee, K.M.; Moon, S.K.; et al. Predictive value of progression-related gene classifier in primary non-muscle invasive bladder cancer. *Mol. Cancer* **2010**, *9*, 3. [CrossRef] [PubMed]

11. Lee, J.S.; Leem, S.H.; Lee, S.Y.; Kim, S.C.; Park, E.S.; Kim, S.B.; Kim, S.K.; Kim, Y.J.; Kim, W.J.; Chu, I.S. Expression signature of E2F1 and its associated genes predict superficial to invasive progression of bladder tumors. *J. Clin. Oncol.* **2010**, *28*, 2660–2667. [CrossRef] [PubMed]

12. Sanchez-Carbayo, M.; Socci, N.D.; Lozano, J.; Saint, F.; Cordon-Cardo, C. Defining molecular profiles of poor outcome in patients with invasive bladder cancer using oligonucleotide microarrays. *J. Clin. Oncol.* **2006**, *24*, 778–789. [CrossRef] [PubMed]

13. Sjodahl, G.; Lauss, M.; Lovgren, K.; Chebil, G.; Gudjonsson, S.; Veerla, S.; Patschan, O.; Aine, M.; Ferno, M.; Ringner, M.; et al. A molecular taxonomy for urothelial carcinoma. *Clin. Cancer Res.* **2012**, *18*, 3377–3386. [CrossRef] [PubMed]

14. Choi, W.; Porten, S.; Kim, S.; Willis, D.; Plimack, E.R.; Hoffman-Censits, J.; Roth, B.; Cheng, T.; Tran, M.; Lee, I.L.; et al. Identification of distinct basal and luminal subtypes of muscle-invasive bladder cancer with different sensitivities to frontline chemotherapy. *Cancer Cell* **2014**, *25*, 152–165. [CrossRef] [PubMed]

15. Cancer Genome Atlas Research Network. Comprehensive molecular characterization of urothelial bladder carcinoma. *Nature* **2014**, *507*, 315–322. [CrossRef] [PubMed]

16. Breyer, J.; Otto, W.; Wirtz, R.M.; Wullich, B.; Keck, B.; Erben, P.; Kriegmair, M.C.; Stoehr, R.; Eckstein, M.; Laible, M.; et al. ERBB2 Expression as Potential Risk-Stratification for Early Cystectomy in Patients with pT1 Bladder Cancer and Concomitant Carcinoma in situ. *Urol. Int.* **2016**, *98*, 282–289. [CrossRef] [PubMed]

17. Hedegaard, J.; Lamy, P.; Nordentoft, I.; Algaba, F.; Hoyer, S.; Ulhoi, B.P.; Vang, S.; Reinert, T.; Hermann, G.G.; Mogensen, K.; et al. Comprehensive Transcriptional Analysis of Early-Stage Urothelial Carcinoma. *Cancer Cell* **2016**, *30*, 27–42. [CrossRef] [PubMed]

18. Robertson, A.G.; Kim, J.; Al-Ahmadie, H.; Bellmunt, J.; Guo, G.; Cherniack, A.D.; Hinoue, T.; Laird, P.W.; Hoadley, K.A.; Akbani, R.; et al. Comprehensive Molecular Characterization of Muscle-Invasive Bladder Cancer. *Cell* **2017**, *171*, 540–556. [CrossRef] [PubMed]

19. Rinaldetti, S.; Rempel, E.; Worst, T.S.; Eckstein, M.; Steidler, A.; Weiss, C.A.; Bolenz, C.; Hartmann, A.; Erben, P. Subclassification, survival prediction and drug target analyses of chemotherapy-naive muscle-invasive bladder cancer with a molecular screening. *Oncotarget* **2018**, *9*, 25935–25945. [CrossRef] [PubMed]

20. Dadhania, V.; Zhang, M.; Zhang, L.; Bondaruk, J.; Majewski, T.; Siefker-Radtke, A.; Guo, C.C.; Dinney, C.; Cogdell, D.E.; Zhang, S.; et al. Meta-Analysis of the Luminal and Basal Subtypes of Bladder Cancer and the Identification of Signature Immunohistochemical Markers for Clinical Use. *EBioMedicine* **2016**, *12*, 105–117. [CrossRef] [PubMed]

21. Breyer, J.; Wirtz, R.M.; Otto, W.; Erben, P.; Kriegmair, M.C.; Stoehr, R.; Eckstein, M.; Eidt, S.; Denzinger, S.; Burger, M.; et al. In stage pT1 non-muscle-invasive bladder cancer (NMIBC), high KRT20 and low KRT5 mRNA expression identify the luminal subtype and predict recurrence and survival. *Virchows Arch.* **2017**, *470*, 267–274. [CrossRef] [PubMed]

22. Moch, H.; Humphrey, P.A.; Ulbright, T.M.; Reuter, V.E. WHO Classification of Tumours of the Urinary System and Male Genital Organs. 2016. Available online: https://www.ncbi.nlm.nih.gov/pubmed/26935559 (accessed on 28 February 2018).

23. Eckstein, M.; Wirtz, R.M.; Pfannstil, C.; Wach, S.; Stoehr, R.; Breyer, J.; Erlmeier, F.; Gunes, C.; Nitschke, K.; Weichert, W.; et al. A multicenter round robin test of PD-L1 expression assessment in urothelial bladder cancer by immunohistochemistry and RT-qPCR with emphasis on prognosis prediction after radical cystectomy. *Oncotarget* **2018**, *9*, 15001–15014. [CrossRef] [PubMed]

24. Tramm, T.; Sorensen, B.S.; Overgaard, J.; Alsner, J. Optimal reference genes for normalization of qRT-PCR data from archival formalin-fixed, paraffin-embedded breast tumors controlling for tumor cell content and decay of mRNA. *Diagn. Mol. Pathol.* **2013**, *22*, 181–187. [CrossRef] [PubMed]

25. Kriegmair, M.C.; Balk, M.; Wirtz, R.; Steidler, A.; Weis, C.A.; Breyer, J.; Hartmann, A.; Bolenz, C.; Erben, P. Expression of the p53 Inhibitors MDM2 and MDM4 as Outcome Predictor in Muscle-invasive Bladder Cancer. *Anticancer Res.* **2016**, *36*, 5205–5213. [CrossRef] [PubMed]

26. Chan, K.S.; Espinosa, I.; Chao, M.; Wong, D.; Ailles, L.; Diehn, M.; Gill, H.; Presti, J., Jr.; Chang, H.Y.; van de Rijn, M.; et al. Identification, molecular characterization, clinical prognosis, and therapeutic targeting of human bladder tumor-initiating cells. *Proc. Natl. Acad. Sci. USA* **2009**, *106*, 14016–14021. [CrossRef] [PubMed]

27. Ho, P.L.; Kurtova, A.; Chan, K.S. Normal and neoplastic urothelial stem cells: Getting to the root of the problem. *Nat. Rev. Urol.* **2012**, *9*, 583–594. [CrossRef] [PubMed]

28. Reis-Filho, J.S.; Simpson, P.T.; Martins, A.; Preto, A.; Gartner, F.; Schmitt, F.C. Distribution of p63, cytokeratins 5/6 and cytokeratin 14 in 51 normal and 400 neoplastic human tissue samples using TARP-4 multi-tumor tissue microarray. *Virchows Arch.* **2003**, *443*, 122–132. [PubMed]

29. Guo, C.C.; Dadhania, V.; Zhang, L.; Majewski, T.; Bondaruk, J.; Sykulski, M.; Wronowska, W.; Gambin, A.; Wang, Y.; Zhang, S.; et al. Gene Expression Profile of the Clinically Aggressive Micropapillary Variant of Bladder Cancer. *Eur. Urol.* **2016**, *70*, 611–620. [CrossRef] [PubMed]

30. Comperat, E.; Roupret, M.; Yaxley, J.; Reynolds, J.; Varinot, J.; Ouzaid, I.; Cussenot, O.; Samaratunga, H. Micropapillary urothelial carcinoma of the urinary bladder: A clinicopathological analysis of 72 cases. *Pathology* **2010**, *42*, 650–654. [CrossRef] [PubMed]

31. Ghoneim, I.A.; Miocinovic, R.; Stephenson, A.J.; Garcia, J.A.; Gong, M.C.; Campbell, S.C.; Hansel, D.E.; Fergany, A.F. Neoadjuvant systemic therapy or early cystectomy? Single-center analysis of outcomes after therapy for patients with clinically localized micropapillary urothelial carcinoma of the bladder. *Urology* **2011**, *77*, 867–870. [CrossRef] [PubMed]

32. Kamat, A.M.; Gee, J.R.; Dinney, C.P.; Grossman, H.B.; Swanson, D.A.; Millikan, R.E.; Detry, M.A.; Robinson, T.L.; Pisters, L.L. The case for early cystectomy in the treatment of nonmuscle invasive micropapillary bladder carcinoma. *J. Urol.* **2006**, *175*, 881–885. [CrossRef]

33. Bertz, S.; Wach, S.; Taubert, H.; Merten, R.; Krause, F.S.; Schick, S.; Ott, O.J.; Weigert, E.; Dworak, O.; Rodel, C.; et al. Micropapillary morphology is an indicator of poor prognosis in patients with urothelial carcinoma treated with transurethral resection and radiochemotherapy. *Virchows Arch.* **2016**, *469*, 339–344. [CrossRef] [PubMed]

34. Christoph, F.; Muller, M.; Schostak, M.; Soong, R.; Tabiti, K.; Miller, K. Quantitative detection of cytokeratin 20 mRNA expression in bladder carcinoma by real-time reverse transcriptase-polymerase chain reaction. *Urology* **2004**, *64*, 157–161. [CrossRef] [PubMed]

35. Gazquez, C.; Ribal, M.J.; Marin-Aguilera, M.; Kayed, H.; Fernandez, P.L.; Mengual, L.; Alcaraz, A. Biomarkers vs conventional histological analysis to detect lymph node micrometastases in bladder cancer: A real improvement? *BJU Int.* **2012**, *110*, 1310–1316. [CrossRef] [PubMed]

36. Retz, M.; Rotering, J.; Nawroth, R.; Buchner, A.; Stockle, M.; Gschwend, J.E.; Lehmann, J. Long-term follow-up of bladder cancer patients with disseminated tumour cells in bone marrow. *Eur. Urol.* **2011**, *60*, 231–238. [CrossRef] [PubMed]

37. Wirtz, R.M.; Sihto, H.; Isola, J.; Heikkila, P.; Kellokumpu-Lehtinen, P.L.; Auvinen, P.; Turpeenniemi-Hujanen, T.; Jyrkkio, S.; Lakis, S.; Schlombs, K.; et al. Biological subtyping of early breast cancer: A study comparing RT-qPCR with immunohistochemistry. *Breast Cancer Res. Treat.* **2016**, *157*, 437–446. [CrossRef] [PubMed]

38. Atmaca, A.; Al-Batran, S.E.; Wirtz, R.M.; Werner, D.; Zirlik, S.; Wiest, G.; Eschbach, C.; Claas, S.; Hartmann, A.; Ficker, J.H.; et al. The validation of estrogen receptor 1 mRNA expression as a predictor of outcome in patients with metastatic non-small cell lung cancer. *Int. J. Cancer* **2014**, *134*, 2314–2321. [CrossRef] [PubMed]

39. Sikic, D.; Breyer, J.; Hartmann, A.; Burger, M.; Erben, P.; Denzinger, S.; Eckstein, M.; Stöhr, R.; Wach, S.; Wullich, B.; et al. High androgen receptor mRNA expression is independently associated with prolonged cancer-specific and recurrence-free survival in stage T1 bladder cancer. *Transl. Oncol.* **2017**, *10*, 340–345. [CrossRef] [PubMed]

40. Wilson, T.R.; Xiao, Y.; Spoerke, J.M.; Fridlyand, J.; Koeppen, H.; Fuentes, E.; Huw, L.Y.; Abbas, I.; Gower, A.; Schleifman, E.B.; et al. Development of a robust RNA-based classifier to accurately determine ER, PR, and HER2 status in breast cancer clinical samples. *Breast Cancer Res. Treat.* **2014**, *148*, 315–325. [CrossRef] [PubMed]

41. Le, D.T.; Durham, J.N.; Smith, K.N.; Wang, H.; Bartlett, B.R.; Aulakh, L.K.; Lu, S.; Kemberling, H.; Wilt, C.; Luber, B.S.; et al. Mismatch repair deficiency predicts response of solid tumors to PD-1 blockade. *Science* **2017**, *357*, 409–413. [CrossRef] [PubMed]

42. Iyer, G.; Balar, A.V.; Milowsky, M.I.; Bochner, B.H.; Dalbagni, G.; Donat, S.M.; Herr, H.W.; Huang, W.C.; Taneja, S.S.; Woods, M.; et al. Multicenter Prospective Phase II Trial of Neoadjuvant Dose-Dense Gemcitabine Plus Cisplatin in Patients With Muscle-Invasive Bladder Cancer. *J. Clin. Oncol.* **2018**, *36*, 1949–1956. [CrossRef] [PubMed]

12

ITIH5 and ECRG4 DNA Methylation Biomarker Test (EI-BLA) for Urine-Based Non-Invasive Detection of Bladder Cancer

Michael Rose [1,2,*], Sarah Bringezu [1], Laura Godfrey [1], David Fiedler [1], Nadine T. Gaisa [1], Maximilian Koch [1], Christian Bach [3], Susanne Füssel [4], Alexander Herr [5], Doreen Hübner [4], Jörg Ellinger [6], David Pfister [3,7], Ruth Knüchel [1], Manfred P. Wirth [4], Manja Böhme [5] and Edgar Dahl [1,2,*]

[1] Institute of Pathology, RWTH Aachen University, 52074 Aachen, Germany; bringezu.sarah@gmail.com (S.B.); laura.dierichs@rwth-aachen.de (L.G.); david@fiedler.online (D.F.); ngaisa@ukaachen.de (N.T.G.); maximilian.koch@uk-koeln.de (M.K.); rknuechel-clarke@ukaachen.de (R.K.)

[2] RWTH Centralized Biomaterial Bank (RWTH cBMB), Medical Faculty, RWTH Aachen University, 52074 Aachen, Germany

[3] Department of Urology, RWTH Aachen University, 52074 Aachen, Germany; chbach@ukaachen.de (C.B.); david.pfister@uk-koeln.de (D.P.)

[4] Department of Urology, University Hospital Carl Gustav Carus, Technische Universität Dresden, 01307 Dresden, Germany; Susanne.Fuessel@uniklinikum-dresden.de (S.F.); Huebner-Doreen@gmx.de (D.H.); Manfred.Wirth@uniklinikum-dresden.de (M.P.W.)

[5] Biotype GmbH, 01109 Dresden, Germany; alx.herr@gmail.com (A.H.); m.boehme@biotype.de (M.B.)

[6] Department of Urology, University Hospital Bonn, 53105 Bonn, Germany; joerg.ellinger@ukb.uni-bonn.de

[7] Department of Urology, Uro-Oncology, Robot Assisted and Reconstructive Urologic Surgery, University Hospital Cologne, 50937 Cologne, Germany

* Correspondence: mrose@ukaachen.de (M.R.); edahl@ukaachen.de (E.D.)

Abstract: Bladder cancer is one of the more common malignancies in humans and the most expensive tumor for treating in the Unites States (US) and Europe due to the need for lifelong surveillance. Non-invasive tests approved by the FDA have not been widely adopted in routine diagnosis so far. Therefore, we aimed to characterize the two putative tumor suppressor genes ECRG4 and ITIH5 as novel urinary DNA methylation biomarkers that are suitable for non-invasive detection of bladder cancer. While assessing the analytical performance, a spiking experiment was performed by determining the limit of RT112 tumor cell detection (range: 100–10,000 cells) in the urine of healthy donors in dependency of the processing protocols of the RWTH cBMB. Clinically, urine sediments of 474 patients were analyzed by using quantitative methylation-specific PCR (qMSP) and Methylation Sensitive Restriction Enzyme (MSRE) qPCR techniques. Overall, ECRG4-ITIH5 showed a sensitivity of 64% to 70% with a specificity ranging between 80% and 92%, i.e., discriminating healthy, benign lesions, and/or inflammatory diseases from bladder tumors. When comparing single biomarkers, ECRG4 achieved a sensitivity of 73%, which was increased by combination with the known biomarker candidate NID2 up to 76% at a specificity of 97%. Hence, ITIH5 and, in particular, ECRG4 might be promising candidates for further optimizing current bladder cancer biomarker panels and platforms.

Keywords: bladder cancer detection; urinary biomarkers; DNA methylation; ECRG4; ITIH5

1. Introduction

Bladder cancer is the most frequent urogenital malignant tumor concerning both sexes worldwide, with an estimated ~549,400 new cases and 200,000 deaths in 2018 [1], which causes the highest costs of all cancers per patient [2]. In the European Union (EU) alone, the costs were €4.9 billion, with health care accounting for €2.9 billion in 2012 [3] due to long-term survival with the need for lifelong surveillance by cost-intensive diagnostically tools [2]. Cystoscopy, the "gold standard" for the detection of bladder cancer, is an invasive and time-consuming procedure, achieving an operator-dependent sensitivity and specificity of approximately 90% [4]. In particular, repeating cystoscopy for patients with non-muscle invasive bladder cancer (NMIBC) to determine whether their disease has recurred or progressed to muscle invasive bladder cancer (MIBC) represents a major cost associated with treating bladder cancer patients [5]. Nevertheless, only 10% of haematuria patients are faced with a diagnosis of bladder cancer [6], a fact that did not increase the compliance of undergoing cystoscopy. Complementary to these procedures, the current guidelines recommend completion by non-invasive urine cytology, which, however, is characterized by poor sensitivity varying between 20 to 53% [7]. Additional non-invasive urinary assays have been developed, which could help to minimize the invasive procedure of cystoscopy and reduce its economic burden (for an overview see: [8]). Although such assays have been shown to increase the sensitivity of urine cytology, they have not been widely adopted in routine practice: either they are characterized by cost-intensive performances, like UroVysion [9], or failed as point of-care tests due to limited sensitivity or specificity, such as the NMP22-based "BladderCheck^{TM} Test" [10,11]. Given that, none of the currently available urinary biomarkers that have been approved by the FDA can absolutely be recommended as a stand-alone test to replace cystoscopy in the clinic. Recently, several commercially available tests have been developed with improved sensitivity and specificity by using mRNA (e.g., "Xpert BC" [12]) or protein-based ELISA assay technology (e.g., "UBC" [13]), but these data must be independently be confirmed in further studies. Therefore, it is still of great interest to identify novel tumor biomarkers for urine-based early detection of bladder cancer, which might optimize existing panels and platforms to improve both the initial detection of bladder cancer and detection of its recurrence.

For several decades now, epigenetic alterations are an excellent source of biomarker candidates for cancer detection, diagnosis, and prognosis [14]. In particular, aberrant DNA hypermethylation of putative tumor suppressor genes emerged as a potential biomarker source for assessing early cancer detection, which has recently moved towards clinical practice, for instance, in colorectal cancer [15]. For non-invasive detection of bladder cancer, promising DNA methylation biomarkers have been described in various studies [16], but the FDA has approved none of the presented methylation biomarkers (panels) for routinely diagnostic procedures so far. In the presented study, we focused on two putative tumor suppressor genes in bladder cancer that may also hold a prognostic impact, namely inter-α-trypsin inhibitor heavy chain 5 (*ITIH5*) and esophageal cancer-related gene 4 (*ECRG4* or *C2orf40*). *ITIH5* has previously been shown to be epigenetically silenced in various cancer entities [17–19], including bladder cancer [20], where its expression was associated with tumor recurrence of the clinical important group of high-grade pT1 patients. In addition, *ITIH5* was characterized as a putative metastasis suppressor gene in breast [21,22] and pancreatic cancers [23]. *ECRG4* has also been described to be a candidate tumor suppressor gene that is inactivated by DNA methylation in cancers, like esophageal squamous cell carcinoma [24,25], breast cancer [26], renal cell cancer [27], and colorectal cancer [28,29], but not in bladder cancer so far.

We now provide evidence that *ECRG4* and *ITIH5* DNA methylation could be useful as urinary biomarkers for non-invasive bladder cancer detection. Biomarkers were assessed by comparing different techniques, i.e., bisulfite-pyrosequencing, qMSP, and MSRE qPCR in comprehensive cohorts of patients with bladder diseases and controls, overall composing 474 urine samples, including a significant number of benign and inflammatory diseases. In particular, we demonstrate strong biomarker performance for *ECRG4*, which might be a suitable candidate to complete and improve current non-invasive biomarker panels and platforms.

2. Results

2.1. Analytical Performance of ITIH5 and ECRG4 qMSP and Pyrosequencing Biomarker Assays

ITIH5 and ECRG4 have been previously identified as putative class II tumor suppressor genes, which are epigenetically silenced in various tumor entities. In the presented study, we aimed to assess the biomarker quality of both candidates to detect bladder tumors *via* urine samples. The analytical performance of quantitative methylation-specific PCR (qMSP) and pyrosequencing assays was assessed involving standard biobank processing procedure of the RWTH cBMB biobank prior to assessing the biomarker performance of ECRG4 and ITIH5 by patient materials.

For *ECRG4*, Figure 1A shows the genomic location of the qMSP and pyrosequencing assays. Both of the assays spanned CpG sites, which were characterized by strong median hypermethylation in bladder tumors within the TCGA data set [30] as compared to normal controls. CpG sites of the *ECRG4* target region showed a significant inverse correlation between DNA methylation and *ECRG4* mRNA expression (Figure 1A). Subsequently, a spiking experiment was performed to assess both sensitivity and reproducibility in dependence on a distinct number of RT112 tumor cells (range: 100–10,000 cells), i.e., RT112 bladder cancer cells harboring methylated *ECRG4* (see Supplementary Figure S1) and *ITIH5* [20] genes were spiked into 20 mL pooled urine of healthy donors ($n = 4$), respectively. Urine samples that were spiked with RT112 cells were processed according to the standard operating protocol of the RWTH cBMB. Urine pellets were either directly used for DNA extraction (probe set A) or urine sediments were stored according to the RWTH cBMB conditions (-80 °C) for two weeks (probe set B) (Figure 1B). We found that DNA yield was significantly higher in freshly processed samples when compared to those processed after two weeks of storage at -80 °C (probe set B, Figure 1C). However, this was not associated with significant changes in the detection sensitivity of *ECRG4* methylation by both assays, qMSP and pyrosequencing). Overall, the *ECRG4* qMSP assay showed the highest sensitivity with a detection limit of 25 tumor cells/ml (equivalent to 89.75 pg tumor DNA), whereas pyrosequencing-based detection of *ECRG4* methylation required 45 tumor cells/ml (161.55 pg tumor DNA) urine (Figure 1D). Furthermore, the *ECRG4* qMSP assay exhibited a robust reproducibility when comparing methylation detection rates of the two storage time points, i.e., the qMSP assay convinced with high sensitivity and strong reliability (Spearman r: 0.955, $p < 0.001$) (Figure 1E). In contrast, pyrosequencing missed a significant correlation of *ECRG4* methylation levels of spiking samples, which were directly used for DNA extraction and those processed after two weeks (Supplementary Figure S2).

qMSP and pyrosequencing assays for the detection of the *ITIH5* promoter methylation were established similar to *ECRG4*. In Figure 2A, the relative location of qMSP and pyrosequencing primers are indicated. TCGA BLCA data analyses confirmed differences in median DNA methylation level for the targeted region of the *ITIH5* qMSP and pyrosequencing assay, which spanned the CpG site (#10119075), showing an inverse correlation between *ITIH5* DNA methylation and corresponding gene expression (Figure 2A). Of clinical significance, *ITIH5* hypermethylation of the CG site #10119075 was associated with shorter overall survival in advanced (pT > 2) bladder tumors (Figure 2B). In concordance with the results that were observed for *ECRG4*, pyrosequencing-based detection of *ITIH5* methylation failed to perform with a suitable reproducibility when using samples of both storage time points (directly processed vs. two weeks biobank storage). The *ITIH5* qMSP assay achieved strong reliability (Spearman correlation: 0.902, $p < 0.001$, Figure 2C,D) and high sensitivity being characterized by a detection limit that ranged between 25 and 30 tumor cells/mL (89.75 pg/107.70 pg tumor DNA), whereas a robust detection of *ITIH5* methylation by pyrosequencing required at least 125 tumor cells/mL (448.75 pg tumor DNA) urine (Supplementary Figure S2). Hence, qMSP assays of both genes were selected for assessment in a clinical cohort setting.

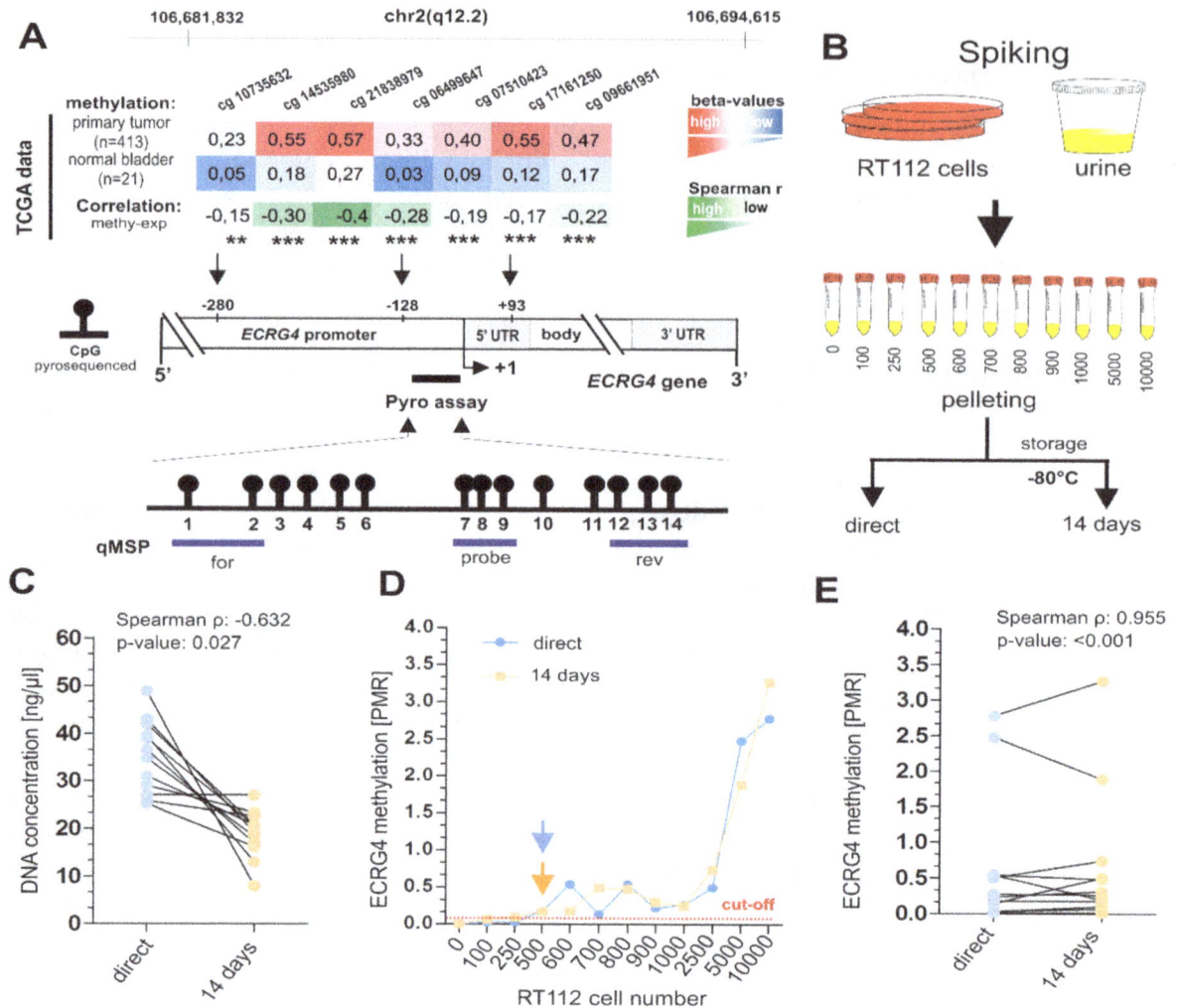

Figure 1. Analytical performance of the Quantitative Methylation-Specific PCR (qMSP) *ECRG4* DNA methylation biomarker assay. (**A**) Schematic map of the human *ECRG4* gene, including the relative positions and median β-values (of normal and tumor samples) of seven CpG sites based on 450K methylation arrays of the bladder cancer (BLCA) TCGA data set and corresponding Spearman correlation between *ECRG4* methylation (colored scale bar red to white; red: high methylation, white: low methylation) and *ECRG4* mRNA expression (colored scale bar green to white; green: strong correlation, white: no correlation) for each CpG site; ** $p \leq 0.01$, *** $p \leq 0.001$. +1: *ECRG4* transcription start site (TSS). Relative position of the promoter area analyzed by bisulfite-pyrosequencing that comprises 14 single CpG sites (black dots) is shown as a black line. CpG sites analyzed by qMSP (blue lines) were indicated covering the pyrosequenced promoter region close to the TSS. (**B**) Cartoon illustrating the spiking experiment using cultured RT112 tumor cells and urine pooled from four healthy donors. Distinct cell numbers of RT112 tumor cells (100-10,000) were spiked into 20 mL urine, respectively. Afterwards, urine samples were processed according to the standard operating protocol of the RWTH cBMB biobank. Pellets of probe set A were directly used for DNA extraction while urine sediments of probe set B were stored according to the RWTH cBMB conditions (−80 °C) for two weeks before further processing. (**C**) Comparison of DNA concentrations (=yield) achieved of samples from probe set A (direct processing) and B (after 14 days). DNA yield was significantly higher in freshly processed urine samples. (**D**) *ECRG4* promoter methylation determined by using qMSP of spiked urines samples. Red dotted line: threshold value for positive detection; orange and blue arrow: stably exceeding the threshold (detection limit) (**E**) Correlation of *ECRG4* DNA methylation for spiked urine samples of probe set A and B.

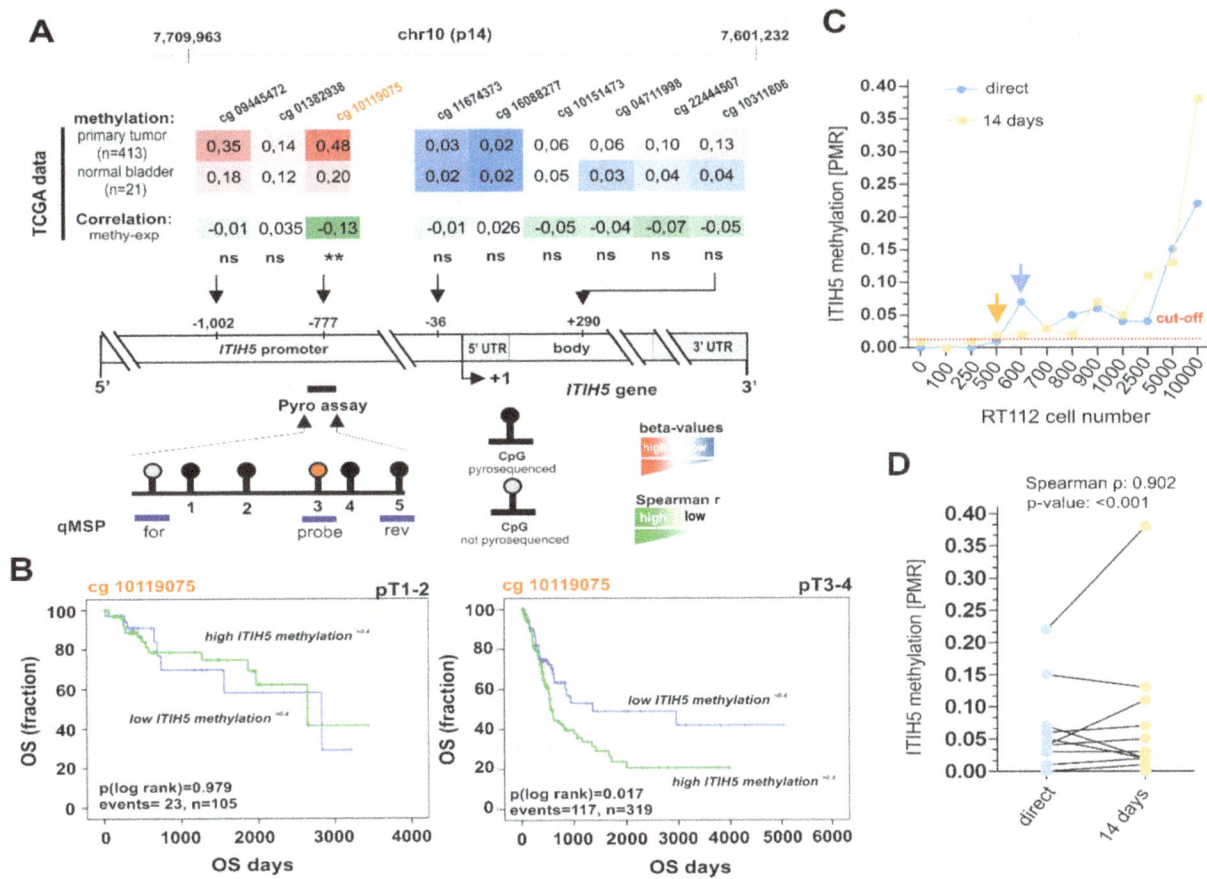

Figure 2. Analytical performance of the qMSP *ITIH5* DNA methylation biomarker assay. (**A**) Schematic map of the human *ITIH5 gene* including the relative positions and median median β-values (of normal and tumor samples) of nine CpG sites based on 450K methylation arrays of the BLCA TCGA data set and corresponding Spearman correlation between *ITIH5* methylation (colored scale bar red to white; red: high methylation, white: low methylation) and *ITIH5* mRNA expression (colored scale bar green to white; green: strong correlation, white: no correlation) for each CpG site; ** $p \leq 0.01$. +1: *ITIH5* transcription start site (TSS). Relative position of the upstream promoter area analyzed by bisulfite-pyrosequencing that comprises five single CpG sites (black dots) is shown as a black line. CpG sites analyzed by qMSP (blue lines) were indicated largely covering the pyrosequenced promoter region. (**B**) Kaplan–Meier survival curves display overall survival (OS) of patients with high ITIH5 methylation (β-value of CG #10119075 > 0.4, green curve) compared to low ITIH5 methylation (β-value of CG #10119075 ≤ 0.4, blue curve) based on TCGA data. (**C**) *ITIH5* promoter methylation determined by using qMSP of spiked urine samples. Red dotted line: threshold value for positive detection; orange and blue arrow: stably exceeding the threshold (detection limit) (**D**) Correlation of *ITIH5* DNA methylation for spiked urine samples of probe set A and B.

2.2. Clinical Biomarker Performance of the ECRG4-ITIH5 qMSP Test for Accurate Non-Invasive Detection of Bladder Cancer

ECRG4 and *ITIH5* performance was initially assessed in a clinical cohort of urine samples (total $n = 263$) comprising 116 urine samples that were derived from bladder cancer patients. Patients with urological malignancies of other origin (testis, prostate, kidney) as well as benign and inflammatory urological-diseases (prostate hyperplasia, renal stones, chronic cystitis) and healthy (without pathological finding) donors that were included as controls (cohort 1a: benign - inflammatory, cohort 1b: all controls including urological cancers). *ECRG4* and *ITIH5* methylation for each urine sample is shown as the mean percentage of methylated reference (PMR) in the scatter plots of Figure 3A,B. *ECRG4* and *ITIH5* methylation were both significantly increased in the urine samples from patients with cancers of the bladder (*ECRG4* mean PMR: 5.011, 95% CI: 2.118–7.905; *ITIH5* mean PMR: 2.634, 95% CI: 0.730–4.539), the prostate (*ECRG4* mean PMR: 1.306, 95% CI: 0.178–2.434; *ITIH5* mean PMR: 1.018, 95% CI: 0.441–1.720), and the kidney (*ECRG4* mean PMR: 0.985, 95% CI: 0.188–1.781, *ITIH5* mean PMR: 1.311, 95% CI: 0.147–2.475) when compared to healthy controls (*ECRG4* mean PMR: 0.017, 95% CI: <0.001–0.033, *ITIH5* mean PMR: 0.031, 95% CI: 0.009–0.070). In benign and inflammatory diseases, a single statistical outlier was detected, respectively, however, diagnosis had been done in a clinical setting and, thus, a true malignancy in this few cases cannot be completely excluded. No associations were found between both *ECRG4* and *ITIH5* promoter methylation and clinical-pathological characteristics, including tumor size, histological grade, age at diagnosis, and gender (Supplementary Table S1 and S2). Calculating the optimal cut-off value for a combined *ECRG4-ITIH5* (EI-BLA) qMSP application with robust specificity by using ROC statistics (Table 1), we demonstrated significant discrimination of bladder cancer patients from non-malignant controls (control cohort 1a) with a sensitivity of 64.3% and a specificity of 81.5% (AUC: 0.783, 95% CI: 0.716–0.850, $p < 0.0001$) (Figure 3C).

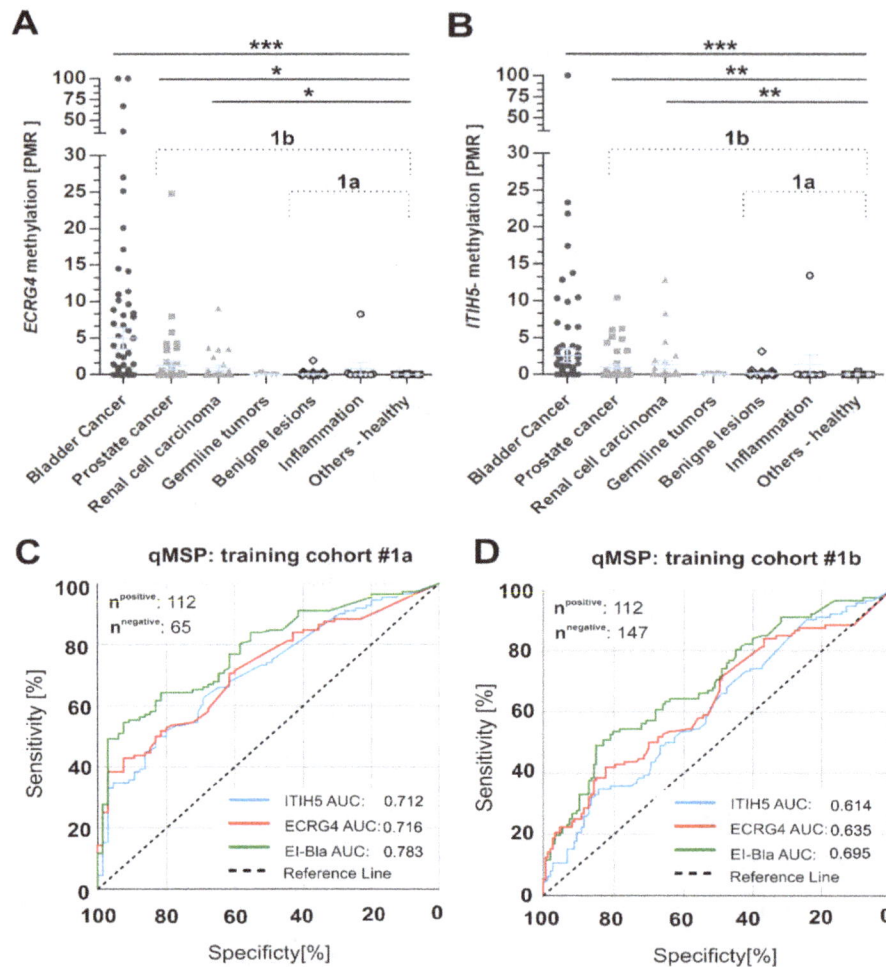

Figure 3. Performance of the *ECRG4* and *ITIH5* biomarker panel using qMSP technique and training cohort #1. (**A,B**) Scatterplots show the PMR methylation values for *ECRG4* (**A**) and *ITIH5* (**B**) in urine sediments of urological tumors, benign lesions, inflammatory diseases and healthy samples; *** $p < 0.001$, ** $p < 0.01$, * $p < 0.05$. 1a: training cohort excluding other urological malignancies 1b: training cohort including other urological malignancies. (**C,D**) ROC-curve analysis illustrating *ECRG4* (red curve), *ITIH5* (blue curve) and *ECRG4-ITIH5* (green curve) biomarker performance based on qMSP in cohort 1a (being and inflammatory controls (**C**)) and cohort 1b (further urological cancer entities as controls (**D**)), *AUC*: Area under the curve.

Table 1. EI-BLA biomarker performance based on training cohort #1 as compared to different control groups.

		EI-BLA qMSP			
Cut-Off	**Specificity**	**Sensitivity**	**AUC**	**p-Value**	**Control Group**
0.54	81.5%	64.3%	0.783	<0.001	1a
0.38	81.6%	50.9%	0.695	<0.001	1b

Additionally, *ECRG4-ITIH5* in combination were able to distinguish bladder cancer patients from patients with neoplasms of other urological origin (control cohort 1b) with similar specificity (81.6%, AUC: 0.695, 95% CI: 0.631–0.760, $p < 0.0001$) but reduced sensitivity (50.9%) (Figure 3D). The application of both biomarker candidates in combination achieved the most reliable results as compared with single biomarker performances.

Next, the biomarker quality of *ECRG4* and *ITIH5* promoter methylation was tested and then compared to a known putative bladder cancer methylation biomarker (*NID2*) by Methylation Sensitive Restriction Enzyme (MSRE) qPCR at the independent laboratories of Biotype GmbH (Dresden, Germany). The independent urine cohort (overall $n = 211$) included 130 urines of patients that were diagnosed with primary bladder cancer as well as 81 control urines (benign lesions, inflammatory diseases, and healthy controls). *ECRG4-ITIH5* methylation was found to be significantly increased in the urines of bladder cancer patients (mean methylation: 10.31, 95% CI: 6.132–14.50) as compared to all control groups, i.e., benign lesions (mean methylation: 0.143), inflammatory diseases (mean methylation: 2.900), and healthy donors (mean methylation: 0.203) (Figure 4A). In this independent cohort, a close association of both *ECRG4* and *ITIH5* with increased tumor size (pTa vs. pT1-4) and age at diagnosis was determined by Fisher's exact test (Tables 2 and 3).

Table 2. Clinico-pathological parameters in relation to ITIH5 methylation in training cohort #2.

		ITIH5 Methylation [b]		
	n [a]	Low	High	p-Value [c]
Age at diagnosis				
≤70 years	111	65	46	**0.001**
>70 years	106	39	67	
Gender				
male	143	57	56	0.150
female	42	22	20	
Histological tumor grade [d]				
low grade	19	4	15	0.174
high grade	113	42	71	
Tumor stage [d]				
pTa	76	33	43	**0.024**
pT1-pT4	54	13	41	

[a] Urines of cohort #2; [b] cut-off level MSRE = 0.22 representing >90% specificity in ROC curve statistic; [c] Fisher's exact test; [d] According to WHO 2004 classification; Significant p-values are marked in bold face.

Table 3. Clinico-pathological parameters in relation to ECRG4 methylation in training cohort #2.

| | n [a] | ECRG4 Methylation [b] | | |
		Low	High	p-Value [c]
Age at diagnosis				
<70 years	111	84	27	**<0.001**
≥70 years	106	55	51	
Gender				
male	143	82	61	0.802
female	42	25	17	
Histological tumor grade [d]				
low grade	19	10	9	0.645
high grade	113	53	60	
Tumor stage [d]				
pTa	76	45	31	**0.007**
pT1-pT4	54	19	35	

[a] Urines of cohort #2; [b] cut-off level MSRE = 0.52 representing >90% specificity in ROC curve statistic; [c] Fisher's exact test; [d] According to WHO 2004 classification; Significant p-values are marked in bold face.

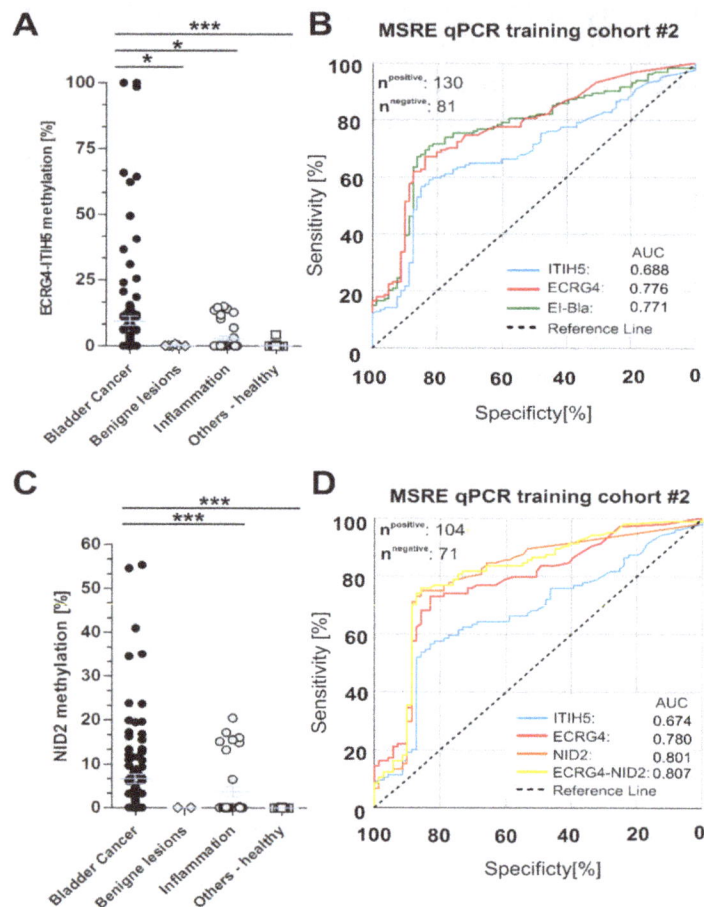

Figure 4. Biomarker performance of ECRG4, ITIH5, and the ECRG4-ITIH5 panel assessed by an independent urine cohort (training cohort #2) and compared to NID2 using MSRE qPCR. (**A**) Scatter plot illustrates significant increased methylation levels for ECRG4 and ITIH5 in urine sediments of bladder cancer compared to benign lesions, inflammatory and healthy samples; *** $p < 0.001$, *$p < 0.05$. (**B**) ROC-curve analysis illustrating ECRG4 (red curve), ITIH5 (blue curve) and ECRG4-ITIH5 (green curve) biomarker performance based on MSRE qPCR in cohort #2. (**C**) Scatter plot showed significant increased methylation values for NID2 in urine sediments of bladder cancer compared to benign lesions, inflammatory and healthy samples; *** $p < 0.001$. (**D**) ROC-curve analysis compares ECRG4 (red curve), ITIH5 (blue curve), and NID2 (orange curve) and combined ECRG4-NID2 biomarker performance based on MSRE qPCR in cohort #2. AUC: Area under the curve.

The ROC analyses showed that *ECRG4-ITIH5* combination achieved a sensitivity of 71.6% at a specificity of 80.2% (AUC: 0.771, 95% CI: 0.706–0.836) in a cohort that included benign lesions and inflammatory diseases of the urinary tract (Figure 4B), whereas specificity was increased up to 92% with minimally decreased sensitivity (69%) focusing on healthy controls. When comparing our single biomarkers, i.e., *ITIH5* and *ECRG4*, with the recently proposed biomarker candidate *NID2* [31], we revealed a similar biomarker performances of *ECRG4* and *NID2*, achieving a sensitivity of 73.1% (AUC: 0.780, 95% CI: 0.709–0.851) and 75% (AUC: 0.801, 95% CI: 0.729–0.873) at a specificity of 83.1%, respectively (Table 4).

Table 4. Biomarker performances based on training cohort #2.

EI-BLA MRSE qPCR					
Cut-Off	Specificity	Sensitivity	AUC	*p*-Value	Control Group
0.52	80.2%	71.6%	0.771	<0.001	all
0.53	91.9%	69.2%	0.850	<0.001	healthy
Single markers MSRE qPCR (control group "all")					
Cut-Off	Specificity	Sensitivity	AUC	*p*-Value	Marker
0.94	83.1%	73.1%	0.780	<0.001	*ECRG4*
0.77	83.1%	56.7%	0.674	<0.001	*ITIH5*
0.11	83.1%	75.0%	0.801	<0.001	*NID2*
Combined ECRG4-NID2 MSRE qPCR					
Cut-Off	Specificity	Sensitivity	AUC	*p*-Value	Control Group
0.49	85.9%	75.0%	0.807	<0.001	all
0.49	97.3%	76.0%	0.884	<0.001	healthy

According to that, *ITIH5* was characterized by reduced sensitivity (56.7%, AUC: 0.674, 95% CI: 0.592–0.755), which did not lead to improved biomarker performance when combining with ECRG4. While considering that, we were able to increase sensitivity for bladder cancer detection up to 75% with improved specificity (85.9%; AUC: 0.807, 95% CI: 0.737–0.877) in a cohort comprising benign lesions and inflammatory diseases of the urinary tract when combining *ECRG4* with the known biomarker *NID2* (Figure 4C,D). In comparison to healthy controls, the panel set of *ECRG-NID2* achieved 76% sensitivity with 97.3% specificity (AUC: 0.884, 95% CI: 0.831–0.937) (Table 4).

3. Discussion

The field of liquid biopsy-based cancer detection systems is rapidly evolving, as novel (epi)genetic biomarkers have been characterized, which can be detected in biological fluids, like blood or urine, offering an easy and non-invasive application for cancer detection, prognosis, and therapy prediction. In colorectal cancer (CRC), for instance, a blood-based screening was realized by targeting Septin 9 (*SEPT9*) hypermethylation, whose Epi proColon®test has been approved by the FDA in 2016 [32]. In bladder cancer, liquid biopsy still needs improvement [33], as various molecular (epi)genetic biomarker candidates and signatures have been described, but none of those assays are FDA-approved for routine diagnostic so far.

In the current study, we present two novel biomarker candidates, *ITIH5* and *ECRG4*, which show strong potential for improving or even completing existing non-invasive biomarker panels and platforms. Already in the year 2010, Renard and colleagues identified *TWIST1* and *NID2* as putative biomarker candidates while using qMSP [31]. In the same year, Costa et. al. showed three novel gene loci, i.e., *GDF15*, *TMEFF2*, and *VIM*, whose DNA methylation could be suitable for detecting bladder cancers in urine samples [34]. Meanwhile, many more putative candidates have been presented [16], but most of the studies were characterized by small sample cohorts without taking into account crucial cohorts of non-malignant diseases like chronic inflammation. Hence, only a handful of biomarkers such as *TMEFF2*, *NID2* and *TWIST1* meet to some degree the needed requirements and, thus, were independently studied and validated [35]. Therefore, we took great care to implement suitable steps and criteria for biomarker validation from the beginning of the study. In the first step, established biomarker assays were assessed by comparing the reliability of different detection methods (qMSP and pyrosequencing) in dependency on the urine sample processing *in vitro*. Of importance, we demonstrated that the regular procedure of urine processing analogue to SOPs of the centralized biomaterial bank (cBMB) of the RWTH Aachen University (i.e., storage at −80 °C) did not impair biomarker detection. However, the DNA yield was considerably higher when fresh urine samples were processed. Beyond that, the qMSP technique showed both the highest sensitivity and reproducibility, which is in line with previous studies demonstrating high levels of accuracy and lower rates of false negatives as compared with other techniques [36]. In a second step, we validated the clinical performance of both biomarkers by independent cohorts and laboratories. In this setting, we included high numbers of urological benign and inflammatory diseases as controls that can be endemically and frequently found in larger population groups, thereby reflecting a much more real-world scenario. We achieved a sensitivity ranging between 64 to 72% at a specificity of over 80% by combined performance of the *ECRG4-ITIH5* DNA methylation biomarker panel. Importantly, we still detect approximately 50% of bladder tumors with a robust true-negative rate (>80% specificity) by including urological malignancies of other origins supporting a liquid biopsy application in the field of bladder cancer. However, a putative benefit of both biomarker candidates being further useful for future assays dealing with the non-invasive detection of other urothelial malignancies, like prostate or renal cell carcinomas, should not be excluded at this stage. Interestingly, in our independent training cohort from Dresden, *ECRG4* reached a sensitivity of over 73% as single biomarker. Hence, a suitable impact was suggested, in particular for *ECRG4*, for discriminating BPH or urocystitis from bladder tumors, which is comparable with proposed biomarker candidates, like *NID2* or *TWIST1* [33]. *CFTR*, *SAL3*, and *TWIST1* have been recently shown to be useful for monitoring bladder cancer in a real clinical scenario, as a sensitivity of 96% was achieved by pyrosequencing in combination with urine cytology—however with low specificity (40%) [35]. In our cohort, the ECRG4-ITIH5 biomarker performance also reached over 90% sensitivity at a specificity of 40%, however, we finally focused on the best panel according to their specificity: combining *ECRG4* and *NID2* led to an increased sensitivity (76%) at a specificity of 97% when compared to healthy controls, encouraging validation studies of this biomarker setting in the future.

In view of novel diagnostic platforms, *ECRG4* and *ITIH5* could also be part of NGS-based gene signatures, which are currently considered to be at the cutting edge of the technical development of future diagnostic applications. In 2017, the multiplex bisulfite NGS-based sequencing concept "UroMark" was described achieving 98% sensitivity and 97% specificity [37]. However, this NGS assay should be confirmed in comprehensive cohorts and the usability of a 150 CpG loci comprising biomarker assay for routinely and cost-effective diagnosis, in particular as a population-based screening tool, in a real-world scenario must be further considered. So far, real-world application of available urinary markers has not reduced any bladder cancer treatment costs, as predicted by decision-analytic economic models [2]. Still, biomarkers are missing, which serve as the basis for decision-making of risk stratification. According to that, DNA methylation of our markers, in particular *ITIH5*, might hold a prognostic impact, as both candidates have been characterized as putative tumor suppressor genes whose silencing could be triggered by DNA promoter hypermethylation [20]. In 2008, *ITIH5* was described to be epigenetically silenced in breast cancer [17] and five years later *ITIH5* DNA methylation has been identified as a putative blood-based biomarker for the early detection of breast cancer [38]. Since then functionally studies revealed, for instance, ITIH5 mediated suppression of breast [21,22] and pancreatic cancer metastases [23] *in vitro* and *in vivo*. Interestingly, in aggressive mammary cancer cells, ITIH5 triggered an epigenetic reprogramming which was associated with a demethylation of various promoter regions, including that of *DAPK1*, a tumor suppressor gene and putative blood-based biomarker in several tumor entities [21]. In bladder carcinogenesis, the downregulation of ITIH5 was also associated with worse prognosis while functionally high-grade bladder cancer cells showed reduced growth *in vitro* after ITIH5 overexpression [20]. Of clinical interest, ITIH5 protein expression was shown to predict tumor relapse of the clinical important subgroup of pT1 high-grade patients [20], of which 30% never displayed recurrence after transurethral resection of the bladder, while a further 30% died due to metastatic disease [39]. In the present study, we now confirmed a putative prognostic impact as *ITIH5* promoter hypermethylation was associated with poor patients' outcome in the subgroup of advanced tumors (pT > 2) of the TCGA bladder cancer data set, while increased *ITIH5* methylation was further shown to correlate with a higher pT status in our second urine cohort. These findings may support our hypothesis that *ITIH5* could be a useful biomarker for risk stratification, helping to monitor patients for the recurrence and/or progression of bladder tumors.

In conclusion, we provide two novel DNA methylation biomarkers for non-invasive detection of bladder carcinomas. As *ITIH5* might keep prognostic information for bladder cancer risk stratification, while *ECRG4* showed a convincing diagnostic performance, in particular in combination with the known biomarker candidate *NID2*, both biomarkers, *ECRG4* and *ITIH5*, may be promising candidates to complete and improve current biomarker panels and platforms. For instance, the "Bladder EpiCheck^{TM}" urine assay that combines 15 DNA methylation biomarkers leading to an overall sensitivity of 68.2% and a specificity of 80.0% [40] may benefit from our biomarker candidates to reduce the number of biomarkers while also improving the overall performance. Future studies should be conducted to clarify which of our biomarkers, is suitable for which clinical application, e.g. as a guidance tool for early detection, risk stratification, surveillance, and/or therapeutic management.

4. Materials and Methods

4.1. Cell Line

The bladder cancer cell line J82 was originally obtained from the American Type Culture Collection (ATCC, Manassas, VA, USA). The urothelial bladder cancer cell line RT112 was used for studies of the analytical performance, a gift from Dr. Alexander Buchner (LMU München, München, Germany). All of the cell lines successfully underwent an identity check (Multiplexion GmbH, Immenstadt, Germany) prior to the experiments.

4.2. Urine Samples

In total, 474 urine samples were assessed in this study. The Departments of Urology of the University Hospitals of Aachen, Bonn, and Dresden provided the voided urine samples. The samples that were collected in Aachen were obtained from the RWTH centralized biomaterial bank (RWTH cBMB). The collection of tissue samples was performed within the framework of the Biobank of the Center for Integrated Oncology Köln Bonn. All of the patients gave written consent for asservation and analysis of their samples according to local Institutional Review Board (IRB)-approved protocols of the Medical Faculty of RWTH Aachen University (EK 206/09, 05 Jan 2010), the University of Bonn (EK 205/13, 16 Mar 2013), and the University of Dresden (EK 96032012, 15 Jul 2014). The urine samples derived from patients diagnosed with a primary bladder tumor ($n = 246$) were used to assess biomarker performance, while samples with a known second malignancy, such as prostate cancer, were excluded from this study. Urines from healthy donors ($n = 49$) and samples derived from patients with inflammatory (chronic cystitis), benign (benign prostate hyperplasia), and urological malignant diseases of other tissue origin (testicular tumors, prostate cancer, renal cell carcinoma) served as the controls (overall $n = 179$). For the characteristics of training cohort I (Aachen–Bonn) and training cohort II (Dresden) see Table 5. Unless otherwise stated, 10–20 mL of urines were centrifuged for 10 min. at $2000 \times g$, washed with PBS and sediments were stored at $-80\ °C$.

Table 5. The clinico-pathological parameters of 474 patients whose urine samples were analyzed in this study.

	Categorization	*n*	% Analyzable
Controls		228	100%
Age (median 61.0; range: 23–82 years)			
	<61.0 years	72	31.6%
	≥61.0 years	80	35.1%
	na	76	33.3%
Gender			
	male	96	42.1%
	female	24	10.5%
	na	108	47.4%
Diagnosis			
	Healthy	49	21.5%
	Uro-stones	13	5.7%
	Inflammatory—Uro-cystitis	38	16.7%
	Inflammatory—other	8	3.5%
	Benign—BPH	23	10.1%
	Benign—other	17	7.5%
	PCa	48	21.1%
	GTR	5	2.2%
	RCC	27	11.8%
BCa-Asscociated [a]		246	100%
Age (median 70; range: 27–89 years)			
	<70 years	119	48.4%
	≥70 years	127	51.6%
Gender			
	male	195	79.3%
	female	51	20.7%
Histological tumor grade [b]			
	low grade	42	17.1%
	high grade	172	69.9%
	na	32	13.0%
Tumor stage [b]			
	pTa	106	43.1%
	pTis	8	3.3%
	pT1	54	22.0%
	pT2	37	15.0%
	pT3	19	7.7%
	pT4	8	3.3%
	pTx	8	3.3%
	na	6	2.4%

[a] Only urine samples of patients preoperatively diagnosed with primary, bladder cancer (BCa, without any other malignancy) were included; [b] According to WHO 2004 classification; BPH: prostate hyperplasia; PCa: prostate cancer; GRT: germline tumor; RCC: renal cell carcinoma; na: not available

4.3. DNA Extraction from Urines

The urine sediments of training cohort I (Aachen–Bonn) stored at −80 °C were subjected to DNA extraction by using the ZR Urine DNA Isolation Kit (ZR, Zymo Research, Freiburg, Germany), following the manufacturer's instructions. DNA extraction from the urine sediments of training cohort II (Dresden) stored at −80 °C in RLT buffer was performed by using the QIAamp DNA Mini Kit (Qiagen, Hilden, Germany), according to the manufacturer's instructions. The DNA yield (ng/mL urine) and purity (A_{260}/A_{280}) were determined by using the NanoDrop (Thermo Fisher Scientific, Waltham, MA, USA). Only extractions from urines with a minimal total amount of 100 ng genomic DNA and a ratio of ≥1.5 were finally used for qMSP, pyrosequencing, and MSRE qPCR analyses.

4.4. DNA Bisulfite Conversion

100 to 250 ng of the genomic DNA (training cohort I) were bisulfite-converted for 14 to 16 h by using the EZ DNA Methylation™ kit (Zymo Research) according to the manufacturer's instructions. Bisulfite-converted DNA was eluted in 20 µL of TRIS-EDTA buffer.

4.5. Bisulfite-Pyrosequencing

The pyrosequencing of bisulfite-converted DNA was performed by using the PyroMark PCR Kit, the PyroMark96 ID device, and the PyroGoldSQA reagent Kit (Qiagen), as reported previously [20]. ECRG4 and ITIH5 pyrosequencing assays were designed by using the Pyromark Assay Design Software (Qiagen), and Supplementary Table S3 lists all of the primers. Primers and sequence of interest meet the following criteria: Based on TCGA data analyses, sequences of interest should cover promoter regions that a) are characterized by strong differences in mean DNA methylation between urothelial normal and bladder cancer samples and b) are located in important gene regulatory sequences, i.e., a statistically significant inverse correlation between ECRG4/ITIH5 gene expression and the corresponding DNA methylation had to be observed. The EpiTect®PCR Control DNA Set (Qiagen) was used as the positive controls for unmethylated and methylated DNA in each run.

4.6. Quantitative Methylation-Specific PCR (qMSP)

Bisulfite-modified DNA was used as a template for fluorescence-based real-time PCR amplified in an iCycler iQ5 (Biorad, Munich, Germany), as previously described [37] with slight modifications: The designed primers and probes were specific for amplifying bisulfite-converted DNA for the genes of interest (ECRG4 and ITIH5) (for cycle conditions, primer sequences, and annealing temperatures, see Supplementary Table S4). The reference gene GAPDH was used for internal normalization. Eight calibration dilutions of in vitro methylated human leukocyte DNA (0.1%, 1%, 5%, 10%, 20%, 30%, 50%, 100%) and unmethylated sequence (human leukocyte DNA from a healthy donor), as well as multiple water blanks were included in each run. The gene of interest was called methylated if the cycle threshold (Ct) of at least two of three qPCR replicates for each specimen had a value of less than 45 cycles. The amount of methylated DNA (percentage of methylated reference, PMR) at a specific locus was calculated by dividing the GENE/GAPDH ratio of a sample by the GENE/GAPDH ratio of SssI-treated human leukocyte DNA and multiplying by 100, as specified [37]. The primer binding sites of the qMSP assays were located in the same genomic promoter region as covered by pyrosequencing. The efficiencies of real time MSP were calculated according to the equation: $E = 10^{[-1/\text{slope of calibration dilutions}]}$ [41] and the mean efficacy of ECRG4 and ITIH5 qMSP was 76.57% and 77.76%, respectively.

4.7. Methylation Sensitive Restriction Enzyme qPCR (MSRE) qPCR

Isolated genomic DNA (125 ng) was used for double restriction digest. Methylation-sensitive restriction enzymes AciI and HpaII (New England Biolabs, NEB, MA, USA) were selected based on their capacity to distinguish methylated from unmethylated DNA sequences. Two independent digestion reactions (test reaction and control) were prepared for each patient DNA. Restriction digest was performed within a total volume of 25 µL in CutSmart Buffer (NEB) for 1 h at 37 °C and followed by heat inactivation for 20 min. at 80 °C. The control samples were treated in the same way but without the addition of the enzymes, 50% glycerol was added instead. Finally, DNA digest was diluted with 1x TE buffer before MSRE qPCR. The designed primers and probes for MSRE qPCR are specific for amplifying unrestricted DNA for the genes of interest (ECRG4, ITIH5, and NID2).

MSRE qPCRs were carried out while using the Roche LightCycler 480 II Real-Time PCR detection system. Mono color hydrolysis probe detection (FAM) was used. All of the samples were done in duplicate in 25 µL reactions containing 5 µL Reaction Mix B (Biotype GmbH, Dresden), 3 U Multi Taq 2 (Biotype), 1.5 µL primers and probes (5 µM each), nuclease-free water (Biotype), and 2 µL of digested DNA (2.5 ng/µL, test or control template). For *ECRG4* and *NID2*, the addition of Combinatorial Enhancer Solution (1× CES, [42]) was necessary due to the very high GC content of the amplified region.

For cycle conditions, primer sequences and annealing temperatures, see Supplementary Table S5. Ct values were analyzed while using LightCycler 480 Software (Hoffmann-La Roche AG, Basel, Switzerland).

Undetected Ct values were normalized to 47 for calculations. The methylation level of the amplified region was calculated by using the following equation: percent methylation = $100 \times 2^{-\Delta Ct}$, where ΔCt is the average Ct value from the test reaction minus the average Ct values from the control reaction. Methylation values exceeding 100% were set to 100%.

4.8. Analytical Assay Performances

RT112 wildtype bladder cancer cells harboring a methylated *ECRG4* and *ITIH5* promoter were cultured for two weeks. After cell counting RT112 cells were spiked into pooled urine of healthy donors ($n = 4$). Serial dilutions (10 to 10.000) of RT112 cells were added to 20 mL pooled urine, respectively, which was subsequently processed at the RWTH cBMB laboratories according to its standard operating protocol. Afterwards, urine pellets were either directly used for DNA extraction (probe set A) or urine sediments were stored according to the RWTH cBMB conditions by using two-dimensional (2D) barcoded LVL tubes (LVL technologies, Crailsheim, Germany) at −80 °C for two weeks (probe set B). Pooled urines without any spiked RT112 cells served as the control for normalization and threshold calculation by defining methylation cut-offs. Next, DNA was bisulfite-treated, as mentioned earlier, and the *ECRG4* and *ITIH5* qMSP as well as pyrosequencing assays were performed for *ECRG4* and *ITIH5*, respectively. The gene of interest was called methylated if the PMR (qMSP) or mean percent of CpG methylation (pyrosequencing) stably exceed the background noise and certainly maintained this threshold (=cut-off).

4.9. TCGA BLCA Data Set

Infinium HumanMethylation450 BeadChip data (level 2) and RNASeqV2 data (level 3) of the tumor and normal tissue samples were obtained from the TCGA data portal [30] and analyzed, as previously described [43].

4.10. Statistical Data Acquisition

Two-sided p-values that were less than 0.05 were considered to be significant. The non-parametric Mann–Whitney U-test was applied in order to compare two groups, whereas, in the case of more than two groups, the Dunn's multiple comparison test was used. Correlation analysis was performed by calculating a non-parametric *Spearman's rank* correlation coefficient. Statistical associations between clinico-pathological parameters and DNA methylation of *ITIH5* and *ECRG4* were determined by Fisher's exact test by using SPSS software version 25.0 (SPSS Inc., Chicago, IL, USA). Survival curves for overall survival (OS) were calculated using the Kaplan–Meier method with log-rank statistics. OS was measured from surgery until death and it was censored for patients alive without evidence of death at the last follow-up date. The receiver operating characteristics (ROC) curves and AUC values were calculated to assess the biomarker performance of *ECRG4* and *ITIH5* methylation similar to our previous report [43]. The ROC curves of combined biomarkers were based on the binary logistic regression model using the probability as test variable.

Author Contributions: Conceptualization, M.R., N.T.G., M.B. and E.D.; Methodology, M.R., S.B., L.G., D.F., M.K., A.H., M.B.; Software and Statistics, M.R.; Resources, C.B., S.F., D.H., J.E., D.P.; Writing—Original Draft Preparation, M.R.; Writing–Editing, S.F. and M.B.; Writing—Review, all authors; Visualization, M.R.; Supervision, M.R., R.K., M.B., M.P.W. and E.D. All authors have read and agreed to the published version of the manuscript.

Acknowledgments: The authors appreciate the excellent technical support of Sonja von Sérenyi. Genomic 450K methylation and RNA seq. data used in this study were provided by the TCGA Research Network BLCA datasets (http://cancergenome.nih.gov). This work was supported by a grant from the Medical Faculty of the RWTH Aachen University (START program project 149/08).

References

1. Ferlay, J.; Colombet, M.; Soerjomataram, I.; Mathers, C.; Parkin, D.M.; Piñeros, M.; Znaor, A.; Bray, F. Estimating the global cancer incidence and mortality in 2018: GLOBOCAN sources and methods. *Int. J. Cancer* **2019**, *144*, 1941–1953. [CrossRef]

2. Yeung, C.; Dinh, T.; Lee, J. The health economics of bladder cancer: An updated review of the published literature. *Pharmacoeconomics* **2014**, *32*, 1093–1104. [CrossRef]

3. Leal, J.; Luengo-Fernandez, R.; Sullivan, R.; Witjes, J.A. Economic Burden of Bladder Cancer Across the European Union. *Eur. Urol.* **2016**, *69*, 438–447. [CrossRef]

4. Schlake, A.; Crispen, P.L.; Cap, A.P.; Atkinson, T.; Davenport, D.; Preston, D.M. NMP-22, urinary cytology, and cystoscopy: A 1 year comparison study. *Can. J. Urol.* **2012**, *19*, 6345–6350.

5. National Collaborating Centre for Cancer (UK). *Bladder Cancer: Diagnosis and Management*; National Institute for Health and Care Excellence: London, UK, 2015. Available online: https://www.ncbi.nlm.nih.gov/books/NBK305022/ (accessed on 5 February 2020).

6. Sarosdy, M.F.; Kahn, P.R.; Ziffer, M.D.; Love, W.R.; Barkin, J.; Abara, E.O.; Jansz, K.; Bridge, J.A.; Johansson, S.L.; Persons, D.L.; et al. Use of a multitarget fluorescence in situ hybridization assay to diagnose bladder cancer in patients with hematuria. *J. Urol.* **2006**, *176*, 44–47. [CrossRef]

7. Lotan, Y.; Roehrborn, C.G. Sensitivity and specificity of commonly available bladder tumor markers versus cytology: Results of a comprehensive literature review and meta-analyses. *Urology* **2003**, *61*, 109–118. [CrossRef]

8. Bhat, A.; Ritch, C.R. Urinary biomarkers in bladder cancer: Where do we stand? *Curr. Opin. Urol.* **2019**, *29*, 203–209. [CrossRef] [PubMed]

9. Bubendorf, L. Multiprobe fluorescence in situ hybridization (UroVysion) for the detection of urothelial carcinoma - FISHing for the right catch. *Acta Cytol.* **2011**, *55*, 113–119. [CrossRef] [PubMed]

10. Behrens, T.; Stenzl, A.; Brüning, T. Factors influencing false-positive results for nuclear matrix protein 22. *Eur. Urol.* **2014**, *66*, 970–972. [CrossRef]

11. Wang, Z.; Que, H.; Suo, C.; Han, Z.; Tao, J.; Huang, Z.; Ju, X.; Tan, R.; Gu, M. Evaluation of the NMP22 BladderChek test for detecting bladder cancer: A systematic review and meta-analysis. *Oncotarget* **2017**, *8*, 100648–100656. [CrossRef]

12. Pichler, R.; Fritz, J.; Tulchiner, G.; Klinglmair, G.; Soleiman, A.; Horninger, W.; Klocker, H.; Heidegger, I. Increased accuracy of a novel mRNA-based urine test for bladder cancer surveillance. *BJU Int.* **2018**, *121*, 29–37. [CrossRef] [PubMed]

13. Ecke, T.H.; Weiß, S.; Stephan, C.; Hallmann, S.; Arndt, C.; Barski, D.; Otto, T.; Gerullis, H. UBC®Rapid Test-A Urinary Point-of-Care (POC) Assay for Diagnosis of Bladder Cancer with a focus on Non-Muscle Invasive High-Grade Tumors: Results of a Multicenter-Study. *Int. J. Mol. Sci.* **2018**, *19*, 3841. [CrossRef] [PubMed]

14. Baylin, S.B.; Jones, P.A. A decade of exploring the cancer epigenome-biological and translational implications. *Nat. Rev. Cancer.* **2011**, *11*, 726–734. [CrossRef] [PubMed]

15. Molnár, B.; Tóth, K.; Barták, B.K.; Tulassay, Z. Plasma methylated septin 9: A colorectal cancer screening marker. *Expert Rev. Mol. Diagn.* **2015**, *15*, 171–184. [CrossRef]

16. Larsen, L.K.; Lind, G.E.; Guldberg, P.; Dahl, C. DNA-Methylation-Based Detection of Urological Cancer in Urine: Overview of Biomarkers and Considerations on Biomarker Design, Source of DNA, and Detection Technologies. *Int. J. Mol. Sci.* **2019**, *20*, 2657. [CrossRef]

17. Veeck, J.; Chorovicer, M.; Naami, A.; Breuer, E.; Zafrakas, M.; Bektas, N.; Dürst, M.; Kristiansen, G.; Wild, P.J.; Hartmann, A.; et al. The extracellular matrix protein ITIH5 is a novel prognostic marker in invasive node-negative breast cancer and its aberrant expression is caused by promoter hypermethylation. *Oncogene* **2008**, *27*, 865–876. [CrossRef]

18. Kloten, V.; Rose, M.; Kaspar, S.; von Stillfried, S.; Knüchel, R.; Dahl, E. Epigenetic inactivation of the novel candidate tumor suppressor gene ITIH5 in colon cancer predicts unfavorable overall survival in the CpG island methylator phenotype. *Epigenetics* **2014**, *9*, 1290–1301. [CrossRef]

19. Dötsch, M.M.; Kloten, V.; Schlensog, M.; Heide, T.; Braunschweig, T.; Veeck, J.; Petersen, I.; Knüchel, R.; Dahl, E. Low expression of ITIH5 in adenocarcinoma of the lung is associated with unfavorable patients' outcome. *Epigenetics* **2015**, *10*, 903–912. [CrossRef]

20. Rose, M.; Gaisa, N.T.; Antony, P.; Fiedler, D.; Heidenreich, A.; Otto, W.; Denzinger, S.; Bertz, S.; Hartmann, A.; Karl, A.; et al. Epigenetic inactivation of ITIH5 promotes bladder cancer progression and predicts early relapse of pT1 high-grade urothelial tumours. *Carcinogenesis* **2014**, *35*, 727–736. [CrossRef]

21. Rose, M.; Kloten, V.; Noetzel, E.; Gola, L.; Ehling, J.; Heide, T.; Meurer, S.K.; Gaiko-Shcherbak, A.; Sechi, A.S.; Huth, S.; et al. ITIH5 mediates epigenetic reprogramming of breast cancer cells. *Mol. Cancer* **2017**, *16*, 44. [CrossRef]

22. Rose, M.; Meurer, S.K.; Kloten, V.; Weiskirchen, R.; Denecke, B.; Antonopoulos, W.; Deckert, M.; Knüchel, R.; Dahl, E. ITIH5 induces a shift in TGF-β superfamily signaling involving Endoglin and reduces risk for breast cancer metastasis and tumor death. *Mol. Carcinog.* **2018**, *57*, 167–181. [CrossRef] [PubMed]

23. Sasaki, K.; Kurahara, H.; Young, E.D.; Natsugoe, S.; Ijichi, A.; Iwakuma, T.; Welch, D.R. Genome-wide in vivo RNAi screen identifies ITIH5 as a metastasis suppressor in pancreatic cancer. *Clin. Exp. Metastasis* **2017**, *34*, 229–239. [CrossRef] [PubMed]

24. Yue, C.M.; Deng, D.J.; Bi, M.X.; Guo, L.P.; Lu, S.H. Expression of ECRG4, a novel esophageal cancer-related gene, downregulated by CpG island hypermethylation in human esophageal squamous cell carcinoma. *World J. Gastroenterol.* **2003**, *9*, 1174–1178. [CrossRef] [PubMed]

25. Li, L.W.; Yu, X.Y.; Yang, Y.; Zhang, C.P.; Guo, L.P.; Lu, S.H. Expression of esophageal cancer related gene 4 (ECRG4), a novel tumor suppressor gene, in esophageal cancer and its inhibitory effect on the tumor growth in vitro and in vivo. *Int. J. Cancer* **2009**, *125*, 1505–1513. [CrossRef]

26. Tang, G.Y.; Tang, G.J.; Yin, L.; Chao, C.; Zhou, R.; Ren, G.P.; Chen, J.Y.; Zhang, W. ECRG4 acts as a tumor suppressor gene frequently hypermethylated in human breast cancer. *Biosci. Rep.* **2019**, *39*, BSR20190087. [CrossRef]

27. Luo, L.; Wu, J.; Xie, J.; Xia, L.; Qian, X.; Cai, Z.; Li, Z. Downregulated ECRG4 is associated with poor prognosis in renal cell cancer and is regulated by promoter DNA methylation. *Tumour Biol.* **2016**, *37*, 1121–1129. [CrossRef]

28. Götze, S.; Feldhaus, V.; Traska, T.; Wolter, M.; Reifenberger, G.; Tannapfel, A.; Kuhnen, C.; Martin, D.; Müller, O.; Sievers, S. ECRG4 is a candidate tumor suppressor gene frequently hypermethylated in colorectal carcinoma and glioma. *BMC Cancer* **2009**, *9*, 447. [CrossRef]

29. Cai, Z.; Liang, P.; Xuan, J.; Wan, J.; Guo, H. ECRG4 as a novel tumor suppressor gene inhibits colorectal cancer cell growth in vitro and in vivo. *Tumour Biol.* **2016**, *37*, 9111–9120. [CrossRef]

30. Cancer Genome Atlas Research Network. Comprehensive molecular characterization of urothelial bladder carcinoma. *Nature* **2014**, *507*, 315–322. [CrossRef]

31. Renard, I.; Joniau, S.; van Cleynenbreugel, B.; Collette, C.; Naômé, C.; Vlassenbroeck, I.; Nicolas, H.; de Leval, J.; Straub, J.; Van Criekinge, W.; et al. Identification and validation of the methylated TWIST1 and NID2 genes through real-time methylation-specific polymerase chain reaction assays for the noninvasive detection of primary bladder cancer in urine samples. *Eur. Urol.* **2010**, *58*, 96–104. [CrossRef]

32. Song, L.; Jia, J.; Peng, X.; Xiao, W.; Li, Y. The performance of the SEPT9 gene methylation assay and a comparison with other CRC screening tests: A meta-analysis. *Sci. Rep.* **2017**, *7*, 3032. [CrossRef] [PubMed]

33. Lodewijk, I.; Dueñas, M.; Rubio, C.; Munera-Maravilla, E.; Segovia, C.; Bernardini, A.; Teijeira, A.; Paramio, J.M.; Suárez-Cabrera, C. Liquid Biopsy Biomarkers in Bladder Cancer: A Current Need for Patient Diagnosis and Monitoring. *Int. J. Mol. Sci.* **2018**, *19*, 2514. [CrossRef]

34. Costa, V.L.; Henrique, R.; Danielsen, S.A.; Duarte-Pereira, S.; Eknaes, M.; Skotheim, R.I.; Rodrigues, A.; Magalhães, J.S.; Oliveira, J.; Lothe, R.A.; et al. Three epigenetic biomarkers, GDF15, TMEFF2, and VIM, accurately predict bladder cancer from DNA-based analyses of urine samples. *Clin. Cancer Res.* **2010**, *16*, 5842–5851. [CrossRef] [PubMed]

35. Van der Heijden, A.G.; Mengual, L.; Ingelmo-Torres, M.; Lozano, J.J.; van Rijt-van de Westerlo, C.C.M.; Baixauli, M.; Geavlete, B.; Moldoveanud, C.; Ene, C.; Dinney, C.P.; et al. Urine cell-based DNA methylation classifier for monitoring bladder cancer. *Clin. Epigenetics* **2018**, *10*, 71. [CrossRef] [PubMed]

36.   Hernández, H.G.; Tse, M.Y.; Pang, S.C.; Arboleda, H.; Forero, D.A. Optimizing methodologies for PCR-based DNA methylation analysis. *Biotechniques* **2013**, *55*, 181–197. [CrossRef] [PubMed]

37.   Feber, A.; Dhami, P.; Dong, L.; de Winter, P.; Tan, W.S.; Martínez-Fernández, M.; Paul, D.S.; Hynes-Allen, A.; Rezaee, S.; Gurung, P.; et al. UroMark-a urinary biomarker assay for the detection of bladder cancer. *Clin. Epigenetics* **2017**, *9*, 8. [CrossRef] [PubMed]

38.   Kloten, V.; Becker, B.; Winner, K.; Schrauder, M.G.; Fasching, P.A.; Anzeneder, T.; Veeck, J.; Hartmann, A.; Knüchel, R.; Dahl, E. Promoter hypermethylation of the tumor-suppressor genes ITIH5, DKK3, and RASSF1A as novel biomarkers for blood-based breast cancer screening. *Breast Cancer Res.* **2013**, *15*, R4. [CrossRef]

39.   Shahin, O.; Thalmann, G.N.; Rentsch, C.; Mazzucchelli, L.; Studer, U.E. A retrospective analysis of 153 patients treated with or without intravesical bacillus Calmette-Guerin for primary stage T1 grade 3 bladder cancer: Recurrence, progression and survival. *J. Urol.* **2003**, *169*, 96–100. [CrossRef]

40.   Witjes, J.A.; Morote, J.; Cornel, E.B.; Gakis, G.; van Valenberg, F.J.P.; Lozano, F.; Sternberg, I.A.; Willemsen, E.; Hegemann, M.L.; Paitan, Y.; et al. Performance of the Bladder EpiCheck™ Methylation Test for Patients Under Surveillance for Non-muscle-invasive Bladder Cancer: Results of a Multicenter, Prospective, Blinded Clinical Trial. *Eur. Urol. Oncol.* **2018**, *1*, 307–313. [CrossRef]

41.   Pfaffl, M.W. A new mathematical model for relative quantification in real-time RT-PCR. *Nucleic Acids Res.* **2001**, *29*, e45. [CrossRef]

42.   Ralser, M.; Querfurth, R.; Warnatz, H.J.; Lehrach, H.; Yaspo, M.L.; Krobitsch, S. An efficient and economic enhancer mix for PCR. *Biochem. Biophys. Res. Commun.* **2006**, *347*, 747–751. [CrossRef] [PubMed]

43.   Mijnes, J.; Veeck, J.; Gaisa, N.T.; Burghardt, E.; de Ruijter, T.C.; Gostek, S.; Dahl, E.; Pfister, D.; Schmid, S.C.; Knüchel, R.; et al. Promoter methylation of DNA damage repair (DDR) genes in human tumor entities: RBBP8/CtIP is almost exclusively methylated in bladder cancer. *Clin. Epigenetics* **2018**, *10*, 15. [CrossRef] [PubMed]

13

UBC® *Rapid* Test—A Urinary Point-of-Care (POC) Assay for Diagnosis of Bladder Cancer with a focus on Non-Muscle Invasive High-Grade Tumors: Results of a Multicenter-Study

Thorsten H. Ecke [1,*], **Sarah Weiß** [2], **Carsten Stephan** [2,3], **Steffen Hallmann** [1], **Christian Arndt** [4], **Dimitri Barski** [4], **Thomas Otto** [4] and **Holger Gerullis** [5]

[1]   HELIOS Hospital, Department of Urology, Bad Saarow D-15526, Germany; steffen.hallmann@helios-gesundheit.de

[2]   Department of Urology, Charité University Hospital, Berlin D-10117, Germany; sarah.weiss2@helios-gesundheit.de (S.W.); carsten.stephan@charite.de (C.S.)

[3]   Berlin Institute for Urological Research, Berlin D-10115, Germany

[4]   Department of Urology, Lukas Hospital Neuss, Neuss D-41464, Germany; arndt_christian@web.de (C.A.); barskidimitri@gmail.com (D.B.); thomas_otto@lukasneuss.de (T.O.)

[5]   University Hospital for Urology, Klinikum Oldenburg, School of Medicine and Health Sciences Carl von Ossietzky University Oldenburg, Oldenburg D-26133, Germany; holger.gerullis@gmx.net

*   Correspondence: thorsten.ecke@helios-kliniken.de

Abstract: Objectives: UBC® *Rapid* Test measures soluble fragments of cytokeratins 8 and 18 in urine. We present results of a multicenter study using an updated version of UBC® *Rapid* Test in bladder cancer patients, patients with urinary bladder cancer positive history, and healthy controls. Material and Methods: In total 530 urine samples have been included in this study. Clinical urine samples were used from 242 patients with tumors of the urinary bladder (134 non-muscle-invasive low-grade tumors (NMI-LG), 48 non-muscle-invasive high-grade tumors (NMI-HG), and 60 muscle-invasive high-grade tumors (MI-HG)), 62 patients with non-evidence of disease (NED), and 226 healthy controls. Urine samples were analyzed by the UBC® Rapid point-of-care (POC) assay and evaluated by Concile Omega 100 POC Reader. All statistical analyses have been performed using R version 3.2.3. Results: Elevated levels of UBC® Rapid Test in urine are higher in patients with bladder cancer in comparison to the control group ($p < 0.001$). The sensitivity for the whole bladder cancer cohort was 53.3% (positive predictive value (PPV) 90.2%, negative predictive value (NPV) 65.2%) and was 38.8% (PPV 78.8%, NPV 72.1%) for non-muscle-invasive low-grade bladder cancer; 75.0% (PPV 72.0%, NPV 94.7%) for non-muscle-invasive high-grade bladder cancer and 68.3% (PPV 74.6%, NPV 91.8%) for muscle-invasive high-grade bladder cancer. The specificity for the statistical calculations was 93.8%. The cut-off value (10 µg/L) was evaluated for the whole patient cohort. The area under the curve of the quantitative UBC® Rapid Test using the optimal threshold obtained by receiver operating characteristics (ROC) analysis was 0.774. Elevated values of UBC® *Rapid* Test in urine are higher in patients with high-grade bladder cancer in comparison to low-grade tumors and the healthy control group. Conclusions: UBC® *Rapid* Test has potential to be a clinically valuable urinary protein biomarker for detection of high-grade bladder cancer patients and could be added in the management of NMI-HG tumors. UBC® *Rapid* results generated in both study centers in the present multicenter study are very similar and reproducible. Furthermore UBC® *Rapid* Test is standardized and calibrated and thus independent of used batch of test as well as study site.

Keywords: bladder cancer; tumor markers; urinary based diagnostics

1. Introduction

In Europe bladder cancer (BCa) is the fifth most frequent cancer. Its incidence rate was 151,200 and its annual mortality rate was 51,400 cases in 2012 [1]. Around 30% of bladder cancer patients suffered from muscle-invasive bladder cancer (MIBC) at the time of first diagnosis [2]. Radical cystectomy (RC) is the gold standard to treat patients with MIBC.

Non-muscle invasive high-grade bladder cancer has a particularly high rate of recurrence and will progress to muscle-invasive disease. The ideal urine-soluble marker should be used for primary diagnosis, follow-up, and screening of high-risk populations; replacing cystoscopy during follow-up or decreasing the number of control cystoscopies during follow-up would be a worthwhile goal. Due to its contact with urine, malignant cells are shed into the urine, and this urine contains the carcinogens producing the malignancy. Some of these urinary based tests have a higher specificity and sensitivity than classical urine cytology and could be important for screening and case findings [3].

Intermediate filaments of the cytoskeleton of epithelial cells containing cytokeratins are often overexpressed in urothelial tumors. In humans twenty different cytokeratins have been identified, and cytokeratins 8, 18, and 19 are known to be important in urothelial cells [4]. The expressions of cytokeratins such as 8, 18, and 19 are higher in urothelial cells and may be elevated because of a higher cell turnover rate [5,6]. Immunohistochemical features of urothelial dysplasia include aberrant cytokeratin 20 expression at different levels of the urothelium, however, there is also usually overexpression of p53 and high Ki-67 index [7].

UBC® *Rapid* Test is based upon an immunochromatographic method and measures fragments of cytokeratin 8 and 18 qualitatively. The measured levels are lower in low-grade tumors and benign urological diseases [8,9]. Cytokeratins 8 and 18 are soluble in urine and can be detected quantitatively with monoclonal antibodies using sandwich ELISA as well as UBC® *Rapid* assay with a photometric reader. It is important to highlight that this version of UBC® *Rapid* Test is a modified and updated version of fast cytokeratin determination in urine in comparison to the assay introduced 15 years ago. Furthermore this new version of UBC® *Rapid* Test is used in combination with a reader to quantitate the signal quite comparably with an ELISA assay, but it is a point-of-care (POC) assay. Previous UBC Rapid assays were only assays for visual evaluation of results.

In the last publication of our group we had a focus on carcinoma in situ (CIS), and we could show excellent results for UBC® *Rapid* Test for detecting CIS [10]. Regarding these facts, it is mandatory to include new tests into bladder cancer diagnostics, specifically a test that could detect flat, high-risk tumors difficult to detect in cystoscopy would be a step to ameliorate the finding of these tumors. The aim of this multicenter study is to report the final results with the highest number of measured samples for UBC® *Rapid* Test and to evaluate the usefulness of UBC® *Rapid* Test in patients with urinary bladder cancer with a focus on non-muscle invasive high-grade (NMI-HG) tumors and compare with healthy individuals.

2. Results

A total of 530 patients were included in the study; 242 with confirmed bladder cancer, 62 with non-evidence of disease (NED), and 226 healthy controls with no history of bladder cancer. The median age of the study population was 73 (range 26–98) years. Of these patients, 391 (73.8%) were men and 139 (26.3%) were women. Among the 242 patients with confirmed bladder cancer, 134 had non-muscle-invasive low-grade (NMI-LG), 48 had NMI-HG, and 60 had muscle-invasive high-grade (MI-HG) BCa; 182 (75.2%) had non-muscle-invasive bladder cancer (pTa and pT1 tumors), 60 (24.8%) had stage pT2–4. Carcinoma in situ (CIS) was detected in 23 cases (9.5%). A detailed analysis of the CIS patients in this study had already been published [10].

The number of patients and healthy controls are listed in Table 1 for study center I (HELIOS Hospital Bad Saarow) and study center II (Lukaskrankenhaus Neuss). Both groups enrolled a similar number of patients in the study. Table 2 shows all relevant data for center 1 and center 2 separately.

We could show that elevated concentrations of UBC® *Rapid* Test are detectable in urine of bladder cancer patients (Tables 1 and 2). Elevated levels of UBC® *Rapid* Test in urine are higher in patients with bladder cancer in comparison to the control group. In 134 NMI-LG tumors the mean value of UBC® *Rapid* Test was 30.9 µg/L, for NMI-HG tumors 95.5 µg/L, for MI-HG tumors 66.9 µg/L, for NED patients 10.0 µg/L, and for the healthy individuals 7.7 µg/L. Elevated levels of UBC® *Rapid* Test in urine are statistically significantly higher in patients with bladder cancer in comparison to the control group ($p < 0.0001$). The high-risk group showed a markedly higher UBC® *Rapid* signal than the low-risk group. The area under the curve (AUC) of the quantitative UBC® *Rapid* Test using the optimal threshold obtained by receiver operating characteristics curve (ROC) analysis (cut-off 10.0 µg/L) was 0.774 as shown in Figure 1. ROC analyses of patients from center 1, center 2, and all patients together is shown in Figure 2, and demonstrated very similar outcomes. Figure 3 shows the distribution of UBC® *Rapid* values in boxplots in the different patient groups (overall $p < 0.001$). It shows also that most of the elevated values are definitely higher than the cut-point, especially for NMI-HG tumors.

Table 1. Patient characteristics and results of UBC® *Rapid*. Abbreviations: non-muscle-invasive low grade (NMI-LG), non-muscle-invasive high grade (NMI-HG), muscle-invasive high grade (MI-HG), non-evidence of disease (NED), positive predictive value (PPV), negative predictive value (NPV).

	NMI-LG	NMI-HG	MI-HG	NED	Control	*p*-Value
n	134	48	60	62	226	
Age						
Mean	71.0	73.8	73.6	70.8	68.9	
(SD)	(11.9)	(10.6)	(10.0)	(11.4)	(12.2)	0.036
Median	73.5	75	74.5	72	71	
Range	26–92	51–94	52–98	46–88	31–93	
Sex						
Female (%)	34 (25.4)	6 (12.5)	19 (31.7)	10 (16.1)	70 (31.0)	0.021
Male (%)	100 (74.6)	42 (87.5)	41 (68.3)	52 (83.9)	156 (69.0)	
Diabetes	25 (18.7%)	8 (16.7%)	12 (20%)	10(16.1%)	34 (15%)	0.849
Erythrocyte (urine dipstick)	83 (61.9%)	44 (91.7%)	58 (96.7%)	38 (61.3%)	73 (32.3%)	<0.001
Leucocytes (urine dipstick)						
Mean	84.6	109.9	229.7	127.8	64.3	
(SD)	(172.6)	(167.6)	(228.1)	(206.6)	(150.3)	<0.001
Median	0	25	100	20	0	
Range	0–500	0–500	0–500	0–500	0–500	
Nitrite pos.	5 (3.7%)	5 (10.4%)	8 (13.3%)	3 (4.8%)	12 (5.3%)	0.085
Cystoscopy	100 (74.6%)	33 (68.8%)	42 (70%)	49 (79%)	36 (15.9%)	<0.001
UBC (µg/L)						
Mean	30.9	95.5	66.9	10	7.7	
(SD)	(63.4)	(104.6)	(90.1)	(9.79)	(13.92)	<0.001
Median	6.4	46	24.85	5	5	
Range	5–300	5–300	5–300	5–56.5	5–166	
Sensitivity	38.8%	75.0%	68.3%	22.6%		
Specificity	93.8%	93.8%	93.8%	93.8%		
PPV	78.8%	72.0%	74.6%	50%		
NPV	72.1%	94.6%	94.6%	81.5%		

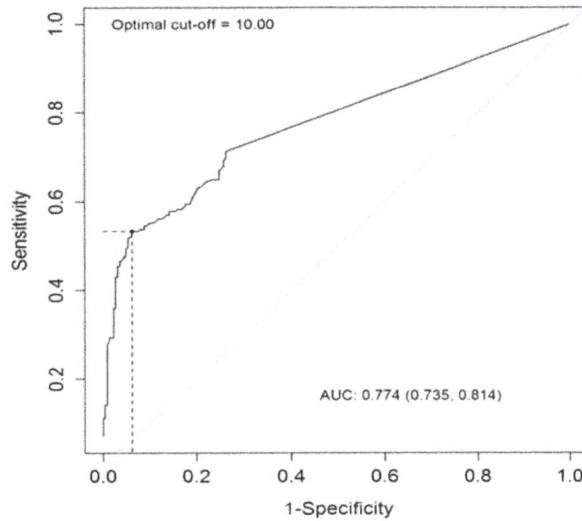

Figure 1. Analysis of the predictive ability—receiver operating (ROC) curve analysis for UBC® Rapid at cut-off value 10.0 µg/L with AUC 0.774 for the whole population.

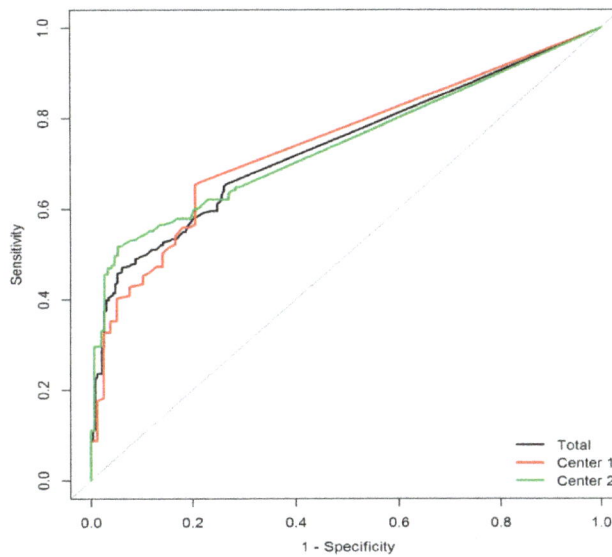

Figure 2. Analysis of the predictive ability—ROC curve analysis for UBC® Rapid at cut-off value 10.0 µg/L for the center 1 (red), center 2 (green), and whole population (black). *p*-value for comparison between centers = 0.874.

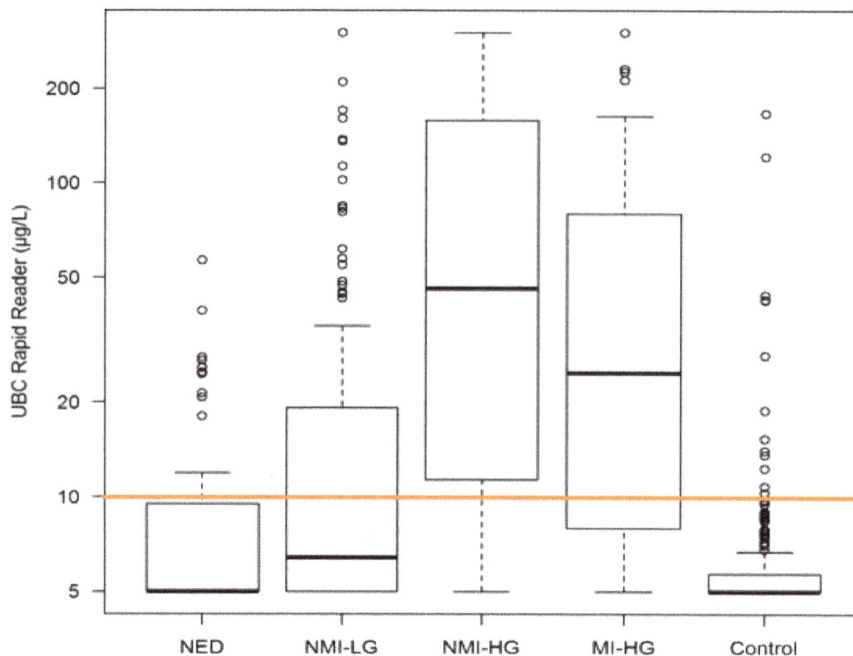

Figure 3. Box plot for non-evidence of disease (NED), non-muscle-invasive low grade (NMI-LG), non-muscle-invasive high grade (NMI-HG), muscle-invasive high grade (MI-HG), control. Orange line for cut-off at 10 µg/L.

Sensitivity was calculated as 38.8% for NMI-LG, 75.0% for NMI-HG, and 68.3% for MI-HG bladder cancer, and the UBC® *Rapid* specificity was 93.8% for all calculations.

Data of sensitivity, specificity, positive, and negative predictive values using a cut-off 10.0 µg/L for UBC® *Rapid* Test including the 95% confidence interval are also listed in Tables 1 and 2.

The data, which were generated in the two centers separately and reported in Figure 2, show impressively that ROC analysis is very similar and the sensitivity and specificity in both centres demonstrate no significant differences (Table 2). In the clinical data base it is obvious that center 1 has a higher rate of patients with diabetes and the rate of cystoscopies is higher in center 2. Though the rate of nitrite positive urine samples in center 2 is higher, the mean value of leucocytes is similar in both centers. Nevertheless, the results for UBC© *Rapid* Test are very similar in both centers demonstrating the robustness and stability of UBC® *Rapid* Test POC assay.

Table 2. Patient characteristics and results of UBC® *Rapid* separated for center 1 and center 2.

	NMI-LG		NMI-HG		MI-HG		NED		Control		p-Value	
	Center 1	Center 2	Center 1	Center 2	Center 1	Center 2	Center 1	Center 2	Center 1	Center 2	Center 1	Center 2
n	78	56	26	22	25	35	30	32	78	148		
Age												
Mean	71.1	70.8	74.9	72.5	74.2	73.2	73.0	68.8	67.6	69.6	0.042	0.554
(SD)	(11.6)	(12.4)	(11.6)	(9.4)	(11.0)	(9.3)	(8.8)	(13.1)	(12.64)	(11.94)		
Median	74	72	78.5	75	75	74	73.5	70.5	69.5	71.5		
Range	33–90	26–92	52–94	51–92	52–98	53–88	46–88	46–88	31–86	33–93		
Gender												
Female (%)	20 (25.6)	14 (25.0)	4 (15.4)	2 (9.1)	6 (24.0)	13 (37.1)	3 (10.0)	7 (21.9)	23 (29.5)	47 (31.8)	0.220	0.127
Male (%)	58 (74.4)	42 (75.0)	22 (84.6)	20 (90.9)	19 (76.0)	22 (62.9)	27 (90.0)	25 (78)	55 (70.5)	101 (68.2)		
Diabetes	22 (28.2%)	3 (5.4%)	6 (23.1%)	2 (9.1%)	6 (24%)	6 (17.1%)	5 (16.7%)	5 (15.6%)	13 (16.7%)	21 (14.2%)	0.469	0.337
Erythrocyte pos.	45 (57.7%)	38 (67.9%)	24 (92.3%)	20 (91.0%)	24 (96.0%)	34 (97.1%)	17 (56.7%)	21 (65.6%)	34 (43.6%)	39 (26.4%)	<0.001	<0.001
Leucocytes												
Mean	79.17	92.39	142.3	71.6	249.0	215.4	142.50	113.55	76.6	57.7	<0.001	<0.001
(SD)	(165.2)	(183.8)	(182.04)	(143.4)	(229.41)	(229.5)	(220.1)	(195.2)	(165.60)	(141.68)		
Median	0	0	100	25	100	100	25	0	0	0		
Range	0–500	0–500	0–500	0–500	0–500	0–500	0–500	0–500	0–500	0–500		
Nitrite pos.	3 (3.8%)	2 (3.6%)	4 (5.1%)	1 (1.8%)	2 (8%)	6 (17.1%)	1 (3.3%)	2 (6.3%)	3 (3.8%)	9 (6.1%)	0.199	0.185
Cystoscopy	47 (60.3%)	53 (94.6%)	11 (42.3%)	22 (100%)	11 (44%)	31 (88.6%)	20 (66.7%)	29 (90.6%)	16 (20.5%)	20 (13.5%)	<0.001	<0.001
UBC [µg/L]												
Mean	21.1	44.6	83.9	109.3	61.4	70.9	7.48	12.37	7.8	7.6	<0.001	<0.001
(SD)	(43.7)	(81.9)	(94.8)	(115.8)	(80.9)	(97.1)	(7.06)	(11.4)	(13.9)	(14.0)		
Median	6.5	6.2	41.4	59.4	28.9	20.7	5	6.5	5	5		
Range	5–300	5–300	5–300	5–300	5–300	5–300	5–39.1	5–56.5	5–121	5–166		
Sensitivity	38.5%	39.3%	73.1%	77.3%	68.0%	68.6%	6.7%	37.5%				
Specificity	92.3%	94.6%	92.3%	94.6%	92.3%	94.6%	92.3%	94.6%				
PPV	83.3%	73.3%	76.0%	68.0%	73.9%	75.0%	25%	60%				
NPV	60.0%	80.5%	91.1%	96.6%	90.0%	92.7%	72%	87.5%				

3. Discussion

The main purpose of this multi-center study was to evaluate the clinical usefulness of UBC® *Rapid* Test for diagnosis of bladder cancer with a specific focus on patients with NMI-HG tumors of the urinary bladder compared with healthy individuals. The results of the present study show that cytokeratin concentrations determined by UBC® *Rapid* Test measured by POC reader are statistically significant for patients with bladder cancer and healthy controls. Values of UBC® *Rapid* Test in high-grade tumors are significantly higher than in low-grade tumors, NED patients, and healthy individuals. The AUC as a parameter of diagnostic quality was calculated with 0.774. UBC® *Rapid* Test determined quantitatively could be applied to determine the risk for bladder cancer, but also the risk of having a high-grade tumor with increased risk for recurrence. The need for quantitative urinary markers like UBC® *Rapid* Test had also been published before [11]. The results of this study are showing again high values for UBC® *Rapid* Test especially for patients with high-grade bladder cancer [9,12–14]. Following from a previously published study with a high number of samples, the results of this study show that this test could be useful for combination in a diagnostic panel for patients of the high-risk group for bladder cancer. In previous reports of UBC® *Rapid*, a sensitivity of 65% and a specificity of 92% was calculated [15,16]. In the study of Mian et al. [16] only the older version UBC® *Rapid* with only visual evaluation was available. In our study, the new version of UBC® *Rapid* Test as cytokeratin assay was used; an improved lateral flow method resulted in a clearer test and control bands to evaluate. In this study UBC® *Rapid* Test was used with the Omega 100 reader to quantify the results.

Data presented in newer UBC® *Rapid* studies reported a cut-off of 12.3 µg/L, a sensitivity, specificity, PPV, and NPV of 60.7%, 70.1%, 46.8%, and 79.3%, respectively, and with an AUC of 0.68 [9]. According to other previous reported UBC® *Rapid* studies in the literature, the sensitivity of the qualitative UBC® *Rapid* Test ranged from 46.2% to 78.4%, and its specificity from 82.4% to 97.4% [9,12,16–20]. These data concur with our own results, whereas the sensitivity was low with 38.8% for detecting non-muscle invasive low-grade tumors. It increased to 75% for non-muscle invasive high-grade tumors and 68.3% for muscle-invasive tumors at a specificity of 93.8%. Therefore, it achieved the highest sensitivity of a single urinary marker test for detecting high-grade bladder cancer. The diagnostic accuracy of the quantitative UBC® *Rapid* Test POC system has been assessed in just five studies, which reported a sensitivity of 46.6% to 64.5% and a specificity ranging from 70.1% to 86.3%, respectively [9,12,17,19,20]. In this multicenter study, we could measure a high number of samples and the results for UBC© *Rapid* Test are very similar in both study centers. There is no significant difference in the ROC analyses, showing that the test is very stable and reproducible.

Currently, many different urinary POC test systems are available on the market, permitting non-invasive and rapid determination of urinary markers. Their diagnostic accuracy, however, is mostly controversially discussed in a small number of studies [21,22]. The sensitivities are usually higher than those reported for urinary cytology alone, but at a lower specificity [5,22]. Nevertheless, additional costs of urinary markers in surveillance protocols are ultimately not justified [23].

According to EAU guidelines, the examination of voided urine to detect cancer cells by cytology has a high sensitivity in high-grade tumors and CIS [2]. The major limitations for cytology are that specimens could be hampered by low cellular yield, urinary tract infections, stones, or intravesical instillations. Regardless, experienced readers can exceed specificity of up to 90% [5,24]. However, negative cytology does not exclude a tumor. As method cytology is subjective, on the other side UBC® *Rapid* Test is an objective method that is standardized and reproducible [22].

The use of those urinary markers for routine follow-up is not recommended in clinical practice by current guidelines and remains a debated issue [22,25]. The use of urine markers is only recommended as an adjunct to cystoscopy in current guidelines [26–28]. Other tests like Fluorescence in situ hybridization (FISH) and immunocytology have shown improved sensitivity compared with cytology [29–31]. These tests are complex and difficult to perform and they require specialized laboratory facilities.

It is common that new urine tests are compared with the results of cytology. Across a large number of studies, the results varied a lot. Sensitivity for G1-tumors is lower than 30%, for G2-tumors around 60%, and for G3-tumors 90%. Specificity is around 90–95% [32]. In the study of Ritter et al., UBC® *Rapid* Test was also compared with cytology, showing better results for UBC® *Rapid* Test [9]. One limitation of our study is that we had no comparison to cytology, mainly due to the focus on high-grade bladder cancer. But it is also known that urinary cytology is of limited diagnostic value for detecting low-grade bladder tumors compared to high-grade tumors (up to 84% [33]). In the reported study by Pichler et al., the sensitivity of bladder wash cytology was only 21.4%; the sensitivity of high-grade tumors can reach sensitivities of up to 84% [33]. Urinary cytology had been evaluated in many studies previously, and sensitivities and specificities are limited by the experience of the pathologists. This well-known fact has also been reported in recent references. Furthermore, it could also be interesting to include a combination of different tumor markers into BCa diagnostics. How to combine UBC® *Rapid* with other markers has been shown by Gleichenhagen et al. [13]. In this study a combination of UBC® *Rapid* and survivin increased the sensitivity to 66% with a specificity of 95%. For high-grade tumors, the combination showed a sensitivity of 82% and a specificity of 95%. A combination of both assays confirmed the benefit of using marker panels.

In contrast to dichotomized urinary tests, the quantitative character of the UBC® *Rapid* Test enables risk stratification for bladder cancer based on the absolute UBC® *Rapid* Test value. UBC® *Rapid* Test might not only contribute to improved detection of bladder cancer, but also to improved prediction of high-risk tumors. This has also been shown for other quantitative protein-based urinary tests [34]. An approach to objectify risk stratification should include a number of different parameters including quantitative UBC® *Rapid* Test, grade of haematuria, smoking status, age, and gender for developing a nomogram [35].

Of course, there are many other markers on the market, and genetic testing looks especially promising. Regardless, at the moment these markers are a rapid diagnostic tool too complicated to be included into basic and fast diagnostics. Currently, we still must stick to the proteins when we discuss quick testing. However, the "ideal urine-based marker" for detecting bladder cancer recurrence during surveillance would be rapid, non-invasive, and easy to perform and interpret. Furthermore, the assay should possess not only a high specificity to reduce superfluous cystoscopies on oncological follow-up, but also a high sensitivity so that no patient with low-grade and high-grade bladder cancer will be missed [34].

4. Materials and Methods

4.1. Patients

For this prospective study, 530 urine samples from bladder cancer patients and healthy controls have been collected between January 2014 and October 2015 at the Department of Urology, HELIOS, Hospital Bad Saarow (study center 1), and Lukas Hospital Neuss (study center 2), Germany. The study was approved by the local Institutional Review Board of national Medical Association Brandenburg (AS 147(bB)/2013). All patients with confirmed bladder cancer underwent cystoscopy, bladder ultrasound, and transurethral resection of bladder tumor in case of abnormal findings. Exclusion criteria were any kind of mechanical manipulation (cystoscopy, transrectal ultrasound, and catheterization) within 10 days before urine sampling. Other exclusion criteria were benign prostate enlargement, urolithiasis, other tumor diseases, severe infections, and pregnancy. All these criteria could influence the test to produce false positive results. Less than 10% of the possible study cohort had to be excluded based on exclusion criteria.

4.2. Procedure

Voided urine samples were collected in a sterile plastic container and subsequently processed. Urine samples were analyzed by the UBC® *Rapid* Test (Concile GmbH, Freiburg/Breisgau, Germany).

All tests were carried out as recommended by the manufacturer's instructions. The presence of a test band after 10 minutes of incubation was checked. After visual evaluation, the test cartridges were analyzed by the photometric point-of-care (POC) system Concile Omega 100 reader (Concile GmbH, Freiburg/Breisgau, Germany) for quantitative analysis. The cut-off value used for calculation of statistical parameters was based upon the evaluation of the receiver operating characteristics curve (ROC) and defined as 10.0 μg/L. The Omega 100 reader illuminates the test field with a complementary colored light to reduce interference in the analysis. The built-in charge-coupled device–matrix sensor takes a photograph of the light reflected, which is analyzed by the device.

4.3. Statistical Analysis

All statistical analyses have been performed using R version 3.2.3 (R Core Team (2015). R: A language and environment for statistical computing. R Foundation for Statistical Computing, Vienna, Austria. URL https://www.R-project.org/). Data are presented descriptively using means and standard deviations for numerical variables and absolute and relative frequencies for categorical variables. Comparison between groups at baseline has been performed using analysis of variance (ANOVA) for numerical variables and chi-square tests for categorical variables.

The predictive ability of UBC® Rapid Test measurements to detect bladder cancer was evaluated using Receiver Operating Characteristics (ROC) analysis, where the optimal cut-point was determined using the Youden index [36]. Sensitivity, specificity, positive, and negative predictive value was then calculated for the optimal cut-off and presented with exact 95% confidence intervals.

4.4. Ethics

The study was performed according to the Declaration of Helsinki. The study was approved by the local Institutional Review Board of National Medical Association Brandenburg (No. AS 147(bB)/2013 dated by 17 November 2013). Written and informed consent was obtained from each participant.

5. Conclusions

Elevated values of UBC® Rapid Test in urine are higher in patients with non-muscle invasive high-grade bladder cancer in comparison to low-grade tumors and the healthy control group. Sensitivity for non-muscle invasive high-grade tumors is very high with 75% at a specificity of 93.8%. Thus, UBC® Rapid Test has the potential to be a more sensitive and specific urinary protein biomarker to identify patients with high-grade tumors that are difficult to detect in cystoscopy. Results for UBC® Rapid Test in both study centers of the present multicenter study are very similar and reproducible. UBC® Rapid Test is standardized and calibrated, and thus independent of use, batch of test, as well as study site. UBC® Rapid Test should be added in the diagnostics and follow-up for NMI-HG tumors of urinary bladder cancer, though cystoscopy is still an important part of monitoring of bladder cancer.

Author Contributions: T.H.E. and H.G. conceived and designed the experiments; T.H.E., C.A. and D.B. performed the experiments; T.H.E. and C.S. analyzed the data; S.W., S.H. and T.O. contributed analysis tools; T.H.E. wrote the paper.

Acknowledgments: We thank the staff of the Urological Departments at HELIOS Hospital Bad, Saarow and Lukas Hospital Neuss, Germany, for their excellent help while collecting the samples. Statistical calculations have been performed by Marcus Thuresson from Statisticon, Uppsala, Sweden. The test systems were sponsored by Concile GmbH, Freiburg/Breisgau, Germany, and IDL Biotech AB, Bromma, Sweden.

References

1. Ferlay, J.; Steliarova-Foucher, E.; Lortet-Tieulent, J.; Rosso, S.; Coebergh, J.W.; Comber, H.; Forman, D.; Bray, F. Cancer incidence and mortality patterns in Europe: Estimates for 40 countries in 2012. *Eur. J. Cancer* **2013**, *49*, 1374–1403. [CrossRef] [PubMed]

2. Witjes, J.A.; Comperat, E.; Cowan, N.C.; de Santis, M.; Gakis, G.; Lebret, T.; Ribal, M.J.; Van der Heijden, A.G.; Sherif, A. EAU guidelines on muscle-invasive and metastatic bladder cancer: Summary of the 2013 guidelines. *Eur. Urol.* **2014**, *65*, 778–792. [CrossRef] [PubMed]

3. Lotan, Y.; Roehrborn, C.G. Sensitivity and specificity of commonly available bladder tumor markers versus cytology: Results of a comprehensive literature review and meta-analyses. *Urology* **2003**, *61*, 109–118. [CrossRef]

4. Southgate, J.; Harnden, P.; Trejdosiewicz, L.K. Cytokeratin expression patterns in normal and malignant urothelium: A review of the biological and diagnostic implications. *Histol. Histopathol.* **1999**, *14*, 657–664. [PubMed]

5. Lokeshwar, V.B.; Habuchi, T.; Grossman, H.B.; Murphy, W.M.; Hautmann, S.H.; Hemstreet, G.P., III; Bono, A.V.; Getzenberg, R.H.; Goebell, P.; Schmitz-Drager, B.J.; et al. Bladder tumor markers beyond cytology: International Consensus Panel on bladder tumor markers. *Urology* **2005**, *66*, 35–63. [CrossRef] [PubMed]

6. Siracusano, S.; Niccolini, B.; Knez, R.; Tiberio, A.; Benedetti, E.; Bonin, S.; Ciciliato, S.; Pappagallo, G.L.; Belgrano, E.; Stanta, G. The simultaneous use of telomerase, cytokeratin 20 and CD4 for bladder cancer detection in urine. *Eur. Urol.* **2005**, *47*, 327–333. [CrossRef] [PubMed]

7. Hodges, K.B.; Lopez-Beltran, A.; Davidson, D.D.; Montironi, R.; Cheng, L. Urothelial dysplasia and other flat lesions of the urinary bladder: Clinicopathologic and molecular features. *Hum. Pathol.* **2010**, *41*, 155–162. [CrossRef] [PubMed]

8. Schroeder, G.L.; Lorenzo-Gomez, M.F.; Hautmann, S.H.; Friedrich, M.G.; Ekici, S.; Huland, H.; Lokeshwar, V. A side by side comparison of cytology and biomarkers for bladder cancer detection. *J. Urol.* **2004**, *172*, 1123–1126. [CrossRef] [PubMed]

9. Ritter, R.; Hennenlotter, J.; Kuhs, U.; Hofmann, U.; Aufderklamm, S.; Blutbacher, P.; Deja, A.; Hohneder, A.; Gerber, V.; Gakis, G.; et al. Evaluation of a new quantitative point-of-care test platform for urine-based detection of bladder cancer. *Urol. Oncol.* **2014**, *32*, 337–344. [CrossRef] [PubMed]

10. Ecke, T.H.; Weiss, S.; Stephan, C.; Hallmann, S.; Barski, D.; Otto, T.; Gerullis, H. UBC® Rapid Test for detection of carcinoma in situ for bladder cancer. *Tumour Biol.* **2017**, *39*, 1010428317701624. [CrossRef] [PubMed]

11. Shariat, S.F.; Casella, R.; Wians, F.H., Jr.; Ashfaq, R.; Balko, J.; Sulser, T.; Gasser, T.C.; Sagalowsky, A.I. Risk stratification for bladder tumor recurrence, stage and grade by urinary nuclear matrix protein 22 and cytology. *Eur. Urol.* **2004**, *45*, 304–313, author reply 313. [CrossRef] [PubMed]

12. Ecke, T.H.; Arndt, C.; Stephan, C.; Hallmann, S.; Lux, O.; Otto, T.; Ruttloff, J.; Gerullis, H. Preliminary Results of a Multicentre Study of the UBC Rapid Test for Detection of Urinary Bladder Cancer. *Anticancer Res.* **2015**, *35*, 2651–2655. [PubMed]

13. Gleichenhagen, J.; Arndt, C.; Casjens, S.; Meinig, C.; Gerullis, H.; Raiko, I.; Bruning, T.; Ecke, T.; Johnen, G. Evaluation of a New Survivin ELISA and UBC® Rapid for the Detection of Bladder Cancer in Urine. *Int. J. Mol. Sci.* **2018**, *19*, 226. [CrossRef] [PubMed]

14. Styrke, J.; Henriksson, H.; Ljungberg, B.; Hasan, M.; Silfverberg, I.; Einarsson, R.; Malmstrom, P.U.; Sherif, A. Evaluation of the diagnostic accuracy of UBC® Rapid in bladder cancer: A Swedish multicentre study. *Scand. J. Urol.* **2017**, *51*, 293–300. [CrossRef] [PubMed]

15. Sanchez-Carbayo, M.; Herrero, E.; Megias, J.; Mira, A.; Soria, F. Initial evaluation of the new urinary bladder cancer rapid test in the detection of transitional cell carcinoma of the bladder. *Urology* **1999**, *54*, 656–661. [CrossRef]

16. Mian, C.; Lodde, M.; Haitel, A.; Vigl, E.E.; Marberger, M.; Pycha, A. Comparison of the monoclonal UBC-ELISA test and the NMP22 ELISA test for the detection of urothelial cell carcinoma of the bladder. *Urology* **2000**, *55*, 223–226. [CrossRef]

17. Hakenberg, O.W.; Fuessel, S.; Richter, K.; Froehner, M.; Oehlschlaeger, S.; Rathert, P.; Meye, A.; Wirth, M.P. Qualitative and quantitative assessment of urinary cytokeratin 8 and 18 fragments compared with voided urine cytology in diagnosis of bladder carcinoma. *Urology* **2004**, *64*, 1121–1126. [CrossRef] [PubMed]

18. Sanchez-Carbayo, M.; Herrero, E.; Megias, J.; Mira, A.; Espasa, A.; Chinchilla, V.; Soria, F. Initial evaluation of the diagnostic performance of the new urinary bladder cancer antigen test as a tumor marker for transitional cell carcinoma of the bladder. *J. Urol.* **1999**, *161*, 1110–1115. [CrossRef]

19. Babjuk, M.; Kostirova, M.; Mudra, K.; Pecher, S.; Smolova, H.; Pecen, L.; Ibrahim, Z.; Dvoracek, J.; Jarolim, L.; Novak, J.; et al. Qualitative and quantitative detection of urinary human complement factor H-related protein (BTA stat and BTA TRAK) and fragments of cytokeratins 8, 18 (UBC rapid and UBC IRMA) as markers for transitional cell carcinoma of the bladder. *Eur. Urol.* **2002**, *41*, 34–39. [CrossRef]

20. Pichler, R.; Tulchiner, G.; Fritz, J.; Schaefer, G.; Horninger, W.; Heidegger, I. Urinary UBC Rapid and NMP22 Test for Bladder Cancer Surveillance in Comparison to Urinary Cytology: Results from a Prospective Single-Center Study. *Int. J. Med. Sci.* **2017**, *14*, 811. [CrossRef]

21. Chou, R.; Gore, J.L.; Buckley, D.; Fu, R.; Gustafson, K.; Griffin, J.C.; Grusing, S.; Selph, S. Urinary Biomarkers for Diagnosis of Bladder Cancer: A Systematic Review and Meta-analysis. *Ann. Intern. Med.* **2015**, *163*, 922–931. [CrossRef] [PubMed]

22. Van Rhijn, B.W.; van der Poel, H.G.; van der Kwast, T.H. Urine markers for bladder cancer surveillance: A systematic review. *Eur. Urol.* **2005**, *47*, 736–748. [CrossRef] [PubMed]

23. Kamat, A.M.; Karam, J.A.; Grossman, H.B.; Kader, A.K.; Munsell, M.; Dinney, C.P. Prospective trial to identify optimal bladder cancer surveillance protocol: Reducing costs while maximizing sensitivity. *BJU Int.* **2011**, *108*, 1119–1123. [CrossRef] [PubMed]

24. Raitanen, M.P.; Aine, R.; Rintala, E.; Kallio, J.; Rajala, P.; Juusela, H.; Tammela, T.L. Differences between local and review urinary cytology in diagnosis of bladder cancer. An interobserver multicenter analysis. *Eur. Urol.* **2002**, *41*, 284–289. [CrossRef]

25. Babjuk, M.; Bohle, A.; Burger, M.; Capoun, O.; Cohen, D.; Comperat, E.M.; Hernandez, V.; Kaasinen, E.; Palou, J.; Roupret, M.; et al. EAU Guidelines on Non-Muscle-invasive Urothelial Carcinoma of the Bladder: Update 2016. *Eur. Urol.* **2017**, *71*, 447–461. [CrossRef]

26. Babjuk, M.; Oosterlinck, W.; Sylvester, R.; Kaasinen, E.; Bohle, A.; Palou-Redorta, J.; Roupret, M. EAU guidelines on non-muscle-invasive urothelial carcinoma of the bladder, the 2011 update. *Eur. Urol.* **2011**, *59*, 997–1008. [CrossRef]

27. Sturgeon, C.M.; Duffy, M.J.; Hofmann, B.R.; Lamerz, R.; Fritsche, H.A.; Gaarenstroom, K.; Bonfrer, J.; Ecke, T.H.; Grossman, H.B.; Hayes, P.; et al. National Academy of Clinical Biochemistry Laboratory Medicine Practice Guidelines for use of tumor markers in liver, bladder, cervical, and gastric cancers. *Clin. Chem.* **2010**, *56*, e1–e48. [CrossRef]

28. Hall, M.C.; Chang, S.S.; Dalbagni, G.; Pruthi, R.S.; Seigne, J.D.; Skinner, E.C.; Wolf, J.S., Jr.; Schellhammer, P.F. Guideline for the management of nonmuscle invasive bladder cancer (stages Ta, T1, and Tis): 2007 update. *J. Urol.* **2007**, *178*, 2314–2330. [CrossRef]

29. Banek, S.; Schwentner, C.; Tager, D.; Pesch, B.; Nasterlack, M.; Leng, G.; Gawrych, K.; Bonberg, N.; Johnen, G.; Kluckert, M.; et al. Prospective evaluation of fluorescence-in situ-hybridization to detect bladder cancer: Results from the UroScreen-Study. *Urol. Oncol.* **2013**, *31*, 1656–1662. [CrossRef]

30. Friedrich, M.G.; Hellstern, A.; Hautmann, S.H.; Graefen, M.; Conrad, S.; Huland, E.; Huland, H. Clinical use of urinary markers for the detection and prognosis of bladder carcinoma: A comparison of immunocytology with monoclonal antibodies against Lewis X and 486p3/12 with the BTA STAT and NMP22 tests. *J. Urol.* **2002**, *168*, 470–474. [CrossRef]

31. Van Rhijn, B.W.; Catto, J.W.; Goebell, P.J.; Knuchel, R.; Shariat, S.F.; van der Poel, H.G.; Sanchez-Carbayo, M.; Thalmann, G.N.; Schmitz-Drager, B.J.; Kiemeney, L.A. Molecular markers for urothelial bladder cancer prognosis: Toward implementation in clinical practice. *Urol. Oncol.* **2014**, *32*, 1078–1087. [CrossRef] [PubMed]

32. Ecke, T.H. Focus on urinary bladder cancer markers: A review. *Ital. J. Urol. Nephrol.* **2008**, *60*, 237–246.

33. Yafi, F.A.; Brimo, F.; Steinberg, J.; Aprikian, A.G.; Tanguay, S.; Kassouf, W. Prospective analysis of sensitivity and specificity of urinary cytology and other urinary biomarkers for bladder cancer. *Urol. Oncol.* **2015**, *33*, 66.e25–66.e31. [CrossRef] [PubMed]

34. Shariat, S.F.; Karam, J.A.; Lotan, Y.; Karakiewizc, P.I. Critical evaluation of urinary markers for bladder cancer detection and monitoring. *Rev. Urol.* **2008**, *10*, 120–135. [PubMed]

35. Lotan, Y.; Capitanio, U.; Shariat, S.F.; Hutterer, G.C.; Karakiewicz, P.I. Impact of clinical factors, including a point-of-care nuclear matrix protein-22 assay and cytology, on bladder cancer detection. *BJU Int.* **2009**, *103*, 1368–1374. [CrossRef] [PubMed]

36. Youden, W.J. Index for rating diagnostic tests. *Cancer* **1950**, *3*, 32–35. [CrossRef]

14

Extracellular Vesicles in Bladder Cancer: Biomarkers and Beyond

Yu-Ru Liu [1], Carlos J. Ortiz-Bonilla [1,2] and Yi-Fen Lee [1,2,*]

[1] Department of Urology, University of Rochester Medical Center, Rochester, NY 14642, USA;
yu-ru_liu@urmc.rochester.edu (Y.-R.L.); Carlos_ortizbonilla@urmc.rochester.edu (C.J.O.-B.)

[2] Department of Pathology and Lab Medicine, University of Rochester Medical Center,
Rochester, NY 14642, USA

* Correspondence: yifen_lee@urmc.rochester.edu

Abstract: Tumor-derived extracellular vesicles (TEVs) are membrane-bound, nanosized vesicles released by cancer cells and taken up by cells in the tumor microenvironment to modulate the molecular makeup and behavior of recipient cells. In this report, we summarize the pivotal roles of TEVs involved in bladder cancer (BC) development, progression and treatment resistance through transferring their bioactive cargos, including proteins and nucleic acids. We also report on the molecular profiling of TEV cargos derived from urine and blood of BC patients as non-invasive disease biomarkers. The current hurdles in EV research and plausible solutions are discussed.

Keywords: extracellular vesicle; exosome; bladder cancer; biomarkers

1. Introduction

In the past decade, a heterogeneous population of nanograde membrane particles in biological fluids, termed extracellular vesicles (EVs), gained newfound meaning in cancer therapy and diagnosis. EVs is a broad term which generally indicates the heterogeneous vesicles released from cells. In fact, most cells, if not all, shed vesicles constantly. Diverse names have been used to refer to various sorts of EVs, including ectosome, microparticle, exosome and microvesicle. Among them, the biogenesis, specific markers and functions of exosomes and microvesicles have been studied relatively thoroughly. As summarized in Figure 1, the release as well as uptake of EVs occurs simultaneously between cells. Exosomes are 50–100 nm in diameter and their biogenesis starts with the inward budding of a late endosomal membrane which forms a multi-vesicular body (MVB) containing a number of intraluminal vesicles (ILVs) [1]. In contrast, microvesicles (100–1000 nm in diameter) are larger than exosomes and formed by outward budding of the cell membrane. Both exosomes and microvesicles act as "intercellular postal service" [2] since they encapsulate a wide variety of bioactive molecules, including proteins, lipids and nucleic acids (DNA, micro-RNA, mRNA and other noncoding RNA species), and they transport this cargo to recipient cells locally or at a distance, consequently altering their behavior. The uptake of EVs by recipient cells is mediated through fusion, phagocytosis, macropinocytosis and receptor raft-mediated endocytosis. However, the mechanisms by which EV cargo is selected are not yet known.

EVs gained biologists' interest following the groundbreaking finding in 1996 that exosomes transfer Major Histocompatibility Complex (MHC) class II molecules from B cells to T cells, thus mediating activation of the adaptive immune response [3]. Later studies reported on the identification of various functional miRNAs encapsulated in EVs of immune cells. In view of the extensive regulatory capacity of miRNA, Valadi and colleagues in 2007 discovered for the first time that EVs have been exploited by cells as a tool to exchange genetic information [4]. This finding reveals a novel mechanism of gene-based communication between cells via EV cargo transfer. The pivotal roles of EVs are found not only in mediating the immune system but also in regulating various physiological and pathological cellular functions. The urinary bladder is susceptible to diverse EV-containing biological fluids, such as blood, lymphatic fluid and urine, reason why there has been an increased interest in EV roles in bladder cancer (BC) and study of their potential clinical applications. In this review article, we will focus on recent research on EVs derived from BC (BCEVs) and their roles in tumorigenesis and disease progression, as well as emerging applications in therapeutics and diagnostics.

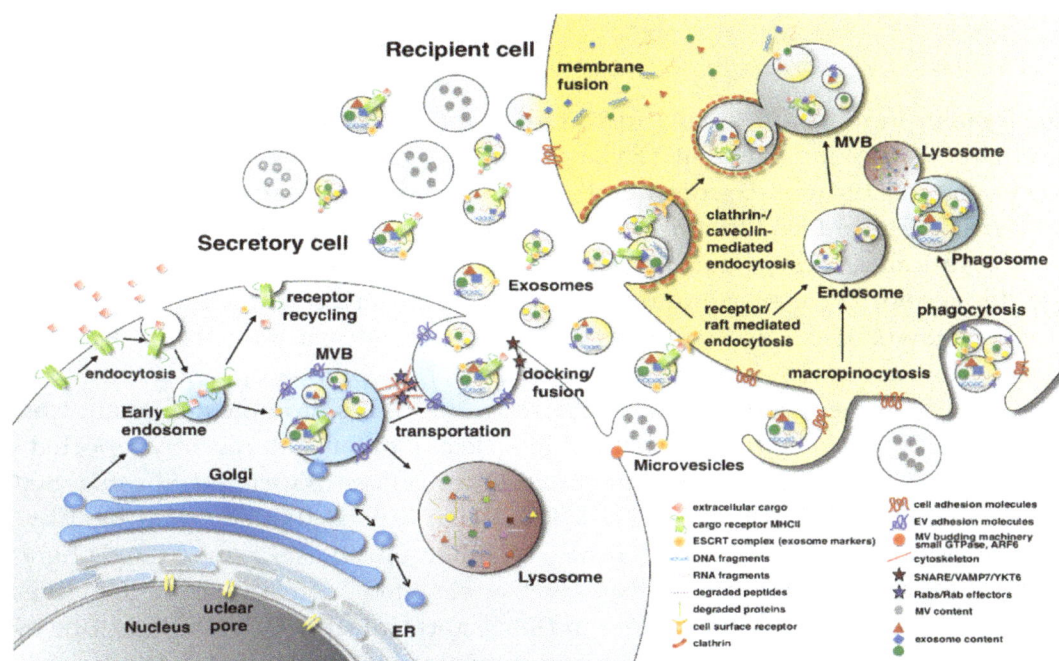

Figure 1. Extracellular vesicles (EV) biogenesis. The EV contents come from three sources: extracellular, intracellular and plasma membrane. Extracellular and plasma membrane molecules enter the early endosome through endocytosis either selectively by cargo receptor (ubiquitinated MHC-II) recognition or non-selectively. In the late endosome, the endosomal sorting complexes required for transport, ESCRT and their associated proteins such as TSG101, Alix, α-arrestin1 and CHMP4 mediate membrane inward invagination and form exosomes within multi-vesicular body (MVB). During the vesicle forming process, certain cytosolic components such as DNA, RNA and proteins are included in the exosome. MVBs can turn into lysosomes and degrade their contents or dock and fuse with the plasma membrane to release their contents to the extracellular space. The transportation and docking of MVBs is mediated by cytoskeleton remodeling which is regulated by Rab GTPase proteins (e.g., Rab27α, Rab27β and Rab7) and their effectors (e.g., SYTL4 and SLAC2B), whereas the fusion of MVBs with the plasma membrane is mediated by SNARE, VAMP7 and YKT6. In contrast, microvesicles are formed by outward budding of the plasma membrane which involves actin-myosin machinery, small GTPase and ARF6. The content sorting in microvesicles also involves TSG101. EV uptake is initiated by adhesion of EVs to the surface adhesion molecules on recipient cells, such as integrins, ICAM-1/LFA-1, CD11a, CD49d, CD44, CD169, heparin sulfate proteoglycans and by CD9, CD81 on EVs. EVs are then internalized through fusion, phagocytosis, macropinocytosis and endocytosis. ESCRT: Endosomal sorting complexes required for transport; TSG101: Tumor susceptibility gene 101; Alix: ALG-2-interacting protein X; CHMP4: Chromatin-modifying protein/charged multivesicular body protein; SYTL4: Synaptotagmin like 4; SLAC2B: Slp homolog lacking C2 domain B; SNARE: SNAP receptor; VAMP7: Vesicle associated membrane protein 7; YKT6: v-SNARE homolog (*S. cerevisiae*); ARF6: ADP-ribosylation factor 6; ICAM1: Intercellulare adhesion molecule 1; LFA1: Lymphocyte function-associated antigen 1.

2. Oncogenic Properties of BCEVs

Cancer cells are known to secrete more EVs than normal cells. The blood plasma of a cancer patient contains approximately 4000 trillion EVs, roughly twice the amount contained in a healthy individual [5]. Numerous studies have shown that EV-mediated cargo transfer to recipient cells affects many stages of cancer progression through communication between the cancer and the surrounding microenvironment, consequently promoting neoplastic transformation, BC proliferation, migration, invasion and angiogenesis. The EV cargo contents and their effects on cancer progression are summarized below.

2.1. BCEVs in Neoplastic Transformation

The transformation of healthy cells into malignant cancer cells involves several pathologic processes and many studies indicate that TEVs participate by transferring oncogenic cargo molecules to recipient cells [6]. A study by Urciuoli et al. [7] reported that treating NIH3T3 fibroblasts with osteosarcoma-derived EVs induced tumor-like phenotypes. Cells gained survival capacity by enhanced proliferation, migration, adhesion and 3D sphere formation and acquired the ability to grow in an anchorage dependent manner. Similar findings were reported in a study by Panagopoulos et al. [8], where they showed that EVs isolated from DU145 prostate cancer cells induced the malignant transformation of non-malignant prostate epithelial cells, possibly via up-regulation of pro-survival protein STAT3 [9,10]. Together, these results demonstrate that TEVs promote malignant transformation.

In the BC field, TEV's role in tumorigenesis is less clear. Goulet et al. recently reported that BCEVs can promote "transformation" of healthy fibroblasts into cancer-associated fibroblasts (CAFs) [11]. They isolated EVs from RT4, T24 and SW1710 BC cells and used them to treat healthy fibroblasts isolated from human bladder biopsies. As a result, recipient fibroblasts gained CAF phenotypes with increased proliferation and migration capacity as well as elevated expression of CAF markers—smooth muscle actin (SMA), fibroblast activation protein (FAP) and Galectin. Interestingly, our unpublished data (12,24,60) reveal that chronically exposing non-malignant immortalized urothelial cells to BCEVs leads to malignant transformation in vitro and in vivo. This might be due to the selection of cells with resistance to a BCEV-induced cellular stress response [12].

2.2. BCEVs Promote Cancer Cell Progression by Mediating Communication between Tumor Cells

2.2.1. Proliferation

The proliferation of tumor cells is an indispensable process for cancer progression, mostly relying on tumor-derived soluble growth factors. TEVs have been shown to promote cancer cell proliferation in leukemia, gastric cancer, glioblastoma, melanoma and prostate cancer, among others [13]. In BC, treating human 5637 and T24 BC cells with BCEVs was shown to stimulate their proliferation, possibly through activation of protein kinase B (Akt) and extracellular signal–regulated kinase (ERK) pathways [14]. Recent research delineating BC proliferation under hypoxia conditions found pivotal roles for BCEVs in transferring long non-coding RNA-urothelial cancer-associated 1 (lncRNA-UCA1) [15]. In this study, Xue et al. demonstrated that BCEVs derived from hypoxic 5637 cells contain high levels of lncRNA-UCA1 which stimulated proliferation, mobility and invasion in human UMUC2 BC recipient cells. In a xenograft model, lncRNA-UCA1-containing EVs facilitated bladder tumor growth and metastasis to the lymph nodes. Knockdown of lncRNA-UCA1 in hypoxic BCEVs increased the expression of E-cadherin while reducing vimentin and MMP9 expression, thereby triggering epithelial-mesenchymal transition (EMT) in the recipient BC cells.

2.2.2. Migration and Invasion

The essential step of tumor progression to metastasis is gaining the ability to migrate and invade. Our previous study showed that EVs derived from high grade TCC-SUP BC cells as well as urinary EVs from patients with muscle invasive bladder cancer (MIBC) facilitated migration and invasion in low grade 5637 BC cells. Two TCC-SUP EV-enriched proteins, EGF-like repeats and discoidin I-like domain-3 (EDIL-3) [16] and periostin [17], were identified. They can activate the ERK1/2 MAP kinase signal pathway in recipient low grade BC cells, thereby promoting migration and invasion and knocking down EDIL-3 and periostin by shRNA disrupted this action. Similar results were reported by other group [18], which showed that EVs derived from T24 and UMUC3 BC cells enhanced urothelial cell migration and invasion. Also, blocking the EV uptake of recipient cells by heparin remarkably reduced BCEV's impact.

In addition to carrying and transferring oncogenic cargos, BCEVs have been found to serve as an apparatus to dispose tumor-suppressor miRNAs (miR23b, miR224 and miR921) [19]. In this study, miRNAs previously identified to possess tumor-suppressor functions, such as miR23b, miR224 and miR921, were identified in BCEVs, implying a cancer character-sustaining mechanism. Silencing of Rab27α and Rab27β, two major EV secretion regulators, indeed halted the tumor-suppressing miRNA secretion. However, the miRNA retained in the cell might be inactivated by sequestration in the MVBs. Suppression of EV release resulted in reduced cellular invasion, which provides a possible explanation for the poor prognosis in BC patients with high expression of RAB27β. The levels of highly exocytosed tumor-suppressor miRNAs were found to be reduced in metastatic lymph nodes relative to primary tumors.

2.3. BCEVs Promote Cancer Cell Progression by Mediating Tumor-Stroma Communication

The tumor microenvironment is composed of a complex and heterogeneous network of different cell types and the extracellular matrix (ECM). Tumor-associated stromal cells arise from various cellular origins: fibroblasts, pericytes, bone marrow mesenchymal stem cells, adipocytes and endothelial cells [20]. The communication between tumor cells and the tumor microenvironment is pivotal to both primary tumor growth and metastatic evolution and this is mediated through direct cell-cell contact as well as via tumor-secreted factors including EVs. One of the most characterized pro-cancer properties of TEVs is their ability to facilitate new growth in vascular networks within tumor microenvironments to sustain the rapidly growing tumor mass during metastasis. TEVs have long been known to be exploited to induce angiogenesis; however, the underlying mechanism was only revealed very recently in a breast cancer study [21]. TEVs derived from breast cancer MDAMB231 cells were reported to contain a unique vascular endothelial growth factor isoform, VEGF$_{90K}$, that was crosslinked with Hsp90 and catalyzed by acyl transferase tissue transglutaminase (tTG). This EV-borne VEGF$_{90K}$-Hsp90 complex stimulates tubulogenesis in HUVEC endothelial cells and this effect was diminished by the use of the HSP90 inhibitor 17AAG to force the release of VEGF$_{90K}$ from the complex. Our group found that EVs from high grade BC cells contain EDIL-3 [16], which is known to promote tumor vascularization through an Arg-Gly-Asp (RGD) motif that interacts with integrin αvβ3 [22]. We demonstrated that the pro-angiogenic property of these BCEVs was abolished when EDIL-3 was suppressed by shRNA, confirming that EV-borne EDIL-3 mediates recipient endothelial angiogenesis.

Another key event mediated by TEVs during cancer progression is the establishment of a pre-metastatic niche (PMN) in favor of future circulating tumor cell (CTC) adhesion and colonization, which eventually leads to metastatic outgrowth. Growing evidence indicates that TEVs play central roles in PMN establishment and maintenance processes such as vascular remodeling, immune modulation, metabolic environment modification, fibroblast differentiation into CAF, ECM re-organization and organotropic homing [23]. However, the difficulty of obtaining pre-metastatic tissues from cancer patients and the lack of metastatic BC animal models have limited clinical investigation into the significance of this phenomenon. Our laboratory has succeeded in isolating metastasis-prone MB49 sub-lines and we have found that pre-conditioning mice with sub-line EVs promotes lung metastases (manuscript in preparation). A broad panel of ECM components is enriched in MB49 sub-line EVs, suggesting that they may participate in PMN formation principally through ECM re-organization [24].

3. Regulation of Immune Responses by BCEVs

Recent global profiling of the genetic and epigenetic landscape of BC has revealed it to be one of the most mutated cancers after lung cancer and melanoma [25,26]. Many new mutations have been identified; interestingly, many of them coincide with mutations that have been discovered previously in BC. This demonstrates that progressive tumors are heterogeneous, making it difficult to predict their outcome and the signatures of some of these molecular alteration patterns seem to have a prognostic impact [27]. With such a high mutation rate, BC can produce many tumor-associated antigens (TAAs) that are either mutated cellular proteins or molecules with different post-translational modifications [28]. The formation of TAAs leads to the generation of TAA-derived peptides, which are then presented through MHC on the surface of cancer cells to activate immunological surveillance. Since EVs have been known to modulate immune responses by directly or indirectly presenting MHC-antigen peptide complex on their surface, it is likely that these TAA-derived peptides can also be loaded into BCEVs to mediate immune response. In this section, we will discuss BCEVs functional roles in regulating the immune system.

3.1. Immune System Activation by BCEVs

While the activation of the immune system by cancer cell-derived EVs is not a well-studied phenomenon, there are a few reports that support this claim. For example, Rao et al. reported that TEVs elicited an antitumor immune response in a murine hepatocellular carcinoma (HCC) model in vivo [29]. They isolated TEVs from the murine HCC cell line hepa1-6 and used them to activate DC2.4, a murine dendritic cell (DC) line. These TEV-pulsed DCs were orthotopically injected into HCC tumor-bearing C57BL/6 mice, which resulted in increasing infiltration of T lymphocytes and elevated levels of interferon-γ (IFN-γ), consequently suppressing tumor growth. A similar finding was reported by Bu et al., who found that TEV-pulsed DCs elicited a tumor-specific $CD8^+$ cytotoxic T cell response in glioma patients [30]. In this study, they applied patient-derived T cells and $CD14^+$ DC precursor cells and found that EVs from the tumors of the same patients can activate T cell-mediated cytotoxicity. In the context of BC, Zhang et al. found that BCEV-educated DCs elicit T cell cytotoxic activity in vitro [31]. This evidence supports the possibility that BCEVs can promote immune system activation to facilitate the anti-tumor immune response.

3.2. Immune System Suppression by BCEVs

TEVs are known to be able to suppress the immune surveillance system, allowing tumor cells to escape the immune barriers and grow. This role of TEVs has been extensively studied using various cell types involved in the immune surveillance of tumors. In one immune escape strategy, cancer cells downregulate their MHC class I surface expression. However, natural killer (NK) cells are known to recognize and eliminate those non- or low-expressing MHC class I cells [32], so as a defense mechanism cancer cells can secrete EVs bearing transforming growth factor $\beta1$ (TGF$\beta1$) to deactivate NK cells and decrease their cytotoxic activity, resulting in the suppression of the anti-tumor immune response [33].

Shinohara et al. reported that the presence of miR145 in colorectal cancer TEVs can polarize classic (M1) type macrophages into M2 type macrophages, thereby supporting cancer cell growth in vitro and in vivo [34]. Further mechanistic dissection revealed that miR145 directly binds to the 3'untrasnlated region (UTR) of *HDACII*, a histone deacetylase, silencing its expression and promoting interleukin 10 (IL-10) production.

TEV suppression of DC function was demonstrated by Salimu et al. [35]. They treated DC cells with TEVs isolated from DU145 prostate cancer cells and co-cultured them with $CD8^+$ T cells. TEV-educated DCs triggered significantly stronger tumor-antigen-specific T cell responses as determined by IL-2 and IFN-γ production.

TEVs also allow immune escape by inactivating T lymphocytes directly. Rong et al. discovered that breast cancer cells secrete TEVs capable of suppressing T lymphocytes [36]. A similar phenomenon was found in head and neck cancer patients, where TEVs suppressed T lymphocytes, allowing tumor progression [37].

In BC, an important question that remains unanswered is whether EVs have an immunosuppressive character as seen in other cancer types. Last year, Lee et al. found that EVs derived from BC patient urine present an altered protein composition [38]. They found significant upregulation of mucin-1 (MUC1), carcinoembryonic antigen (CEA) and moesin. MUC1 has been reported to contribute to NK cell evasion by cancer cells [39] and its expression level has been associated with BC prognosis [40]. CEA has been correlated with tumor angiogenesis [41] and can inhibit NK cell targeting of cancer cells [42]. Moesin has been associated with metastasis and poor prognosis in a number of different cancers, including pancreatic, colon and laryngeal carcinomas [43–46]. These findings suggest that BCEVs might have immunosuppressive roles and open a new avenue for future research.

3.3. BCEVs in Promoting Inflammation

BCEVs may also have a role in controlling inflammation. We reported that MIBC patient urinary EVs are enriched in transaldolase (TALDO1) [47], an enzyme linked to oxidative stress, inflammation and carcinogenesis [46]. ApoB is another BCEV protein with a functional link to the inflammation process [48]. ApoB is another BCEV protein with a functional link to the inflammation process [49]. Andreu et al. compared the urinary EV protein profiles of BC patients versus healthy non-smokers and found that ApoB expression was significantly increased in BC patient-derived EVs. ApoB is involved in a wide range of biological processes including secretion associated with exosomes [50] and EVs [51]. ApoB has also been reported to play important roles in angiogenesis [52] and inflammation [53].

In summary, our understanding of BCEVs' functional roles in regulation of immune response is still in its initial stage. With recent progress made in cancer immunotherapy and the emerging evidence of BCEVs mediating communication between tumor and immune cells, we anticipate that further research will reveal pathological roles of BCEVs and their cargos in the regulation of immune responses, especially in response to checkpoint inhibitors.

4. Therapeutic Application of BCEVs

4.1. EV-Mediated Delivery of Therapeutic Agents in BC

Nanomedicine was introduced in cancer therapy during the 1990s [54]. With the benefit of small size (usually less than 200 nm), nanoparticles are able to escape from being engulfed by macrophages and neutrophils (which eliminate particles about 250–1000 nm) and then diffuse into the blood circulation and be transported to their target sites. With EVs' small size, various cell origins and low cytotoxicity, EVs have become an ideal nanoparticle drug carrier [55].

EVs were first used as a drug delivery vehicle to transport curcumin, an anti-inflammatory drug, to treat brain inflammatory disease [56]. Administration of exosomes encapsulating curcumin resulted in 5–10 fold higher plasma concentrations than curcumin alone and more effective inhibition of LPS-induced brain inflammation. BC cells are known to take-up EVs in a dose-dependent manner [57]. A recent study also found robust EV internalization in BC cells [58] where human BC cell lines (SW780 and UMUC3) showed 20–50 fold higher EV internalization rates than normal urothelial cells. Such high uptake rates make EV-nanoparticles an attractive method of drug delivery to BC cells. Moreover, the membrane structure of EVs encapsulates and protects vulnerable molecular contents, in particular various RNA species, such as siRNA, miRNA and lncRNA. In a recent study, EVs were exploited as a vector to deliver the designed siRNA to BC cells [58]. EVs were loaded with artificially synthesized siRNAs targeting polo-like kinase-1 (PLK1) by electroporation and then used to treat UMUC3 cells. As a result, the UMUC3 expression of PLK1 was significantly decreased, consequently inducing apoptosis and necrosis.

Chemotherapy following removal of the primary tumor is the standard treatment in many cancers. While chemotherapy is often capable of inducing cell death in tumors, many patients develop more advanced tumor growth due to the appearance of chemo-resistance, which remains one of most challenging problems in cancer research today. A recent study reported an innovative approach of using TEVs to sensitize BC cells to chemotherapeutic agents [59]. In a mouse model, intravesical instillation of TEVs prior to instillation of drugs including doxorubicin, mitomycin C, hydroxycamptothecin and gemcitabine, significantly reduced hematuria and tumor incidence. These TEVs were initially collected from UV-treated tumor cells and ranged in size from 100–1000 nm (microparticles). The recipient BC cells internalized the EVs into lysosomes, increasing lysosomal pH from 4.6 to 5.6, thereby promoting transportation of the lysosome to the nucleus over exocytosis and subsequently retaining drug bioactivity in the BC cells.

In the context of immunotherapy for BC, our group found that Bacillus Calmette–Guérin (BCG) infection stimulated BC cells to release EVs that could activate T lymphocytes, bone marrow-derived DCs and macrophages in vitro. This unpublished data suggests that TEVs are capable of mediating the anti-tumor immune response, possibly from transferring immune-active cargos [60].

4.2. Prognosis and Diagnosis of BC Using EVs

There is a growing trend towards exploring the use of minimally invasive liquid biopsy for early cancer detection and TEVs are attractive sources of cancer diagnostic and prognostic biomarkers for the following reasons: (1) EVs contain a specific cargo of proteins and RNAs that might reflect the status of the originating cells, (2) EVs are membranous structures that can protect the cargo contents from degradation, [61] EVs are relatively accessible as they are found in clinical specimens that can be obtained through non-invasive methods. Apart from plasma/serum, urine is considered the most relevant body fluid in terms of its physical contact with bladder tumor mass. Although EVs compose only 3% of excreted urinary protein [62], with proper isolation methodology and proteomic analysis, many urinary exosomal proteins have been identified to have pathophysiologic significance [61,63–69]. Nawaz et al. in 2014 published a comprehensive review of EVs as biomarkers for urogenital cancers which addressed the great potential of utilizing EVs in prognosis and diagnosis [70].

To define appropriate baselines, proteomic investigation of EVs derived from healthy donors is needed. The first comprehensive study of urinary EV protein contents was performed by Pisitkun et al. in 2004 using liquid chromatography-tandem MS (LC-MS/MS) [71]. Soon after, more detailed proteomic analyses were reported which determined protein profiles for urinary EVs of bladder and prostate gland origin [68,72–76].

Cell-free urine has been used to predict treatment response, recurrence, prognosis and diagnosis by detecting DNA level, methylation, mutation and integrity [77,78]. In BC, DNA level and integrity in cell-free urine were found to be significantly elevated relative to controls [79–81]. Urinary EV profiling of quantity as well as miRNA and protein content has been reported to serve as a prognostic and diagnostic biomarker. Recently, Liang et al. developed an integrated double-filtration microfluidic device to measure EV concentration at the point-of-care. They found higher amounts of EVs in the urine of BC patients compared to healthy controls and this result further suggests that urinary EVs have great potential to be used as a disease biomarker for BC [82]. Profiling miRNAs in cell-free urine was demonstrated to have >80% sensitivity and specificity in detecting different stages of BC [83]. Proteomic analysis of urinary EV cargo provides another prospect for disease prediction. Lin et al. collected urine EVs and analyzed the proteomic data from 129 BC patients versus 62 healthy participants and found SERPINA1 and H2B1K as promising BC biomarkers for prognosis Proteomic analysis of urinary EV cargo provides another prospect for disease prediction. Lin et al. collected urine EVs and analyzed the proteomic data from 129 BC patients versus 62 healthy participants and found alpha-1 antitrypsin (SERPINA1) and Histone H2B type 1-K (H2B1K) as promising BC biomarkers for prognosis [84]. We have searched the cargo contents of EVs derived from BC cells and urine of BC patients from the past 10-year publication and summarized the list of miRNAs and proteins encapsulated in EV cargos in Tables 1 and 2, respectively. The BC patient urinary EVs are a mixture of the whole body EVs and BCEVs, which reflects the clinical reality and relevance. Note that most of the reported cargo molecules are based on global screening that identified differentially displayed miRNAs and proteins between BC samples and controls but their functional roles in BC have not been verified.

Table 1. List of miRNAs identified in BC urinary EVs and/or BC cells EVs.

miRNA	Regulation	Sample Sources	Reference
miR-21	up	urine & BC cells lines	[85–89]
miR-200c	up	urine	[85,86,88]
miR-23b	up	urine	[19,90]
miR-513b-5p	up	urine	[90,91]
miR-183	up	urine	[88,92]
miR-205	up	urine from NMIBC patients	[86,88]
miR-16-1-3p, miR-28-5p, miR-92a-2-5p, miR-142-3p, miR-195-3p, miR-196b-5p, miR-299-3p, miR-492, miR-601, miR-619-5p, miR-3155a, miR-3162-5p, miR-3678-3p, miR-4283, miR-4295, miR-4311, miR-4531, miR-5096, miR-5187-5p	up	urine	[90]
miR-155-5p, miR-132-3p, miR-31-5p, miR-15a-5p	up	urine	[87]
miR-93, miR-940	up	urine	[85]
miR-16, miR-96	up	urine	[92]
miR-486-5p, miR-205-5p, let-7i-5p	up	urine from NMIBC/(G1 + G2)	[88]
miR-106b-3p, let-7c-5p, miR-486-5p, miR-151a-3p, miR-200c-3p, miR-183-5p, miR-185-5p, miR-224-5p	up	urine from NMIBC/G3	
miR-4454, miR-720/3007a, miR-29-3p	up	urine from NMIBC	[86]
miR-214	up	urine from NMIBC	[93]
miR-503-5p, miR-145-5p, miR-3158-3p, miR-30a-3p	up	urine from MIBC	[91]
miR-106b-3p, miR-486-5p, miR-205-5p, miR-451a, miR-25-3p, miR-7-1-5p, miR-146a-5p	up	urine from MIBC	[88]
miR-1, miR-99a, miR-125b, miR-133b, miR-143, miR-1207-5p	down	urine	[92]
let-7f-2-3p, miR-520c-3p, miR-4783-5p	down	urine	[90]
miR-30c-2-5p, miR-30a-5p	down	urine from NMIBC/(G1 + G2)	[88]
miR-30a-5p, miR-30c-2-5p, miR-10b-5p	down	urine from NMIBC/G3	
miR-30a-5p, let-7c-5p	down	urine from MIBC	
miR-27b-3p	down	BC cells	[91]
miR-let-7i-3p	down	BC cells	[89]
miR-29c-5p, miR-146b-5p, miR-200a-3p, miR-200b-3p, miR-141-3p	down	BC cells	[91]

Table 2. List of proteins identified in BC urinary EVs and/or BC cells EVs.

Protein ID	Sample Sources	Validated	Proteomic Detection
EHD4	urine and BC cells	[47]	[16,38,94]
HEXB	urine and BC cells		[16,38]
ANXA; SND1	urine and BC cells		[16,95]
S100A4	urine and BC cells		[16]
TALDO1	urine and BC cells		[16]
MUC1	urine and BC cells	[38,96]	[95]
EPS8	urine	[38]	[94]
CEAM5	urine		
CD44; BSG	BC cells	[96]	
ITGB1; ITGA6; CD36; CD73; CD10; CD147; 5T4	BC cells		

Table 2. *Cont.*

Protein ID	Sample Sources	Validated	Proteomic Detection
NRAS; MUC4	urine	[94]	
SERPINA1 H2B1K	urine	[84]	
TACSTD2	urine	[74]	
EDIL3	urine and BC cells	[16]	
POSTN	urine and BC cells	[17]	
CTNNB1; CDC42	urine and BC cells		[95,97]
14-3-3; ALIX; B2M; EGFR; EZR; FSCN1; LGALS; GST; MSN; PRDX1; PTGFRN; RDX; TAGLN2	BC cells		[95]

5. Current Challenges and Future Prospects

5.1. Current Challenges

Researchers have used dozens of names for various secreted vesicles (including exosomes, microvesicles and EVs), which have been broadly used and are sometimes interchangeable. However, exosomes and microvesicles are functionally and structurally distinct; there are differences in charge, size and molecular composition [98]. Importantly, the size distributions of exosomes and microvesicles overlap significantly and the identity of EVs between 100–150 nm in diameter is ambiguous [12]. Therefore, size alone cannot always be used to distinguish these EV subpopulations from one another. While "extracellular vesicle" is a widely accepted generic term for all secreted vesicles, there is a need for consensus about how to apply the other terms appropriately to different EV subpopulations in terms of vesicle size.

The conflicting names for different EV subpopulations are largely due to the different procedures used in individual laboratories to obtain and sort biological fluids to isolate EVs. Currently, with the rapid increase in the understanding of EV biology, including their function in numerous aspects of human disease and their potential significance in clinical applications, there is a growing demand for simple, efficient and reliable techniques to isolate EVs. Until now, the most standard EV isolation procedure combines filtration and ultracentrifugation, which purify particles based on their size and density [99]. To further purify exosomes from EVs, a common technique uses a continuous sucrose gradient during ultracentrifugation, which distributes particles according to density (exosomes float at densities ranging from 1.15–1.19 g/mL) [100]. In addition, microfluidic techniques combining immune-affinity, sieving and trapping have been applied to concentrate exosomes [101–103]. However, the unavoidable damage to the exosome structure and the low recovery narrows the application of this technique. Another common EV isolation method that has also been widely used for exosome purification is immune-affinity precipitation. This technique captures exosomes using antibodies against exosome surface markers. However, this method is limited by the exclusion of some EV subpopulations that do not carry the well-known markers. Therefore, the identification of general markers for EVs, such as lipid composition, pH value and electrical properties might be useful for capturing whole EV populations [104]. With the rapidly growth of the field, more and more isolation methods are proposed, the most updated EV isolation technic were comprehensively covered by recent reviews [1,12]. The recent launched EV-TRACK database encourages researchers to report their EV isolation details for developing a standardized protocol. (http://evtrack.org).

One of the hurdles to urinary EV isolation is the aggregation of highly abundant non-exosomal proteins, such as Tamm-Horsfall protein (THP), which tends to form fibrillary aggregates at low temperature. This aggregation during the EV isolation process was proposed to be reduced by a disulfide bond reducer, such as dithiothreitol (DTT), or a mild solubilizing detergent, such as CHAPS (3-[(3-cholamidopropyl) dimethylammonio]-1-propanesulfonic), which can separate THP from EVs during differential centrifugation [99,105–107]. However, DTT treatment can cause changes in the extracellular domains of EV proteins that would affect their stability and function. CHAPS treatment is better at preserving EV features but requires longer preparation [99].

The major challenge of EV-based biomarker discovery is the lack of a validated and standardized approach to normalize body-fluid concentrations among patients, especially in urine samples due to variation of water excretion in each individual. Urinary creatinine (UCr) excretion in the renal system is considered to be constant across and within individuals and is commonly used to normalize urinary biomarker concentrations against variations in urine flow rate in the evaluation of chronic kidney disease and prediction of acute kidney injury [108,109]. However, creatinine excretion rates vary widely among individuals with different age, sex, race, diet, physical activity, muscle mass, emotional stress and disease state [110,111], thus potentially masking the true value of EV proteins. Alternatively, specific exosome markers such as TSG101 and Alix can be used for normalization of urinary EV proteins [112]. More studies are needed to evaluate these normalization techniques and/or identify new ones.

Urinary EVs originate from cells throughout the urinary system; therefore, it is important to distinguish BC-specific EVs from the heterogeneous population of urinary EVs shed from other sources such as kidney and prostate. A recent study was able to increase the purity of podocyte-derived exosome isolation using immune-absorption with antibodies against the podocyte-specific complement receptor type 1 (CR1). Proteomic analysis of the podocyte EVs identified 14 new podocyte EV-enriched proteins that can potentially be used as kidney-specific EV markers to distinguish them from the broader urinary EV population [113]. This finding encourages similar efforts to identify BC-specific EV markers that are greatly needed to improve the diagnostic utility of urinary EVs.

5.2. Future Prospects

With accumulating evidence of TEVs' functional roles in cancer progression, depletion of the TEVs in circulation while retaining normal and healthy EVs becomes an ideal therapeutic approach. In 1989, Lentz conducted a primary experiment to remove low molecular weight (<120 kDa) proteins from cancer patients' blood by ultrapheresis, which resulted in tumor size reduction in 6 out of 16 patients [114]. At that time, serum cytokine receptors were proposed to be the key factors in blocking the antineoplastic immune response. However, this therapeutic effect might be because the process also results in the elimination of EVs. Previously, plasmapheresis combined with an affinity matrix containing *Galanthus nivalis* agglutinin to capture hepatitis C viruses has been applied clinically [115]. A similar plasmapheresis system was adapted to capture TEVs using a specific antibody-conjugated cartridge [116]. Therefore, identifying TEV-specific surface markers is the crucial step to take this approach to the next stage.

Another TEV targeting strategy is the inhibition of EV biogenesis and uptake. Amiloride, an endocytic vesicle recycling inhibitor, reduces the EV amount in the circulation and increases chemotherapy effects in mice [117]. Interference with the key proteins in EV biogenesis, such as Rab27β, also results in inhibition of EV release and reduction of tumor progression [118,119]. Theoretically, inhibiting EV uptake can be achieved by blocking surface phosphatidylserine. However, such inhibition can also affect microvesicle uptake by normal cells that might cause off-target side effects. Further dissection of EV machinery might lead to the identification of regulatory pathways in EV biogenesis or internalization that are specifically utilized by cancers.

The mechanisms by which secreted EVs are targeted to recipient cells are not yet well understood. It has been suggested that various integrins expressed on the surface of EVs might determine that they will interact with specific recipients through ligand-receptor binding [56,120,121]. A study by Hoshino et al. found that EVs from a variety of cancer cell types were preferentially taken up by specific cells in various organs depending on their integrin expression [122] This finding raises the possibility of utilizing EVs as therapeutic vectors to deliver RNA, protein or drug cargos to specific targeted cells by genetically engineering the EV integrins [123]. As more understating of the physical and pathological role of EV, more applicable areas of BCEV will be proposed.

6. Conclusions

In this review article, we have discussed various functional roles of BCEVs in mediating BC pathogenesis. As summarized in Figure 2, BCEVs can drive normal urothelial cell malignant transformation, promote BC progression via stimulation of proliferation, invasion and migration of recipient neighboring BC cells and modify the tumor stroma to support tumor growth. BCEVs have been further suggested to have roles in mediating cancer-related immunity, either by promoting inflammation favorable to tumors or by participating in the immune surveillance mechanism. Finally, potential clinical applications of BCEVs, mainly in diagnosis or prognosis or as drug-delivery vehicles, are discussed. However, the normal physiological functions of EVs should not be neglected, so that the off-target side effects of EV-based therapy can be reduced. As to EV-based liquid biopsy development, the identification of tissue/disease-specific EV markers is necessary to facilitate sorting of TEVs from the heterogeneous EV populations in patient specimens. Further investigation of EV biogenesis, content packing and uptake is also critical for future applications.

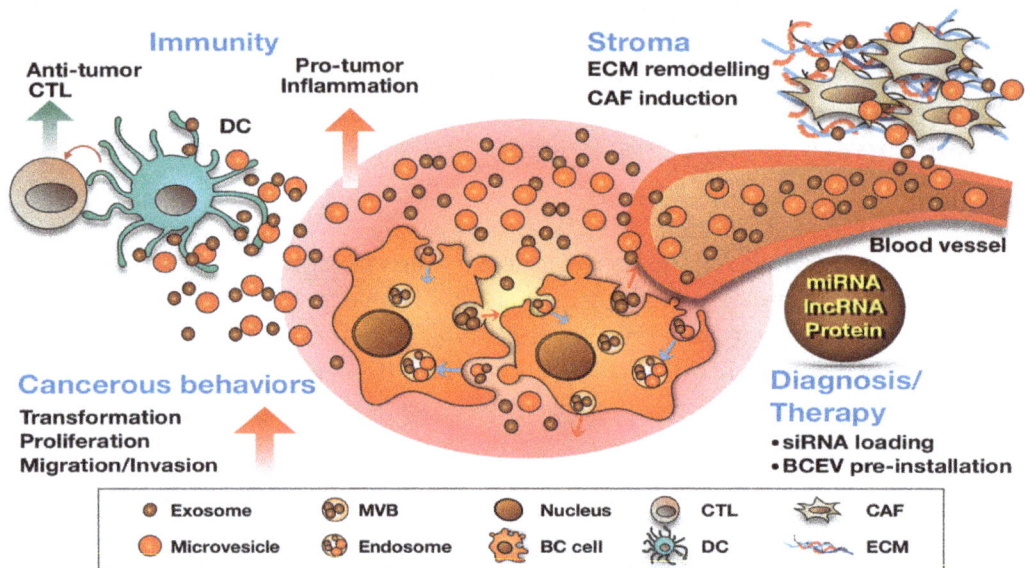

Figure 2. Summary of the roles of BCEVs in cancer, the tumor microenvironment and therapeutic applications. BCEVs are involved in many aspects of cancer development and progression. Like other cancer cells, BC cells release EVs into extracellular spaces and can be received by urothelial cells and immune cells, consequently modifying their behavior to support or suppress tumor growth (red and blue arrows indicate the migrating direction of intracellular vesicles). On the one hand, BCEVs can promote neighboring recipient cells' cancerous behaviors, including malignant transformation, proliferation, migration and invasion, as well as modify the tumor microenvironment in favor of tumor outgrowth, including promoting inflammation, ECM remodeling and fibroblast differentiation to cancer-associated fibroblasts (CAF). In contrast, BCEVs also participate in the immune surveillance system by presenting tumor antigens to provoke dendritic and cytotoxic T cell anti-tumor immunity. With specific cargoes carried by BCEVs such as miRNA, lncRNA and proteins, their clinical application, particularly in disease biomarkers, has rapidly expanded. Moreover, researching the utilization of BCEVs as vesicles to deliver therapeutic materials is also underway.

References

1. Ramirez, M.I.; Amorim, M.G.; Gadelha, C.; Milic, I.; Welsh, J.A.; Freitas, V.M.; Nawaz, M.; Akbar, N.; Couch, Y.; Makin, L.; et al. Technical challenges of working with extracellular vesicles. *Nanoscale* **2018**, *10*, 881–906. [CrossRef] [PubMed]

2. Yellon, D.M.; Davidson, S.M. Exosomes: Nanoparticles involved in cardioprotection? *Circ. Res.* **2014**, *114*, 325–332. [CrossRef] [PubMed]

3. Aalberts, M.; Stout, T.A.; Stoorvogel, W. Prostasomes: Extracellular vesicles from the prostate. *Reproduction* **2014**, *147*, R1–R14. [CrossRef] [PubMed]

4. Valadi, H.; Ekstrom, K.; Bossios, A.; Sjostrand, M.; Lee, J.J.; Lotvall, J.O. Exosome-mediated transfer of mRNAs and microRNAs is a novel mechanism of genetic exchange between cells. *Nat. Cell Biol.* **2007**, *9*, 654. [CrossRef] [PubMed]

5. Kalluri, R. The biology and function of exosomes in cancer. *J. Clin. Investig.* **2016**, *126*, 1208–1215. [CrossRef] [PubMed]

6. Choi, D.; Lee, T.H.; Spinelli, C.; Chennakrishnaiah, S.; D'Asti, E.; Rak, J. Extracellular vesicle communication pathways as regulatory targets of oncogenic transformation. *Semin. Cell Dev. Biol.* **2017**, *67*, 11–22. [CrossRef] [PubMed]

7. Urciuoli, E.; Giorda, E.; Scarsella, M.; Petrini, S.; Peruzzi, B. Osteosarcoma-derived extracellular vesicles induce a tumor-like phenotype in normal recipient cells. *J. Cell. Physiol.* **2018**, *233*, 6158–6172. [CrossRef] [PubMed]

8. Panagopoulos, K.; Cross-Knorr, S.; Dillard, C.; Pantazatos, D.; Del Tatto, M.; Mills, D.; Goldstein, L.; Renzulli, J.; Quesenberry, P.; Chatterjee, D. Reversal of chemosensitivity and induction of cell malignancy of a non-malignant prostate cancer cell line upon extracellular vesicle exposure. *Mol. Cancer* **2013**, *12*. [CrossRef] [PubMed]

9. Barton, B.E.; Karras, J.G.; Murphy, T.F.; Barton, A.; Huang, H.F.S. Signal transducer and activator of transcription 3 (STAT3) activation in prostate cancer: Direct STAT3 inhibition induces apoptosis in prostate cancer lines. *Mol. Cancer Ther.* **2004**, *3*, 11–20. [PubMed]

10. Bromberg, J. Stat proteins and oncogenesis. *J. Clin. Investig.* **2002**, *109*, 1139–1142. [CrossRef] [PubMed]

11. Goulet, C.R.; Bernard, G.; Tremblay, S.; Chabaud, S.; Bolduc, S.; Poulit, F. Exosomes induce fibroblast differentiation into cancer-associated fibroblasts through TGFβ signaling. *Mol. Cancer Res.* **2018**. [CrossRef]

12. Mateescu, B.; Kowal, E.J.; van Balkom, B.W.; Bartel, S.; Bhattacharyya, S.N.; Buzas, E.I.; Buck, A.H.; de Candia, P.; Chow, F.W.; Das, S.; et al. Obstacles and opportunities in the functional analysis of extracellular vesicle RNA—An ISEV position paper. *J Extracell. Vesicles* **2017**, *6*, 1286095. [CrossRef] [PubMed]

13. Maia, J.; Caja, S.; Strano Moraes, M.C.; Couto, N.; Costa-Silva, B. Exosome-Based Cell-Cell Communication in the Tumor Microenvironment. *Front. Cell Dev. Biol.* **2018**, *6*, 18. [CrossRef] [PubMed]

14. Yang, L.; Wu, X.H.; Wang, D.; Luo, C.L.; Chen, L.X. Bladder cancer cell-derived exosomes inhibit tumor cell apoptosis and induce cell proliferation in vitro. *Mol. Med. Rep.* **2013**, *8*, 1272–1278. [CrossRef] [PubMed]

15. Xue, M.; Chen, W.; Xiang, A.; Wang, R.Q.; Chen, H.; Pan, J.J.; Pang, H.; An, H.L.; Wang, X.; Hou, H.L.; et al. Hypoxic exosomes facilitate bladder tumor growth and development through transferring long non-coding RNA-UCA1. *Mol. Cancer* **2017**, *16*. [CrossRef] [PubMed]

16. Beckham, C.J.; Olsen, J.; Yin, P.N.; Wu, C.H.; Ting, H.J.; Hagen, F.K.; Scosyrev, E.; Messing, E.M.; Lee, Y.F. Bladder cancer exosomes contain EDIL-3/Del1 and facilitate cancer progression. *J. Urol.* **2014**, *192*, 583–592. [CrossRef] [PubMed]

17. Silvers, C.R.; Liu, Y.R.; Wu, C.H.; Miyamoto, H.; Messing, E.M.; Lee, Y.F. Identification of extracellular vesicle-borne periostin as a feature of muscle-invasive bladder cancer. *Oncotarget* **2016**, *7*, 23335–23345. [CrossRef] [PubMed]

18. Franzen, C.; Greco, K.; Blackwell, R.; Foreman, K.; Gupta, G. Urothelial Cells Undergo Epithelial to Mesenchymal Transition after Exposure to Muscle Invasive Bladder Cancer Exosomes. *J. Urol.* **2015**, *193*, E605–E606. [CrossRef]

19. Ostenfeld, M.S.; Jeppesen, D.K.; Laurberg, J.R.; Boysen, A.T.; Bramsen, J.B.; Primdal-Bengtson, B.; Hendrix, A.; Lamy, P.; Dagnaes-Hansen, F.; Rasmussen, M.H.; et al. Cellular Disposal of miR23b by RAB27-Dependent Exosome Release Is Linked to Acquisition of Metastatic Properties. *Cancer Res.* **2014**, *74*, 5758–5771. [CrossRef] [PubMed]

20. Bussard, K.M.; Mutkus, L.; Stumpf, K.; Gomez-Manzano, C.; Marini, F.C. Tumor-associated stromal cells as key contributors to the tumor microenvironment. *Breast Cancer Res.* **2016**, *18*. [CrossRef] [PubMed]

21. Feng, Q.Y.; Zhang, C.L.; Lum, D.; Druso, J.E.; Blank, B.; Wilson, K.F.; Welm, A.; Antonyak, M.A.; Cerione, R.A. A class of extracellular vesicles from breast cancer cells activates VEGF receptors and tumour angiogenesis. *Nat. Commun.* **2017**, *8*. [CrossRef] [PubMed]

22. Choi, E.Y.; Chavakis, E.; Czabanka, M.A.; Langer, H.F.; Fraemohs, L.; Economopoulou, M.; Kundu, R.K.; Orlandi, A.; Zheng, Y.Y.; Prieto, D.A.; et al. Del-1, an endogenous leukocyte-endothelial adhesion inhibitor, limits inflammatory cell recruitment. *Science* **2008**, *322*, 1101–1104. [CrossRef] [PubMed]

23. Lobb, R.J.; Lima, L.G.; Moller, A. Exosomes: Key mediators of metastasis and pre-metastatic niche formation. *Semin. Cell Dev. Biol.* **2017**, *67*, 3–10. [CrossRef] [PubMed]

24. Liu, Y.R.; Lee, Y.F. Bladder cancer extracellular vesicle facilitate metastasis. Unpublished; manuscript in preparation.

25. Lawrence, M.S.; Stojanov, P.; Polak, P.; Kryukov, G.V.; Cibulskis, K.; Sivachenko, A.; Carter, S.L.; Stewart, C.; Mermel, C.H.; Roberts, S.A.; et al. Mutational heterogeneity in cancer and the search for new cancer-associated genes. *Nature* **2013**, *499*, 214–218. [CrossRef] [PubMed]

26. Weinstein, J.N.; Akbani, R.; Broom, B.M.; Wang, W.Y.; Verhaak, R.G.W.; McConkey, D.; Lerner, S.; Morgan, M.; Creighton, C.J.; Smith, C.; et al. Comprehensive molecular characterization of urothelial bladder carcinoma. *Nature* **2014**, *507*, 315–322. [CrossRef]

27. Sjodahl, G.; Lauss, M.; Lovgren, K.; Chebil, G.; Gudjonsson, S.; Veerla, S.; Patschan, O.; Aine, M.; Ferno, M.; Ringner, M.; et al. A Molecular Taxonomy for Urothelial Carcinoma. *Clin. Cancer Res.* **2012**, *18*, 3377–3386. [CrossRef] [PubMed]

28. Finn, O.J. Immuno-oncology: Understanding the function and dysfunction of the immune system in cancer. *Ann. Oncol.* **2012**, *23*, 6–9. [CrossRef] [PubMed]

29. Rao, Q.; Zuo, B.F.; Lu, Z.; Gao, X.J.; You, A.B.; Wu, C.X.; Du, Z.; Yin, H.F. Tumor-Derived Exosomes Elicit Tumor Suppression in Murine Hepatocellular Carcinoma Models and Humans In Vitro. *Hepatology* **2016**, *64*, 456–472. [CrossRef] [PubMed]

30. Bu, N.; Wu, H.Q.; Sun, B.Z.; Zhang, G.L.; Zhan, S.Q.; Zhang, R.; Zhou, L. Exosome-loaded dendritic cells elicit tumor-specific CD8(+) cytotoxic T cells in patients with glioma. *J. Neurooncol.* **2011**, *104*, 659–667. [CrossRef] [PubMed]

31. Zhang, J.M.; Wu, X.H.; Zhang, Y.; Xia, Y.G.; Luo, C.L. Exosomes derived form bladder transitional cell carcinoma cells induce CTL cytotoxicity in vitro. *Zhonghua Zhong Liu Za Zhi* **2009**, *31*, 738–741. [PubMed]

32. Ljunggren, H.G.; Karre, K. In search of the "missing self": MHC molecules and NK cell recognition. *Immunol. Today* **1990**, *11*, 237–244. [CrossRef]

33. Whiteside, T.L. Immune modulation of T-cell and NK (natural killer) cell activities by TEXs (tumour-derived exosomes). *Biochem. Soc. Trans.* **2013**, *41*, 245–251. [CrossRef] [PubMed]

34. Shinohara, H.; Kuranaga, Y.; Kumazaki, M.; Sugito, N.; Yoshikawa, Y.; Takai, T.; Taniguchi, K.; Ito, Y.; Akao, Y. Regulated Polarization of Tumor-Associated Macrophages by miR-145 via Colorectal Cancer-Derived Extracellular Vesicles. *J. Immunol.* **2017**, *199*, 1505–1515. [CrossRef] [PubMed]

35. Salimu, J.; Webber, J.; Gurney, M.; Al-Taei, S.; Clayton, A.; Tabi, Z. Dominant immunosuppression of dendritic cell function by prostate-cancer-derived exosomes. *J. Extracell. Vesicles* **2017**, *6*, 1368823. [CrossRef] [PubMed]

36. Rong, L.; Li, R.; Li, S.; Luo, R. Immunosuppression of breast cancer cells mediated by transforming growth factor-beta in exosomes from cancer cells. *Oncol. Lett.* **2016**, *11*, 500–504. [CrossRef] [PubMed]

37. Theodoraki, M.N.; Yerneni, S.S.; Hoffmann, T.K.; Gooding, W.E.; Whiteside, T.L. Clinical Significance of PD-L1(+) Exosomes in Plasma of Head and Neck Cancer Patients. *Clin. Cancer Res.* **2018**, *24*, 896–905. [CrossRef] [PubMed]

38. Lee, J.; McKinney, K.Q.; Pavlopoulos, A.J.; Niu, M.; Kang, J.W.; Oh, J.W.; Kim, K.P.; Hwang, S. Altered Proteome of Extracellular Vesicles Derived from Bladder Cancer Patients Urine. *Mol. Cells* **2018**, *41*, 179–187. [CrossRef] [PubMed]

39. Suzuki, Y.; Sutoh, M.; Hatakeyama, S.; Mori, K.; Yamamoto, H.; Koie, T.; Saitoh, H.; Yamaya, K.; Funyu, T.; Habuchi, T.; et al. MUC1 carrying core 2 O-glycans functions as a molecular shield against NK cell attack, promoting bladder tumor metastasis. *Int. J. Oncol.* **2012**, *40*, 1831–1838. [CrossRef] [PubMed]

40. Nielsen, T.O.; Borre, M.; Nexo, E.; Sorensen, B.S. Co-expression of HER3 and MUC1 is associated with a favourable prognosis in patients with bladder cancer. *BJU Int.* **2015**, *115*, 163–165. [CrossRef] [PubMed]

41. Bramswig, K.H.; Poettler, M.; Unseld, M.; Wrba, F.; Uhrin, P.; Zimmermann, W.; Zielinski, C.C.; Prager, G.W. Soluble carcinoembryonic antigen activates endothelial cells and tumor angiogenesis. *Cancer Res.* **2013**, *73*, 6584–6596. [CrossRef] [PubMed]

42. Stern, N.; Markel, G.; Arnon, T.I.; Gruda, R.; Wong, H.; Gray-Owen, S.D.; Mandelboim, O. Carcinoembryonic antigen (CEA) inhibits NK killing via interaction with CEA-related cell adhesion molecule 1. *J. Immunol.* **2005**, *174*, 6692–6701. [CrossRef] [PubMed]

43. Adada, M.M.; Canals, D.; Jeong, N.; Kelkar, A.D.; Hernandez-Corbacho, M.; Pulkoski-Gross, M.J.; Donaldson, J.C.; Hannun, Y.A.; Obeid, L.M. Intracellular sphingosine kinase 2-derived sphingosine-1-phosphate mediates epidermal growth factor-induced ezrin-radixin-moesin phosphorylation and cancer cell invasion. *FASEB J.* **2015**, *29*, 4654–4669. [CrossRef] [PubMed]

44. Jiang, L.; Phang, J.M.; Yu, J.; Harrop, S.J.; Sokolova, A.V.; Duff, A.P.; Wilk, K.E.; Alkhamici, H.; Breit, S.N.; Valenzuela, S.M.; et al. CLIC proteins, ezrin, radixin, moesin and the coupling of membranes to the actin cytoskeleton: A smoking gun? *Biochim. Biophys. Acta* **2014**, *1838*, 643–657. [CrossRef] [PubMed]

45. Piao, J.; Liu, S.; Xu, Y.; Wang, C.; Lin, Z.; Qin, Y.; Liu, S. Ezrin protein overexpression predicts the poor prognosis of pancreatic ductal adenocarcinomas. *Exp. Mol. Pathol.* **2015**, *98*, 1–6. [CrossRef] [PubMed]

46. Wang, Y.; Yago, T.; Zhang, N.; Abdisalaam, S.; Alexandrakis, G.; Rodgers, W.; McEver, R.P. Cytoskeletal regulation of CD44 membrane organization and interactions with E-selectin. *J. Biol. Chem.* **2014**, *289*, 35159–35171. [CrossRef] [PubMed]

47. Silvers, C.R.; Miyamoto, H.; Messing, E.M.; Netto, G.J.; Lee, Y.F. Characterization of urinary extracellular vesicle proteins in muscle-invasive bladder cancer. *Oncotarget* **2017**, *8*, 91199–91208. [CrossRef] [PubMed]

48. Perl, A.; Hanczko, R.; Telarico, T.; Oaks, Z.; Landas, S. Oxidative stress, inflammation and carcinogenesis are controlled through the pentose phosphate pathway by transaldolase. *Trends Mol. Med.* **2011**, *17*, 395–403. [CrossRef] [PubMed]

49. Andreu, Z.; Otta Oshiro, R.; Redruello, A.; Lopez-Martin, S.; Gutierrez-Vazquez, C.; Morato, E.; Marina, A.I.; Olivier Gomez, C.; Yanez-Mo, M. Extracellular vesicles as a source for non-invasive biomarkers in bladder cancer progression. *Eur. J. Pharm. Sci.* **2017**, *98*, 70–79. [CrossRef] [PubMed]

50. Van Niel, G.; Bergam, P.; Di Cicco, A.; Hurbain, I.; Lo Cicero, A.; Dingli, F.; Palmulli, R.; Fort, C.; Potier, M.C.; Schurgers, L.J.; et al. Apolipoprotein E Regulates Amyloid Formation within Endosomes of Pigment Cells. *Cell Rep.* **2015**, *13*, 43–51. [CrossRef] [PubMed]

51. Sodar, B.W.; Kittel, A.; Paloczi, K.; Vukman, K.V.; Osteikoetxea, X.; Szabo-Taylor, K.; Nemeth, A.; Sperlagh, B.; Baranyai, T.; Giricz, Z.; et al. Low-density lipoprotein mimics blood plasma-derived exosomes and microvesicles during isolation and detection. *Sci. Rep.* **2016**, *6*, 24316. [CrossRef] [PubMed]

52. Avraham-Davidi, I.; Ely, Y.; Pham, V.N.; Castranova, D.; Grunspan, M.; Malkinson, G.; Gibbs-Bar, L.; Mayseless, O.; Allmog, G.; Lo, B.; et al. ApoB-containing lipoproteins regulate angiogenesis by modulating expression of VEGF receptor 1. *Nat. Med.* **2012**, *18*, 967–973. [CrossRef] [PubMed]

53. Rao, L.N.; Ponnusamy, T.; Philip, S.; Mukhopadhyay, R.; Kakkar, V.V.; Mundkur, L. Hypercholesterolemia Induced Immune Response and Inflammation on Progression of Atherosclerosis in Apob(tm2Sgy) Ldlr(tm1Her)/J Mice. *Lipids* **2015**, *50*, 785–797. [CrossRef] [PubMed]

54. Bergin, C.; O'Leary, A.; McCreary, C.; Sabra, K.; Mulcahy, F. Treatment of Kaposi's sarcoma with liposomal doxorubicin. *Am. J. Health Syst. Pharm.* **1995**, *52*, 2001–2004. [PubMed]

55. Sun, D.M.; Zhuang, X.Y.; Zhang, S.Q.; Deng, Z.B.; Grizzle, W.; Miller, D.; Zhang, H.G. Exosomes are endogenous nanoparticles that can deliver biological information between cells. *Adv. Drug Deliv. Rev.* **2013**, *65*, 342–347. [CrossRef] [PubMed]

56. Zhuang, X.Y.; Xiang, X.Y.; Grizzle, W.; Sun, D.M.; Zhang, S.Q.; Axtell, R.C.; Ju, S.W.; Mu, J.Y.; Zhang, L.F.; Steinman, L.; et al. Treatment of Brain Inflammatory Diseases by Delivering Exosome Encapsulated Anti-inflammatory Drugs From the Nasal Region to the Brain. *Mol. Ther.* **2011**, *19*, 1769–1779. [CrossRef] [PubMed]

57. Franzen, C.A.; Simms, P.E.; Van Huis, A.F.; Foreman, K.E.; Kuo, P.C.; Gupta, G.N. Characterization of Uptake and Internalization of Exosomes by Bladder Cancer Cells. *Biomed Res. Int.* **2014**. [CrossRef] [PubMed]

58. Greco, K.A.; Franzen, C.A.; Foreman, K.E.; Flanigan, R.C.; Kuo, P.C.; Gupta, G.N. PLK-1 Silencing in Bladder Cancer by siRNA Delivered With Exosomes. *Urology* **2016**, *91*. [CrossRef] [PubMed]

59. Jin, X.; Ma, J.W.; Liang, X.Y.; Tang, K.; Liu, Y.Y.; Yin, X.A.; Zhang, Y.; Zhang, H.F.; Xu, P.W.; Chen, D.G.; et al. Pre-instillation of tumor microparticles enhances intravesical chemotherapy of nonmuscle-invasive bladder cancer through a lysosomal pathway. *Biomaterials* **2017**, *113*, 93–104. [CrossRef] [PubMed]

60. Ortiz-Bonilla, C.J.; Lee, Y.F. BCG internalization releases increased levels of immune-active extracellular vesicles. Unpublished; manuscript in preparation.

61. Zhou, H.; Cheruvanky, A.; Hu, X.; Matsumoto, T.; Hiramatsu, N.; Cho, M.E.; Berger, A.; Leelahavanichkul, A.; Doi, K.; Chawla, L.S.; et al. Urinary exosomal transcription factors, a new class of biomarkers for renal disease. *Kidney Int.* **2008**, *74*, 613–621. [CrossRef] [PubMed]

62. Moon, P.G.; You, S.; Lee, J.E.; Hwang, D.; Baek, M.C. Urinary exosomes and proteomics. *Mass Spectrom. Rev.* **2011**, *30*, 1185–1202. [CrossRef] [PubMed]

63. Adachi, J.; Kumar, C.; Zhang, Y.; Olsen, J.V.; Mann, M. The human urinary proteome contains more than 1500 proteins, including a large proportion of membrane proteins. *Genome Biol.* **2006**, *7*, R80. [CrossRef] [PubMed]

64. Moon, P.G.; Lee, J.E.; You, S.; Kim, T.K.; Cho, J.H.; Kim, I.S.; Kwon, T.H.; Kim, C.D.; Park, S.H.; Hwang, D.; et al. Proteomic analysis of urinary exosomes from patients of early IgA nephropathy and thin basement membrane nephropathy. *Proteomics* **2011**, *11*, 2459–2475. [CrossRef] [PubMed]

65. Knepper, M.A. Common sense approaches to urinary biomarker study design. *J. Am. Soc. Nephrol.* **2009**, *20*, 1175–1178. [CrossRef] [PubMed]

66. Gonzales, P.; Pisitkun, T.; Knepper, M.A. Urinary exosomes: Is there a future? *Nephrol. Dial. Transplant.* **2008**, *23*, 1799–1801. [CrossRef] [PubMed]

67. Keller, S.; Rupp, C.; Stoeck, A.; Runz, S.; Fogel, M.; Lugert, S.; Hager, H.D.; Abdel-Bakky, M.S.; Gutwein, P.; Altevogt, P. CD24 is a marker of exosomes secreted into urine and amniotic fluid. *Kidney Int.* **2007**, *72*, 1095–1102. [CrossRef] [PubMed]

68. Hogan, M.C.; Manganelli, L.; Woollard, J.R.; Masyuk, A.I.; Masyuk, T.V.; Tammachote, R.; Huang, B.Q.; Leontovich, A.A.; Beito, T.G.; Madden, B.J.; et al. Characterization of PKD protein-positive exosome-like vesicles. *J. Am. Soc. Nephrol.* **2009**, *20*, 278–288. [CrossRef] [PubMed]

69. Zhang, Y.; Li, Y.; Qiu, F.; Qiu, Z. Comprehensive analysis of low-abundance proteins in human urinary exosomes using peptide ligand library technology, peptide OFFGEL fractionation and nanoHPLC-chip-MS/MS. *Electrophoresis* **2010**, *31*, 3797–3807. [CrossRef] [PubMed]

70. Nawaz, M.; Camussi, G.; Valadi, H.; Nazarenko, I.; Ekstrom, K.; Wang, X.; Principe, S.; Shah, N.; Ashraf, N.M.; Fatima, F.; et al. The emerging role of extracellular vesicles as biomarkers for urogenital cancers. *Nat. Rev. Urol.* **2014**, *11*, 688–701. [CrossRef] [PubMed]

71. Pisitkun, T.; Shen, R.F.; Knepper, M.A. Identification and proteomic profiling of exosomes in human urine. *Proc. Natl. Acad. Sci. USA* **2004**, *101*, 13368–13373. [CrossRef] [PubMed]

72. Gonzales, P.A.; Pisitkun, T.; Hoffert, J.D.; Tchapyjnikov, D.; Star, R.A.; Kleta, R.; Wang, N.S.; Knepper, M.A. Large-scale proteomics and phosphoproteomics of urinary exosomes. *J. Am. Soc. Nephrol.* **2009**, *20*, 363–379. [CrossRef] [PubMed]

73. Wang, Z.; Hill, S.; Luther, J.M.; Hachey, D.L.; Schey, K.L. Proteomic analysis of urine exosomes by multidimensional protein identification technology (MudPIT). *Proteomics* **2012**, *12*, 329–338. [CrossRef] [PubMed]

74. Chen, C.L.; Lai, Y.F.; Tang, P.; Chien, K.Y.; Yu, J.S.; Tsai, C.H.; Chen, H.W.; Wu, C.C.; Chung, T.; Hsu, C.W.; et al. Comparative and targeted proteomic analyses of urinary microparticles from bladder cancer and hernia patients. *J. Proteome Res.* **2012**, *11*, 5611–5629. [CrossRef] [PubMed]

75. Principe, S.; Jones, E.E.; Kim, Y.; Sinha, A.; Nyalwidhe, J.O.; Brooks, J.; Semmes, O.J.; Troyer, D.A.; Lance, R.S.; Kislinger, T.; et al. In-depth proteomic analyses of exosomes isolated from expressed prostatic secretions in urine. *Proteomics* **2013**, *13*, 1667–1671. [CrossRef] [PubMed]

76. Principe, S.; Kim, Y.; Fontana, S.; Ignatchenko, V.; Nyalwidhe, J.O.; Lance, R.S.; Troyer, D.A.; Alessandro, R.; Semmes, O.J.; Kislinger, T.; et al. Identification of prostate-enriched proteins by in-depth proteomic analyses of expressed prostatic secretions in urine. *J. Proteome Res.* **2012**, *11*, 2386–2396. [CrossRef] [PubMed]

77. Leiblich, A. Recent Developments in the Search for Urinary Biomarkers in Bladder Cancer. *Curr. Urol. Rep.* **2017**, *18*, 100. [CrossRef] [PubMed]

78. Hauser, S.; Kogej, M.; Fechner, G.; Von Ruecker, A.; Bastian, P.J.; Von Pezold, J.; Vorreuther, R.; Lummen, G.; Muller, S.C.; Ellinger, J. Cell-free serum DNA in patients with bladder cancer: Results of a prospective multicenter study. *Anticancer Res.* **2012**, *32*, 3119–3124. [PubMed]

79. Casadio, V.; Calistri, D.; Tebaldi, M.; Bravaccini, S.; Gunelli, R.; Martorana, G.; Bertaccini, A.; Serra, L.; Scarpi, E.; Amadori, D.; et al. Urine cell-free DNA integrity as a marker for early bladder cancer diagnosis: Preliminary data. *Urol. Oncol.* **2013**, *31*, 1744–1750. [CrossRef] [PubMed]

80. Lu, T.; Li, J. Clinical applications of urinary cell-free DNA in cancer: Current insights and promising future. *Am. J. Cancer Res.* **2017**, *7*, 2318–2332. [PubMed]

81. Berrondo, C.; Flax, J.; Kucherov, V.; Siebert, A.; Osinski, T.; Rosenberg, A.; Fucile, C.; Richheimer, S.; Beckham, C.J. Expression of the Long Non-Coding RNA HOTAIR Correlates with Disease Progression in Bladder Cancer and Is Contained in Bladder Cancer Patient Urinary Exosomes. *PLoS ONE* **2016**, *11*, e0147236. [CrossRef] [PubMed]

82. Liang, L.G.; Kong, M.Q.; Zhou, S.; Sheng, Y.F.; Wang, P.; Yu, T.; Inci, F.; Kuo, W.P.; Li, L.J.; Demirci, U.; et al. An integrated double-filtration microfluidic device for isolation, enrichment and quantification of urinary extracellular vesicles for detection of bladder cancer. *Sci. Rep.* **2017**, *7*, 46224. [CrossRef] [PubMed]

83. Juracek, J.; Peltanova, B.; Dolezel, J.; Fedorko, M.; Pacik, D.; Radova, L.; Vesela, P.; Svoboda, M.; Slaby, O.; Stanik, M. Genome-wide identification of urinary cell-free microRNAs for non-invasive detection of bladder cancer. *J. Cell. Mol. Med.* **2018**, *22*, 2033–2038. [CrossRef] [PubMed]

84. Lin, S.Y.; Chang, C.H.; Wu, H.C.; Lin, C.C.; Chang, K.P.; Yang, C.R.; Huang, C.P.; Hsu, W.H.; Chang, C.T.; Chen, C.J. Proteome Profiling of Urinary Exosomes Identifies Alpha 1-Antitrypsin and H2B1K as Diagnostic and Prognostic Biomarkers for Urothelial Carcinoma. *Sci. Rep.* **2016**, *6*, 34446. [CrossRef] [PubMed]

85. Long, J.D.; Sullivan, T.B.; Humphrey, J.; Logvinenko, T.; Summerhayes, K.A.; Kozinn, S.; Harty, N.; Summerhayes, I.C.; Libertino, J.A.; Holway, A.H.; et al. A non-invasive miRNA based assay to detect bladder cancer in cell-free urine. *Am. J. Transl. Res.* **2015**, *7*, 2500–2509. [PubMed]

86. Armstrong, D.A.; Green, B.B.; Seigne, J.D.; Schned, A.R.; Marsit, C.J. MicroRNA molecular profiling from matched tumor and bio-fluids in bladder cancer. *Mol. Cancer* **2015**, *14*, 194. [CrossRef] [PubMed]

87. Matsuzaki, K.; Fujita, K.; Jingushi, K.; Kawashima, A.; Ujike, T.; Nagahara, A.; Ueda, Y.; Tanigawa, G.; Yoshioka, I.; Ueda, K.; et al. MiR-21-5p in urinary extracellular vesicles is a novel biomarker of urothelial carcinoma. *Oncotarget* **2017**, *8*, 24668–24678. [CrossRef] [PubMed]

88. Pardini, B.; Cordero, F.; Naccarati, A.; Viberti, C.; Birolo, G.; Oderda, M.; Di Gaetano, C.; Arigoni, M.; Martina, F.; Calogero, R.A.; et al. microRNA profiles in urine by next-generation sequencing can stratify bladder cancer subtypes. *Oncotarget* **2018**, *9*, 20658–20669. [CrossRef] [PubMed]

89. Heba Fanous, T.S. Kimberly Rieger-Christ. Distinct exosomalL miRNA profiles in chemoresistant bladder carcinoma cell lines. *J. Urol.* **2017**, *197*, 2.

90. Yasui, T.; Yanagida, T.; Ito, S.; Konakade, Y.; Takeshita, D.; Naganawa, T.; Nagashima, K.; Shimada, T.; Kaji, N.; Nakamura, Y.; et al. Unveiling massive numbers of cancer-related urinary-microRNA candidates via nanowires. *Sci. Adv.* **2017**, *3*, e1701133. [CrossRef] [PubMed]

91. Baumgart, S.; Holters, S.; Ohlmann, C.H.; Bohle, R.; Stockle, M.; Ostenfeld, M.S.; Dyrskjot, L.; Junker, K.; Heinzelmann, J. Exosomes of invasive urothelial carcinoma cells are characterized by a specific miRNA expression signature. *Oncotarget* **2017**, *8*, 58278–58291. [CrossRef] [PubMed]

92. Zhang, D.Z.; Lau, K.M.; Chan, E.S.; Wang, G.; Szeto, C.C.; Wong, K.; Choy, R.K.; Ng, C.F. Cell-free urinary microRNA-99a and microRNA-125b are diagnostic markers for the non-invasive screening of bladder cancer. *PLoS ONE* **2014**, *9*, e100793. [CrossRef] [PubMed]

93. Kim, S.M.; Kang, H.W.; Kim, W.T.; Kim, Y.J.; Yun, S.J.; Lee, S.C.; Kim, W.J. Cell-Free microRNA-214 From Urine as a Biomarker for Non-Muscle-Invasive Bladder Cancer. *Korean J. Urol.* **2013**, *54*, 791–796. [CrossRef] [PubMed]

94. Smalley, D.M.; Sheman, N.E.; Nelson, K.; Theodorescu, D. Isolation and identification of potential urinary microparticle biomarkers of bladder cancer. *J. Proteome Res.* **2008**, *7*, 2088–2096. [CrossRef] [PubMed]

95. Fontana, S.; Saieva, L.; Taverna, S.; Alessandro, R. Contribution of proteomics to understanding the role of tumor-derived exosomes in cancer progression: State of the art and new perspectives. *Proteomics* **2013**, *13*, 1581–1594. [CrossRef] [PubMed]

96. Welton, J.L.; Khanna, S.; Giles, P.J.; Brennan, P.; Brewis, I.A.; Staffurth, J.; Mason, M.D.; Clayton, A. Proteomics analysis of bladder cancer exosomes. *Mol. Cell. Proteom.* **2010**, *9*, 1324–1338. [CrossRef] [PubMed]

97. Kumari, N.; Saxena, S.; Agrawal, U. Exosomal protein interactors as emerging therapeutic targets in urothelial bladder cancer. *J. Egypt. Natl. Cancer Inst.* **2015**, *27*, 51–58. [CrossRef] [PubMed]

98. Alvarez, M.L.; Khosroheidari, M.; Ravi, R.K.; DiStefano, J.K. Comparison of protein, microRNA and mRNA yields using different methods of urinary exosome isolation for the discovery of kidney disease biomarkers. *Kidney Int.* **2012**, *82*, 1024–1032. [CrossRef] [PubMed]

99. Musante, L.; Saraswat, M.; Duriez, E.; Byrne, B.; Ravida, A.; Domon, B.; Holthofer, H. Biochemical and physical characterisation of urinary nanovesicles following CHAPS treatment. *PLoS ONE* **2012**, *7*, e37279. [CrossRef] [PubMed]

100. Thery, C.; Amigorena, S.; Raposo, G.; Clayton, A. Isolation and characterization of exosomes from cell culture supernatants and biological fluids. *Curr. Protoc. Cell Biol.* **2006**, *3*, 3–22. [CrossRef] [PubMed]

101. Liga, A.; Vliegenthart, A.D.B.; Oosthuyzen, W.; Dear, J.W.; Kersaudy-Kerhoas, M. Exosome isolation: A microfluidic road-map. *Lab Chip* **2015**, *15*, 2388–2394. [CrossRef] [PubMed]

102. Kanwar, S.S.; Dunlay, C.J.; Simeone, D.M.; Nagrath, S. Microfluidic device (ExoChip) for on-chip isolation, quantification and characterization of circulating exosomes. *Lab Chip* **2014**, *14*, 1891–1900. [CrossRef] [PubMed]

103. Santana, S.M.; Antonyak, M.A.; Cerione, R.A.; Kirby, B.J. Microfluidic isolation of cancer-cell-derived microvesicles from hetergeneous extracellular shed vesicle populations. *Biomed. Microdevices* **2014**, *16*, 869–877. [CrossRef] [PubMed]

104. Momen-Heravi, F.; Balaj, L.; Alian, S.; Mantel, P.Y.; Halleck, A.E.; Trachtenberg, A.J.; Soria, C.E.; Oquin, S.; Bonebreak, C.M.; Saracoglu, E.; et al. Current methods for the isolation of extracellular vesicles. *Biol. Chem.* **2013**, *394*, 1253–1262. [CrossRef] [PubMed]

105. Fernandez-Llama, P.; Khositseth, S.; Gonzales, P.A.; Star, R.A.; Pisitkun, T.; Knepper, M.A. Tamm-Horsfall protein and urinary exosome isolation. *Kidney Int.* **2010**, *77*, 736–742. [CrossRef] [PubMed]

106. Witwer, K.W.; Buzas, E.I.; Bemis, L.T.; Bora, A.; Lasser, C.; Lotvall, J.; Nolte-'t Hoen, E.N.; Piper, M.G.; Sivaraman, S.; Skog, J.; et al. Standardization of sample collection, isolation and analysis methods in extracellular vesicle research. *J. Extracell. Vesicles* **2013**, *2*. [CrossRef] [PubMed]

107. Lotvall, J.; Rajendran, L.; Gho, Y.S.; Thery, C.; Wauben, M.; Raposo, G.; Sjostrand, M.; Taylor, D.; Telemo, E.; Breakefield, X.O. The launch of Journal of Extracellular Vesicles (JEV), the official journal of the International Society for Extracellular Vesicles—About microvesicles, exosomes, ectosomes and other extracellular vesicles. *J. Extracell. Vesicles* **2012**, *1*. [CrossRef] [PubMed]

108. Waikar, S.S.; Sabbisetti, V.S.; Bonventre, J.V. Normalization of urinary biomarkers to creatinine during changes in glomerular filtration rate. *Kidney Int.* **2010**, *78*, 486–494. [CrossRef] [PubMed]

109. Tang, K.W.A.; Toh, Q.C.; Teo, B.W. Normalisation of urinary biomarkers to creatinine for clinical practice and research—When and why. *Singapore Med. J.* **2015**, *56*, 7–10. [CrossRef] [PubMed]

110. Mattix, H.J.; Hsu, C.Y.; Shaykevich, S.; Curhan, G. Use of the albumin/creatinine ratio to detect microalbuminuria: Implications of sex and race. *J. Am. Soc. Nephrol.* **2002**, *13*, 1034–1039. [PubMed]

111. Mitch, W.E.; Collier, V.U.; Walser, M. Creatinine Metabolism in Chronic Renal-Failure. *Clin. Res.* **1978**, *26*, A636. [CrossRef]

112. Zhou, H.; Yuen, P.S.; Pisitkun, T.; Gonzales, P.A.; Yasuda, H.; Dear, J.W.; Gross, P.; Knepper, M.A.; Star, R.A. Collection, storage, preservation and normalization of human urinary exosomes for biomarker discovery. *Kidney Int.* **2006**, *69*, 1471–1476. [CrossRef] [PubMed]

113. Prunotto, M.; Farina, A.; Lane, L.; Pernin, A.; Schifferli, J.; Hochstrasser, D.F.; Lescuyer, P.; Moll, S. Proteomic analysis of podocyte exosome-enriched fraction from normal human urine. *J. Proteom.* **2013**, *82*, 193–229. [CrossRef] [PubMed]

114. Lentz, M.R. Continuous whole blood UltraPheresis procedure in patients with metastatic cancer. *J. Biol. Response Mod.* **1989**, *8*, 511–527. [PubMed]

115. Tullis, R.H.; Duffin, R.P.; Handley, H.H.; Sodhi, P.; Menon, J.; Joyce, J.A.; Kher, V. Reduction of hepatitis C virus using lectin affinity plasmapheresis in dialysis patients. *Blood Purif.* **2009**, *27*, 64–69. [CrossRef] [PubMed]

116. Marleau, A.M.; Chen, C.S.; Joyce, J.A.; Tullis, R.H. Exosome removal as a therapeutic adjuvant in cancer. *J. Transl. Med.* **2012**, *10*, 134. [CrossRef] [PubMed]

117. Chalmin, F.; Ladoire, S.; Mignot, G.; Vincent, J.; Bruchard, M.; Remy-Martin, J.P.; Boireau, W.; Rouleau, A.; Simon, B.; Lanneau, D.; et al. Membrane-associated Hsp72 from tumor-derived exosomes mediates STAT3-dependent immunosuppressive function of mouse and human myeloid-derived suppressor cells. *J. Clin. Investig.* **2010**, *120*, 457–471. [CrossRef] [PubMed]

118. Jiang, Y.; Wang, X.; Zhang, J.; Lai, R. MicroRNA-599 suppresses glioma progression by targeting RAB27B. *Oncol. Lett.* **2018**, *16*, 1243–1252. [CrossRef] [PubMed]

119. Ostrowski, M.; Carmo, N.B.; Krumeich, S.; Fanget, I.; Raposo, G.; Savina, A.; Moita, C.F.; Schauer, K.; Hume, A.N.; Freitas, R.P.; et al. Rab27a and Rab27b control different steps of the exosome secretion pathway. *Nat. Cell Biol.* **2010**, *12*, 19–30. [CrossRef] [PubMed]

120. Sun, D.; Zhuang, X.; Xiang, X.; Liu, Y.; Zhang, S.; Liu, C.; Barnes, S.; Grizzle, W.; Miller, D.; Zhang, H.G. A novel nanoparticle drug delivery system: The anti-inflammatory activity of curcumin is enhanced when encapsulated in exosomes. *Mol. Ther.* **2010**, *18*, 1606–1614. [CrossRef] [PubMed]

121. Tian, Y.; Li, S.; Song, J.; Ji, T.; Zhu, M.; Anderson, G.J.; Wei, J.; Nie, G. A doxorubicin delivery platform using engineered natural membrane vesicle exosomes for targeted tumor therapy. *Biomaterials* **2014**, *35*, 2383–2390. [CrossRef] [PubMed]

122. Hoshino, A.; Costa-Silva, B.; Shen, T.L.; Rodrigues, G.; Hashimoto, A.; Tesic Mark, M.; Molina, H.; Kohsaka, S.; Di Giannatale, A.; Ceder, S.; et al. Tumour exosome integrins determine organotropic metastasis. *Nature* **2015**, *527*, 329–335. [CrossRef] [PubMed]

123. Xitong, D.; Xiaorong, Z. Targeted therapeutic delivery using engineered exosomes and its applications in cardiovascular diseases. *Gene* **2016**, *575*, 377–384. [CrossRef] [PubMed]

Permissions

List of Contributors

Yasuyoshi Miyata, Tomohiro Matsuo, Kojiro Ohba, Kensuke Mitsunari, Yuta Mukae, Asato Otsubo, Junki Harada, Tsuyoshi Matsuda, Tsubasa Kondo and Hideki Sakai
Department of Urology, Graduate School of Biomedical Sciences, Nagasaki University, Nagasaki 852-8501, Japan

Valentina Pasquale, Giacomo Ducci, Gloria Campioni, Stefano Busti, Marco Vanoni and Elena Sacco
Department of Biotechnology and Biosciences, University of Milano-Bicocca, Piazza della Scienza 2, 20126 Milan, Italy
SYSBIO-ISBE-IT-Candidate National Node of Italy for ISBE, Research Infrastructure for Systems Biology Europe, 20126 Milan, Italy

Adria Ventrici
Department of Biotechnology and Biosciences, University of Milano-Bicocca, Piazza della Scienza 2, 20126 Milan, Italy

Chiara Assalini
Urological Research Institute, Division of Experimental Oncology, IRCCS San Raffaele Hospital, 20132 Milan, Italy

Riccardo Vago
Urological Research Institute, Division of Experimental Oncology, IRCCS San Raffaele Hospital, 20132 Milan, Italy
Università Vita-Salute San Raffaele, 20132 Milan, Italy

Iris Lodewijk, Ester Munera-Maravilla and Cristian Suárez-Cabrera
Molecular Oncology Unit, CIEMAT (Centro de Investigaciones Energéticas, Medioambientales y Tecnológicas), Avenida Complutense n° 40, 28040 Madrid, Spain
Biomedical Research Institute I+12, University Hospital "12 de Octubre", Av Córdoba s/n, 28041 Madrid, Spain

Marta Dueñas, Carolina Rubio, Cristina Segovia, Alejandra Bernardini and Jesús M. Paramio
Molecular Oncology Unit, CIEMAT (Centro de Investigaciones Energéticas, Medioambientales y Tecnológicas), Avenida Complutense n° 40, 28040 Madrid, Spain
Biomedical Research Institute I+12, University Hospital "12 de Octubre", Av Córdoba s/n, 28041 Madrid, Spain
Centro de Investigación Biomédica en Red de Cáncer (CIBERONC), 28029 Madrid, Spain

Alicia Teijeira
Molecular Oncology Unit, CIEMAT (Centro de Investigaciones Energéticas, Medioambientales y Tecnológicas), Avenida Complutense n° 40, 28040 Madrid, Spain

Kyoung-Hwa Lee, Byung-Chan Kim, Chang Wook Jeong, Ja Hyeon Ku and Hyeon Hoe Kim
Department of Urology, Seoul National University Hospital, Seoul 03080, Korea

Seung-Hwan Jeong
Graduate School of Medical Science and Engineering, Korea Advanced Institute of Science and Technology (KAIST), Daejeon 34052, Korea

Cheol Kwak
Department of Urology, Seoul National University Hospital, Seoul 03080, Korea
Department of Urology, Seoul National University College of Medicine, Seoul 03080, Korea

Rui Batista, João Vinagre, ValdemarMáximo and Paula Soares
Instituto de Investigação e Inovação em Saúde (i3S), 4200-135 Porto, Portugal
Instituto de Patologia e Imunologia Molecular da Universidade do Porto (IPATIMUP), 4200-135 Porto, Portugal
Faculdade de Medicina da Universidade do Porto (FMUP), 4200-319 Porto, Portugal

Luís Lima and Lúcio Santos
Grupo de Patologia e Terapêutica Experimental, Instituto Português de Oncologia do Porto FG, EPE (IPO-Porto), 4200-072 Porto, Portugal

Vasco Pinto and Joana Lyra
Instituto de Patologia e Imunologia Molecular da Universidade do Porto (IPATIMUP), 4200-135 Porto, Portugal
Faculdade de Medicina da Universidade do Porto (FMUP), 4200-319 Porto, Portugal

Anja Rabien, Nadine Ratert and Klaus Jung
Department of Urology, Charité—Universitätsmedizin Berlin, Corporate Member of Freie Universität Berlin, Humboldt-Universität zu Berlin, and Berlin Institute of Health, 10117 Berlin, Germany
Berlin Institute for Urologic Research, 10117 Berlin, Germany

Anica Högner
Institute of Pathology, Charité—Universitätsmedizin Berlin, Corporate Member of Freie Universität Berlin, Humboldt-Universität zu Berlin, and Berlin Institute of Health, 10117 Berlin, Germany

Andreas Erbersdobler
Institute of Pathology, University Medicine Rostock, 18055 Rostock, Germany

Ergin Kilic
Institute of Pathology, Charité—Universitätsmedizin Berlin, Corporate Member of Freie Universität Berlin, Humboldt-Universität zu Berlin, and Berlin Institute of Health, 10117 Berlin, Germany
Institute of Pathology, Hospital Leverkusen, 51375 Leverkusen, Germany

Thorsten H. Ecke
Department of Urology, HELIOS Hospital Bad Saarow, DE-15526 Bad Sarrow, Germany
Brandenburg Medical School, DE-14770 Brandenburg, Germany

Adisch Kiani, Thorsten Schlomm and Frank Friedersdorff
Department of Urology, Charité—Universitätsmedizin, Corporate Member of Freie Universität Berlin, Humboldt-Universität zu Berlin, and Berlin Institute of Health, DE-10098 Berlin, Germany

Anja Rabien and Klaus Jung
Department of Urology, Charité—Universitätsmedizin, Corporate Member of Freie Universität Berlin, Humboldt-Universität zu Berlin, and Berlin Institute of Health, DE-10098 Berlin, Germany
Berlin Institute for Urological Research, DE-10098 Berlin, Germany

Peter Boström
Department of Urology, Turku University Hospital, FI-20521 Turku, Finland

Minna Tervahartiala
MediCity Research Laboratory, Department of Medical Microbiology and Immunology, University of Turku

Pekka Taimen
Institute of Pathology, Turku University Hospital, FI-20521 Turku, Finland

Jan Gleichenhagen, Georg Johnen and Thomas Brüning
Institute for Prevention and Occupational Medicine of the German Social Accident Insurance (IPA), Institute of the Ruhr University Bochum, DE-44789 Bochum, Germany

Stefan Koch
Brandenburg Medical School, DE-14770 Brandenburg, Germany
Institute of Pathology, HELIOS Hospital Bad Saarow, DE-15526 Bad Sarrow, Germany

Jenny Roggisch
Institute of Pathology, HELIOS Hospital Bad Saarow, DE-15526 Bad Sarrow, Germany

Ralph M. Wirtz
STRATIFYER Molecular Pathology GmbH, DE-50935 Cologne, Germany

Milena Matuszczak and Maciej Salagierski
Department of Urology, Collegium Medicum, University of Zielona Góra, 65-046 Zielona Góra, Poland

Mirja Geelvink, Armin Babmorad, Angela Maurer, Ruth Knuechel, Michael Rose and Nadine T. Gaisa
Institute of Pathology, RWTH Aachen University, Pauwelsstrasse 30, 52074 Aachen, Germany

Robert Stöhr
Institute of Pathology, University Hospital Erlangen, Friedrich-Alexander University Erlangen-Nürnberg (FAU), 91054 Erlangen, Germany

Tobias Grimm
Department of Urology, Ludwig Maximilian University Munich, 81377 Munich, Germany

Melissa P. Tan and Robert A. Huddart
Division of Radiotherapy & Imaging, Institute of Cancer Research, 15 Cotswold Road, Sutton, Surrey SM2 5NG, UK
Academic Urology Unit, The Royal Marsden NHS Foundation Trust, Downs Road, Sutton, Surrey SM2 5PT, UK

Gerhardt Attard
Research Department of Oncology, UCL Cancer Institute, University College London, 72 Huntley Street, London WC1E 6DD, UK

Markus Eckstein, Robert Stoehr and Arndt Hartmann
Institute of Pathology, University of Erlangen-Nuremberg, 91054 Erlangen, Germany

Ralph Markus Wirtz
STRATIFYER Molecular Pathology GmbH, 50935 Cologne, Germany
Institute of Pathology at the St Elisabeth Hospital Köln-Hohenlind, 50935 Cologne, Germany

Matthias Gross-Weege, Katja Nitschke and Philipp Erben
Department of Urology, University Medical Centre Mannheim, Medical Faculty Mannheim, University of Heidelberg, 68167 Mannheim, Germany

Johannes Breyer and Wolfgang Otto
Department of Urology, University of Regensburg, 93053 Regensburg, Germany

Danijel Sikic and Bastian Keck
Department of Urology and Pediatric Urology, University Hospital Erlangen, 91058 Erlangen, Germany

Sebastian Eidt
Institute of Pathology at the St Elisabeth Hospital Köln-Hohenlind, 50935 Cologne, Germany

Maximilian Burger
Department of Urology, University of Regensburg, 93053 Regensburg, Germany

Christian Bolenz
Department of Urology, University of Ulm, 89081 Ulm, Germany

Stefan Porubsky
Department of Pathology, University Medical Centre Mannheim, Medical Faculty Mannheim, University of Heidelberg, 68167 Mannheim, Germany

Michael Rose
Institute of Pathology, RWTH Aachen University, 52074 Aachen, Germany
RWTH Centralized Biomaterial Bank (RWTH cBMB), Medical Faculty, RWTH Aachen University, 52074 Aachen, Germany

Sarah Bringezu, Laura Godfrey, David Fiedler, Nadine T. Gaisa, Maximilian Koch and Ruth Knüchel
Institute of Pathology, RWTH Aachen University, 52074 Aachen, Germany

Christian Bach
Department of Urology, RWTH Aachen University, 52074 Aachen, Germany

Susanne Füssel and Doreen Hübner
Department of Urology, University Hospital Carl Gustav Carus, Technische Universität Dresden, 01307 Dresden, Germany

Alexander Herr
Biotype GmbH, 01109 Dresden, Germany

Jörg Ellinger
Department of Urology, University Hospital Bonn, 53105 Bonn, Germany

David Pfister
Department of Urology, RWTH Aachen University, 52074 Aachen, Germany
Department of Urology, Uro-Oncology, Robot Assisted and Reconstructive Urologic Surgery, University Hospital Cologne, 50937 Cologne, Germany

Manfred P. Wirth
Department of Urology, University Hospital Carl Gustav Carus, Technische Universität Dresden, 01307 Dresden, Germany

Manja Böhme
Biotype GmbH, 01109 Dresden, Germany

Edgar Dahl
Institute of Pathology, RWTH Aachen University, 52074 Aachen, Germany
RWTH Centralized Biomaterial Bank (RWTH cBMB), Medical Faculty, RWTH Aachen University, 52074 Aachen, Germany

Steffen Hallmann
HELIOS Hospital, Department of Urology, Bad Saarow D-15526, Germany

Sarah Weiß
Department of Urology, Charité University Hospital, Berlin D-10117, Germany

Carsten Stephan
Department of Urology, Charité University Hospital, Berlin D-10117, Germany
Berlin Institute for Urological Research, Berlin D-10115, Germany

Christian Arndt, Dimitri Barski and Thomas Otto
Department of Urology, Lukas Hospital Neuss, Neuss D-41464, Germany

Holger Gerullis
University Hospital for Urology, Klinikum Oldenburg, School of Medicine and Health Sciences Carl von Ossietzky University Oldenburg, Oldenburg D-26133, Germany

Yu-Ru Liu
Department of Urology, University of Rochester Medical Center, Rochester, NY 14642, USA

Carlos J. Ortiz-Bonilla and Yi-Fen Lee
Department of Urology, University of Rochester Medical Center, Rochester, NY 14642, USA
Department of Pathology and Lab Medicine, University of Rochester Medical Center, Rochester, NY 14642, USA

Index

www.ingramcontent.com/pod-product-compliance
Lightning Source LLC
Chambersburg PA
CBHW080503200326
41458CB00012B/4066